# CHRONIC KIDNEY DISEASE

Edited by **Monika Göőz**

**Chronic Kidney Disease**
Edited by Monika Gööz

**Published by InTech**
Janeza Trdine 9, 51000 Rijeka, Croatia





**Publishing Process Manager** Jana Sertic

**Technical Editor** Teodora Smiljanic

**Cover Designer** InTech Design Team

Additional hard copies can be obtained from orders@intechopen.com

Chronic Kidney Disease, Edited by Monika Gööz
p. cm.
ISBN 978-953-51-0171-0

For EU product safety concerns:
IN TECH d.o.o., Prolaz Marije Krucifikse Kozulić 3, 51000 Rijeka, Croatia,
info@intechopen.com or visit our website at intechopen.com.

# Meet the editor

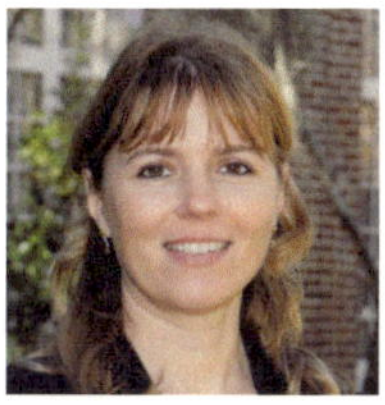

Dr Monika Gööz is an Associate Professor of Medicine in the Division of Nephrology at the Medical University of South Carolina (MUSC). She is also an Associate Member of the College of Graduate Studies at MUSC, and an Affiliate Member of the Hollings Cancer Center. She earned her MD and PhD degrees at the Semmelweis University, Budapest, Hungary, and completed her Fellowships at the Institute of Experimental Medicine of the Hungarian Academy of Sciences, Budapest, at the University of Oulu, Finland, and at MUSC. Dr Gooz is a member of several organizations including the American Physiological Society and the International Nephrology Society. She serves on the editorial board of the American Journal of Physiology: Renal Physiology, and is a special editor of The American Journal of Medical Sciences.

# Contents

# Preface

Chronic kidney disease is an increasing health and economical problem in our world. Obesity and diabetes mellitus, the two most common cause of CKD, are becoming epidemic in our societies. Education on healthy lifestyle and diet is becoming more and more important for reducing the number of type 2 diabetics and patients with hypertension. Education of our patients is also crucial for successful maintenance therapy. There are, however, certain other factors leading to CKD, for instance the genetic predisposition in the case of polycystic kidney disease or type 1 diabetes, where education alone is not enough.

When the first angiotensin converting enzyme inhibitor, Captopril, was developed in 1975 it changed not only the treatment of hypertension, but of diabetic nephropathy and other chronic kidney diseases. In the past forty years we did not have such a breakthrough in the treatment of CKD. However, several valuable discoveries were made which greatly enhanced our understanding of the role of nitric oxide and mechanisms responsible for anemia and CKD-related bone diseases. Most certainly, dialysis techniques have developed greatly over the past seventy years and have become available for a wide range of people. Furthermore, advanced surgical procedures and tools were developed in the past years to resolve ureteral obstructions originating from stones or prostate hypertrophy. These modern techniques are discussed in our book along with currently accepted procedures for kidney cancers.

How can we further improve the treatment of CKD patients? Besides prevention, the most important aim would be to constantly look for, and try to understand the mechanistic details of disease development and progression. Perhaps no other disease is as complex and complicated as CKD since the symptoms result from the constant interaction of multiple organ systems as is the case with cardiorenal syndrome, CKD-related anemia, and bone diseases. Because of the interdisciplinary nature of the disease, we need continuous communication between nephrologists, surgeons, and basic scientists, since only our joint approach can lay down the foundation of the next (bio)medical breakthrough. The chapters of our book introduce readers to this enthusiastic approach.

I would like to thank all of our contributors for their valuable time and expertise and for the high quality chapters which provide a greatly enjoyable reading experience. I also would like to thank my family and friends who supported me during the editing process: my Mom and Dad, Pal and Adam, and Carol of course. I dedicate this book to you.

**Monika Gööz, MD PhD**
Medical University of South Carolina
Charleston, SC,
USA

# 1

# ADAM Proteases as Novel Therapeutic Targets in Chronic Kidney Disease

Monika Göőz
*Medical University of South Carolina, Charleston, SC USA*

## 1. Introduction

More than 20 million Americans suffer, and ultimately die, from chronic kidney disease (CKD). Based on data from the National Institute of Diabetes and Digestive and Kidney Diseases (NIDDK), the yearly cost of dialysis treatment of patients with end stage renal disease (ESRD) is currently $35 billion [1], and this number is predicted to rise as the US population ages and more people develop obesity, metabolic syndrome, and diabetes. CKD is associated with progressive renal fibrosis and inflammation, and currently there is no cure for the disease.

The most common primary illnesses which result in end stage renal disease (ESRD) are diabetes (~37%), hypertension (~24%), glomerulonephritis (~15%), cystic kidney diseases (~4.7%) and urologic diseases (2.5%) [1]. There were 111,000 new ESRD patients diagnosed in 2007 and out of a total of ~500,000 ESRD patients 368,500 people received dialysis treatment in the same year. Dialysis patients have poor quality of life due to high hospitalization rate (458/1000 patients in 2008), high morbidity and mortality (~20%) [1]. Presently, kidney transplant is the only option for these patients to have a close to normal life. According to the US Renal Data System 2010 [1] however, out of the ~85,000 patients awaiting transplant about 18,000 will receive kidney since the amount of available organs did not increase significantly above this number for several years.

Angiotensin converting enzyme inhibitors (ACEIs) and angiotensin receptor blockers (ARBs) are widely used to attenuate the development of cardiovascular diseases and support renal function in CKD patients. However, novel therapeutic targets are desperately needed to effectively treat CKD and slow down disease progression.

Currently, there are about 2,000 clinical trials worldwide addressing some aspects and/or co-morbidities of CKD [2]. These include treatment of anemia, hypertension, secondary hyperparathyroidism, depression and inflammation among others. So far increasing frequency and quality of dialysis did not show advantages in survival rate [2]. Similarly, treatments targeting hypercholesterolemia [3] and hyperhomocysteinemia [4] or the usage of statins [5] failed to increase significantly the survival of ESRD patients.

In recent years, we and others obtained exciting new data on the pathophysiological role of the disintegrin and metalloenzyme ADAMs in renal fibrosis and CKD. This chapter is dedicated to summerize these discoveries and discuss their significance and potential role in the future treatment of patients with renal diseases.

## 2. Physiology of ADAMs and ADAMTS

ADAMs (a disintegrin and metalloenzymes) and ADAMTS (ADAMs with thrombospondin-1-like domains) are membrane-bound multidomain proteins similar to snake venom metalloenzymes and disintegrins. Both groups have pro-, metalloenzyme-like, disintegrin-like and cysteine-rich domains, but compared to ADAMs ADAMTS do not possess cytoplasmic or transmembrane regions. Catalytically active ADAMs are $Zn^{2+}$-dependent endopeptidases and are best known for their sheddase activity. They cleave epidermal growth factor ligands, cytokines and their receptors, adhesion molecules and the infamous amyloid precursor protein among others [6]. ADAMs participate in interreceptor crosstalk between G protein coupled receptors (like angiotensin receptors [7], bradykinin receptors [8] and serotonin receptors [9]) and members of the tyrosine kinase receptors (epidermal growth factors receptor, tumor necrosis factor receptor) by shedding membrane-bound pro-forms of tyrosine kinase ligands (Figure 1). ADAMs are indispensable for normal development, cell proliferation and growth however, at the same time, they can drive pathological cell division and inflammation and have major role in the development of several proliferative and inflammatory diseases [8]. Some of the ADAMs have mutation in their so-called hemopexin-domain (HEXXHXXGXXH) which is responsible for the $Zn^{2+}$-binding of the protein. These ADAMs are catalytically inactive and may have a role in cell-matrix and cell-cell interactions rather than in proteolytic processes [11].

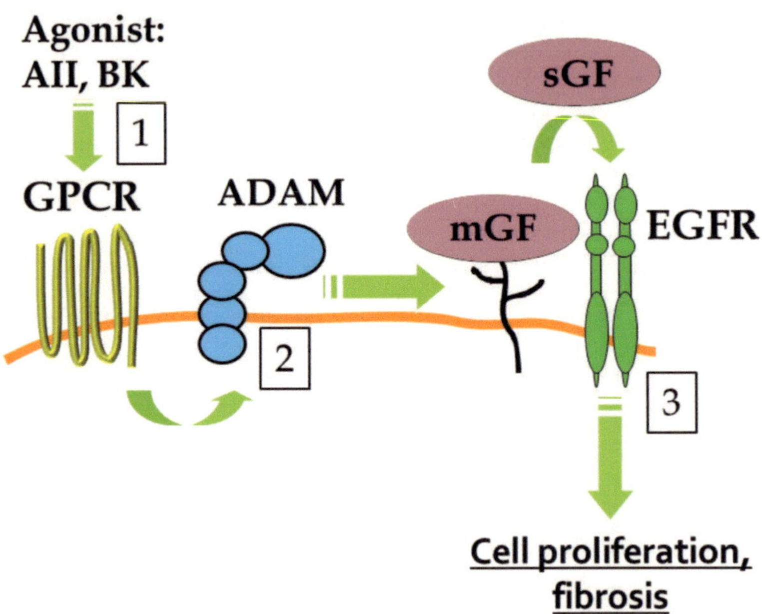


Fig. 1. ADAMs participate in inter-receptor crosstalk: triple membrane spanning signalling. AII: angiotensin-II, BK: bradykinin; GPCR: G protein-coupled receptor; mGF: membrane-bound growth factor, sGF: soluble growth factor; EGFR: epidermal growth factor receptor.

ADAMTSs are secreted proteins which anchor to extracellular matrix molecules through their thrombospondin-1 domain [12] and are involved in proteolytic cleavage of proteoglycans [13], and of the von Willebrand factor [14]. Both protein families can have significant contribution to CKD progression.

### 2.1 Expression of ADAM enzymes in the normal kidney

There are several ADAM and ADAMTS proteins which expression was shown in the human or murine kidney by various techniques. Histochemical analysis showed that ADAM9 was expressed in the nephron: both in the glomerulus and in tubular epithelial cells [15]. Expression of a short form of the enzyme lacking the cytoplasmic region was also reported in the kidney [16]. ADAM10 expression was first shown in chick kidney [17], in mouse kidney of mesenchymal origin [18] and later in humans in the distal tubule, in the connecting tubule, in the principal cells of the collecting duct and in the thick ascending limb of Henle [19]. ADAM11, which is known as a disintegrin metalloenzyme primarily expressed in the central and peripheral nervous system, was also expressed in the epithelial cells of the collecting duct at a low level [20]. Since ADAM11 is differentially expressed during development, it may have an important role in normal kidney morphogenesis. There is also data on the expression of ADAM13 mRNA in the developing mouse kidney [21]. ADAM17 is a disintegrin metalloenzyme which is ubiquitously expressed in almost all mammalian cells. It is present in the kidney [22] and its expression is upregulated in various renal diseases in humans [23]. The mRNA of ADAM19 was present in developing human kidney, and in the endothelial cells and in cell of the distal tubules of the adult kidney [23]. Expression of ADAM31, another proteolytically active disintegrin metalloenzyme was also identified in the epithelium of the convoluted tubuli [24]. High mRNA level of mouse ADAM33 was also shown in the kidney [25]. Since this protein is catalytically inactive, it may have a role in cell-cell interaction and communication.

Of the ADAMTS proteins ADAMTS-1 is expressed at high levels in the adult mice kidney [26], and in situ hybridization showed high level of ADAMTS-1 in the epithelia of the developing kidney [27]. In the rat higher level of ADAMTS-1 was observed in the adult animals compared to newborns, and expression pattern of the protease was restricted to the renal medulla and the principal cells of the collecting ducts in the kidney [28]. ADAMTS-5 was observed in glomerular mesangial cells [29]. ADAMTS-9 [30] and ADAMTS-10 [18] are highly expressed in the developing and adult kidney, respectively, similarly to human ADAMTS-14, -15, -16 [31] with no known function at the present. ADAMTS-13 was shown in healthy human kidney samples and in kidneys of patients with thrombotic thrombocytopenic purpura by real-time PCR and immunohistochemistry. ADAMTS-13 was present in the glomeruli as well as in the tubuli [32]. Also, various transcripts of ADAM16 were shown in the developing human and rat kidneys [33, 34].

#### 2.1.1 ADAM and ADAMTS in kidney development - what we learned from knockout studies

There is very few data available on the role of ADAMs and ADAMTS enzymes in kidney development. There is evidence that expression pattern of ADAMTS-1 [27] and ADAM10 [35] and ADAM13 [21] changes in the kidney during development and that ADAMTS-9 is highly expressed in the mesenchyme of the developing kidney [30]. However, as of present, there is no detail about how knocking down ADAMs influence kidney development.

Targeted knockout of Adamts-1 in mice showed that the enzyme has an important role in kidney development. Deletion of exon 2 (encoding part of the metalloenzyme domain) resulted in lack of ADAMTS-1 protein in mice and high perinatal lethality of the animals due to kidney malfunction [36]. In these animals both the cortical and medullary areas were reduced with concomitant increase in the caliceal space. Another group found that lack of the whole metalloenzyme domain (deletion of exon 2-4) rendered ADAMTS-1 catalytically inactive which resulted in enlarged renal calices and fibrosis of the uteropelvic junction [37]. These animals also developed bilateral hydronephrosis and papillary atrophy shortly after birth [38]. Since normally there is a high level of ADAMTS-1 expressed in the epithelium of the collecting ducts and of the uteropelvic junction, and because the phenotype greatly resembles to symptoms of the human uteropelvic obstruction, these animals can be good models for this genetic disease.

These data also show that targeting strategies can greatly influence the evolving phenotypes.

## 3. ADAMs and ADAMTSs in chronic kidney diseases

### 3.1 ADAMs in diabetic nephropathy

There is increasing evidence on the pathophysiological role of ADAM17 (TACE), ADAM19, ADAMTS-13 in CKD.

ADAM17 is a most well-studied sheddase enzyme. It was originally identified as the tumor necrosis factor (TNF)-α converting (or activating) enzyme [22] or TACE. It cleaves cell surface molecules, most importantly cytokines and growth factors [39]. By activating EGFR ligands and TNF-α ADAM17 has a central role in inflammatory and proliferative processes both of which have crucial role in the development of CKD (Figure 2).

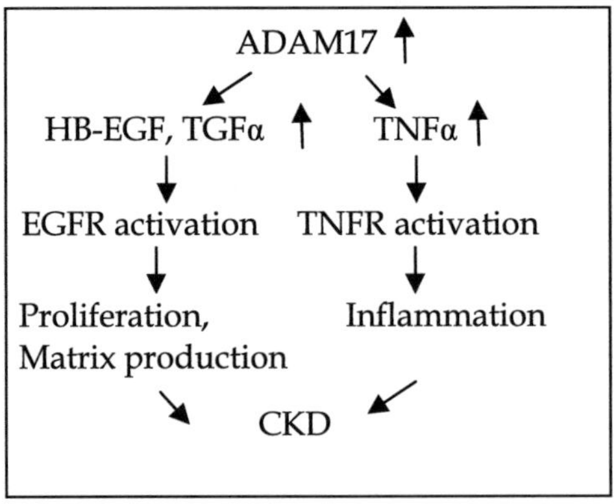


Fig. 2. Role of ADAM17 in CKD.

Besides initiating inflammation, TNFα has important pathophysiological role in insulin resistance (reviewed in [40]). After activation by ADAM17, the soluble homotrimer of TNFα activates the TNF receptor and downstream signaling molecules. Activation of the MAP kinase pathway initiates serine phosphorylation of the insulin receptor substrate (IRS) intracellularly. Being phosphorylated on serine inhibits tyrosine phosphorylation of the IRS which results in insensitivity of the insulin receptor to extracellular insulin and contributes the development of diabetes (Figure 3).

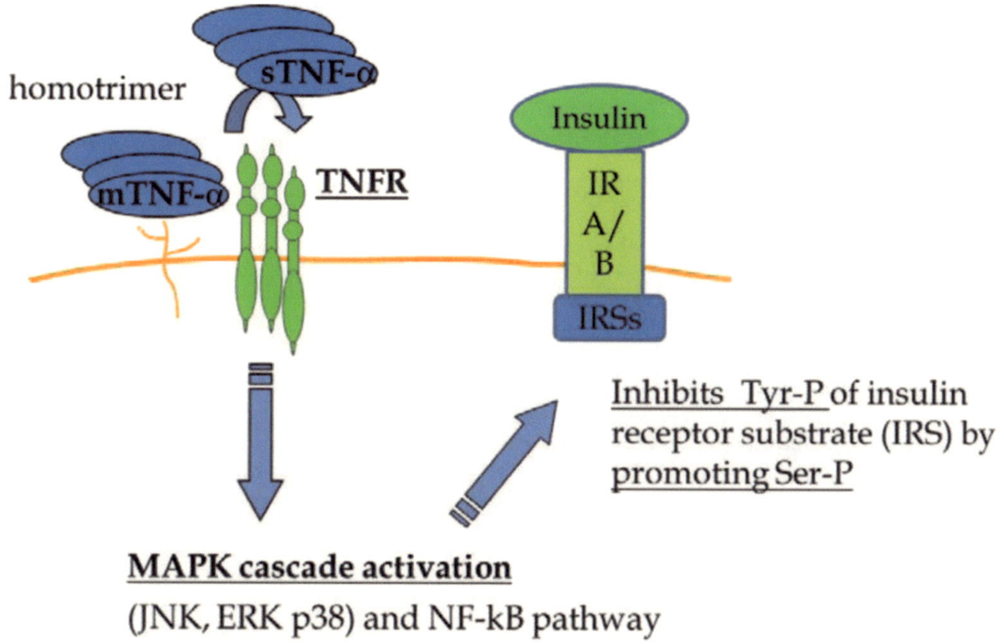


Fig. 3. Mechanism of TNFα-induced insulin resistance

High glucose was also shown to promote heparin-binding growth factor (HB-EGF) shedding through ADAM17 activation, however the exact mechanism is unknown [41].

Since ADAM17 activates secretion of TNFα, pharmacological inhibitors of the enzyme were tested on blood glucose regulation in animal model of non-obesity-related insulin resistance (fructose-fed rats). ADAM17 inhibitor restored the animals' insulin resistance [42]. In another study, animals heterozygous for ADAM17 (+/-) proved to be relatively protected from high-fat diet-induced obesity and diabetes [43].

A close structural relative of ADAM17, ADAM10 is involved in shedding of RAGE: receptor for advanced glycation end products [44]. Since soluble RAGE can block pathophysiological processes initiated by RAGE, ADAM10 activation may slow down development of diabetes.

As of today, we do not have data on the pathophysiological role of ADAMTS enzymes in diabetes mellitus.

### 3.2 ADAMs in renal transplant dysfunction and ischemia reperfusion injury

In vitro studies modelling mechanisms of transplant rejection showed that the mRNA expression of ADAM17 was upregulated in the kidney and that the protein expression of the enzyme was localized next to TNF receptor II. This suggested that ADAM17 may antagonize the effect of TNFα by shedding of its receptor during transplant rejection and therefore higher ADAM17 activity might be beneficial [45]. On the other hand, ADAM17 also co-localized with HB-EGF in experimental ischemia-reperfusion injury which suggested that increased shedding of the growth factor may have contributed to the observed fibrotic injury [46]. Pharmacological inhibitors targeting ADAM17 activity reduced renal tissue injury associated with reperfusion. This confirmed that the increased enzyme activity was a cause rather than the consequence of the tissue injury [47].

Another ADAM enzyme, ADAM19 was also implicated in allograft nephropathy however, we do not know any mechanistic details of its actions [48].

### 3.3 ADAMs in renal fibrosis

Renal fibrosis is a manifestation of several pathological processes. Glomerular fibrosis can be induced by over-activation of the renin-angiotensin system, and the developing fibrosis and inflammation can be successfully attenuated by ADAM17 inhibitors in animal models of the injury [7]. We showed previously that serotonin-induced mesangial cell proliferation, which is an important component of glomerular fibrosis, can be inhibited by knocking down ADAM17 expression and inhibiting the enzyme activity [9]. On the other hand, we also found that ADAM17 can protect glomerular function by decreasing podocyte permeability through inducing re-arrangement of the zonula occludens protein ZO-1 [8]. These data suggest that depending on the cellular context the enzyme can have different effect on the renal function. Nonetheless, inhibitors of ADAM17 decreased infiltration of macrophages both in the glomeruli and in the interstitium in models of kidney fibrosis [7, 46] proving that targeting ADAM17 can be beneficial for preserving renal function.

There is very few data available on ADAMTS enzymes and renal fibrosis. Unilateral ureteral obstruction in rat induced upregulation of ADAMTS-1 in the tubular epithelial cells. Further, secreted ADAMTS-1 of cultured epithelial cells decreased proliferation of a tubular fibroblast cell line which suggested that ADAMTS-1 may have anti-fibrotic effect [49].

### 3.4 ADAMs in polycystic kidney disease (PKD)

Autosomal-recessive polycystic kidney disease (AR-PKD) is one of the most common genetic disorders of the kidney results in end-stage renal disease. This disease leads to rapid enlargement of the kidney through massive cysts formation. The main pathogenic process in cyst development is the overactivation of the mislocalized EGFR in the cystic apical epithelia (for review see [50]). Excessive shedding of the pro-proliferative growth factor, transforming growth factor (TGF)α was also observed. Since secretion of TGFα is regulated by ADAM17, therapeutic potential of ADAM17 inhibitors were explored and established in the *bpk* murine model of AR-PKD [51]. In a later study, the role of TGFα was not confirmed even if ADAM17 inhibitors were beneficial for attenuating cyst development in AR-PKD [52].

### 3.5 Thrombotic thrombocytopenic purpura (TTP)/ haemolytic-uremic syndrome (HUS)

Thrombotic thrombocytopenic purpura/haemolytic uremic syndrome are often considered variants of a disease characterized by microangiopathic haemolytic anaemia [53]. Platelets are consumed by spontaneously developing microscopic thrombosis. ADAMTS-13, the enzyme which normally processes the very large von Willebrand factor (vWF) is missing [54] or disabled [55, 56] in this disease. Therefore, the very large vWF "capture" circulating platelets and initiates microthrombi formation. The red blood cells passing through the damaged arteries experience excessive shear stress which leads to haemodialysis. Besides purpura and anaemia there are often fever and neurologic symptoms present and the disease can lead to both acute kidney failure and CKD [57, 58]. Interestingly, a recent study which investigated plasma level of vWF in patients with chronic kidney disease of different origin found decreased level of vWF-cleaving protease [59]. Level of vWF was higher in stage IV patients compared to stages II and III, but whether the increased vWF contributed to the worsening of CKD is currently not known.

## 4. ADAMs in kidney cancer

Several ADAM enzymes were upregulated at the message level in human renal cell carcinomas. Compared to normal tissue mRNA levels of ADAM8, -17, -19, -28 as well as ADAMTS-2 were upregulated. Interestingly, mRNA level of ADAMTS-1 did not change [60]. In other studies, ADAM10 [61] and ADAM9 expression was increased in renal cancer cells and associated with tumor progression [62] suggesting that expression of these enzyme may be used as tumor markers. ADAM15 and -17 contributed to the migratory potential of kidney cancer cells through activation of the EGFR [63] and ADAM17 silencing disabled the capability of renal carcinoma cells to form in vivo tumors [64]. Therefore these enzymes seem to have direct role in renal cancer pathophysiology.

## 5. Conclusion

ADAM and ADAMTS families include growing number of metalloenzymes which have important role in kidney development and are indispensable to normal kidney function.

Lack or overactivation of certain ADAM enzymes (especially ADAM17 and ADAMTS-13) can have major pathophysiological role in development of various type of CKD. Therefore, targeting these enzymes can be an exciting novel therapeutic approach in the future and a new hope for CKD patients.

## 6. Acknowledgment

This work was partly supported by the Paul Teschan Research Fund of the Dialysis Clinic Incorporated.

## 7. References

[1] National Institutes of Health, National Institute of Diabetes and Digestive and Kidney Diseases. United States Renal Data System: *2010 Atlas of CKD in the United States.* Available from http://www.usrds.org/

[2] *Clinical Trials at the U. S. National Institute of Health.* Available from http://clinicaltrials.gov/

[3] Liu, Y., et al., *Association between cholesterol level and mortality in dialysis patients: role of inflammation and malnutrition.* JAMA : the journal of the American Medical Association, 2004. 291(4): p. 451-9.

[4] Kalantar-Zadeh, K., et al., *A low, rather than a high, total plasma homocysteine is an indicator of poor outcome in hemodialysis patients.* Journal of the American Society of Nephrology : JASN, 2004. 15(2): p. 442-53.

[5] Wanner, C., et al., *Atorvastatin in patients with type 2 diabetes mellitus undergoing hemodialysis.* The New England journal of medicine, 2005. 353(3): p. 238-48.

[6] Blobel, C.P., *ADAMs: key components in EGFR signalling and development.* Nature reviews. Molecular cell biology, 2005. 6(1): p. 32-43.

[7] Lautrette, A., et al., *Angiotensin II and EGF receptor cross-talk in chronic kidney diseases: a new therapeutic approach.* Nature medicine, 2005. 11(8): p. 867-74.

[8] Dey, M., et al., *Bradykinin decreases podocyte permeability through ADAM17-dependent epidermal growth factor receptor activation and zonula occludens-1 rearrangement.* The Journal of pharmacology and experimental therapeutics, 2010. 334(3): p. 775-83.

[9] Gooz, M., et al., *5-HT2A receptor induces ERK phosphorylation and proliferation through ADAM-17 tumor necrosis factor-alpha-converting enzyme (TACE) activation and heparin-bound epidermal growth factor-like growth factor (HB-EGF) shedding in mesangial cells.* The Journal of biological chemistry, 2006. 281(30): p. 21004-12.

[10] Gooz, M., *ADAM-17: the enzyme that does it all.* Critical reviews in biochemistry and molecular biology, 2010. 45(2): p. 146-69.

[11] Schlondorff, J. and C.P. Blobel, *Metalloprotease-disintegrins: modular proteins capable of promoting cell-cell interactions and triggering signals by protein-ectodomain shedding.* Journal of cell science, 1999. 112 ( Pt 21): p. 3603-17.

[12] Kuno, K. and K. Matsushima, *ADAMTS-1 protein anchors at the extracellular matrix through the thrombospondin type I motifs and its spacing region.* The Journal of biological chemistry, 1998. 273(22): p. 13912-7.

[13] Stanton, H., et al., *Proteoglycan degradation by the ADAMTS family of proteinases.* Biochimica et biophysica acta, 2011. 1812(12): p. 1616-29.

[14] Fujikawa, K., et al., *Purification of human von Willebrand factor-cleaving protease and its identification as a new member of the metalloproteinase family.* Blood, 2001. 98(6): p. 1662-6.

[15] Mahimkar, R.M., et al., *Identification, cellular distribution and potential function of the metalloprotease-disintegrin MDC9 in the kidney.* Journal of the American Society of Nephrology : JASN, 2000. 11(4): p. 595-603.

[16] Hotoda, N., et al., *A secreted form of human ADAM9 has an alpha-secretase activity for APP.* Biochemical and biophysical research communications, 2002. 293(2): p. 800-5.

[17] Hall, R.J. and C.A. Erickson, *ADAM 10: an active metalloprotease expressed during avian epithelial morphogenesis.* Developmental biology, 2003. 256(1): p. 146-59.

[18] Somerville, R.P., K.A. Jungers, and S.S. Apte, *Discovery and characterization of a novel, widely expressed metalloprotease, ADAMTS10, and its proteolytic activation.* The Journal of biological chemistry, 2004. 279(49): p. 51208-17.

[19] Schramme, A., et al., *Characterization of CXCL16 and ADAM10 in the normal and transplanted kidney.* Kidney international, 2008. 74(3): p. 328-38.

[20] Rybnikova, E., et al., *Developmental regulation and neuronal expression of the cellular disintegrin ADAM11 gene in mouse nervous system.* Neuroscience, 2002. 112(4): p. 921-34.

[21] Lin, J., C. Redies, and J. Luo, *Regionalized expression of ADAM13 during chicken embryonic development.* Developmental dynamics : an official publication of the American Association of Anatomists, 2007. 236(3): p. 862-70.

[22] Black, R.A., et al., *A metalloproteinase disintegrin that releases tumour-necrosis factor-alpha from cells.* Nature, 1997. 385(6618): p. 729-33.

[23] Melenhorst, W.B., et al., *ADAM17 upregulation in human renal disease: a role in modulating TGF-alpha availability?* American journal of physiology. Renal physiology, 2009. 297(3): p. F781-90.

[24] Liu, L. and J.W. Smith, *Identification of ADAM 31: a protein expressed in Leydig cells and specialized epithelia.* Endocrinology, 2000. 141(6): p. 2033-42.

[25] Gunn, T.M., et al., *Identification and preliminary characterization of mouse Adam33.* BMC genetics, 2002. 3: p. 2.

[26] Miles, R.R., et al., *ADAMTS-1: A cellular disintegrin and metalloprotease with thrombospondin motifs is a target for parathyroid hormone in bone.* Endocrinology, 2000. 141(12): p. 4533-42.

[27] Thai, S.N. and M.L. Iruela-Arispe, *Expression of ADAMTS1 during murine development.* Mechanisms of development, 2002. 115(1-2): p. 181-5.

[28] Gunther, W., et al., *Distribution patterns of the anti-angiogenic protein ADAMTS-1 during rat development.* Acta histochemica, 2005. 107(2): p. 121-31.

[29] McCulloch, D.R., et al., *Adamts5, the gene encoding a proteoglycan-degrading metalloprotease, is expressed by specific cell lineages during mouse embryonic development and in adult tissues.* Gene expression patterns : GEP, 2009. 9(5): p. 314-23.

[30] Jungers, K.A., et al., *Adamts9 is widely expressed during mouse embryo development.* Gene expression patterns : GEP, 2005. 5(5): p. 609-17.

[31] Cal, S., et al., *Cloning, expression analysis, and structural characterization of seven novel human ADAMTSs, a family of metalloproteinases with disintegrin and thrombospondin-1 domains.* Gene, 2002. 283(1-2): p. 49-62.

[32] Manea, M., et al., *Podocytes express ADAMTS13 in normal renal cortex and in patients with thrombotic thrombocytopenic purpura.* British journal of haematology, 2007. 138(5):
p. 651-62.

[33] Surridge, A.K., et al., *Characterization and regulation of ADAMTS-16.* Matrix biology : journal of the International Society for Matrix Biology, 2009. 28(7): p. 416-24.

[34] Joe, B., et al., *Positional identification of variants of Adamts16 linked to inherited hypertension.* Human molecular genetics, 2009. 18(15): p. 2825-38.

[35] Stuart, R.O., K.T. Bush, and S.K. Nigam, *Changes in gene expression patterns in the ureteric bud and metanephric mesenchyme in models of kidney development.* Kidney international, 2003. 64(6): p. 1997-2008.

[36] Mittaz, L., et al., *Neonatal calyceal dilation and renal fibrosis resulting from loss of Adamts-1 in mouse kidney is due to a developmental dysgenesis.* Nephrology, dialysis, transplantation : official publication of the European Dialysis and Transplant Association - European Renal Association, 2005. 20(2): p. 419-23.

[37] Shindo, T., et al., *ADAMTS-1: a metalloproteinase-disintegrin essential for normal growth, fertility, and organ morphology and function.* The Journal of clinical investigation, 2000. 105(10): p. 1345-52.

[38] Yokoyama, H., et al., *A disintegrin and metalloproteinase with thrombospondin motifs (ADAMTS)-1 null mutant mice develop renal lesions mimicking obstructive nephropathy.* Nephrology, dialysis, transplantation : official publication of the European Dialysis and Transplant Association - European Renal Association, 2002. 17 Suppl 9: p. 39-41.

[39] Sunnarborg, S.W., et al., *Tumor necrosis factor-alpha converting enzyme (TACE) regulates epidermal growth factor receptor ligand availability.* The Journal of biological chemistry, 2002. 277(15): p. 12838-45.

[40] Taniguchi, C.M., B. Emanuelli, and C.R. Kahn, *Critical nodes in signalling pathways: insights into insulin action.* Nature reviews. Molecular cell biology, 2006. 7(2): p. 85-96.

[41] Uttarwar, L., et al., *HB-EGF release mediates glucose-induced activation of the epidermal growth factor receptor in mesangial cells.* American journal of physiology. Renal physiology, 2011. 300(4): p. F921-31.

[42] Togashi, N., et al., *Effect of TNF-alpha--converting enzyme inhibitor on insulin resistance in fructose-fed rats.* Hypertension, 2002. 39(2 Pt 2): p. 578-80.

[43] Serino, M., et al., *Mice heterozygous for tumor necrosis factor-alpha converting enzyme are protected from obesity-induced insulin resistance and diabetes.* Diabetes, 2007. 56(10): p. 2541-6.

[44] Zhang, L., et al., *Receptor for advanced glycation end products is subjected to protein ectodomain shedding by metalloproteinases.* The Journal of biological chemistry, 2008. 283(51): p. 35507-16.

[45] Wang, J., et al., *The role of tumor necrosis factor-alpha converting enzyme in renal transplant rejection.* American journal of nephrology, 2010. 32(4): p. 362-8.
[46] Mulder, G.M., et al., *ADAM17 up-regulation in renal transplant dysfunction and non-transplant-related renal fibrosis.* Nephrology, dialysis, transplantation : official publication of the European Dialysis and Transplant Association - European Renal Association, 2011.
[47] Souza, D.G., et al., *Effects of PKF242-484 and PKF241-466, novel dual inhibitors of TNF-alpha converting enzyme and matrix metalloproteinases, in a model of intestinal reperfusion injury in mice.* European journal of pharmacology, 2007. 571(1): p. 72-80.
[48] Melenhorst, W.B., et al., *Upregulation of ADAM19 in chronic allograft nephropathy.* American journal of transplantation : official journal of the American Society of Transplantation and the American Society of Transplant Surgeons, 2006. 6(7): p. 1673-81.
[49] Nakamura, A., et al., *Expression and significance of a disintegrin and metalloproteinase with thrombospondin motifs (ADAMTS)-1 in an animal model of renal interstitial fibrosis induced by unilateral ureteral obstruction.* Experimental and toxicologic pathology : official journal of the Gesellschaft fur Toxikologische Pathologie, 2007. 59(1): p. 1-7.
[50] Torres, V.E. and P.C. Harris, *Mechanisms of Disease: autosomal dominant and recessive polycystic kidney diseases.* Nature clinical practice. Nephrology, 2006. 2(1): p. 40-55; quiz 55.
[51] Dell, K.M., et al., *A novel inhibitor of tumor necrosis factor-alpha converting enzyme ameliorates polycystic kidney disease.* Kidney international, 2001. 60(4): p. 1240-8.
[52] Nemo, R., N. Murcia, and K.M. Dell, *Transforming growth factor alpha (TGF-alpha) and other targets of tumor necrosis factor-alpha converting enzyme (TACE) in murine polycystic kidney disease.* Pediatric research, 2005. 57(5 Pt 1): p. 732-7.
[53] Desch, K. and D. Motto, *Is there a shared pathophysiology for thrombotic thrombocytopenic purpura and hemolytic-uremic syndrome?* Journal of the American Society of Nephrology : JASN, 2007. 18(9): p. 2457-60.
[54] Sasahara, Y., et al., *Deficient activity of von Willebrand factor-cleaving protease in patients with Upshaw-Schulman syndrome.* International journal of hematology, 2001. 74(1): p. 109-14.
[55] Coppo, P., et al., *Severe ADAMTS13 deficiency in adult idiopathic thrombotic microangiopathies defines a subset of patients characterized by various autoimmune manifestations, lower platelet count, and mild renal involvement.* Medicine, 2004. 83(4): p. 233-44.
[56] Veyradier, A., et al., *Severe deficiency of the specific von Willebrand factor-cleaving protease (ADAMTS 13) activity in a subgroup of children with atypical hemolytic uremic syndrome.* The Journal of pediatrics, 2003. 142(3): p. 310-7.
[57] George, J.N., *ADAMTS13, thrombotic thrombocytopenic purpura, and hemolytic uremic syndrome.* Current hematology reports, 2005. 4(3): p. 167-9.
[58] Bramham, K., et al., *ADAMTS-13 deficiency: can it cause chronic renal failure?* Nephrology, dialysis, transplantation : official publication of the European Dialysis and Transplant Association - European Renal Association, 2011. 26(2): p. 742-4.

[59] Lu, G.Y., et al., *Significance of plasma von Willebrand factor level and von Willebrand factor-cleaving protease activity in patients with chronic renal diseases.* Chinese medical journal, 2008. 121(2): p. 133-6.

[60] Roemer, A., et al., *Increased mRNA expression of ADAMs in renal cell carcinoma and their association with clinical outcome.* Oncology reports, 2004. 11(2): p. 529-36.

[61] Doberstein, K., J. Pfeilschifter, and P. Gutwein, *The transcription factor PAX2 regulates ADAM10 expression in renal cell carcinoma.* Carcinogenesis, 2011. 32(11): p. 1713-23.

[62] Fritzsche, F.R., et al., *ADAM9 is highly expressed in renal cell cancer and is associated with tumour progression.* BMC cancer, 2008. 8: p. 179.

[63] Schafer, B., et al., *Distinct ADAM metalloproteinases regulate G protein-coupled receptor-induced cell proliferation and survival.* The Journal of biological chemistry, 2004. 279(46): p. 47929-38.

[64] Franovic, A., et al., *Multiple acquired renal carcinoma tumor capabilities abolished upon silencing of ADAM17.* Cancer research, 2006. 66(16): p. 8083-90.

# 2

# Severity and Stages of Chronic Kidney Disease

Syed Ahmed and Gerard Lowder
*Internal Medicine, Harbor Hospital, Baltimore, USA*

## 1. Introduction

Nearly ten years ago Nephrologists began using asystem of classification for chronic kidney disease (CKD). This was established in 2002 by the Kidney Disease Outcome Quality Initiative (KDOQI) to estimate kidney function in a given patient regardless of the etiology of the primary insult to the kidneys. Physicians were able place their patients in stages from mild disease to end stage renal disease (ESRD).CKD is defined as glomerular filtration rate (GFR) below 60 ml/min per 1.73 $m^2$ for 3 months or more.

Each stage served as a "mile marker" on life's road for the patient with CKD. The natural history of CKD usually is a steady decline in kidney function, as found in the relationship between the reciprocal of serum creatinine values and time. A percentage of patients do not follow this linear pattern, suggesting either worsening or improvement in their kidney function. Factors which may cause worsening of CKD in such individuals are often infections, dehydration, poor control of systemic blood pressure and exposure to nephrotoxins, in particular nonsteroidal anti-inflamatorydrugs and radiocontrast agents. Other individuals who do not follow the steady decline may actually show improvement in their GFR. The potential to improve the natural history of CKD is through tight blood pressure control and inhibition of rennin-angiotensin-aldosterone system.

## 2. Stages of chronic kidney disease

The early stages of kidney dysfunction are often clinically silent, especially when the condition is only slowly progressive and symptoms are nonspecific. Stages 1 & 2 show decreased kidney function without signs or symptoms of disease although the estimated GFR is less than 120 ml/min per 1.73 $m^2$ but greater than 60 ml/min per 1.73 $m^2$. The rate of progression is influenced by a wide range of factors which may or may not have the potential of modification and varies among different individuals and with the underlying cause of nephropathy.When the patient enters Stage 3 he or she has lost approximately half their kidney function. It is less likely for the kidney disease to progress unless more than 50% of the nephron function is lost. For example, individuals with a solitary kidney after unilateral nephrectomy for living kidney donation usually do not progress to CKD.Increased risk of natural progression with less than 50% of nephron loss can occur in persons of African ancestry with hypertensive nephrosclerosis. In 2008, the U.K National Institute of Health and Clinical Excellence (NICE) sub divided the stage 3 into 3A and 3B with estimated GFRs of 45 to 59 ml/min per 1.73 $m^2$ and 44 to 30 ml/min per 1.73 $m^2$

respectively. The NICE CKD guideline also suggested adding the suffix *p* to the stages in proteinuric patients.It has generally been assumed that the majority of patients with CKD stages 3B to 5 eventually progress to ESRD. A Canadian study showed the natural history of CKD stages 3 and 4 to be variable and reflecting the patient's risk factor profile.Stage 4 may present with hyperkalemia or problems with salt and water retention. The kidneys are no longer able to adjust to abrupt changes in sodium, potassium and fluid intake (or loss). Prior to initiation of renal replacement therapy, the patient's appetite may decrease, accompanied by weight loss and a decrease in the serum albumin. In CKD clinics, with patients seen at frequent intervals, the goal is to initiate dialysis before the patient becomes malnourished.

| Stage | Description | GFR (ml/min/1.73m$^2$) |
|---|---|---|
| 1 | Kidney damage with normal or ↑ GFR | ≥ 90 |
| 2 | Kidney damage with mild ↓ GFR | 60-89 |
| 3 | Moderate ↓ GFR | 3A 45 – 59<br>3B 30 - 44 |
| 4 | Severe ↓ GFR | 15-29 |
| 5 | Kidney Failure | < 15 (or dialysis) |
| The suffix p to be added to the stage in patients with proteinuria > 0.5 g/24h | | |

Table 1. Stages of CKD.

Two commonly used formulas to calculate creatinine clearance are the Cockcroft-Gault formula and MDRD formula.

**Cockcroft-Gault formula:** $GFR = \frac{(140 - Age) \times Mass(Kgs) \times (0.85 \ \ if \ \ female)}{72 \times Serum\ Cr}$

**Modification of diet in renal disease (MDRD) formula:**

$$GFR = 186 \times SCr.^{-1.154} \times Age^{-0.203} \times (1.212 \ if \ black) \times (0.742 \ \ if \ \ female)$$

## 3. Risk factors

It is estimated that by 2030,more than 2,000,000 Americans will need dialysis or transplantation. Who are these patients? What risk factors do they have?

Low birth weight individuals with a decreased number of nephrons, the elderly population losing 1 ml/min/year after the age of 30 and Americans of African descent with hypertension, are several groups of individuals at risk.About one half of patients starting dialysis in America have diabetes mellitus, with hypertension the second largest group. Autoimmune disorders, infections, kidney stones, cystic kidneys and toxins/medications round out the list. Microalbuminuria may indicate systemic endothelial dysfunction and may be associated with a prothrombotic state. Insulin resistance is mediated in part by aldosterone; blocking the receptor attenuates cardiovascular and renal injury.

The risk factors can be classified as those that increase the risk of development of kidney disease and those that increase the risk of adverse outcomes associated with CKD. The factors which increase the risk for CKD are further classified into susceptibility and initiation factors; whereas factors which effect adverse outcomes are classified as progression factors and end stage factors. The association between variables and disease may be due to chance, a non-causal relation or may signify a true risk factor.

### 3.1 Risk factors for development of CKD

**1. Susceptibility Factors**

A susceptibility factor is one that increases susceptibility to kidney damage following exposure to an initiation factor. An ideal study design to study these factors would be to identify a population of individuals who are free of kidney disease and are exposed to an initiation factor and follow them for a period of time.

**2. Initiation Factor**

An initiation factor is one that directly initiates kidney damage in an individual who is susceptible to kidney damage. An ideal study design for identification of initiation factors is a prospective cohort study. This would involve identification and follow up of a group of individuals free of kidney disease at baseline, with known susceptibility factors and with or without exposure to initiation factors, for the development of kidney disease.

### 3.2 Risk factors effecting adverse outcome of CKD

**1. Progression Factors**

Progression factors worsen the kidney damage caused by initiation factors and lead to further decline in kidney function. Indicators of progression may include progression of microalbuminuria to overt proteinuria or reduced GFR, rate of decrease of GFR, or development of kidney failure necessitating dialysis or transplantation.

**2. End-Stage Factors**

End -stage factors are those that exacerbate the morbidity and mortality associated with kidney failure. Examples of indicators of mobidity include hospitalizations, poor quality of life measures, and cardiovascular disease complications.

### 3.3 Risk factors for progression of chronic kidney disease

1. Proteinuria

   Proteinuria is associated with faster rates of CKD progression. It contributes to nephron loss; filtered proteins are reabsorbed by the proximal tubular cells. Tubular cell contents may leak into the interstitium. This can cause macrophage infiltration and inflammatory mediators produced by them. The MDRD study showed proteinuria to be the strongest predictor of kidney disease progression in non diabetic patients. The REIN study done in non diabetic patients with proteinuria, showed the protein excretion rate to be the best single predictor of GFR decline to ESRD. This finding was independent of the initial insult.

   The US Collaborative Study in type 1 diabetic patients with >500mg proteinuria/day and serum creatinine values of 2.5mg% or less showed a 50% reduction in the risk of combined endpoints (death, dialysis, transplantation) in patients treated with an ACE inhibitor.

| Risk Factor | Definition | Examples |
|---|---|---|
| Susceptibility factors | Increase susceptibility to kidney damage | Older age, family history of chronic kidney disease, reduction in kidney mass, low birthweight, U.S. racial or ethnic minority status, low income or education |
| Initiation factors | Directly initiate kidney damage | Diabetes, high blood pressure, autoimmune diseases, systemic infections, urinary tract infections, urinary stones, lower urinary tract obstruction, drug toxicity |
| Progression factors | Cause worsening kidney damage and faster decline in kidney function after initiation of kidney damage | Higher level of proteinuria, higher blood pressure, poor glycemic control in diabetes, smoking |
| End-stage factors | Increase morbidity and mortality in kidney failure | Lower dialysis dose (Kt/V), temporary vascular access, anemia, low serum albumin level, late referral |

Table 2. Risk Factors for Chronic Kidney Disease and its Outcomes.

The IDNT Study looked at type 2 diabetic patients treated with placebo, ibesartan or amlodipine. The ARB outperformed the placebo group and calcium channel patients in reaching doubling of the serum creatinine, ESRD, death by 20% and 23% respectively.

2. Hypertension

   Blood pressure should be lowered to <120/80.

   Patients with blood pressure 120-129/80-84 have a 1.6 fold greater risk of developing ESRD and those with pressure >210/120 have a 4.2 fold risk of ESRD.

   The MRFIT study showed that hypertension was an independent risk factor for the development of ESRD.
3. Smoking cessation- smoking is a risk factor in the progession to kidney failure

   Hallan, S & Orth, S. KI 2011.157
4. Glycemic control

   Blood pressure control is more important with progression of CKD in the diabetic patient, whereas hyperglycemia is important with the initiation of diabetic nephropathy.
5. Management of dyslipidemia

   LDL stimulates mesangial cell proliferation and the synthesis of proinflammatory molecules.

   No large study is available to show that control of lipids is effective in slowing the progression of CKD. The SHARP study showed that CKD patients receiving simvastatin and ezetimibe had approximately 15% fewer strokes and MIs.

## 4. Mechanism of progression

The characteristic structural change in CKD is scarring associated with glomerulosclerosis, tubulointerstitial fibrosis, and vascular sclerosis. After this initial insult the kidney goes down on one of the two paths, healing and functional recovery or scarring with loss of kidney function progressing to CKD. It is less known what leads the kidney to which pathway.

Healing primarily occurs in Acute Kidney Injury (AKI) and acute interstitial nephritis, when treatment is instituted early in its course. Healing is also a hallmark of acute post infectious glomerulonephritis. Renal function typically recovers within few weeks of acute nephritic process.Chronic kidney damage on the other hand is usually induced by diabetes, hypertension, chronic glomerulonephritits, or chronic exposure to infections or nephrotoxins, progress to scarring with loss of function and CKD. (Fig. 1)

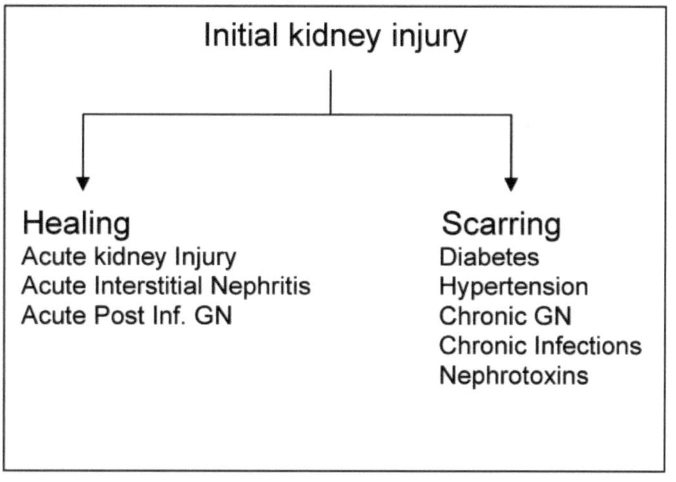


Fig. 1. Progression of initial kidney injury.

Renal cell injury results in loss of glomerular capillaries and cellular elements are replaced by extracellular matrix and fibrous tissue. Acute severe glomerulonephritis damages the capillaries and endothelium whereas sub-acute and chronic glomerulonephritis affect the mesangium or the podocytes. Progressive renal scarring is associated with progressive tubular cell loss and atrophy.

### 4.1 Role of intrinsic renal cells in kidney damage

Endothelium: Damage to the protective anticoagulant and anti-inflamatory endothelial capillary lining in acute glomerulonephritis, transforms it into a pro-inflammatory surface leading to accumulation of inflammatory cells and platelets within golmerular capillaries as well as the stimulation of mesangial proliferation. Glomerular endothelial damage can also be due to a metabolic insult as in diabetes or a physical hemodynamic stress as in hypertension.

Mesangium: Mesangial cells respond to injury either with death, transformation, proliferation and migration,or synthesis and deposition of extracellular matrix (ECM). Scarring is usually characterized by uncontrolled mesangial proliferation and excessive deposition of mesangial matrix. This process is driven by a number of growth factors like transforming growth factor β1 (TGFβ1), platelet derived growth factor (PDGF), and fibroblast growth factor (FGF).

Podocytes: After an injury to the podocytes, the glomerular basement membrane is exposed to the parietal epithelial cells leading to the formation of capsular adhesions and segmental glomerulosclerosis. This may lead to misdirected filtration with accumulation of amorphous material in the glomerular space. Misdirected filtration causes disruption of the glomerular-tubular junction resulting in atubularglomeruli. It may also contribute to tubular atrophy and interstitial fibrosis. Thus podocytes help in conserving the structural integrity of the glomerulus by forming a protective membrane over the basement membrane.

Tubular cells: As mentioned earlier, after the initial insult the tubular cells may undergo healing and recover renal function, but repeated insults stimulate epithelial mesenchymal transformation of tubular cells to myofibroblastic phenotype with excessive deposition of ECM. Thus tubular injury can lead to renal fibrogenesis.

Vascular cells: Vascular sclerosis is an intergral feature of renal scarring and is associated with progressive kidney failure in glomerulonephritis. Hyalinosis of afferent arterioles, in diabetes, and damage to the post-glomerular arteriole and peritubular capillaries cause interstitial ischemia and fibrosis.

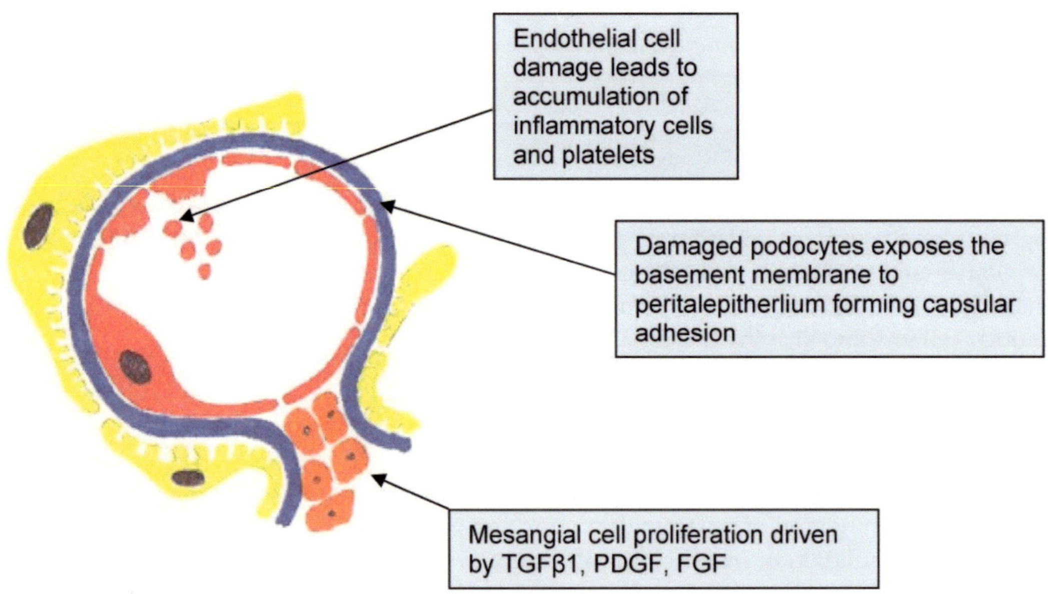


Fig. 2. Role of Intrinsic Cells in Kidney Damage.

### 4.2 Role of extrinsic cells in kidney damage

Infiltration of inflammatory cells into the glomeruli and the renal interstitium is the hallmark of glomerulosclerosis and tubuloiterstitial fibrosis.

Platelets and coagulation: Platelets and their release products within the damaged glomeruli stimulate a coagulation cascade which activate the mesangial cells to induce sclerosis. Thrombin stimulates glomerular TGF-β1 leading to production of mesangial ECM and inhibition of metalloproteinases.

Lymphocytes, Monocytes-Macrophages, Dendritic cells play important role in the formation of glomerulosclerosis by causing inflammation.

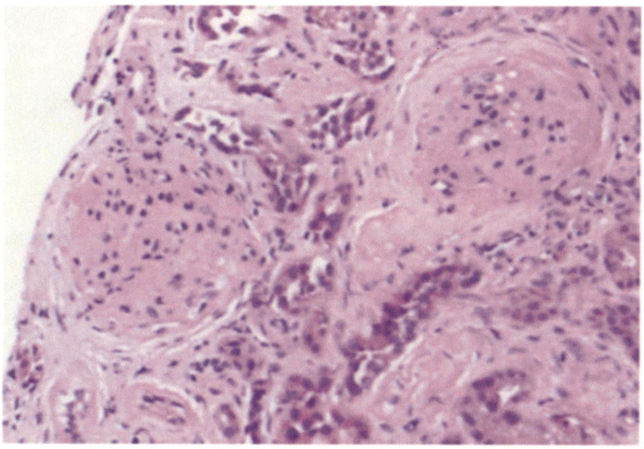

Fig. 3. Deposition on of ECM within and around the glomerulus.

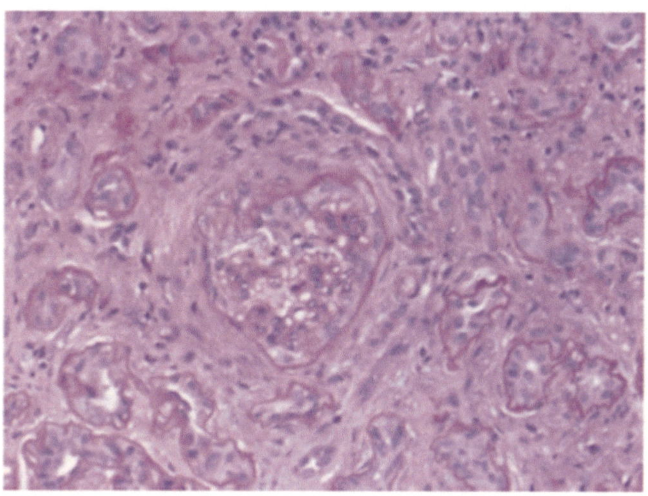

Fig. 4. Glomerular hypercellularity due to proliferation of intrinsic glomerular cells and intracapillary leukocytes.

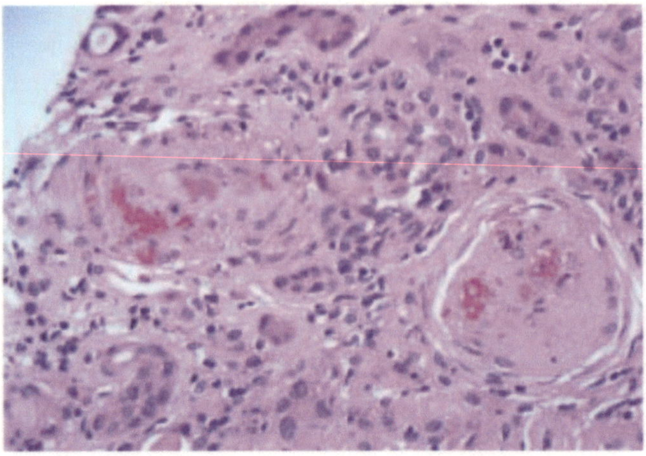

Fig. 5. Capillary tufts almost replaced by the fibous tissue forming glomerular scarring.

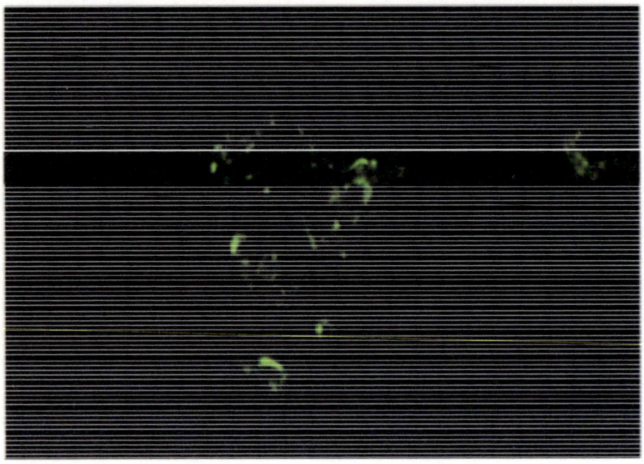

Fig. 6. Immunofluorescent stain shows deposition of coarsely granular deposits of complement C3.

### 4.3 Role of angiotensin II, hypertension and hyperfiltration

With progression of kidney disease the afferent arteriole tone decreases to a much larger extent than the efferent tone. As a result intra-glomerular pressure rises leading to hyperfiltration. Angiotensin II aides in hyperfiltration through its vasoconstrictor effect predominantly on the efferent arteriole. Apart from its hemodynamic effects, Angiotensin II acts directly on the glomerular membrane. It acts on the angiotensin II receptors on the surface of the podocytes, altering their permselective property, by contracting the foot processes. This allows proteins to escape in the urinary space.

Angiotensin II also induces proliferation ofglomerular cells and fibroblasts. It acts on AT1 receptors on tubular cells causing hypertrophy, which results in increased synthesis of collagen type IV. It increases macrophage activation and phagocytosis responsible for the inflammatory component associated with CKD.

### 4.4 Role of proteinuria

Proteinuria is not only a marker of kidney damage, but also contributes to nephron damage. Filtered proteins are reabsorbed from the proximal tubule. Damaged tubular basement membrane causes leakage of tubular content into the interstitium, thereby causing macrophage infiltration. Macrophages produce inflammatory mediators thus mounting an immense inflammatory reaction inside the renal interstitium.

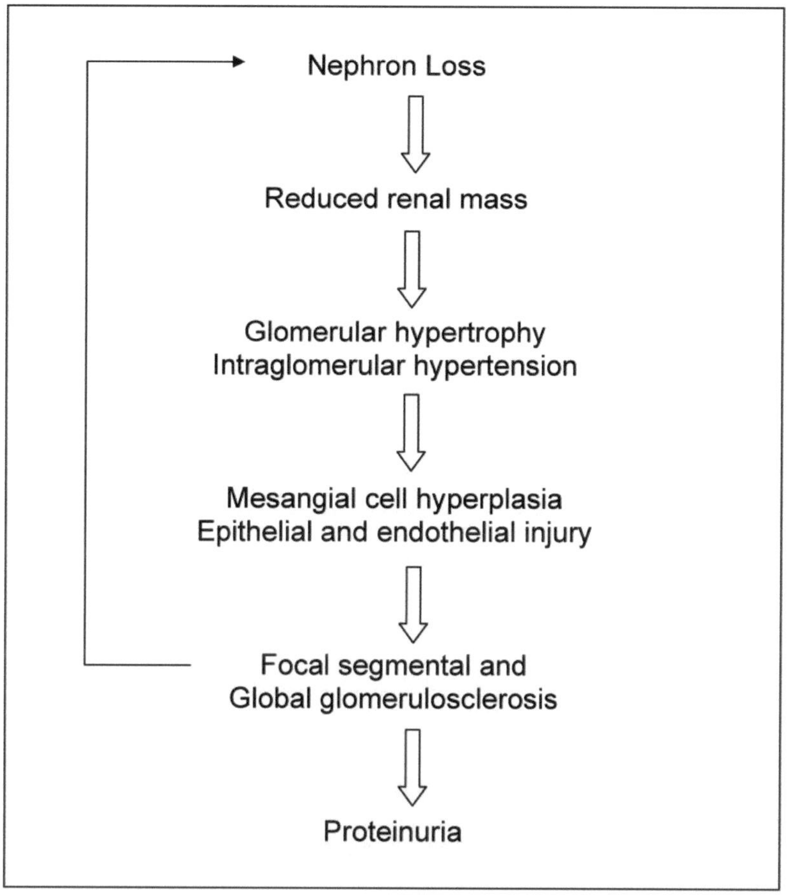


Fig. 7. Focal segmental and global Glomerulosclerosis and nephron loss is a vicious circle ultimately leading to proteinuria.

## 5. Pathology of CKD

Fibrosis in the kidneys initiated by a variety of insults may not be a uniform process.

Progressive disease in diabetic patients may be related to endothelial nitric oxide deficiency with resultant endothelial dysfunction.The eventual pathology of the above mentioned series of events lead to two major histologic characteristic of CKD, focal segmental glomerulosclerosis and tubulointerstitial fibrosis. An initial insult to the kidneys will cause nephron loss.The remaining nephrons work harder to compensate for the lost nephrons (compensatory hypertrophy). This leads to hemodynamic changes including glomerular hypertension and hyperfiltration. There is reduced afferent arteriolar resistance and intraglomerular pressure rises with increased filtration by the remaining nephrons. The intrinsic and extrinsic cells contribute to sclerosis as mentioned above contributing to the focal and segmental glomerulosclerosis.

Tubulointerstitial injury results from ischemia of tubule segments downstream from sclerotic glomeruli. Acute and chronic inflammation in the adjacent interstitium, and damage of pericapillary blood supply also contribute to tubular injury. The above events along with proteinuria eventually lead to tubulointerstitial fibrosis.

Angiotensin II increases vascular tone (predominantly post-glomerular) and affects intraglomerular pressure. The increased pressure alters the structure of the pores in the glomerular basement membrane (GBM) and increases proteinuria.

### 5.1 Clinical manifestation and management

What is the best way to manage these individuals? In the outpatient setting, achecklist for each patient ensures that each individual's needs are met. A list of "ten commandments" for the CKD patient is:

1. Estimate the GFR and stage the patient's CKD.
2. Round up the usual suspects. Diabetes and hypertension account for almost ¾ of the patient population. Urinalysis, serologies, sonography and biopsy (if necessary) to make the diagnosis.
3. Fix what you can. Discontinue NSAIDs, correct volume depletion and treat BPH (men) and bladder dysfunction (women).
4. Treat hypertension. Goal of therapy is <130/80.
   Use ACE, ARB, both, renin blockers, calcium channel blockers, aldosterone antagonists, loop diuretics as needed.
5. Measure (spot urine protein /creatinine) and treat proteinuria. The goal is<300mg/day. Maximize the dose of an ACE inhibitor, then add an ARB at ½ full dose and increase to reach goal. Loop diuretics are essential to manage edema fluid and offset the development of hyperkalemia. Renin blockers and aldosterone antagonists are added with monitoring of the patient's potassium and creatinine. If the potassium rises to greater than 5.5 meq/l or if the serum creatinine increases more than 30% above baseline, dosages will need to be decreased.
6. Treat anemia of CKD with an ESA if there is no blood loss and iron stores are adequate. Check thyroid function, B-12, folic acid levels. The target Hgb is >10g/dl. Parenteral iron may be needed to keep the TSAT > 25%.
7. Give base supplements to correct metabolic acidosis. Untreated acidosis causes osteopenia and muscle catabolism, along with the release of calcium and phosphorous from bone. Sodium bicarbonate is replaced at 0.5-1.0 meq/kg/day.
   Treat hyperurricemia with allopurinol if the eGFR is >30 ml/min.
8. Phosphate binders, precursor vitamin D and active D (when necessary). We are using both calcium and non-calcium containing binders in our clinic. We try to keep serum calcium levels less than or equal to 9.5 mg%. Vitamin D2 and 3 are used in patients with 25(OH)D levels less than 30 ng/ml. Active vitamin D is used to control elevated iPTH levels and the effects of secondary HPT.

9. Have a nutritionist help patients maintain caloric intake. Protein restriction is difficult and may lead to malnutrition in patients with already poor appetites. We encourage protein supplementation in our CKD patients. The phosphorus level will increase, however, we try to maintain the patient's albumin predialysis or pretransplantation. Patients are started on a 2 gram potassium diet and educated about avoidance of foods high in potassium. Loop diuretics + base supplements aid in the management of hyperkalemia. Resin exchange binders are reserved for values greater than 6 as they cause diarrhea, bicarbonate loss and may worsen acidemia and further increase the serum potassium value.
10. Education and preparation for hemodialysis or peritoneal dialysis. See if acandidate is available for transplantation. We encourage patients to have a fistula constructed after they have attended the education class and decide to do in center or home hemodialysis. These are patients generally in late stage 3 CKD.

Diabetic patients should maintain euglycemia, insulin requirements may decrease as CKD progresses. Metformin should be avoided and glipizide isthe preferred oral agentbecause it is not downgraded to a metabolite excreted by the kidneys.

## 6. Summary

CKD will remain a health concern into the future. CKD clinics managing patients in a coordinated fashion with nutritionists and surgeons will improve lives. Better blood pressure control with diminution of proteinuria will slow the progress of established disease. Attention to acidemia and hyperruricemia will also be beneficial. New insights into the pathogenesis and treatment of diabetes may help manage the number one cause of kidney failure in America.

## 7. References

[1] Primer on Kidney Disease, 5th Edition, Greenberg et al. editors, Saunders (2009).
[2] Comprehensive Clinical Nephrology, 4th edition, Jurgen Floege; Richard J. Johnson, John Feehally
[3] Brenner and Rector's The Kidney, 8th Edition.
[4] Pathologic Basis of Diseases, Eighth Edition. Robins and Cotran
[5] Tuttle, K. Relationship between cardiovascular disease and albuminuria in hypertension. The Heart Institute of Spokane, Spokane, Waashington.
[6] Sowers J, Whaley-Connell A, Epstein M. The Emerging Clinical Implications of the Role of Aldosterone in the Metabolic Syndrome and Resistant Hypertension. Annals of Internal Medicine 150,776-783(2009).
[7] Rennke, Helmut.Glomerular Adaptations to Renal Injury: The Role of Capillary Hypertension in the Pathogenesis of Focal and Segmental Glomerulosclerosis. Advances in Nephrology 15,15-26(1988).
[8] Boor, P, Ostendorf, T andFroeje, J. Renal Fibrosis: Novel Insights into Mechanisms and Therapeutic Targets. Nature Reviews in Nephrology 6,643-656 (2011).
[9] Carrero, Juan Jesus and Stenvinkel, Peter. Novel Targets for Slowing CKD Progression. Nature Reviews in Nephrology 7,65-66(2011).

[10] Nakagama T, Tanabe K, Grant MB, Kosugi T, Croker B, Johnson R and Li Qiuhong. Endothelial Dysfunction as a Potential Contributor in Diabetic Nephropathy. Nature Reviews in Nephrology 7,36-44(2011).
[11] Baines R and Brunskill NJ.Tubular Toxicity of Proteinuria.Nature Reviews in Nephrology 7,177-180(2011).
[12] Peralta C.Detection of Chronic Kidney Disease with creatinine,cystatin c and urine albumin-to-creatinine ratio and association with progression to ESRD and mortality. JAMA 305,1545-1552 (2011).
[13] Tonnelli M. Using proteinuria and estimated GFR to classify risk in patients with CKD: a cohort study. Annals of Internal Medicine 154,12-21(2011).
[14] Levin A, Djurdjev O, Beaulieu M, Er L. Longitudinal follow-up and outcomes among a population with chronic kidney disease in a large managed care organization.Arch Intern Med. 2004 Mar 22;164(6):659-63.

# 3

# The New Kidney and Bone Disease: Chronic Kidney Disease – Mineral and Bone Disorder (CKD–MBD)

Igor G. Nikolov[1], Ognen Ivanovski[2] and Nobuhiko Joki[3]
*[1]University Clinic of Nephrology, Medical Faculty - Skopje,*
*[2]University Clinic of Urology, Medical Faculty - Skopje,*
*[3]Division of Nephrology, Toho University Ohashi Medical Center, Tokyo,*
*[1,2]Republic of Macedonia*
*[3]Japan*

## 1. Introduction

Kidney is one of the most important organs in the regulation of mineral metabolism (Fukagawa et al., 2006). Chronic kidney disease (CKD) is a worldwide public health problem that affects 5% to 10% of the world population, with increasing prevalence and adverse outcomes, including progressive loss of kidney function, cardiovascular disease, and premature death (Eknoyan et al., 2004). Calcium and phosphorus are fundamentally important in a wide array of biological functions. Abnormalities in calcium, phosphorus, parathyroid hormone (PTH), and vitamin D metabolism (usually referred to as disordered mineral metabolism) are common in patients with (CKD) (Block et al., 1998). Cardiovascular disease is the leading cause of death in patients with CKD (London et al., 2003). It has been shown that in individuals with kidney failure on maintenance dialysis who are younger than 65 years, cardiovascular mortality is 10 to 500 times higher than in the general population, even after adjustment for sex, race, and presence of diabetes (Foley RN et al., 1998). Disturbances in mineral metabolism are common complications of CKD and an important cause of morbidity and decreased quality of life. Importantly, increasing evidence suggests that these disturbances are associated with changes in arterial compliance, cardiovascular calcification, bone disorders and all-cause and cardiovascular mortality (Palmer SC et al., 2005, Drueke et al., 2010). Traditionally, when defining bone diseases in CKD patients, this group of disorders has been usually termed renal osteodystrophy. However, beside strictly defined, the term renal osteodystrophy means only bone abnormalities. Recently, the KDIGO (Kidney Disease: Improving Global Outcomes) conference group agreed that the definition of renal osteodystrophy should be only specific to bone pathology found in patients with CKD (Moe S. et al., 2006). It has been concluded that renal osteodystrophy is one component of the mineral and bone disorders that occur as a complication of CKD. It has been proposed that the evaluation and definitive diagnosis of renal osteodystrophy requires performing a bone biopsy. Histomorphometry is not essential for clinical diagnosis, but should be performed in research studies. There was an agreement that histomorphometric results are to be reported by use of the standard nomenclature recommended by the American Society for Bone and Mineral Research (Parfitt et al., 1987), and investigators would supply primary measurements used to report any derived parameters. Based on all of this a new term has been proposed and coined "Chronic kidney disease - mineral and bone disorder (CKD-MBD)" willing to describe the systemic consequences of mineral metabolism disturbances in CKD patients which can no longer be considered restricted only to bone disease. CKD-MBD defines a triad of interrelated abnormalities of serum biochemistry, bone and the vasculature associated with CKD. The adverse effects of high serum phosphorus and an increase of serum calcium due to calcium overload which are present late in CKD are important component of CKD-MBD as well as vascular changes. Furthermore, to clarify the interpretation of bone biopsy results in the evaluation of CKD-MBD, it has been proposed to use three key histologic descriptors—bone turnover, bone mineralization, and bone volume (so called TMV system)— with any combination of each of the descriptors possible in a given specimen. The TMV classification scheme provides a clinically relevant description of the underlying bone pathology, as assessed by histomorphometry, which, in turn, helps to define the pathophysiology, and, thereby, probably to guide the therapy (Moe S. et al., 2006).

## 2. CKD – MBD and biochemical abnormalities

The initial evaluation of CKD-MBD should include laboratory for calcium (it has been proposed either ionized or total corrected for albumin), phosphorus, PTH, alkaline phosphatases (total or bone specific), bicarbonate, as well as imaging for soft-tissue calcification. Epidemiologic studies from the early 1990s have demonstrated that an increase in serum phosphorus and in calcium x phosphorus product are associated with poor outcomes in CKD patients. The association of elevated serum phosphorus and calcium and increased mortality in these patients has been confirmed in several recent studies. If inconsistencies exist in the biochemical markers (eg, high PTH but low alkaline phosphatases), unexplained bone pain, or unexplained fractures are present, a bone biopsy would be strongly indicated (London and Drueke, 1997; London *et al., 2003;* Neves et al., 2007; Bucay et al., 1998).

### 2.1 Calcium

Serum calcium is tightly controlled in healthy individuals, within a narrow range, usually 2.2–2.6 mmol/l, with a minimal, diurnal variation. In patients with CKD, serum calcium levels fluctuate more, because of altered homeostasis and concomitant therapies. Serum calcium levels are routinely measured in clinical laboratories using colorimetric methods in automated machines. In patients with CKD stage 5D, there are additional fluctuations in association with dialysis-induced changes, hemoconcentration, and subsequent hemodilution. Moreover, predialysis samples collected from dialysis patients after the longer interdialytic interval during the weekend, as compared with predialysis samples drawn after the shorter interdialytic intervals during the week, often contain higher serum calcium levels (Tentori et al., 2008). It has been shown that the serum calcium level is a poor reflection of overall total body calcium. Only 1% of total body calcium is measurable in the extracellular compartment while the most important part of calcium is stored in the bones. Serum ionized calcium, generally 40–50% of total serum calcium, is physiologically active, while non-ionized calcium is bound to albumin or anions such as citrate, bicarbonate, and phosphate, and is therefore not physiologically active. In the presence of hypoalbuminemia, there is an increase in ionized calcium relative to total calcium; thus, total serum calcium may underestimate the physiologically active (ionized) serum calcium. The most commonly used formula for estimating ionized calcium from total calcium is the addition of 0.2 mmol/l for every 1 g decrease in serum albumin below 40 g/l. Unfortunately, recent data have shown that it offers no superiority over total calcium alone and is less specific than ionized calcium measurements. In addition, the assay used for albumin may affect the corrected calcium measurement.

### 2.2 Phosphorus

It has been shown that inorganic phosphorus is critical for numerous normal physiological functions, including skeletal development, mineral metabolism, cell-membrane phospholipid content and function, cell signaling, platelet aggregation, and energy transfer through mitochondrial metabolism. Owing to its importance, normal homeostasis maintains serum concentrations between 0.81–1.45 mmol/l. The terms, phosphorus and phosphate, are often used interchangeably, but strictly speaking, the term phosphate means the sum of the two physiologically occurring inorganic ions in the serum, and in other body fluids, hydrogenphosphate ($HPO4_2$) and dihydrogenphosphate ($H2PO_4$). However, most laboratories report this measurable, inorganic component as phosphorus. Unlike calcium, a major component of phosphorus is intracellular, and factors such as pH and glucose can cause shifts of phosphate ions into or out of cells, thereby altering the serum concentration without changing the total body phosphorus. Phosphorus is routinely measured in clinical laboratories with colorimetric methods in automated machines. Serum phosphorus levels reach the lowest level in the early hours of the morning, increasing to a plateau at the afternoon, and further increasing to a peak late in the evening (Portale et al., 1987).

Hyperphosphatemia occurs as a consequence of diminished phosphorus filtration and excretion with the progression of CKD. Decreased phosphorus excretion can initially be overcome by increased secretion of parathyroid hormone (PTH), which decreases proximal phosphate reabsorption (Slatopolsky and Delmez, 1994). Hence, phosphorus levels are usually within normal range until the GFR falls below approximately 30 ml/min, or stage IV. CKD according to the National Kidney Foundation Kidney Disease Outcomes Quality Initiative (NKF-K/DOQI) classification (National Kidney Foundation: K/DOQI). In more advanced stages of CKD, the blunted urinary excretion of phosphorus can no longer keep pace with the obligatory intestinal phosphate absorption, resulting in hyperphosphatemia. Therefore, it is not surprising that the majority of patients with CKD stage 4 and stage 5 have a significant hyperphosphatemia (Block et al., 1998). It has been shown that in patients with advanced CKD high serum calcium, phosphate, and calcium-phosphate product levels are associated with unaccountably high rates of cardiovascular disease (Ganesh et al., 2001; Stevens et al., 2004; Slinin et al., 2005). Moreover, it has been shown also that these derangements in mineral metabolism could occur as well during the early stages of CKD (Slatopolsky and Delmez, 1994).

### 2.3 Parathyroid hormone

The parathyroid gland plays an important role in the regulation of mineral homeostasis by effects trough other organs such as the kidney and bone. Fluctuation in extracellular calcium ion levels is sensed by the parathyroid calcium-sensing receptors (CaSRs) and subsequently regulates the synthesis and secretion of parathyroid hormone (PTH) (Felsenfeld et al., 2007). PTH acts on the bone to increase the efflux of calcium and phosphate, and acts on the kidney to reduce urinary calcium excretion, inhibit phosphate reabsorption, and stimulate the production of 1,25-dihydroxyvitamin D (1,25(OH)2D). PTH is cleaved to an 84-amino-acid protein in the parathyroid gland, where it is stored with fragments in secretory granules for release. When it is released, the circulating 1–84-amino-acid protein has a half-life of 2–4 min. The hormone is cleaved both within the parathyroid gland and after secretion into the N-terminal, C-terminal, and middle region fragments of PTH, which are metabolized in the liver and in the kidneys. Enhanced PTH synthesis/secretion occurs in response to hypocalcemia, hyperphosphatemia, and/or a decrease in serum 1,25-dihydroxyvitamin D (1,25(OH)2D), whereas high serum levels of calcium or calcitriol—and, as recently shown, of Fibroblast growth factor 23 (FGF-23)—suppress PTH synthesis/secretion. The extracellular concentration of ionized calcium is the most important determinant of the minute-to-minute secretion of PTH, which is normally oscillatory.

In patients with CKD, this normal oscillation is somehow altered. Over the past few decades there has been a progress in development of sensitive assays in order to measure PTH. Initial measurements of PTH using C-terminal assays were inaccurate in patients with CKD because of the impaired renal excretion of C-terminal fragments (and thus retention) and the measurement of these probably inactive fragments. The development of the N-terminal assay was initially thought to be more accurate but it also detected inactive metabolites. The development of a second generation of PTH assays, the two-site immunoradiometric assay—commonly called an 'intact PTH' assay—improved the detection of full-length (active) PTH molecules. In this assay, a captured antibody binds within the amino terminus and a second antibody binds within the carboxy terminus. Unfortunately, recent data indicate that this 'intact' PTH assay also detects accumulated large C-terminal fragments, commonly referred to as '7–84' fragments; these are a mixture of four PTH fragments that include, and are similar in size to, 7–84 PTH (Gao and D'Amour 2005). In parathyroidectomized rats, the injection of a truly whole 1- to 84-amino-acid PTH was able to induce bone resorption, whereas the 7- to 84-amino-acid fragment was antagonistic, explaining why patients with CKD may have high levels of 'intact' PTH but relative hypoparathyroidism at the bone-tissue level (Slatopolsky et al., 2000; Malluche et al., 2003; Huan et al., 2006). Thus, the major difficulty in accurately measuring PTH with this assay is the presence of circulating fragments, particularly in the presence of CKD. Unfortunately, the different assays measure different types and amounts of these circulating fragments, leading to inconsistent results. More recently, a third generation of assays has become available that truly detect only the 1- to 84-amino-acid, full-length molecule: 'whole' or 'bioactive' PTH assays. There are differences in PTH results when samples are measured in plasma, serum, or citrate, and depending on whether the samples are on ice, or are allowed to sit at room temperature.

PTH and vitamin D have been shown to influence cardiac and vascular growth and function experimentally in human subjects with normal renal function. Because of increased prevalence of hyperparathyroidism and altered vitamin D status in CKD, these alterations have been considered to contribute to the increased prevalence of cardiovascular disease and hypertension seen in this patient population (Slinin Y et al., 2005).

### 2.4 Vitamin D (25(OH)D)

The parent compounds of vitamin D—$D_3$ (cholecalciferol) or $D_2$ (ergocalciferol)—are highly lipophilic. They are difficult to quantify in the serum or plasma. They also have a short half-life in circulation of about 24 h. These parent compounds are metabolized in the liver to $25(OH)D_3$ (calcidiol) or $25(OH)D_2$ (ercalcidiol). Collectively, they are called 25(OH)D or 25-hydroxyvitamin D. The measurement of serum 25(OH)D is regarded as the best measure of vitamin D status, because of its long half-life of approximately 3 weeks. In addition, it is an assessment of the multiple sources of vitamin D, including both nutritional intake and skin synthesis of vitamin D. There is a seasonal variation in calcidiol levels because of an increased production of cholecalciferol by the action of sunlight on skin during summer months. The gold standard of calcidiol measurement is high performance liquid chromatography (HPLC), but this is not widely available clinically. This is because HPLC is time consuming, requires expertise and special instrumentation, and is expensive. In early 1985, Hollis and Napoli developed the first radioimmunoassay (RIA) for total 25(OH)D, which was co-specific for $25(OH)D_2$ and $25(OH)D_3$. The values correlated with those obtained from HPLC analysis, and DiaSorin RIA became the first test to be approved by the Food and Drug Administration for use in clinical settings (Hollis and Napoli, 1985). Another method now carried out is liquid chromatography- tandem mass spectrometry (LC-MS/MS). Similar to HPLC, the LC-MS/MS method also has the ability to quantify $25(OH)D_2$ and $25(OH)D_3$ separately, which distinguishes it from RIA and enzyme-linked immunosorbent assay technologies. This method is very accurate and has been shown to correlate well with DiaSorin RIA (Saenger et al. 2006; Tsugawa et al., 2005). It has been suggested recently that the assays for 25(OH)D are not well standardized, and the definition of deficiency is not yet well validated. At best, clinicians should ensure that patients use the same laboratory for measurements of these levels, if carried out. The most appropriate vitamin D assays presently available seem to be those that measure both $25(OH)D_2$ and $25(OH)D_3$. Presently, approximately 20–50% of the general population has low vitamin D levels, irrespective of CKD status. However, the benefits from replacing vitamin D have not been documented in patients with CKD, particularly if they are taking calcitriol or a vitamin D analog.

### 2.5 Vitamin D ($1,25(OH)_2D$)

$1,25(OH)_2D$ is used to describe both hydroxylated $D_2$ (ercalcitriol) and $D_3$ (calcitriol) compounds, both of which have a short half-life of 4–6 h. Furthermore, in patients with earlier stages of CKD and in the general population, mild-to-moderate vitamin D deficiency, or partly treated vitamin D deficiency, is frequently associated with increased levels of $1,25(OH)_2D$. Thus, even accurate levels can be misleading. The serum levels of $1,25(OH)_2D$ are uniformly low in late stages of CKD–MBD, at least in patients not treated with vitamin D derivatives (Andress et al., 2006). It has not been recommend a routine measurement of $1,25(OH)_2D$ levels, as the assays are not well standardized, the half-life is short, and there are no data indicating that the measurement is helpful in guiding therapy or predicting outcomes (KDIGO).

### 2.6 Alkaline phosphatases

Alkaline phosphatases (ALP) are enzymes that remove phosphate from proteins and nucleotides, functioning optimally at alkaline pH. Measurement of the level of total ALP (t-

ALP) is a colorimetric assay that is routinely used in clinical laboratories in automated machines. The enzyme is found throughout the body in the form of isoenzymes that are unique to the tissue of origin. Highest concentrations are found in the liver and bone, but the enzyme is also present in the intestines, placenta, kidneys, and leukocytes (Iba K et al. 2004). Specific ALP isoenzymes to identify the tissue source can be determined after fractionation and heat inactivation, but these procedures are not widely available in clinical laboratories. Bone-specific ALP (b-ALP) is measured with an immunoradiometric assay. Elevated levels of t-ALP are generally due to an abnormal liver function, an increased bone activity, or bone metastases. Levels are normally higher in children with growing bones than in adults, and often are increased after fracture. In addition, t-ALP and b-ALP can be elevated in both primary and secondary HPT, osteomalacia, and in the presence of bone metastasis and Paget's disease. In patients with CKD–MBD alkaline phosphatise may be used as an adjunct test, but if values are high, then liver function tests should be checked. t-ALP could reasonably be used as a routine test to follow response to therapy. The more expensive testing for b-ALP can be used when the clinical situation is more ambiguous. Testing for t-ALP is inexpensive and therefore may be helpful for following patients' response to therapy or determining bone turnover status when the interpretation of PTH is unclear. The use of b-ALP, an indicator of bone source, may provide additional and more specific information, although it is not readily available (Iba K et al. 2004).

## 3. CKD – MBD and bone abnormalities

Disorders of mineral metabolism are also associated with abnormal bone structure. It has been shown that the gold standard test for bone quality is its ability to resist fracture under strain. In animal models, this resistance can be directly tested with three-point bending mechanical tests. Bone quality is impaired in CKD, as the prevalence of hip fracture is increased in dialysis patients compared with the general population in all age groups. Dialysis patients in their forties have a relative risk of hip fracture that is 80-fold higher than that of age-matched and sex-matched control subjects. Furthermore, hip fracture in dialysis patients is associated with a doubling of the mortality observed in hip fractures in nondialysis patients (Coco M and Rush H., 2000; Alem et al., 2000). It has been shown that risk factors for hip fracture in CKD patients include age, gender, duration of dialysis, and presence of peripheral vascular disease. There are also analyses that found race, gender, duration of dialysis, and low or very high PTH levels as risk factors for hip fracture. It has been reported that both hip and lumbar-spine fractures occur independent of gender and race in CKD patients. Other risk factors for abnormal bone identified in studies from the general population are also common in CKD, including smoking, sedentary lifestyle, and hypogonadism (Alem et al., 2000). These factors are likely to increase the risk of bone fragility and fractures in CKD but have not been well evaluated. Extremes of bone turnover found in patients with CKD have significant impact on fragility and are likely additive to bone abnormalities commonly found in the aging and sedentary general population (Vassalotti et al., 2008; Melamed et al., 2008).

### 3.1 Classification of renal osteodystrophy by bone biopsy

Bone biopsy is performed to understand the pathophysiology and course of bone disease, to relate histological findings to clinical symptoms of pain and fracture, and to determine whether treatments are effective. The traditional types of renal osteodystrophy have been defined on the basis of turnover and mineralization as follows: mild, slight increase in turnover and normal mineralization; osteitis fibrosa, increased turnover and normal mineralization; osteomalacia, decreased turnover and abnormal mineralization; adynamic, decreased turnover and acellularity; mixed, increased turnover with abnormal mineralization. It has been suggested recently that by performing bone biopsies in patients with CKD the most important parameters which should be determined are bone turnover, bone mineralization, and bone volume (TMV) (Moe et al., 2009).

#### 3.1.1 Bone turnover

In CKD patients a spectrum of bone formation rates varies from abnormally low to very high. Other measurements that help to define a low or high turnover (such as eroded surfaces, number of osteoclasts, fibrosis, or woven bone) tend to be associated with the bone-formation rate as measured by tetracycline labeling. This is the most definite dynamic measurement, hence it was chosen to represent bone turnover. It should be noted that an improvement of a bone biopsy cannot be determined on the basis of a simple change in the bone-formation rate, because the restoration of normal bone may require either an increase or a decrease in bone turnover, depending on the starting point (Melsen and Moselkilde, 1978).

#### 3.1.2 Bone mineralization

It is a parameter which reflects the amount of unmineralized osteoid. Mineralization is measured by the osteoid maturation time or by mineralization lag time, both of which depend heavily on the osteoid width as well as on the distance between tetracycline labels. The classic disease with an abnormality of mineralization is osteomalacia, in which the bone-formation rate is low and the osteoid volume is high. Some patients have a modest increase in osteoid, which is a result of high bone formation rates. They do not have osteomalacia because the mineralization lag time remains normal. The overall mineralization, however, is not normal because unmineralized osteoid is increased.

#### 3.1.3 Bone volume

Bone volume contributes to bone fragility and is separate from the other parameters. The bone volume is the end result of changes in bone-formation and resorption rates: if the overall bone formation rate is higher than the overall bone resorption rate, the bone is in positive balance and the bone volume will increase. If mineralization remains constant, an increase in bone volume would also result in an increase in BMD and should be detectable by dual-energy X-ray absorptiometry (DXA). Although both cortical and cancellous bone volumes decrease in typical idiopathic osteoporosis, these compartments are frequently different in patients with CKD. In dialysis patients with high PTH levels, the cortical bone volume is decreased but the cancellous volume is increased. (Lindergard et al., 1985).

### 3.2 Bone markers

Generally, two different types of bone markers are used to determine the bone patophysiology:

### 3.2.1 Collagen based bone markers

Active osteoblasts secrete pro-collagen type I, and the pro-peptides at both C-terminal and N-terminal ends are immediately cleaved and can be measured in the circulation. The collagen molecules are then covalently bonded through pyridinoline cross-linking. The fragments containing these pyridinoline links (at both the C-terminal and N-terminal ends of the peptides) are released during bone resorption: carboxyterminal (CTX) and aminoterminal (NTX) cross-linking telopeptide of bone collagen, respectively. These collagen-based markers have been studied in normal populations, where there are significant but moderate correlations with bone-formation/resorption rates. These markers are usually increased after bone fracture (Ureña and De Vernejoul, 1999; Ivaska et al., 2007).

### 3.2.2 Non collagen type of bone markers

Osteoblasts secrete other proteins that have been used to assess their function, including b-ALP, osteocalcin, osteoprotegerin, and receptor activator for nuclear factor kB ligand. Osteoclasts secrete tartrate-resistant acid phosphatase. Osteocytes secrete FGF-23 in response to phosphate and calcitriol. High levels of FGF-23 are seen in patients with CKD, but this is a new measurement, and clinical significance remains to be determined. Some of these markers are excreted by the kidneys, so in CKD, the serum concentrations may merely represent accumulation instead of bone turnover (Rogers and Eastell, 2005).

Renal phosphate excretion is physiologically regulated mainly by proximal tubular cells, which express Na/Pi Type II cotransporters at their apical membrane that control phosphate reclamation. Renal phosphate reabsorption is mediated primarily through the Na/Pi IIa co-transporter, whereas approximately one-third of phosphate ions are reabsorbed through the Na/Pi IIc cotransporter. FGF-23 mediates its phosphaturic effect by reducing the abundance of the Na/Pi IIa cotransporter in proximal tubular cells (Baum et al., 2005). In animal studies, transgenic mice over-expressing human or mouse FGF-23 have severe renal phosphate wasting because of suppression of renal Na/Pi cotransporter activity, whereas FGF-23 inactivation leads to hyperphosphatemia (Liu et al., 2006). In addition, FGF-23 may inhibit gastrointestinal phosphate absorption by reducing intestinal Na/Pi IIb cotransporter activity in a vitamin D dependent manner (Liu et al., 2006). In CKD patients, circulating FGF-23 levels gradually increase with renal function declining. Although the increase in FGF-23 is most pronounced in patients with advanced CKD, it may begin at a very early stage. Apparently, FGF-23 and PTH stimulate phosphaturia in a similar manner by reducing phosphate reclamation through Na/Pi IIa cotransporters. Nonetheless, PTH is not indispensable for FGF-23 activity, as the phosphaturic effects of FGF-23 are maintained in animals after parathyroidectomy (Liu et al., 2006). In CKD patients, the increase in FGF-23 starts with modestly impaired estimated glomerular filtration rate, when serum phosphate levels are still within the normal range CKD (KDOQI stages 2–3), whereas FGF-23 levels increase by more than 100-fold in advanced CKD (KDOQI stage 5) compared with healthy controls (Imanishi et al., 2004). However, this is inconsistent with the observation that there is no increase in the accumulation of degraded FGF-23 in advanced CKD. These data instead favor a mechanism involving increased FGF-23 secretion as the cause of elevated FGF-23 levels. Instead of decreased renal clearance, an end organ resistance to the phosphaturic stimulus of FGF-23 may exist because of a deficiency of the necessary Klotho cofactor (Kurosu et al., 2006). Moreover, higher FGF-23 levels in CKD may reflect a physiological compensation to stabilize serum phosphate levels as the number of intact nephrons declines. As a result, FGF-23 increases urinary phosphate excretion and decreases gastrointestinal phosphate absorption directly and through inhibition of 1a-hydroxylase and reduction of circulating calcitriol levels indirectly. Oversecretion of FGF-23 allows the body to maintain phosphate levels within a 'physiological' range until very advanced CKD stages (Miyamoto K et al. 2004).

## 4. CKD – MBD – and vascular calcification

Tissue calcification is a complex and highly regulated process in bone and teeth, and also at extraosseous sites. The most threatening localization of unwanted calcification is at vascular sites, where it may manifest as both medial and intimal calcification of arteries. Studies in the general population have identified calcification in most of atherosclerotic plaques. Calcification seems to be a part of the natural development of atherosclerotic plaques, with extensive calcification associated with late-stage atherosclerosis. In the general population, atherosclerotic plaque calcification is associated with cardiovascular events such as myocardial infarction, symptomatic angina pectoris, and stroke. Medial calcification causes arterial stiffness, resulting in an elevated pulse pressure and increased pulse wave velocity, thereby contributing to left ventricular hypertrophy, dysfunction, and heart failure. Furthermore, an advanced calcification of the heart valves may lead to dysfunction contributing to heart failure and a risk of endocarditis development (Vliegenthart et al. 2002; Vliegenthart et al. 2002).

### 4.1 Different types of vascular calcification

It is generally well recognized that the prevalence of calcification increases with progressively decreasing kidney function and is greater than that in the general population. Cardiovascular calcification is associated with increased frequency of major cardiovascular diseases, and could be of predictive importance for adverse clinical outcomes, including cardiovascular events and death (Foley RN et al., 1998). There is an increased prevalence of cardiovascular calcification in patients even at early stages of CKD. Thus, an important percentage of CKD patients are at high risk of cardiovascular events from vascular calcification. Two patterns of vascular calcification have been described: namely intimal and medial calcification. In the general population, an elevated coronary artery calcium (CAC) score almost exclusively reflects the atherosclerotic disease burden. In two small autopsy studies, it became apparent that, in dialysis patients, CAC is also predominantly localized in the coronary intima, whereas the medial calcifications observed in a minority of such patients seemed to be adjacent to plaque areas just beneath the internal elastic lamina. Although the coronary vascular bed may differ considerably from other arteries with regard to the calcification process and its manifestations, the same group observed a 'pure' medial calcification in the coronary arteries during the early stages of CKD (Schwarz et al., 2000). A 'pure' medial calcification, in the absence of intimal disease, was also observed in epigastric arteries obtained from dialysis patients at the time of renal transplantation (Amann K., 2008;).

### 4.2 Promoters and inhibitors of calcification

Vascular calcification is the result of passive and active processes, as is bone mineralization. It has been shown that that normal extracellular phosphate concentration is required for bone mineralization, while lowering this concentration prevents mineralization of any extracellular matrix. However, simply raising extracellular phosphate concentration is not sufficient to induce pathological mineralization, because of the presence in all extracellular matrices of pyrophosphate, an inhibitor of mineralization (Riser et al., 2011). They further showed that extracellular matrix mineralization normally occurs only in bone because of the exclusive coexpression in osteoblasts of Type I collagen and of tissue non-specific alkaline phosphatase (Tnap), an enzyme that cleaves pyrophosphate. Pyrophosphate probably is the most important non-protein inhibitor of vascular calcification. Its extracellular concentration is strictly regulated by several enzymes. It is generated by PC-1 nucleotide triphosphate pyrophosphohydrolase and metabolized to inorganic phosphate by nucleotide pyrophosphatase/phosphodiesterase (NPP1), in addition to Tnap. Its hydrolysis to inorganic phosphate actually transforms it from a calcification inhibitor to a promoter. In addition to pyrophosphate other inhibitors are also present locally in VSMCs, including matrix-gla protein (MGP) and Smad6 proteine (Lomashvili et al., 2008; Rutsch et al., 2001; Johnson et al., 2005).

### 4.3 Contribution of experimental models in vascular calcification

Arterial calcification assessed by all the available imaging studies cannot accurately differentiate calcification that is localized to the intima from calcification in the media adjacent to the internal elastic lamina, or in the medial layer (Figure 1 and 2). Thus, there is neither definitive evidence to suggest that isolated medial calcification is distinct from the calcification that occurs in the natural history of atherosclerosis nor is there definite proof against it. Experimental and ex vivo studies suggest that the vascular smooth muscle cell may be critical in the development of calcification by transforming into an osteoblast-like phenotype (Giachelli CM, 2004). Elevated phosphorus, elevated calcium, oxidized low-density lipoprotein cholesterol, cytokines, and elevated glucose, among others, stimulate this transformation of vascular smooth muscle cells into osteoblast-like cells in vitro using cell-culture techniques. These factors likely interact at the patient level to increase and/or accelerate calcification in CKD. Given the potential complexity of the pathogenesis and the inability of radiological techniques to differentiate the location of calcification, the approach to all patients with calcification should be to minimize atherosclerotic risk factors and control biochemical parameters of CKD–MBD. In addition, the pericyte in the media and adventitia may have a role in the secretion of vascular calcification-inducing factors (Giachelli et al., 2004). The stimulus for such a transformation may depend on the location of calcification within the artery wall (Figure 2A and 2B). For example, in intimal lesions, atherosclerosis may be the most important stimulus. However, in patients with CKD and medial calcification, there may be additional, or additive, factors potentially explaining why medial calcification of the peripheral arteries can be seen without intimal changes and is more common in CKD than in the non-CKD population (Moe et al., 2003).

Over the past decade, several animal studies have provided evidence for an accelerated progression of atherosclerosis in association with the uremic state. We and others have used the apolipoprotein e knockout (*Apoe*–/–) mouse with superimposed CKD and observed that in this experimental model of severe hypercholesterolemia the development of atheromatous lesions was greatly enhanced compared with the rate of lesion development in nonuremic *Apoe*–/– mice (Massy et al., 2005; Ivanovski et al., 2005). Additionally, in our

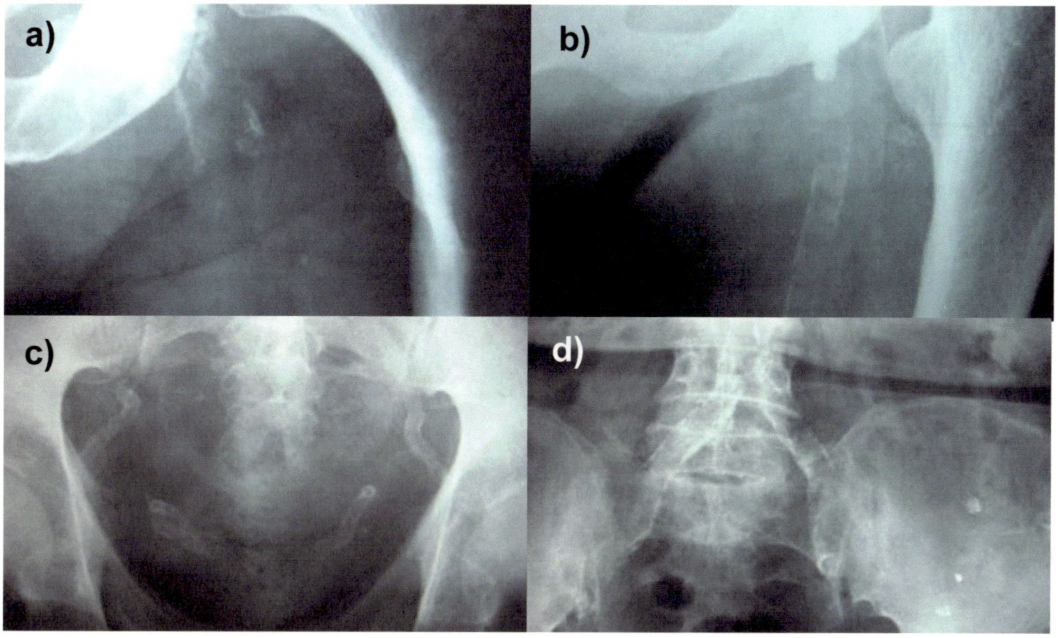


Fig. 1A. Intima and media calcification by radiography. a) Femoral artery intimal calcification; b) Femoral artery medial calcification; c) Pelvic artery medial calcification; d) Iliac arteries mixed calcification. (London et al. 2003).

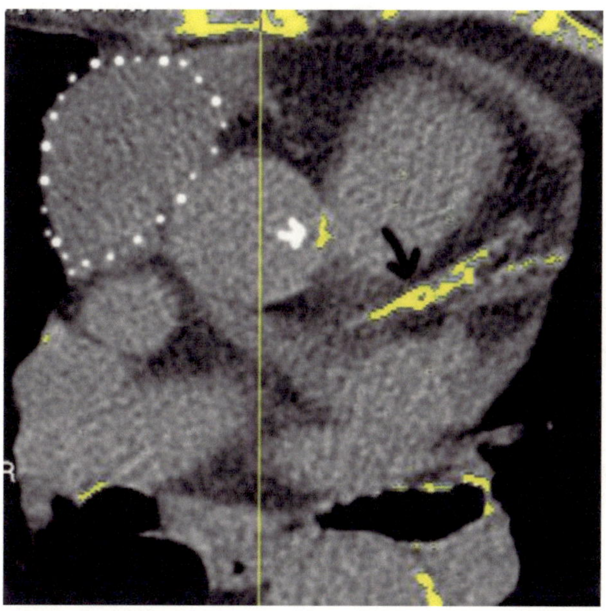

Fig. 1B. Coronary artery calcification by Electron beam computed tomography (EBCT), (scan courtesy of Pr P. Raggi).

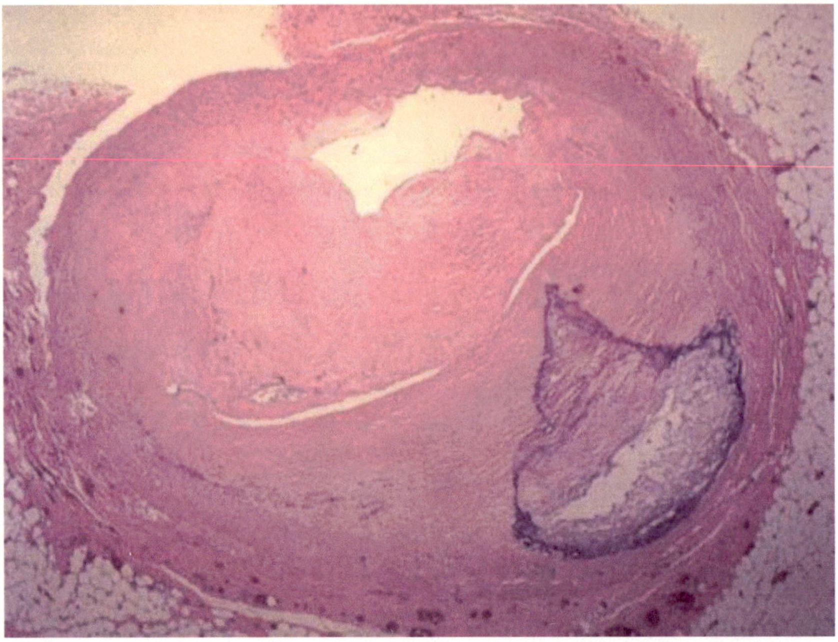

A

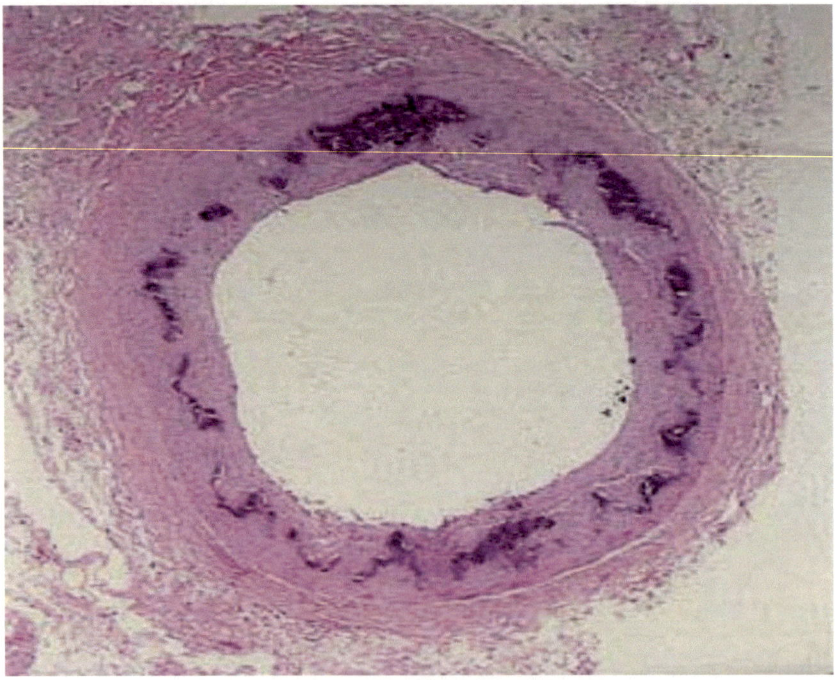

B

Fig. 2. Localization of different types of vascular calcification in humans. A) Intimal; B) Medial; (London et al. 2003).

model, accelerated calcification of the aortic wall both in the intima and the media, (Figure 3A and 3B, respectively) occurred in the absence of hypertension, and fetuin a deficiency greatly enhanced intimal calcification. Similar observations have been made using another hyper cholesterolemic animal model of severe atherosclerosis with superimposed CKD, namely the LDL receptor knockout mouse model (Mathew et al. 2007; Davies et al. 2005). Of note, the first cardiovascular changes observed in early stages of CKD in *Apoe-/-* mice as well as in wild type mice were left ventricular hypertrophy, altered left ventricular relaxation and increased aortic stiffness in the absence of identifiable morphological changes of the vessel wall. The observed cardiac and aortic abnormalities were not associated with the degree of aortic calcification or the level of serum total cholesterol, but with the extent of subendothelial dysfunction and the severity of CKD. Our findings have revealed that the cardio vascular lesions observed in early stage of acute kidney injury are likely functional. Although the above experimental findings need to be confirmed by additional studies in the clinical setting, they open up the possibility of attenuation of atherosclerosis and even reversal by adequate therapeutic strategies. Findings from experimental observations favor the existence of two different types of vascular disease linked to CKD, namely early arteriosclerosis, in the absence of atherosclerosis, and the acceleration of already existing or subsequently developing atherosclerosis by the uremic state (Drueke and Massy, 2010).

Finally, a rare but very severe form of medial calcification of small (cutaneous) arteries is calciphylaxis, also called calcific uremic arteriolopathy. This complication is strongly associated with CKD-related disturbances of mineral metabolism, including secondary HPT, in approximately one-third of cases. It is characterized by ischemic, painful skin ulcerations followed by superinfections, and is associated with high mortality. Relationships with dysregulated calcification inhibitors (fetuin-A and matrix Gla protein) have been implicated in the pathogenesis of calciphylaxis (Schoppet et al., 2008; Suliman et al., 2008), but because of the relatively low incidence of the disease, no conclusive data are available to firmly comment on the nature of the disease process or to allow generalizable treatment options to be recommended.

### 4.4 Management of patients with vascular/valvular calcification

Recently it has been confirmed that cardiovascular calcification development and progression can be influenced by treatment. Given that vascular calcification is associated with increased cardiovascular risk, and that the pathogenesis seems to be related to CKD-MBD abnormalities and atherosclerosis, it is appropriate to evaluate and modify both. CKD-MBD longitudinal studies have also shown that the progression of vascular calcification to be modifiable by the choice of phosphate binders. Aluminum-containing phosphate binders have been widely abandoned because of serious adverse effects including adynamic bone disease, microcytic anemia, dementia, and death (Alfrey et al., 1976). They were initially replaced by calcium-containing, aluminum-free phosphate binders. Subsequently, several studies showed that the high amounts of calcium ingested with these binders were associated with vascular calcification whose progression could be slowed by the calcium-free, aluminum-free binder sevelamer (Block et al., 2005; Chertow et al., 2002; London et al., 2008). The Treat-to-Goal study compared sevelamer-HCl to calcium-containing phosphate binders, analyzing the progression of coronary artery and aortic calcification (by EBCT) in prevalent HD patients over 1 year. Although calcification scores progressed with calcium-

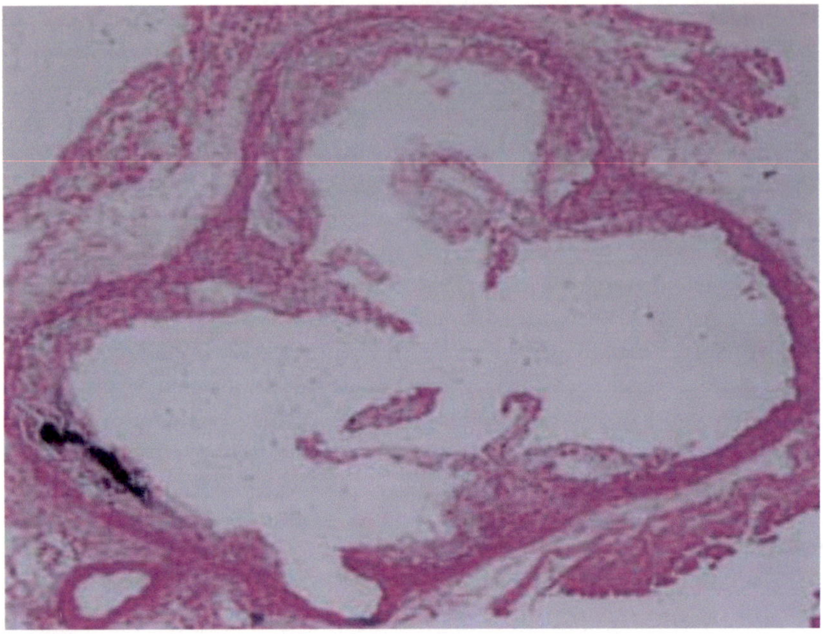

(a)

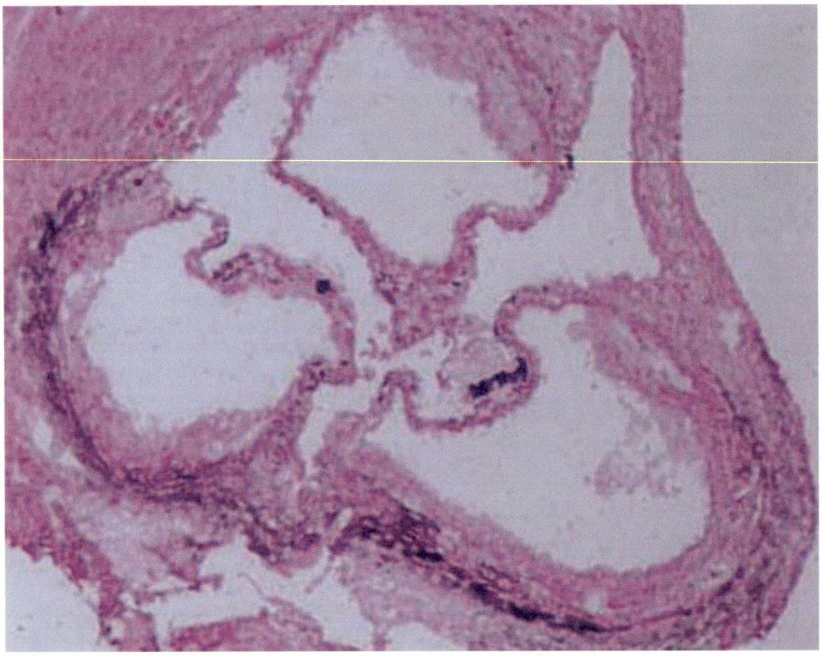

(b)

Fig. 3. Extent and localization of different types of atherosclerotic lesion calcification in apoE−/− mice with CRF. von Kossa staining. a) solid type of plaque calcification, magnification ×25; b) non-plaque calcification, magnification×25. (Phan et al. 2008).

containing phosphate binders, treatment with sevelamer-HCl was associated with a lack of calcification progression (Chertow et al., 2002). A similar design was used, and the results showed more calcification progression in patients treated with calcium based binders compared with sevelamer-HCl in the Renagel in New Dialysis Patients study, which studied incident HD patients who were randomized within 90 days after starting dialysis treatment (Block et al., 2005). The Calcium Acetate Renagel Evaluation-2 study showed that the use of sevelamer-HCl and calcium acetate was associated with equal progression of CAC when statins were used to achieve a similar control of the serum low-density lipoprotein cholesterol in the two study arms (Qunibi et al., 2008). Interestingly, in Calcium Acetate Renagel Evaluation-2, the combination of sevelamer- HCl and atorvastatin was actually associated with a higher progression rate of CAC than that in Treat-to-Goal, instead of showing an amelioration of CAC progression with the combination of calcium acetate and statin. It is difficult to reconcile these differences, although one potential explanation is that the Calcium Acetate Renagel Evaluation- 2 study patient population had a higher number of cardiovascular risk factors than did that of the Treat-to-Goal study (Floege J., 2008).

Although abnormalities of calcium phosphate homeostasis have long been linked with dysfunction of large arteries in these patients, more recent studies have suggested a role in the pathogenesis of atherosclerosis in smaller, critical arteries, most notably the coronary arteries (London et al., 2003). Coronary artery calcification (CAC) is a strong predictor of atherosclerotic disease in the general population. It has been recognized that most population studies measuring CAC did not necessarily exclude individuals on the basis of kidney function and thus include variable numbers of CKD patients. In general, this literature evaluating the general population supports the view that CAC is part of the development of atherosclerosis and occurs almost exclusively together with atherosclerosis in human arteries. It seems that calcification occurs early in the atherosclerotic process; however, the amount of calcification per lesion has a variable relationship with the associated severity of luminal stenosis. The relationship between the degree of calcification in an individual lesion and the probability of plaque rupture is unknown. In the general population, the overall coronary calcium score can be considered as a measure of the overall burden of coronary atherosclerosis. The American College of Cardiology/American Heart Association document indicates that the relationship between CAC and cardiovascular events in the CKD population is less clear than that in the non-CKD population because of a relative lack of informative studies and the possibility that medial calcification may not be indicative of atherosclerotic disease severity. The almost exclusive relationship between magnitude of calcification and atherosclerosis burden is controversial in CKD patients (Amann, 2008), in contrast to the situation in the general population. Antiatherosclerotic strategies using statin treatment have been shown to have a beneficial impact on the atherogenic profile, atheroma progression, and cardiovascular events in patients with no known CKD (Nissen et al. 2004). In our experimental model, we have shown that statins had a beneficial effect on uremia enhanced vascular calcification in apoE knock out mice with chronic kidney disease. This effect was observed despite the absence of changes in uremia accelerated atherosclerosis progression, serum total cholesterol levels or osteopontin and alkaline phosphatase expression. This observation opened the possibility of a cholesterol independent action of statins on vascular calcification via a decrease in oxidative stress (Ivanovski et al., 2008). In CKD patients, there are no data on the effects of statins on arterial calcification, as compared with those of placebo. Even worse, the 4D study failed to show a benefit of atorvastatin treatment on the outcome of diabetic dialysis patients. Studies in progress like SHARP (Study of Heart and Renal Protection) and AURORA (A Study to Evaluate the Use of Rosuvastatin in Subjects on Regular Hemodialysis: An Assessment of Survival and Cardiovascular Events) failed to show a better understanding of the benefits of correcting atherosclerotic risk factors on cardiovascular events and mortality in patients with CKD stages 3–5 and 5D (Baigent et al., 2003).

An association of vascular calcification with high phosphate intake has so far not been directly demonstrated in uremic patients, probably owing to the fact that it is difficult, if not impossible, to assess phosphate (protein) intake in a quantitative manner over prolonged time periods. Indirect evidence for a role of oral phosphate, however, has recently been provided by Russo et al (Russo et al., 2007). They showed that in patients with CKD stage 3-5, coronary artery calcification score progressed significantly over a time period of 2 years, in association with a significant increase in phosphaturia. Many pharmaco-epidemiologic studies have shown a survival benefit in CKD patients receiving active vitamin D derivatives, as compared to those who did not receive such treatments. Finally, let us not forget that association does not imply causation. We clearly need randomized prospective trials showing that active reduction of serum phosphorus, PTH, or alkaline phosphatases and normalization of serum calcium leads to an improvement in patient outcomes, and that specific treatments given to the patients improve outcome, as compared to either placebo or other treatments (Drueke and McCarron, 2003).

To date, there are no published prospective studies in humans that have evaluated the impact of calcimimetics or calcitriol and vitamin D analogs on arterial calcification. However, a recent observational study showed a U-curve type of relationship between serum 1,25(OH)2D3 and arterial calcification in children and adolescents with CKD stage 5D. No such association existed between serum 25(OH)D and arterial calcification. In one study in adult patients with CKD stage 5, no independent association of serum 25(OH)D or 1,25(OH)2D3 levels with arterial calcification was observed, (London et al., 2007). Although the authors of another report identified an association between 25(OH)D deficiency and the magnitude of vascular calcification (Matias et al., 2009). The experimental data supporting less toxicity of vitamin D analogs compared with calcitriol are not completely consistent across studies, but, in general, support the claim that there is reduced calcification with equivalent PTH lowering with different vitamin D analogs (Lopez et al., 2008**).** Experimental studies showed differential effects of calcimimetics and calcitriol on extraosseous calcification, the former being neutral or protective, the latter being a dose-dependent risk factor for calcification. In our studies, we have analysed the role of chronic renal failure (CRF) on the arterial wall changes including atherosclerosis and vascular calcifications in CRF apoE-/- mice experimental model (Massy, Ivanovski et al. 2005). Furthermore, we have studied the effect of different non-calcium (Phan et al., 2005) and calcium phosphate binders (Phan et al., 2008) and role of control of phosphatemia on vascular calcification and atherosclerosis (Ivanovski et al. 2009). We have also showed for the first time that the phosphate binder La carbonate is capable of preventing both uremia-enhanced vascular calcification and atherosclerosis in experimental model of CKD (Nikolov et al., 2011). These effects were comparable to those of sevelamer on vascular calcification and atherosclerosis, as previously reported by us for sevelamer-HCl in this model (Phan et al., 2008).

## 5. CKD – MBD summary

Mineral and bone disorders are complex abnormalities that cause morbidity and decreased quality of life in patients with CKD. To enhance communication and facilitate research, a new term has been established, CKD–Mineral and Bone Disorder (CKD-MBD), to describe the syndrome of biochemical, bone, and extraskeletal calcification abnormalities that occur in patients with CKD. Also, it has been recommended that the term renal osteodystrophy be used exclusively to define alterations in bone morphology associated with CKD. The latter can be further assessed by histomorphometry, with results reported on the basis of a classification system that includes parameters of turnover, mineralization, and volume. The international adoption of the proposed uniform terminology, definition, and classification to describe these two disorders caused by CKD enhanced communication, facilitated clinical decision making, and can promote the evolution of evidence based clinical-practice guidelines worldwide. This issue of Advances in CKD further describes the clinical manifestations and pathophysiology of CKD-MBD. The optimal management of CKD-MBD (Chronic Kidney Disease - Mineral and Bone Disorder) should be achieved without increasing the risk of metastatic calcification, including that of blood vessels.

## 6. References

Andress DL. (2006). "Vitamin D in chronic kidney disease: a systemic role for selective vitamin D receptor activation". Kidney Int.; 69(1): 33-43.

Alem AM, Sherrard DJ, et al., (2000). "Increased risk of hip fracture among patients with end-stage renal disease". Kidney Int.; 58(1): 396-9.

Alfrey AC, LeGendre GR, et al. (1976). "The dialysis encephalopathy syndrome. Possible aluminum intoxication. " N Engl J Med. 22;294(4):184-8.

Amann K. (2008). "Media calcification and intima calcification are distinct entities in chronic kidney disease". Clin J Am Soc Nephrol.: 3: 1599-605.

Baigent C, Landry M. (2003). "Study of Heart and Renal Protection (SHARP)." Kidney Int Suppl.; (84): S207-10.

Baum M, Schiavi S, et al. (2005). "Effect of fibroblast growth factor-23 on phosphate transport in proximal tubules. " Kidney Int; 68: 1148–1153.

Block GA, Hulbert-Shearon TE et al. (1998). "Association of serum phosphorus and calcium x phosphate product with mortality risk in chronic hemodialysis patients: a national study." Am J Kidney Dis.; 31(4): 607-17.

Block GA, Spiegel DM et al. (2005). "Effects of sevelamer and calcium on coronary artery calcification in patients new to hemodialysis.", Kidney Int. 2005 Oct;68(4):1815-24.

Bucay N, Sarosi I et al. (1998). "Osteoprotegerin-deficient mice develop early onset osteoporosis and arterial calcification." *Genes Dev;* 12:1260-1268

Chertow GM, Burke SK,. (2002). "Sevelamer attenuates the progression of coronary and aortic calcification in hemodialysis patients." Kidney Int.; 62(1): 245-52.

Coco M, Rush H. (2000). Increased incidence of hip fractures in dialysis patients with low serum parathyroid hormone. Am J Kidney Dis.; 36(6): 1115-21.

Davies, M. R., Lund, R. J., et al. (2005). Low turnover osteodystrophy and vascular calcification are amenable to skeletal anabolism in an animal model of chronic kidney disease and the metabolic syndrome. *JASN.* 16, 917–928.

Drüeke TB, McCarron DA. (2003). "Paricalcitol as compared with calcitriol in patients undergoing hemodialysis." N Engl J Med. 31; 349(5): 496-9.

Drüeke, TB., (2008) "Arterial intima and media calcification: distinct entities with different pathogenesis or all the same?" Clin J Am Soc Nephrol. 3(6):1583-4.

Drüeke TB, Massy ZA. (2010). "Atherosclerosis in CKD: differences from the general population". Nat Rev Nephrol.; 6: 723-35.

Eknoyan G, Lameire N, et al., (2004). The burden of kidney disease: improving global outcomes. Kidney Int.; 66(4): 1310-4.

Felsenfeld AJ, Rodríguez M et al. (2007). "Dynamics of parathyroid hormone secretion in health and secondary hyperparathyroidism." CJASN; 2(6):1283-305.

Floege J. (2008). "Calcium-containing phosphate binders in dialysis patients with cardiovascular calcifications: should we CARE-2 avoid them?" NDT.; 23(10):3050-2.

Foley RN, Parfrey PS et al. (1998). "Clinical epidemiology of cardiovascular disease in chronic renal disease. Am J Kidney Dis; 32 (5 Suppl 3):S112-9.

Fukagawa, M., Y. Hamada, et al. (2006). "The kidney and bone metabolism: Nephrologists' point of view". J Bone Miner Metab. 24(6): 434-8.

Ganesh SK, Stack AG et al. (2001). "Association of elevated serum PO(4), Ca x PO(4) product, and parathyroid hormone with cardiac mortality risk in chronic hemodialysis patients." J Am Soc Nephrol.;12(10): 2131-8.

Gao P, and D'Amour P (2005). "Evolution of the parathyroid hormone (PTH) assay--importance of circulating PTH immunoheterogeneity and of its regulation.", Clin Lab.; 51(1-2): 21-9.

Giachelli CM. (2004). "Vascular calcification mechanisms." J Am Soc Nephrol.;15(12): 2959-64.

Hollis BW and Napoli JL. (1985). "Improved radioimmunoassay for vitamin D and its use in assessing vitamin D status." Clin Chem.; 31(11): 1815-9.

Huan J, Olgaard K, et al. (2006). "Parathyroid hormone 7-84 induces hypocalcemia and inhibits the parathyroid hormone 1-84 secretory response to hypocalcemia in rats with intact parathyroid glands." JASN;17(7):1923-30.

Iba K, Takada J et al. (2004). "The serum level of bone-specific alkaline phosphatase activity is associated with aortic calcification in osteoporosis patients." J Bone Miner Metab.; 22(6): 594-6.

Ivaska KK, Gerdhem P et al. (2007). "Effect of fracture on bone turnover markers: a longitudinal study comparing marker levels before and after injury in 113 elderly women." J Bone Miner Res.; 22(8):1155-64.

Ivanovski, O., I.G. Nikolov, et al. (2009). "The calcimimetic R-568 retards uremia-enhanced vascular calcification and atherosclerosis in apolipoprotein E deficient (apoE-/-) mice." Atherosclerosis. 205(1):55-62.

Ivanovski O, Szumilak D, et al., (2005). "The antioxidant N-acetylcysteine prevents accelerated atherosclerosis in uremic apolipoprotein E knockout mice. " Kidney Int. 2005 Jun;67(6):2288-94.

Ivanovski O, Szumilak D, et al. (2008). "Effect of simvastatin in apolipoprotein E deficient mice with surgically induced chronic renal failure. " J Urol.; 179(4):1631-6.

Imanishi Y, Inaba M, et al., (2004). "FGF-23 in patients with end-stage renal disease on hemodialysis." Kidney Int.; 65(5): 1943-6.

Johnson K, Polewski M et al. (2005). "Chondrogenesis mediated by PPi depletion promotes spontaneous aortic calcification in NPP1-/- mice." Arterioscler Thromb Vasc Biol.;25(4):686-91.

Kurosu H, Ogawa Y, et al. (2006). "Regulation of fibroblast growth factor-23 signaling by klotho." J Biol Chem; 281: 6120–6123.

Lindergård B, Johnell O et al. (1985). "Studies of bone morphology, bone densitometry and laboratory data in patients on maintenance hemodialysis treatment. ", Nephron. 1985; 39(2): 122-9.

Liu S, Tang W, et al. (2006) "Fibroblast growth factor 23 is a counter-regulatory phosphaturic hormone for vitamin D. " J Am Soc Nephrol.;17(5):1305-15.

Lomashvili KA, Garg P et al. (2008). "Upregulation of alkaline phosphatase and pyrophosphate hydrolysis: potential mechanism for uremic vascular calcification." Kidney Int.; 73(9): 1024-30.

London GM and Drueke TB (1997). "Atherosclerosis and arteriosclerosis in chronic renal failure." *Kidney Int;* 51:1678-1695

London GM, Guerin AP *et al. (2003).* "Arterial media calcification in end-stage renal disease: impact on all-cause and cardiovascular mortality." *Nephrol Dial Transplant;* 18:1731-1740

London GM, Marchais SJ, et al., (2008). "Association of bone activity, calcium load, aortic stiffness, and calcifications in ESRD."; JASN; 19(9): 1827-35.

London GM, Guérin AP et al. (2007). "Mineral metabolism and arterial functions in end-stage renal disease: potential role of 25-hydroxyvitamin D deficiency."; JASN.; 18(2):613-20.

Lopez I, Mendoza FJ et al. (2008). "The effect of calcitriol, paricalcitol, and a calcimimetic on extraosseous calcifications in uremic rats.", Kidney Int.; 73(3):300-7.

Massy, Z.A., O. Ivanovski, et al. (2005). "Uremia accelerates both atherosclerosis and arterial calcification in apolipoprotein E knockout mice". J Am Soc Nephrol. 16(1):109-16.

Malluche HH, Mawad H, et al. (2003). "Parathyroid hormone assays--evolution and revolutions in the care of dialysis patients." Clin Nephrol.; 59(5):313-8.

Mathew, S., Lund R.J., et al. (2007). "Reversal of the adynamic bone disorder and decreased vascular calcification in chronic kidney disease by sevelamer carbonate therapy." JASN. 18, 122–130.

Matias PJ, Ferreira C et al. (2009). "25-Hydroxyvitamin D3, arterial calcifications and cardiovascular risk markers in haemodialysis patients."; 24(2): 611-8.

Melamed ML, Eustace JA et al. (2008). "Third-generation parathyroid hormone assays and all-cause mortality in incident dialysis patients: the CHOICE study. ", NDT; 23(5): 1650-8.

Melsen F and Moselkilde L. (1978). Tetracycline double labeling of iliac trabecular bone in 41 normal adults. Calcif Tiss Res; 26: 99–102.

Moe, S., T. Drüeke, et al. (2006). "Definition, evaluation, and classification of renal osteodystrophy: a position statement from Kidney Disease: Improving Global Outcomes (KDIGO)". Kidney Int. 69(11): 1945-53.

Moe SM, Drüeke TB, et al. (2009). "KDIGO clinical practice guideline for the diagnosis, evaluation, prevention, and treatment of Chronic Kidney Disease-Mineral and Bone Disorder (CKD-MBD).". Kidney Int Suppl.; (113): S1-130.

Moe SM, Duan D et al. (2003). "Uremia induces the osteoblast differentiation factor Cbfa1 in human blood vessels."; Kidney Int.; 63(3):1003-11.

Miyamoto K, Segawa H et al. (2004). "Physiological regulation of renal sodium-dependent phosphate cotransporters." Jpn J Physiol.; 54(2): 93-102.

Neves KR, Graciolli FG et al. (2007). "Vascular calcification: contribution of parathyroid hormone in renal failure." *Kidney Int;* 71:1262-1270

Nikolov, I.G., N. Joki, et al. (2010). "Chronic kidney disease bone and mineral disorder (CKD-MBD) in apolipoprotein E-deficient mice with chronic renal failure". Bone. 47(1):156-63.

Nikolov I.G, N. Joki et al., (2011). Lanthanum carbonate, like sevelamer-HCl, retards the progression of vascular calcification and atherosclerosis in uremic apolipoprotein E-deficient mice. Nephrol Dial Transplant. In press.

Nissen SE, Tuzcu EM et al. (2004). "Effect of intensive compared with moderate lipid-lowering therapy on progression of coronary atherosclerosis: a randomized controlled trial." JAMA. 3; 291(9): 1071-80.

Palmer SC, Strippoli GF et al. (2005). "Interventions for preventing bone disease in kidney transplant recipients: a systematic review of randomized controlled trials." Am J Kidney Dis.;45(4): 638-49.

Parfitt AM, Drezner MK et al. (1987). "Bone histomorphometry: standardization of nomenclature, symbols, and units". Report of the ASBMR Histomorphometry Nomenclature Committee. J Bone Miner Res.;2 (6): 595-610.

Phan, O., O. Ivanovski, et al. (2005). "Sevelamer prevents uremia-enhanced atherosclerosis progression in apolipoprotein E-deficient mice". Circulation. 1;112(18):2875-82.

Phan, O., O. Ivanovski, et al. (2008). "Effect of oral calcium carbonate on aortic calcification in apolipoprotein E-deficient (apoE-/-) mice with chronic renal failure." Nephrol Dial Transplant. 23(1):82-90.

Portale AA, Halloran BP et al. (1987). "Dietary intake of phosphorus modulates the circadian rhythm in serum concentration of phosphorus. Implications for the renal production of 1,25-dihydroxyvitamin D." J Clin Invest.; 80(4): 1147-54.

Qunibi W, Moustafa M, et al. (2008). "A 1-year randomized trial of calcium acetate versus sevelamer on progression of coronary artery calcification in hemodialysis patients with comparable lipid control: the Calcium Acetate Renagel Evaluation-2 (CARE-2) study." AJKD.; 51(6): 952-65.

Riser BL, Barreto FC, et al., (2011). Daily peritoneal administration of sodium pyrophosphate in a dialysis solution prevents the development of vascular calcification in a mouse model of uraemia. Nephrol Dial Transplant. 2011, in press.

Rogers A and Eastell R. (2005). "Circulating osteoprotegerin and receptor activator for nuclear factor kappaB ligand: clinical utility in metabolic bone disease assessment." J Clin Endocrinol Metab.; 90(11):6323-31.

Rutsch F, Vaingankar S et al. (2001). "PC-1 nucleoside triphosphate pyrophosphohydrolase deficiency in idiopathic infantile arterial calcification." Am J Pathol.; 158(2): 543-54.

Russo D, Miranda I et al. (2007). "The progression of coronary artery calcification in predialysis patients on calcium carbonate or sevelamer." KI; 72(10): 1255-61.

Saenger AK, Laha TJ, et al. (2006). "Quantification of serum 25-hydroxyvitamin D(2) and D(3) using HPLC-tandem mass spectrometry and examination of reference intervals for diagnosis of vitamin D deficiency."Am J Clin Pathol.; 125(6): 914-20.

Schwarz U, Buzello M et al. (2000). "Morphology of coronary atherosclerotic lesions in patients with end-stage renal failure."Nephrol Dial Transplant.; 15(2): 218-23.

Schoppet M, Shroff RC, et al. (2008). "Exploring the biology of vascular calcification in chronic kidney disease: what's circulating? " Kidney Int.; 73(4): 384-90.

Slatopolsky E and Delmez JA. (1994). "Pathogenesis of secondary hyperparathyroidism." Am J Kidney Dis.; 23(2):229-36.

Slatopolsky E, Finch J et al. (2000). "A novel mechanism for skeletal resistance in uremia." Kidney Int; 58(2): 753-61

Slinin Y, Foley RN et al. (2005). "Calcium, phosphorus, parathyroid hormone, and cardiovascular disease in hemodialysis patients: the USRDS waves 1, 3, and 4 study." J Am Soc Nephrol.;16(6): 1788-93.

Stevens LA, Djurdjev O, et al. (2004). "Calcium, phosphate, and parathyroid hormone levels in combination and as a function of dialysis duration predict mortality: vidence for the complexity of the association between mineral metabolism and outcomes." JASN; 15(3):770-9.

Suliman ME, García-López E, et al., (2008). Vascular calcification inhibitors in relation to cardiovascular disease with special emphasis on fetuin-A in chronic kidney disease. Adv Clin Chem. 2008;46:217-62.

Tentori F, Blayney MJ et al. (2008). "Mortality risk for dialysis patients with different levels of serum calcium, phosphorus, and PTH: the Dialysis Outcomes and Practice Patterns Study (DOPPS)." Am J Kidney Dis.;52(3): 519-30.

Tsugawa N, Suhara Y, et al. (2005). "Determination of 25-hydroxyvitamin D in human plasma using high-performance liquid chromatography--tandem mass spectrometry." Anal Chem.; 77(9): 3001-7.

Ureña P and De Vernejoul MC. (1999). "Circulating biochemical markers of bone remodeling in uremic patients." Kidney Int.; 55(6): 2141-56.

Vassalotti JA, Uribarri J, et al. (2008). "Trends in mineral metabolism: Kidney Early Evaluation Program (KEEP) and the National Health and Nutrition Examination Survey (NHANES) 1999-2004." Am J Kidney Dis.; 51(4 Suppl 2): S56-68.

Vliegenthart R, Hollander M et al. (2002). "Stroke is associated with coronary calcification as detected by electron-beam CT: the Rotterdam Coronary Calcification Study." Stroke.;33(2):462-5.

Vliegenthart R, Oudkerk M et al. (2002). Coronary calcification detected by electron-beam computed tomography and myocardial infarction. The Rotterdam Coronary Calcification Study. Eur Heart J.; 23(20): 1596-1603.

4

# The Prevalence of Renal Osteodystrophy in Chronic Renal Failure Patients in Urban Niger Delta of Nigeria

U. R. Onyemekeihia[1], C. O. Esume[2], E. Unuigbe[3], E. Oviasu[3], L. Ojogwu[3]
[1]*Renal Unit, Department of Medicine, Central Hospital Warri, Delta State*
[2]*Department of Pharmacology and Therapeutics, Delta State University, Abraka*
[3]*Department of Medicine, University of Benin Teaching Hospital, Benin City*
*Nigeria*

## 1. Introduction

Chronic renal failure (CRF) is defined as a progressive and persistent deterioration in renal function with serum creatinine consistently greater than 175µmol (Adelakun and Akinsola, 1988). It occurs as the termination of many chronic renal diseases, and is an important cause of morbidity and mortality in Africa (Kadiri, 2001). End stage renal failure may be defined as creatinine clearance of less than 10mls/minute or sustained plasma creatinine concentration above 500pmol/l (Ojogwu, 2001).

In United Kingdom the prevalence of chronic renal failure is approximately 600 individuals per million population per year (0.06%). The incidence of end-stage renal failure is of the order of 200 per million population per year (0.02%) (Baker, 1999).

In Nigeria, although accurate figures are not available, the size of the problem has been estimated using hospital admission records (Kadiri, 2001). Hospital admission rates of CRF in South West Nigeria were reported as between 6.7%-8% (Akinsola et al, 1989; Kadiri and Arije, 1999). However, much earlier reports by Adetuyibi *et al* showed that CRF accounted for 11.4% of deaths on the medical wards of a major teaching hospital in the region (Adetuyibi et al, 1976).

Chronic glomerulonephritis and hypertension account for majority of CRF cases in Nigeria, with diabetes mellitus, obstructive uropathy and autosomal dominant polycystic kidney disease accounting for smaller proportions (Akinsola et al, 1989). Chronic interstitial nephritis is thought not to be a common cause of CRF in Nigeria and other parts of Africa (Gold et al 1990, Ojogwu 1990, Mate-Kole et al 1990). Once established, chronic renal impairment tends to progress inexorably to end-stage renal failure, but the rate of progression depends on the underlying aetiology: for example chronic glomerulonephritis leads to a more rapid deterioration compared with chronic tubulointerstitial nephropathies (Baker, 1999). Chronic renal failure is associated with widespread complications, and renal osteodystrophy (ROD) is one of such complications (Hartmut and Marie-Claude 1990). ROD develops in the early stages of loss of the excretory functions of the kidney, and can begin many years before its symptoms and radiological changes appear in adults (Hartmut and

Marie-Claude 1990). Symptoms of ROD are seen only in about 10% of pre-dialysis patients, but when they have been on dialysis for several years, 90% of them will have symptoms (Sanchez 2001). When glomerular filtration rate (GFR) falls to 50% of normal, more than 50% of patients exhibit abnormal bone histology. As much as 90% of patients with end-stage renal failure on maintenance haemodialysis have abnormal bone history.

The bone disorders associated with chronic renal failure are; Osteitis Fibrosa cystica due to secondary hyperparathyroidism, osteomalacia, osteoporosis. Adynamic osteopathy, skeletal microglobulin amyloid deposit, aluminum related low turnover bone disease and mixed forms of ROD. Osteitis Fibrosa is the commonest form of ROD (Hartmut and Marie-Claude 1990). All these increase the morbidity and mortality in patients with CRF. The prevalence of the different types of ROD may vary depending on aluminum exposure, treatment with Vitamin D metabolites, dietary intake, and whether or not is undergoing dialysis (Hartmut and Marie-Claude 1990).

The diagnosis of ROD can either be by invasive or non invasive methods. The invasive methods include: bone biopsy after double tetracycline labeling, scintigraphical scan studies, computed tomography and bone densitometry (Sanchez 2001). A definitive diagnosis of ROD can only be made with bone biopsy. The non invasive methods employ the use of serum markers of bone metabolism, including bone-specific alkaline phosphatase (bap), pre collagen type 1 carboxy1- terminal extension peptide (PICP), osteocalcin, pyridinoline (PYD), tartrate resistance acid phospatase (TRAPE) and intact parathyroid hormone (IPTH), and skeletal x-ray (Sanchez 2001). Indeed, detection of biochemical makers such as serum bap can predict the presence of ROD. Serum bap is a specific and sensitive marker that is used to evaluate the degree of bone remodeling in uraemic patients (Sanchez 2001, Urena et al, 1991). Also intact PTH and several relatively new bone markers such as PYD and PICP are of immense value in the non-invasive diagnosis of ROD. In patients that do not have liver disease, parathyroid hormone and alkaline phosphatase are less expensive and non-invasive alternatives for evaluation of ROD (Urena et al, 1991). These biochemical markers have the added advantage of allowing for repeated measurements, and therefore make possible the study of short term changes in bone turn over and the effect of treatment (Coen et al 1998). They may be used to predict the risk of fracture (independently of bone loss), Rate of bone loss and also the response to therapy (Coen et al 1998).

In developing countries like Nigeria, these non-invasive and relatively less expensive methods for evaluating bone changes in CRF patients will be a very useful alternative to the invasive and relatively more expensive method used in developed counties.

Because of paucity of data, the prevalence of ROD in Nigeria is not known, however the prevalence of ROD in University of Nigeria Teaching Hospital Enugu using skeletal x-ray was reported to be 3.35% (Odenigbo, 2003). With the increase in the number of patients with CRF requiring or undergoing dialysis across Nigeria, it has becomes necessary to study the extent of ROD in CRF patient with or without dialysis.

## 2 Methodology

### 2.1 Place of study

The study was done at the University of Benin Teaching Hospital (UBTH)) Benin City, which is a 420-bedded tertiary hospital with Renal Unit that offers dialysis. Majority of patients come from Edo State (where the hospital is situated), Delta, Anambra, Ondo, and Oyo States.

### 2.2 Type of study

The study was prospective, descriptive, Clinico-pathological and hospital based.

### 2.3 Subjects

The study group was made up of consecutive chronic renal failure patients attending the University of Benin Teaching Hospital (UBTH).

### 2.4 Inclusion criteria

1. Ultrasonographic findings of bilaterally shrunken kidneys of less than 9cm bipolar diameter.
2. Persistently elevated serum creatinine concentration above 175 µmol/l.
3. Patients aged between 18years and 65years.

The subjects were recruited after obtaining informed consent from them (and /or relations when necessary). Also ethical approval was sought and obtained from the Ethical Committee of the UBTH.

### 2.5 Exclusion criteria

Exclusion from the study included:

1. Patients aged below 18years
2. Those who have had or are on vitamin D therapy
3. Those with chronic liver disease
4. Those who indulge in excessive alcohol intake
5. Post menopausal women.
6. Bed ridden patients.
7. Patient with metastatic bone disease.

### 2.6 Sample size

Fisher's formula for determining sample size was used. This is:

$$N = \frac{Z2Pq}{d2}$$

n= number of sample size
p= prevalence of the problem =0.06%
q= 1-P
z= 95% confidence interval =1.96
d= level of precision =0.05
n= 86.7=87
However since this was a pilot study, sample size of approximately 50% of above (that is 50) was used.

A total of 115 patients were screened by:

Taking of a detailed history and physical examination at the initial contact with the patients with view to determining whether the patients had features suggestive of CRF and also whether patients met the inclusion criteria. Those with obvious exclusion criteria were dropped from the study at this level. This resulted in the exclusion of 55 subjects.

Twenty-four hours urine was collected and used for estimation of creatinine clearance and 24hours urinary calcium. On the morning of the test (8.00am), patients emptied their bladder and discarded the urine. Subsequently, urine passed was put into a clean container until 8.00am the next day. At the end of the urine collection, 5mls of blood was collected from the patients for estimation of serum creatinine. The creatinine clearance was calculated by using the formula: UV/P, where V is the urine flow rate (mls/min). Normal values of creatinine clearance was taken as 105-150mls/min while 24 hours urinary calcium was taken as 100-300 mg/dl. Where it was necessary radiograph of the chest and lumbo-sacral spines were carried out to rule out metastatic bone lesion. An abdominal ultrasonographic scan was carried out. After these evaluations a total of 52 subjects were studied having met the inclusion criteria.

### 2.7 Study design

The eventual 52 subjects who satisfied the inclusion criteria were required to complete a researcher administered questionnaire which includes age, sex, occupation, dietary habits, clinical symptoms of ROD, frequency and regularity of dialysis. Physical examination was performed by the investigator.

Ten milliters (10ml) of venous blood was drawn from the remaining 60 patients from a suitable vein with loose fitting tourniquet. The blood sample was used to assay for serum alkaline phosphatase levels, bone specific alkaline phosphatase levels, serum albumin levels, calcium and phosphate levels.

Osteocalcin, hydroxyproline, parathyroid hormone and calcitriol assays were not carried out because of lack of necessary facilities. However, a surrogate for parathyroid hormone was taken as total serum alkaline phosphatase.

Glomerular filtration rate was determined by 24hour urinary creatinine clearance. Also 24hour urine calcium was determined from the 24 hr urine. Plain x-rays of the wrist/ phalanges of both hands and / or lumbo-sacral spine to include the pelvis was carried out looking out for features of osteodystrophy. Bone histology, though more sensitive in the diagnosis of ROD than radiographic evidence could not be done in live subjects because consent for the procedure was refused. 20 of the CRF patients died during the study. However, out of these, only 14 died in the hospital and the corpse deposited in the mortuary. Post mortem bone biopsies were done on 10 of the 14 bodies whose relations gave consent for the post mortem after obtaining consent from relations.

40 patients without the exclusion criteria and who did not have the have renal failure but attending out -patient clinic of UBTH, whose ages ranged from 18-65years were used as controls.

## MATERIAL AND METHODS

### 2.8 Apparatus

#### 2.8.1 X-ray machine - Watson RO1

This is a standard machine with good resolution quality.

The procedure was carried out by an experienced radiographer using the posterior- anterior positions.

The film was read and reported by an experienced consultant Radiologist.

#### 2.8.2 Ultrasound machine

Sonoace 1500 (Medison) 3.5 MHz sector probe was used. This is a standard machine with good resolution.

Renal ultrasound scan was carried out by an experience Sonographer

### 2.9 Serum phosphate estimation

This was done using Fiske-Subbarow method. This is a colorimetric method using Fiske-Subbarow reagent.

The composition of the reagent is a follows:

| | |
|---|---|
| Ammonium molybdate | -7nM |
| Sulphuric acid | - 1.7N |
| Iron (11) Sulphate | -8Mm |

#### 2.9.1 Principle

The phosphate ion reacts with Molybdate to produce Phosphomolybdate, which is finally reduced to a molybdenum blue, which is photo metrically measured.

#### 2.9.2 Technique

1. Three test tubes were labeled as: Blank -BL
   Standard -ST
   Sample -SA
2. 0.1ml of patient's blood sample was added to SA. 0.1ml of standard was added to ST. To all 3 test tubes were added 3.0ml of the reagent.
3. The content of each of the test tubes were mixed properly and allowed to stand for 10 minutes at room temperature (20-25$^0$C).
4. Reading was done using a spectrophotometer set at 650nM wavelength.
5. The concentration of inorganic phosphate in patient sample was calculated using the formula.

   $$\text{Inorganic phosphate (mg/dl)} = \frac{\text{SA O.D} \times 4}{\text{ST O.D}}$$

   O.D = Optic Density
   Normal value of serum phosphate was taken as 2.4- 4.5 mg/dl.

### 2.10 Measurement of total serum calcium

The Cresolphtalein- Complexone method (CPC) was used for the determination of total serum calcium. This is a standard Colorimetric method. This like most calcium assays measures the total serum calcium although it is only the free calcium which constitutes 50-65% of total calcium that is biologically active.

#### 2.10.1 Principle

CPC forms a violet colored complex with calcium. The absorbance of the colour produced was measured in a colorimeter using a Spectrophotometer at 575nM wavelength measured in a colorimeter using a spectrophotometer at 575nM wave length. Interference from magnesium was reduced by including 8-hydroxquinoline in the working CPC reagent. The Ethanediol in the reagent suppresses the ionization of the 0- Cresolphtalein and helps to give a clear solution. A correction was made when the patient's serum albumin level was below 40g/l using this formula:

$$\text{Corrected serum albumin} = 40 - \frac{\text{albumin g}/1 + \text{Ca}^2}{40}$$

#### 2.10.2 Method

1. Two sets of four tubes were labeled as follows:
   B-reagent blank, standard (2mmol/l)

   C - Control; p - patient.
2. 5mls of CPC reagent was added into each tube using a pipette
3. The following were added into each set of tubes using a pipette as follows:
   B. - 0.05mls distilled water
   S - 0.05mls standard (2mmol/1)
   C- 0.05mls Control serum
   p - 0.05mls patient serum
   The contents of each tube were mixed for several seconds.
4. Using clean Cuvettes, the absorbance of the solution were read in a colorimeter using a spectrophotometer set at 575nM. The instrument was zero with a blank solution in tube B.
5. The concentration of $Ca^{2+}$ in the patients sample was calculated with the following formula:

$$Ca^{2+}\ (\text{mmo1/L}) = \frac{AT}{AS} \times 2$$

   AT= Absorbance of test or control
   AS= Absorbance of standard
   Serum calcium values of 8.5 – 10.5mg/dl was taken as normal.

### 2.11 Measurement of serum alkaline phosphatase

This was done using the kind and king method (1954). This is a standard colorimetric method.

### 2.11.1 Princile

4- amino antipyrine gives a red purple colour with compounds containing a phenolic group in the presence of alkaline oxidizing agents.

### 2.11.2 Technique

2mls of buffer substrate was measured into each of the 2 test tubes and placed in water bath at 37$^0$C for a few minutes. To one of the test tube (patients' test tube) was added 0.lml of serum and the tubes were incubated for exactly 15 minutes. They were removed from the bath and 0.8ml of 0.5M sodium hydroxide and 1.2ml of 0.5M (the blank) was added to both tubes, 1ml of amino- antipyrine reagent and 1ml of potassium ferricyanide were added. For the standard, 1ml of buffer and 1ml of phenol standard containing 0.01mg of phenol was taken. For the standard blank, 1.1ml of buffer and 1ml of water was taken to both tubes, and then sodium hydroxide, bicarbonate amino-antipyrine and ferricyanide was added as above. It was read with a spectrophotometer set at 520 millimicrons. Serum alkaline phosphatase (King- Amstrong unit per 100mls) was derived from the formula:

Serum alkaline phosphatase = Reading of unknown - Reading of blank x 10

Reading of standard - Reading of standard blank

Total serum alkaline phosphatase values of 25-95 IU/L was taken as normal

## 2.12 Determination of bone specific alkaline phospatse

This was done by curve-fitting of inhibition kinetic as popularized by (Statland et al, 1972).

### 2.12.1 Principle

After the determination of the total serum alkaline phosphatase as described above, the serum is heated for 13 minutes at 56$^0$c to inactivate the bone- type isoenzyme. The sera are now read as in the determination of the total serum alkaline phosphatase using a spectrophotometer set at 520 millimicron wavelength.

The concentration of serum alkaline phosphatase excluding the bone isoenzyme was determined as was done for total alkaline phosphatase using a spectrophotometer set at 520millimicron wavelength. The bone isoenzyme was determined by subtracting this value from the total alkaline phosphatase. Values of bone specific alkaline phosphatase level greater than 50% of total serum alkaline phosphatase shows significant contribution from bone iso-enzyme.

## 2.13 Bone histology (post mortem)

### 2.13.1 Procedure

1. The autopsy specimen biopsy was taken from the pelvic bone.
2. Decalcification: The piece of bone biopsied was decalcified by emersion in 10% nitric acid for 2 days.
3. Dehydration: the decalcified bone was dehydrated by passing the bone through ascending grades of alcohol. (70%, 90%, 100%) respectively.

4. Clearing of excess alcohol: to rinse off excess alcohol that could be in the tissue, it was rinsed with xylene or toluene.
5. Impregnation with paraffin wax: the tissue was then impregnated with paraffin wax, and subsequently embedded into paraffin block.
6. Cutting into sections: the tissue embedded into paraffin block was cut into section of about 5 micron thick.
7. The cut section was then placed on a slide and allowed to dry for a minimum of 30 min.
8. Staining process: heamatin and eosin stains were used.
9. Reading of slide: the slide was read and reported by an experienced histopathologist.

### 2.14 Statistical analysis

Data analysis was done using SPSS package, and the storage was in Microsoft excel. Data are expressed in tabular, bar chart and prose forms. Mean standard deviation and percentages of all data were derived. Odd ratio was used to measure strength of association between ROD and their relative risk.

The t-test and chi-squared test were used to determine the differences in means of the CRF group and control.

P value of less than 0.05 was regarded as significant.

## 3. Results

### 3.1 Characteristics of subjects studied

A total of 115 patients were screened for the study. 52 of them were studied, having met the inclusion criteria. This was made up of 30 (58%) males and 22 (42%) females. 40 age and sex matched controls, made up of 22 (55%) males and 18 (45%) females were also studied. The age range of the study population was 18 - 65 years. 3 (5%) of the CRF patients were in the age range less than 30 years, 16 (30%) were in the 31 - 40 years age range, 13 (25%) and 14 (26%) were in the age range 41 - 50 years and 51 - 60 years respectively, while 6 (11%) were in the age range greater than 60 years. The peak incidence of CRF was in the 31 - 40 years age range. The mean age of the CRF patients and controls were 42.5 $\pm$ 11.6 years and 40.4 $\pm$ 11.3 years respectively (refer to table 1).

| AGE (YEARS) | CRF GROUP (n = 52) | CONTROL GROUP (n = 40) |
|---|---|---|
| | Frequency (%) | Frequency (%) |
| <30 | 3 (5%) | 7 (17%) |
| 31 -40 | 16 (30%) | 12 (30%) |
| 41 - 50 | 13 (25%) | 10 (25%) |
| 51 - 60 | 14 (26%) | 7 (17%) |
| >60 | 6 (11%) | 4 (10%) |

Table 1. Age and sex distribution of both CRF and control groups.

| Characteristics | CRF Group (n=52) Mean ± SD | Control Group (n=40) Mean ±SD | P Value |
|---|---|---|---|
| Sex | M (30), F (22) | M (22), F (18) | |
| Age (Yrs) | 42.5 ± 11.6 | 40.38 ± 11.3 | >0.05 |
| Renal sizes (cm) | | | |
| Right | 8.33 ± 0.5 | 11.99 ± 0.32 | <0.05 |
| Left | 8.16 ± 0.5 | 11.92 ± 0.33 | <0.05 |
| Creatinine clearance (mls/min) | 9.8 ± 6.7 | 126 ± 7.3 | <0.05 |
| Total alkaline phosphatase (iu/l) | 129.4 ± 21.6 | 43.73 ± 8.31 | <0.05 |
| BAP (iu/l) | 83.12 ± 21.6 | 21.8 ± 4.11 | <0.05 |
| Serum calcium (mg/dl) | 6.9 ± 2.3 | 9.12 ± 0.5 | <0.05 |
| Serum phosphate (mg/dl) | 6.1 ± 1.9 | 3.20 ± 0.6 | <0.05 |
| 24 hours urine calcium (mg/dl) | 1.7 ± 2.37 | 3.8 ± 1.76 | >0.05 |
| Serum creatinine (mg/dl) | 7.16 ± 2.4 | 0.8 ± 0.15 | <0.05 |
| Blood urea (mg/dl) | 123.8 ± 39.8 | 24.4 ± 5.6 | <0.05 |
| Serum protein (gm/dl) | 3.2 ± 0.60 | 4.46 ± 0.52 | >0.05 |

Table 2. Characteristics of CRF and control group.

In the age ranges <30 years and 31 - 40 years, the mean creatinine clearance were 7 ± 1.83 mls/min and 12.6 ± 2.16 mls/min respectively. In the age ranges 41 - 50 years and 51 - 60 years, the mean creatinine clearances were 8.6 ± 3.2mls/min and 8.2 ± 2.6mls/min respectively. In the age range >60 years, the mean creatinine clearance was 11.8 ± 5.2mls/min. Creatinine clearance was lowest in the <30 years age range. This is represented in figure1.

### 3.2 Symptoms of renal osteodydtrophy (ROD)

The symptoms suggestive of ROD in the study population include bone pain and pruritus. 7(14%) of the CRF group had symptoms. This was made up of 5(71%) that had bone pain and 2(29%) that had pruritus. 5(12%) of the control group had bone pain. None had pruritus. The symptom of bone pain was commoner in males compared to females. Of those that had bone pain, 4 (80%) were males while 1 (20%) was a females. Pruritus was equally as common in both sexes (1 male and 1 female).

The entire patients that had pruritus in the CRF group had elevated serum alkaline phosphatase, hyperphosphataemia and elevated calcium-phosphate product. There was a statistically significant correlation between bone pain and creatinine clearance (r =-0.3), such that bone pain occurred more commonly in patients with end stage renal disease (ESRD).

Only 1(1%) patient in the CRF group had radiological evidence of Rugger Jersey Spine. Radiological evidence of osteoarthritis was found in 3(60%) and 2(40%) of the patients that had bone pain in the CRF and control group respectively (see Table 3).

| Patients | | | | | Characteristics | | | | |
|---|---|---|---|---|---|---|---|---|---|
| | Sex | Age (Yrs) | Serum Ca (mg/dl) | Serum P04 (mg/dl) | Serum Alk Phosp (iu/l) | Ca x P04 $mg^2/dl^2$ | X-ray Findings | Crcl (mls/min) | Symptoms |
| 1. | M | 40 | 9.8 | 14 | 142 | 137.2 | - | 12 | Pruritus |
| 2. | M | 46 | 6.4 | 9.9 | 156 | 64.4 | RJS | 10.6 | Pain |
| 3. | M | 52 | 4 | 5.4 | 128 | 21.6 | OA | 12.6 | Pain |
| 4. | F | 48 | 10.2 | 9 | 106 | 19.8 | OA | 9.6 | Pruritus |
| 5. | F | 56 | 4.5 | 13 | 136 | 58.5 | OA | 7.2 | Pain |
| 6. | M | 62 | 5.6 | 9.9 | 99 | 64.4 | OA | 8.5 | Pain |
| 7. | M | 64 | 7.7 | 6.5 | 127 | 48.1 | * | 16 | Pain |

RJS = Rugger Jersey spine, $PO_4$ = Phosphate, Ca = Calcium, Alk Phosp = Alkaline phosphate, Crcl = Creatinine clearance, OA = Osteoarthritis.

Table 3. Characteristics of CRF patients symptomatic of ROD.

### 3.3 Creatinine clearance of subjects

The mean creatinine clearance in the CRF and control groups was 9.8 ± 6.7mls/min and 126.2 ± 7.4 mls/min respectively. There was a statistically significant difference between both means ($p < 0.05$).

Table 4 shows the distribution of subjects according to creatinine clearance. In the CRF group, 47 (90%) had ESRD, with creatinine clearance < 15mls/min, 4 (8%) had creatinine clearance of 15 - 29mls/min, and 1 (2%) had creatinine clearance 30 - 59mls/min. All controls had creatinine clearance > 95mls/min (see Table 4).

| Creatinine clearance (mls/min) | Frequency | | | |
|---|---|---|---|---|
| | CRF group n = 52 | | Control group n = 40 | |
| | Frequency | % | Frequency | % |
| > 95 | - | - | 40 | 100% |
| 30 - 59 | 1 | 2 | - | - |
| 15 - 29 | 4 | 8 | - | - |
| <15 | 47 | 90 | - | - |

Table 4. Distribution of subjects according to creatinine clearance.

### 3.4 Renal ultrasonographic scan of subjects

The mean kidney sizes in the CRF group was 8.2 $\pm$ 0.5cm and 8.3 + 0.5cm for the right and left kidneys respectively, while that of the control was 12.10 $\pm$ 0.33cm and 12.02 $\pm$ 0.33cm for the right and left kidneys respectively. 52 (100%) patients in the CRF group had shrunken kidneys (<11cm).

There was a weak positive correlation between renal sizes and creatinine clearance, with r = 0.12 and r = 0.17 for the right and left kidneys respectively (see Table 5).

| Renal sizes (cm) | Frequency | | | |
|---|---|---|---|---|
| | CRF GROUP (n = 52) | | CONTROL GROUP (n = 40) | |
| | Right | Left | Right | Left |
| Small size (<9cm) | 51 | 51 | - | - |
| 9 - 10.9cm | 1 | 1 | - | - |
| Normal size (11 - 12cm) | - | - | 40 | 40 |
| Large size >12cm | - | - | - | - |

Table 5. Renal sizes of subjects on abdominal ultrasonographic scan.
Normal kidney size: 11 - 12cm (Brenner and Rector. The kidney vol.1, 6th edition 2000).

### 3.5 Serum calcium of subjects

The mean serum calcium in the CRF and control groups was 6.9 $\pm$ 2.3mg/dl and 9.12 $\pm$ 0.53mg/dl respectively. This difference between the means was statistically significant ($p<0.05$).

Table 6 shows the pattern of serum calcium concentration in the study population. In the CRF group, 37 (71%) patients had hypocalcaemia (<8.5mg/dl), 3 (6%) had hypercalcaemia (>10.5mg/dl, while 12 (23%) had normal calcium levels (8.5 - 10.5mg/dl). In the control group, 39 (97%) patients had normal calcium levels, while only 1 (3%) had hypocalcaemia. None in the control group had hypercalcaemia. There was a weak positive correlation between serum calcium and total alkaline phosphate in the CRF group (r = 0.04), such that as the serum alkaline phosphate was increasing, the serum calcium was decreasing. Amongst the CRF patients with total serum alkaline phosphate of <25iu/l, the mean serum calcium was 6.4 $\pm$ 1.6mg/dl, while in the group with total serum alkaline phosphate of 25 - 95iu/l, the mean serum calcium was 7.9 $\pm$ 3.0mg/dl, and in the group with total serum alkaline phosphate of >95iu/l, the mean serum calcium was 6.8 $\pm$ 1.8mg/dl. There was an insignificant correlation between serum calcium and creatinine clearance (r = 0.007). Amongst the CRF patients with creatinine clearance of <15mls/min, the mean serum calcium was 5.2 $\pm$ 2.4mg/dl, while in the group that had creatinine clearance of 15 - 29mls/min, the mean serum calcium was 6.3 $\pm$ 2.1mg/dl, and in the group with creatinine clearance of >30mls/min, the mean serum calcium was 8.4 $\pm$ 1.6mg/dl. Mean serum calcium tends to be lower in ESRD patients (see table 6).

| Serum Calcium (mg/dl) | CRF group n = 52 | Control group n = 40 |
|---|---|---|
| Hypocalcaemia (<8.5mg/dl) | 37 (71%) | 1 (3%) |
| Normal levels (8.5 - 10.5mg/dl) | 12 (23%) | 39 (97%) |
| Hypercalcaemia (>10.5mg/dl) | 3 (6%) | - |

Table 6. The distribution of subjects according to serum calcium.

### 3.6 Serum phosphate of subjects

The mean serum phosphate in the CRF group was 6.1 $\pm$ 2.0mg/dl, and this was significantly higher than the mean serum phosphate of 3.2 $\pm$ 0.6mg/dl in the control group ($p<0.05$). Table 7 shows the pattern of serum phosphate in both the CRF and control groups. In the CRF group, 41 (79%) patients had hyperphosphataemia, while 11 (21%) had normal serum phosphate levels. No patient had hypophosphataemia. In the control group, all the 40 (100%) patients had normal serum phosphate levels. There was insignificant but positive correlation between serum phosphate and creatinine clearance ($r = 0.1$) and bone pain ($r = 0.4$). (See Table 7)

| Serum phosphate (mg/dl) | CRF group n = 52 | Control group n = 40 |
|---|---|---|
| Hypophosphataemia (<2.4mg/dl) | - | - |
| Normal phosphate Level (2.4 - 4.5mg/dl) | 11 (21%) | 40 (100%) |
| Hyperphosphataemia (>4.5mg/dl) | 41 (79%) | - |

Table 7. Pattern of serum phosphate in subjects.

Amongst the CRF patients with serum alkaline phosphatase of <25iu/l, the mean serum phosphate was 5.1 $\pm$ 0.9mg/dl, while in the group with serum alkaline phosphatase of 25 – 95iu/l, serum phosphate was 6.5 $\pm$ 1.2mg/dl, and in the group with serum alkaline phosphatase of >95iu/l the mean serum phosphate was 6.2 $\pm$ 1.4mg/dl. Thus, there was a weak but negative correlation between serum phosphate and total serum alkaline phosphatase (r - 0.15), such that when total serum alkaline phosphatase was increasing, the serum phosphate also increased.

Amongst the CRF patients with creatinine clearance of >30mls/min, the mean serum phosphate was 4.4 $\pm$ 1.2mg/dl, while in the groups with creatinine clearance of 15 – 29mls/min and <15mls/min (ESRD), the mean serum phosphate was 6.6 $\pm$ 1.1mg/dl and 6.2 $\pm$ 1.3mg/dl respectively. As the creatinine clearance tended towards ESRD, the serum phosphate rises. There was a positive correlation between serum phosphate and creatinine clearance ($r = 0.10$).

### 3.7 Serum alkaline phosphatase of subjects

The mean total serum alkaline phosphatase in the CRF group was 129.4 $\pm$ 21.6iu/l, while that of the control was 43.73 $\pm$ 8.3iu/l. There was a statistically significant difference between both means ($p<0.05$). 41 (79%) of the CRF group had elevated total serum alkaline phosphatase levels, 8 (15%) had normal levels, 3 (6%) had low levels, while all controls had normal levels. Of the 41 CRF patients that had elevated total serum alkaline phosphatase levels, all (100%) had >50% of their alkaline phosphatase levels, from bone isoenzyme (bone specific alkaline phosphatase). Only 1 (2%) CRF patient had radiological evidence of ROD (Rugger Jersey Spine). Total serum alkaline phosphatase correlated positively with creatinine clearance ($r = 0.06$) and bone pain ($r = 0.4$).

Amongst the CRF group with creatinine clearance of >30mls/min the mean total alkaline phosphatase was 105 $\pm$ 6.1iu/l, while in the groups with creatinine clearance of 15 - 29mls/min and <15mls/min (ESRD), the mean alkaline phosphatase were 124 $\pm$ 4.6iu/l and 143 + 5.6iu/l respectively (see Table 8).

| Total serum alkaline phosphatase (iu/l) | CRF group, n = 52 Frequency (%) | Control group, n = 40 Frequency (%) |
|---|---|---|
| Increased levels (>95iu/l) | 41 (79%) | - |
| Normal levels (25 - 95iu/l | 8 (15%) | 40 (100%) |
| Decreased levels (<25iu/l) | 3 (6%) | - |

Table 8. Distribution of CRF and control groups according to serum alkaline phosphatase.

### 3.8 Calcium and phosphate products of CRF subjects

The mean calcium x phosphate products in the CRF group was 42.8 $\pm$ 21.6mg$^2$/dl$^2$ while that of the control was 28.21 $\pm$ 2.4mg$^2$/dl$^2$. There was a statistically significant difference in both means ($p<0.05$). Table 9 shows distribution of calcium x phosphate product amongst the CRF patients. 3 (5%) of the CRF patients had calcium x phosphate product >70mg$^2$/dl$^2$. This was made up of 2 (66%) males and 1 (34%) female. 6 (11%) patients had their calcium x phosphate product between 52 - 70mg$^2$/dl$^2$. This was made up of 2 (33%) males and 4 (67%) females. 43 (82%) patients had their calcium x phosphate products <52mg$^2$/dl$^2$. This was made up of 26 (60%) males and 17 (40%) females. All 3 patients who had calcium x phosphate product >70mg$^2$/dl$^2$ died during the period of study and showed evidence of ROD on postmortem bone biopsy.

Normal Ca x P04 product = <70mg$^2$/dl$^2$.

### 3.9 Urinary calcium excretion in study group

The mean 24 hours urinary calcium in the CRF group was 68.4$\pm$ 12.8mg/dl, and 162 $\pm$ 40.4mg/dl in the control group. This difference in means is statistically significant ($p<0.05$). There was an insignificant correlation between 24hours urinary calcium and creatinine clearance, and serum calcium ($r =-0.16$) and ($r =0.02$) respectively. There was a statistically significant correlation between 24hours urinary calcium and total serum alkaline phosphatase ($r= 0.38$) but no significant correlation with sex ($r =0.79$), age ($r=0.46$) or bone paint ($r =0.23$).

| MALES | | | | FEMALES | | | |
|---|---|---|---|---|---|---|---|
| Serial number | Serum P04 (mg/dl) | Serum Ca (mg/dl) | Ca x P04 product ($mg^2/dl^2$) | Serial number | Serum Ca (mg/dl) | Serum P04 (mg/dl) | Ca x P04 product ($mg^2/dl^2$) |
| 1. | 6 | 5.1 | 30.6 | 1 | 6 | 5.2 | 31.2 |
| 2. | 5 | 4.8 | 24.0 | 2 | 8.7 | 3.8 | 33.1 |
| 3. | 4.2 | 5.8 | 24.4 | 3 | 5 | 6.5 | 32.5 |
| 4. | 6 | 7.3 | 43.8 | 4 | 9.8 | 5.8 | 56.8 |
| 5. | 8.9 | 4.9 | 43.6 | 5 | 10.6 | 6.4 | 67.8 |
| 6. | 8.5 | 5.3 | 45.1 | 6 | 9.2 | 7.5 | 69.0 |
| 7. | 3 | 4.1 | 12.3 | 7 | 4 | 11.1 | 44.4 |
| 8. | 6.2 | 5.8 | 36.0 | 8 | 5.6 | 4.9 | 27.4 |
| 9. | 9.7 | 4.8 | 46.6 | 9 | 3.7 | 4.4 | 16.3 |
| 10 | 6.8 | 3.2 | 21.8 | 10 | 6 | 6.4 | 38.4 |
| 11. | 5 | 2.7 | 13.5 | 11 | 6.2 | 7.4 | 45.9 |
| 12. | 5.4 | 8.7 | 47.0 | 12 | 6.5 | 8.6 | 55.9 |
| 13. | 9.9 | 6.5 | 64.4 | 13 | 5.7 | 7.8 | 44.5 |
| 14. | 6.5 | 7 | 45.5 | 14 | 6.8 | 7 | 47.6 |
| 15. | 5.4 | 4 | 21.6 | 15 | 7.6 | 4.8 | 36.5 |
| 16. | 7.3 | 4.3 | 31.4 | 16 | 7.8 | 4.2 | 32.8 |
| 17. | 8.6 | 6 | 51.6 | 17 | 4.8 | 6.4 | 30.7 |
| 18. | 8.6 | 3 | 25.8 | 18 | 5.8 | 6.5 | 37.7 |
| 19. | 4.9 | 7.3 | 48.1 | 19 | 10.2 | 5.8 | 53.4 |
| 20. | 5.4 | 7.1 | 34.8 | 20 | 4.6 | 10.2 | 91.8 |
| 21. | 5.4 | 3.2 | 17.3 | 21 | 7.1 | 4.6 | 35.0 |
| 22. | 14 | 9.8 | 17.3 | 22 | 4.9 | 7.1 | 34.8 |
| 23. | 7 | 6.9 | 137.2 | | | | |
| 24. | 13 | 4.5 | 48.3 | | | | |
| 25. | 9 | 12.5 | 58.5 | | | | |
| 26. | 6.5 | 5.9 | 112.5 | | | | |
| 27. | 8.3 | 60.1 | 38.4 | | | | |
| 28. | 3 | 6.1 | 50.6 | | | | |
| 29. | 5.6 | 5.8 | 17.4 | | | | |
| 30. | 5.4 | 5.9 | 37.0 | | | | |
| Mean | 6.99 | 5.83 | 42.02 | | 6.84 | 6.47 | 43.79 |
| Std Dev. | 2.5 | 2.1 | 26.4 | | 1.9 | 1.9 | 16.8 |

Table 9. Serum Calcium, Serum phosphate and calcium x phosphate product of CRF patients.

### 3.10 Radiological evidence of ROD

Of the patient that had symptoms of ROD, 5 (71%) had bone pain while 2 (29%) had pruritus. Only 1 (20%) of the 5 patients that had bone pain showed radiological evidence of Rugger-Jersey spine (see appendix 1), constituting 9%of the CRF group. Table 10 shows the characteristics of the only patient with radiological evidence of Rugger Jersey spine. In the control group, 5 (21%) had bone pain. Of these, 2 (40%) constituting 5% of the control group, had radiological evidence of osteoarthritis while Radiological evidence of osteoarthritis was found in 3(60%) patients that had bone pain in the CRF group.

APPENDIX 1: X-RAY OF THE SPINE SHOWING RUGER-JERSEY APPEARANCE.

NOTE THE ALTERNATING BANDS OF HYPO-DENSITY AND HYPERDENSITY INDICATING OSTEOPOROSIS AND OSTEOSCLEROSIS RESPECTIVELY.

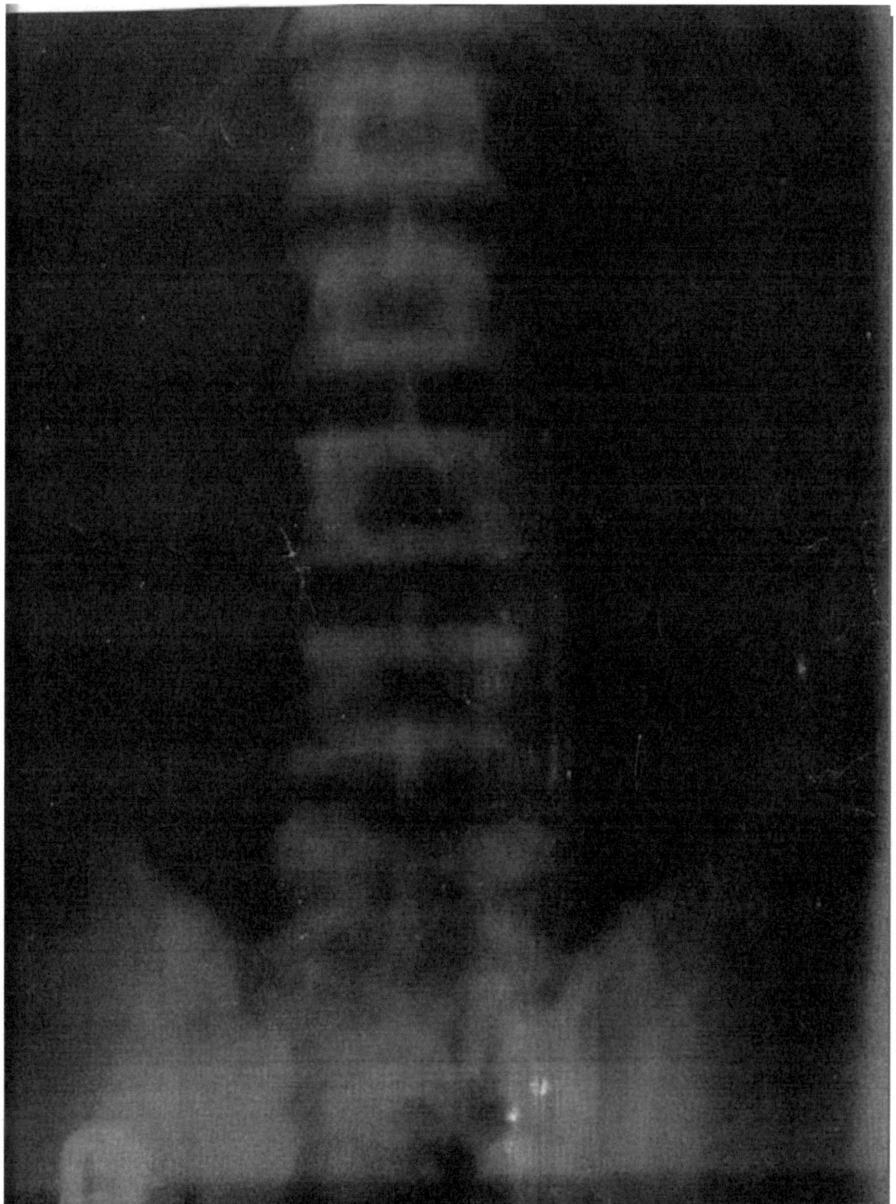

| Age (Years) | Sex | RS (cm) Left | Right | Serum Ca (mg/dl) | Alk Phosp (iu/l) | Serum P04 (mg/dl) | Ca x P04 ($mg^2/dl^2$) | Crcl (mls/min) |
|---|---|---|---|---|---|---|---|---|
| 54 | M | 7.8 | 7.6 | 6.5 | 156 | 9.9 | 64.4 | 6.0 |

(Rugger Jersey Spine).
Crcl = Creatinine clearance, Alk phosp = Alkline phosphatase,
P04 = Phosphate, Ca = Calcium, RS = Renal Size.

Table 10. Characteristics of the only patient with radiological evidence of ROD.

### 3.11 Histological evidence of rod on postmortem bone biopsy

10 Postmortem bone biopsies were carried out. This was made up of 7 (70%) males and 3 (30%) females. 9 (90%) had histological evidence of ROD, while 1 had normal bone histology. Of the 9 that had histological evidence, 6 (66%) were males while 3 (34%) were females. 6 (66%) had Osteitis Fibrosa. This was made up of 4 (50%) males and 2 (34%) females. 2 (22%) had Osteomalacia, 1 each (50%) of male and female, while 1 (12%) male had evidence of mixed type ROD (see Appendices 2-4). All the patients who had histological evidence of ROD had their creatinine clearance < 15mls/min (ESRD). 8 (88%) of the patient with histological evidence of ROD did not have any radiological evidence of ROD.

All the patients that had bone histological evidence of ROD had elevated total serum alkaline phosphatase and serum phosphatase. There is a positive correlation between histological evidence of ROD and total serum alkaline phosphatase and serum phosphate, (r = 0.04) and (r = 0.036) respectively. There was no correlation between histological evidence of ROD and symptoms of ROD (r = 0.48), see table 11.

| Patients | Gender | Age (Year) | Histological type | Calcium (mg/dl) | Phosp (mg/dl) | Ca x P04 ($mg^2/dl^2$) | Total Alk. Phosp (iu/L) |
|---|---|---|---|---|---|---|---|
| 1 | M | 46 | OF | 6.8 | 9.9 | 64.4 | 156 |
| 2 | M | 48 | OM | 12.5 | 9.0 | 112.5 | 140 |
| 3 | M | 52 | OF | 5.3 | 8.5 | 45.1 | 122 |
| 4 | F | 46 | OM | 7.5 | 9.2 | 69.0 | 134 |
| 5 | M | 39 | Mixed type | 8.7 | 5.4 | 47.0 | 138 |
| 6 | M | 36 | OF | 9.8 | 14.0 | 137.5 | 152 |
| *7 | F | 48 | OF | 10.2 | 9.0 | 91.8 | 98 |
| 8 | M | 40 | OF | 6.1 | 8.3 | 50.6 | 106 |
| 9 | F | 54 | OF | 6.4 | 10.6 | 67.8 | 146 |

* Patient 7 had normal histology
OF = Osteitis Fibrosa, OM = Osteomalacia

Table 11. Characteristics of patients with bone histological evidence of ROD.

APPENDIX 2: PHOTOMICROGRAMS OF BONE HISTOLOGY SHOWING OSTEITIS FIBROSA, OSTEOMALACIA AND OSTEITIS FIBROSA IN PATIENTS 1, 2 AND 3 RESPECTIVELY.

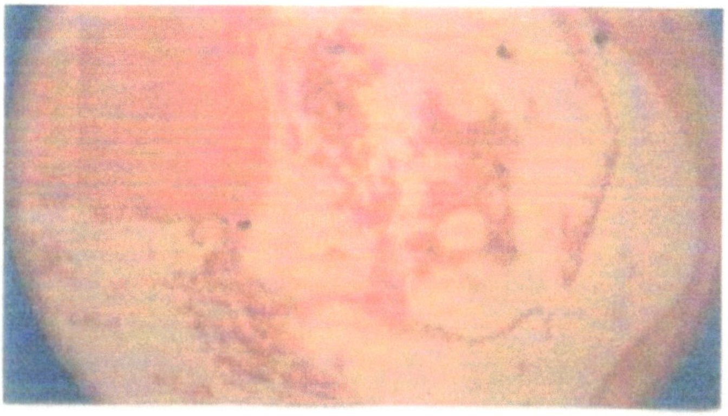

1

**Osteitis fibrosa**

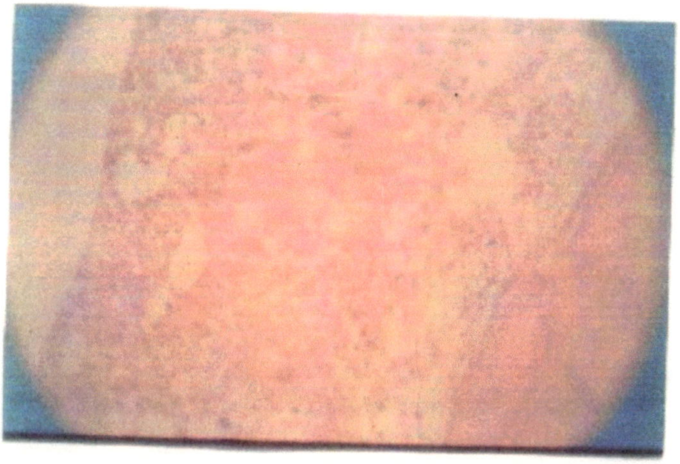

2

**Osteomalacia**

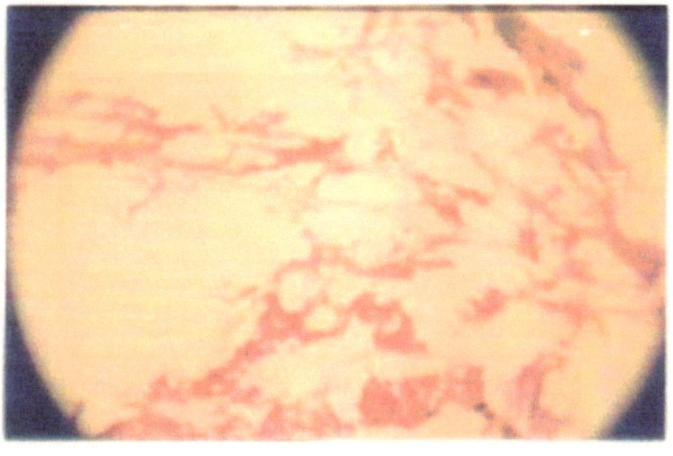

3

**Osteitis fibrosa**

APPENDIX 3: PHOTOMICROGRAMS OF BONE HISTOLOGY SHOWING OSTEOMALACIA, MIXED TYPE ROD AND OSTEITIS FIBROSA IN PATIENT4, 5 AND 6 RESPECTIVELY.

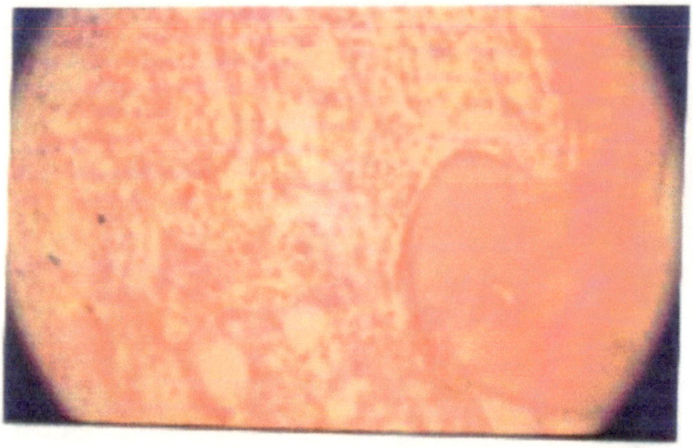

4
Osteomalacia

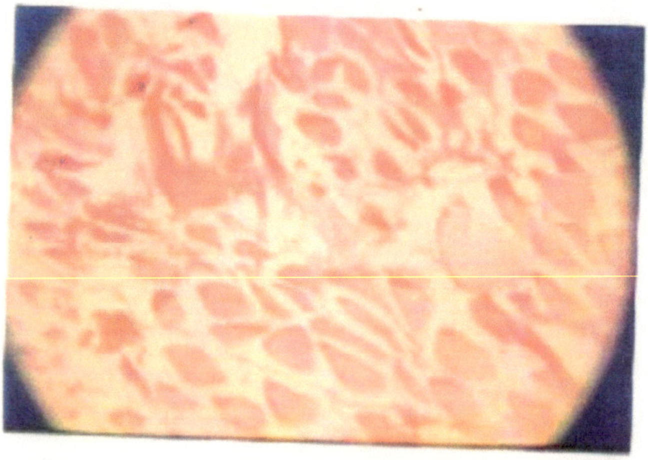

5
Mixed type ROD

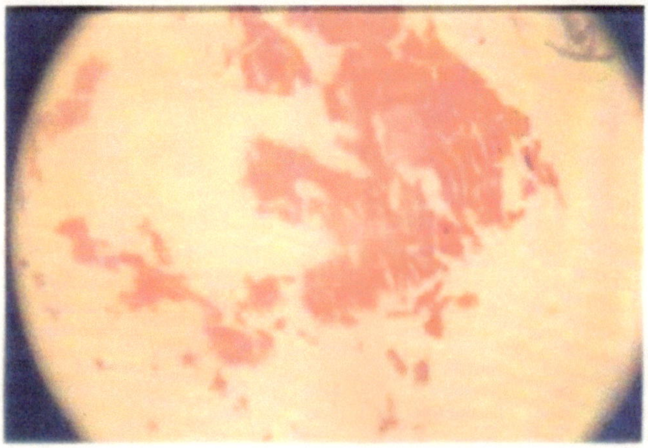

6
OSTEITIS FIBROSA

APPENDIX 4: PHOTOMICROGRAMS OF BONE HISTOLOGY SHOWING NORMAL HISTOLOGY, OSTEITIS FIBROSA, OSTEITIS FIBROSA AND OSTEITIS FIBROSA IN PATIENT 7, 8, 9 AND 10 RESPECTIVELY.

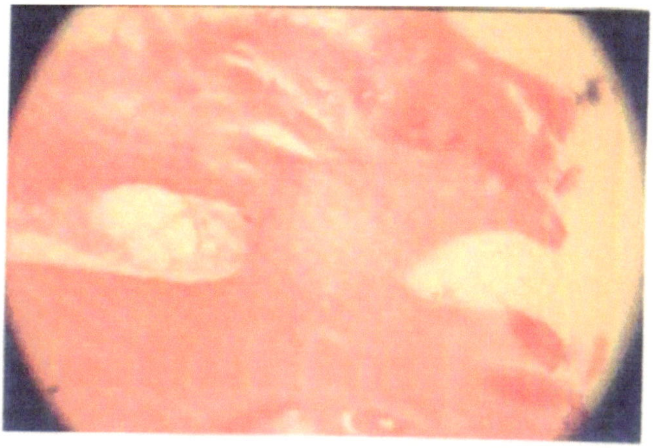

7
**Normal**

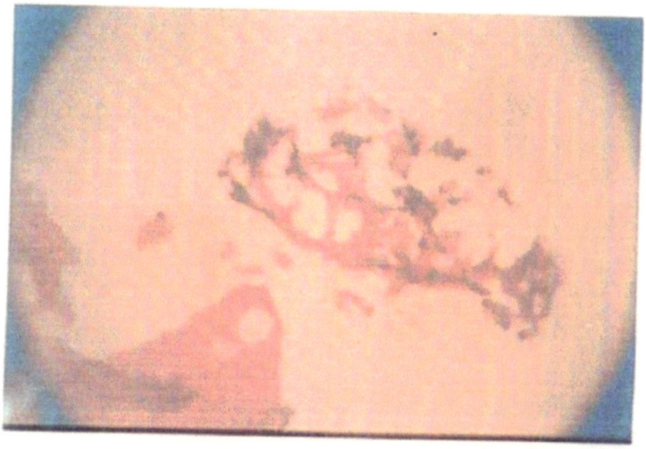

8
**Osteitis fibrosa**

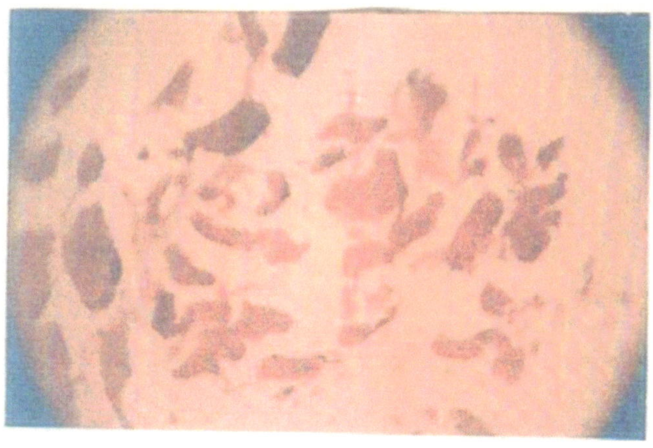

9
**Osteitis fibrosa**

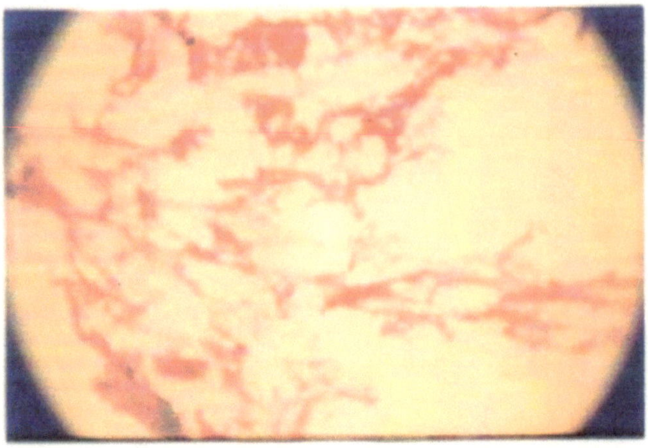

10

OSTEITIS FIBROSA

| Patients | Gender | Age (Year) | Histological type | Calcium (mg/dl) | Phosp (mg/dl) | Ca x P04 ($mg^2/dl^2$) | Total Alk. Phosp (iu/L) |
|---|---|---|---|---|---|---|---|
| 1 | M | 46 | OF | 6.8 | 9.9 | 64.4 | 156 |
| 2 | M | 48 | OM | 12.5 | 9.0 | 112.5 | 140 |
| 3 | M | 52 | OF | 5.3 | 8.5 | 45.1 | 122 |
| 4 | F | 46 | OM | 7.5 | 9.2 | 69.0 | 134 |
| 5 | M | 39 | Mixed type | 8.7 | 5.4 | 47.0 | 138 |
| 6 | M | 36 | OF | 9.8 | 14.0 | 137.5 | 152 |
| *7 | F | 48 | OF | 10.2 | 9.0 | 91.8 | 98 |
| 8 | M | 40 | OF | 6.1 | 8.3 | 50.6 | 106 |
| 9 | F | 54 | OF | 6.4 | 10.6 | 67.8 | 146 |

* Patient 7 had normal histology
OF = Osteitis Fibrosa, OM = Osteomalacia

Table 11. Characteristics of patients with bone histological evidence of ROD.

## 4. Dicussion

### 4.1 Findings of the study

This study was carried out to determine the prevalence of ROD in chronic renal failure in Benin City.

The main findings of the study suggest that:

1. Osteitis Fibrosa is the commonest type of ROD.
2. There is a correlation between histological evidence of ROD and biochemical maker (Alkaline Phosphatase).
3. The yield of ROD using radiological examination is low in our chronic renal patients.

4. Radiological and biochemical evidence of ROD seems to be more prevalent in severe chronic renal failure (ESRD).
5. ROD may be more prevalent in males.
6. There is no correlation between symptoms of ROD and biochemical or radiological evidence of ROD. This suggests that many patients may have ROD with no symptoms.
7. Hypocalcaemia and hyperphosphataemia is prevalent in our CRF patients.

### 4.2 Osteitis fibrosa is the commonest type of rod

Osteitis Fibrosa is a form of high turnover bone disease as a result of hyperparathyroidism. PTH assay was not done because of lack of facility in our center. However serum alkaline phosphatase was used as a surrogate. 78% of the CRF patients had raised levels of total serum alkaline phosphatase which correlate well with PTH levels and histological features of secondary hyperparathyroidism. This is in agreement with the work done by Duursma et al, (1975); Ritz et al (1974) and Hruska et al (1978). 66% of patients had Osteitis Fibrosa on histology. This finding agrees with the work of Jarava et al (1996) who found bone histological evidence of Osteitis Fibrosa cystica in 17 (85%) out of 20 haemodialysis patients in England. Our findings also agrees with that of shin et al (1999) who found Osteitis Fibrosa as the commonest type of ROD in predialysis patients in Canada (44%). This finding contradicts that if Coen et al (1996) who found mixed type ROD as the commonest type in predialysis CRF patient in England.

### 4.3 There is correlation between histological evidence of rod and serum alkaline phoshatase

In this study, it was found that 90% of patient had histological evidence of ROD on postmortem bone biopsy. This agrees with the finding Sanchez (2001), who found that 90% of patients with ESRD on maintenance dialysis have abnormal bone histology. Majority of patients are either predialysis or those who were not dialyzing adequately. It is known that once a patient start on maintenance, the prevalence of ROD increases. One of the contributing factors being aluminum deposition (from dialysate fluid), it means that the prevalence may even be higher if our patients are dialyzed adequately. In our study we found that all the patients that had histological evidence of ROD had elevated serum alkaline phosphatase levels. This finding may possibly be pointing to the fact that serum alkaline phosphatase can be used as a surrogate of parathyroid hormone as a predictor of ROD in our patients. This agrees with the finding of Urena et al, (1991) that in the absence of liver disease, serum alkaline phosphatase can be used to predict the presence of ROD. The finding is also in agreement with that of Duursma et al and Ritz et al who found that plasma alkaline phosphatase levels correlates with histological features of secondary hyperparathyroidism (HPTH).

### 4.4 The yield of rod using radiological examination is low in our chronic renal failure patients

In our study, we found only 2% of ROD using radiological examination. This agrees with Odenigbo (2003) who found 3.35% of ROD in Enugu using radiological examination. In this study, radiological evidence of ROD was not found in all 9(100%) patients who had histological evidence of ROD on postmortem bone biopsy. This agrees with the finding of

Hodsons et al, (1981) that there is a disparity between the radiological and histological evidence of ROD. In a study in Germany, Hodsons et al found only 7(41%) patients with radiological evidence of ROD out of 17 with histological evidence of ROD. Micheal et al (1998) found radiological features of ROD in 35% of CRF patients in ESRD.

There are some reasons for the low prevalence of ROD using x-rays. Firstly, the conventional techniques for x-ray contribute. Meama et al (1972) noted the phalanges to be normal in 67% if uremic patients using conventional techniques for X-ray films, and only 8% showed subperiosteal erosion. With the introduction of better films and the use of magnification techniques, only 26% appeared normal while 29% for exhibited subperiosteal erosion. There is no facility for magnification technique in the center where the study was done. Secondly, it has been reported that more than 50% of bone can be lost without any evidence in a radiograph, because only the cortical bone is clearly noted, and an important loss of cancellous bone should occur before radiological feature of ROD can be appreciated (Poznanki, 1993). Perhaps the fact that CRF patients in our environment have infrequent haemodialysis and do not live long enough for these changes to be detected on x-ray studies may be contributory to the low yield of ROD using radiological examination.

### 4.5 Radiological and biochemical evidence of rod is more prevalent in esrd patients

In our study, the only patient who had radiological evidence of ROD had a creatinine clearance of 6mls/min. 90% of the CRF patients had creatinine clearance <15mls/min (ESRD). The entire patients who had creatinine clearance <15mls/min had elevated serum alkaline phosphatase levels. Theses finding agree with the findings of Coen et al (1996) that adynamic bone disease is commoner n early stages of renal failure, while Osteomalacia and Osteitis Fibrosa cystica tend to occur as resistance to PTH develops, a situation which occurs in ESRD.

### 4.6 ROD may be more prevalent in males

In this study, the one patient who had radiological evidence of ROD was a male. Also, of the 9 patients that had histological evidence of ROD, 6(66%) were males, while 3(34%) were females, with a male- female ratio of 2:1, this finding is in contrast to the finding of Odenigbo et al (2003) in a study carried out at Enugu where ROD was found to be more prevalent in females. The finding also contradicts that of Couttenye et al (1997) who showed that women seem to develop hyperparathyroidism whereas men seems to more frequently develop aplastic bone disease. The reason why men in this study showed evidence of ROD more than women may be due to the fact that there were more men in this study, particularly in the group of 10 patients that had postmortem biopsy. However, the number of patients studied was small for a general statement to be made on gender difference.

### 4.7 There is no correlation between symptoms of rod and biochemical or radiological evidence

In the study, 7 (14%) of the CRF subjects had symptoms suggestive of ROD. Of these, 5(71%) had bone pain while 2 (29%) had radiological evidence of ROD ('Rugger Jersey" spine), while 3 (80%) had radiological features of osteoarthritis. This agrees with the finding of Odenigbo, who reported that out of the 11 patients who had bone pain, none had radiological evidence of ROD, but all patients who had radiological evidence of

Osteoarthritis (Odenigbo 2003). This study also agrees with the work of Harowin et al (1987) who found a high incidence of joint symptoms and radiological abnormalities in his group of Canadian patient, not necessarily due osteodystrophy.

### 4.8 Hypocalcaemia and hyperphosphataemia is prevalent in our crf patients

In the study the mean serum calcium of CRF subject was 5.83± 2.1mg/dl. 37(71%) of CRF subjects had hypocalcaemia (<8.5mg/dl). This finding agrees with that of Slatoposky et al (1986). Calcium supplementation is a known modality for the treatment of hypocalcaemia. The mean serum phosphate of CRF patients in this was 6.1±2.0mg/dl. 41 (79%) had hyperphosphataemia (>4.5mg/dl). This agrees with finding of Slotoposky et al (1986) who demonstrated hyperphosphataemia even in moderate CRF. Dietary phosphate restriction and phosphate binding are effective methods of control of hyperphosphataemia.

### 4.9 Conclusion and recommendations

#### 4.9.1 Conclusion

The findings of this study suggest that ROD which is a complication of chronic renal failure does exist in our environment. The study has also shown that Osteitis Fibrosa is the commonest type of ROD, and that ROD may be commoner in males. The study showed that in majority of patients with ESRD there is biochemical evidence. This finding may possibly be pointing to the fact that clinical features are a poor guide to the presence of ROD. Before now, it was thought that ROD hardly existed in our chronic renal failure patients, because they did not live long enough to manifest it. Though the findings of this study they agree with that, going by the low incidence of ROD using clinical symptoms and radiological methods, it is possible that in the nearest future, ROD may become more prevalent in on society. This is because there is now an increase in the availability of dialysis in many centers across the Nation, with possibility that many CRF patients may live long enough to develop ROD. The findings of this study suggest that serum alkaline phosphatase assay, a surrogate of parathyroid hormone, may be a good guide to the presence of ROD in our CRF patients. Majority of patients had hypocalcaemia and hyperphosphataemia.

#### 4.9.2 Recommendations

It is hereby recommended that:

1. In all chronic renal failure patients, ROD should be anticipated. Serum calcium, phosphate, alkaline phosphatase should be done routinely.
2. Dietary restrictions of phosphate should be enforced in our chronic renal failure patient as well as the use of phosphate binders,
3. Calcium supplementation should be routinely part of the management of our chronic renal failure patients.
4. Control of hyperparathyroidism in our chronic renal failure patient will be an integral part of management of CRF patients.

#### 4.9.3 Limitation of the study

This study was faced with some limitations. It was not possible to carry out bone biopsies for live patients because of lack of consent from the patients. However, postmortem bone biopsy was carried out instead; it was also not possible to assay parathyroid hormone because of lack of facility for its assay. In its place, serum alkaline phosphatase was used as a surrogate. There is no doubt that alkaline phosphatase is influenced by several factors and so is non-specific. It was also not possible to measure serum and tissue aluminum in the study.

## 5. References


Adelejun T.A., Akinsola. Hypertension induced chronic renal failure: clinical features, management and prognosis. WAJM . 1988 17(2): 104-108.

Adetuyibi A, Akinsanya J.B, Onadeko BO. Analysis of the cause of death on the medical wards of the UCH, Ibadan over 14years period (1960-1973). Trans. Roy. Soc. Trop.Med. Hyp. 1976; 70: 466-73.

Akinsola, W, Odesanmi WO, Ogunniyi JO, Ladipo G.O.A. Diseases causing renal failure in Nigeria - a prospective study of 100 cases. Afr. J. med. Sc. 1989, 18: 131-5

Baker LRL. Renal Disease. In: Kumar P, Clark M(eds). Clinical medicine, 4th edn. W.B Saunders. Philadelphia. 1999: 572-573.

Brenner and Rector. The kidney vol.1, 6th edition 2000

Gold CH, Isaacson C, Levin J. The pathological bases of end stage renal disease in Blacks. South Africa Med. J. 1990; 19: 103-6.

Coen G, Ballantini P, Bonucci E. Bone Markers in the diagnosis of low turnover ostrodystrohy in haemodialysis patients. Nephrol Dial transplant. 1996, 11: A41.

Coen G, Ballanti P, Bonucci E, Calabria S, Centorrino M, Fassino V. Bone markers in the diagnosis of low turnover osteodystrophy in haemodialysis patients. Nephrol-Dial-transplant. 1998; 13(9): 2294-302.

Couttenye M M, D' Haese PC., Deng J T, High prevalence of a dynamic bone disease diagnosed European CAPD population. Nephrol. Dial. Transplant 1997; 12: 2144-2150.

Cottenye M.M. D'Haese P.C, Verschoren W J, Behets G.J, Schrooten I, De-Broe M.E. Low bone tunrnover in patients with renal failure. Kid. Int. 1999; 56 Suppl. 73: 70-6.

Duursma S,A, Vonkesteren R.G., Visser W J. serum alkaline phosphate: its relationship to bone cell and its Significance as an indicator for vit D treatment in Patients with renal insufficiency. In Norman WW, Schaefer K, Grigoleit HG (eds): vit D and problems related to uremic bone disease. Walter de Gruyter, Berlin 1975; 167.

Jarava C, Armas J R, Sagueria M, Palma A. Bone alkaline phosphatase isoenzyme in renal osteodystrophy. Nephrol dial transplant 1996: 11: 43-46.

Kadiri S, Arijie A. Temporal variations and meterological factors in hospital admission of chronic renal failure in South West Nigeria. West Africa J. Med. 1999, 18: 49-51.

Kadiri S. towards reducing the impact of chronic renal failure. Africa Health 2001; 23(2): 9-10.

Harowin P, lecomte - Houcke M, Flipo RM. Current aspects of osteoarticular pathology in patients undergoing haemodialysis. Study of 80 patients. Laboratory and pathologic analysis. Discussion of the pathogenic mechanism J. Rheumafol. 1987; 14: 748-9.

Hartmut M; Marie-Claude F. Renal bone diease: An unmet challenge for the nephrologist: Kidney Int. 1990; 38(2): 193-205.

Hodsons E M, Howman - Gilles RB, Evans RB, The diagnosis of renal oesteodystrophy; A comparison of technetium99. Pyrophosphate bone scintigraph with other techniques. Chine Nephrol 1981; 16:24-28.

Hruska K A, Teitelbaum SL, Kopelman R: The predictability of the histologic features of uremic bone disease by non-invasive techniques. Metab bone Dis Relat. Res 1978; 12: 393.

Mate-Kole M, Affram K, Lee SJ et al. Hypertension and end-Stage renal failure in tropical Africa. J. Hum. Hypertens. 1993; 7: 443-6.

Meema HE, Robinovich S, Meama S et al. Improved radiological diagnosis of azotemic osteodystrophy. Radiology. 1972; 102: 1-10.

Michael L J, Brenner BM, Bone, phosphate and calcium abnormalities in chronic renal failure: In 15th ed; Harrisons principles of internal medicine; E. Braunwald, A Facuci, D Kasper et al. Mc Graw Hill Medical Publishing Division, Jackson W Y, USA 1998: 1517.

Odenigbo C.U. The prevalence and radiological markers of ROD in patients with chronic renal failure in Enugu FMCP, National Postgraduate Medical College of Nigeria May 2003.

Ojogwu L.I. The Pathological Basis of end-stage renal disease in Nigerians: experience from Benin City. West Afr.J. Med.1990;9: 193-6.

Ojogwu L.I. The Clinical assessment of Heamodialysis Machine in the management of kidney failure. Nig. J.Biomedical Engineering 2001;(1):19-26.

Poznanki A K, Radiological Evaluation of bone mineral in children. In Favus M J (ed) primer on metab bone diseases and disorders of mineral metabolism. Raven press New-York 1993; 115.

Ritz E, Malluche H H, Bommer J: Metabolic bone disease in patients on haemodialysis. Nephron. 1974; 12:393.

Slatoposky EA, Weerts C, Lopez –Hilker S et al: Calcium Carbonate as a phosphate binder in patients with chronic renal failure undergoing dialysis. N Engl J med. 1986, 315: 157-161.

Sanchez OP. Prevention and treatment of renal osteodystrophy in children with chronic renal insufficiency and end stage renal diaseses; Semin Nepphrol 2001;21 (5): 441-50.

Shin SK, Kim Hs, et al. Renal osteodystrophy in predialysis patients: Ethic difference? Perit – Dial int. 1999; 19(suppl): S402-7.

Statland BE, Nishi HH, Young DS. Serum alkaline phosphatase: total activity and iso-enzyme determination made by use of the centrifugal fast analyzer. Clin chem. 1972; 18: 1488-74.

Urena P, De-Vernejoul MC. Circulating biochemical markers of bone remodeling in uremic patients. Kid.Int. 1991; 55(6): 2141-56

Mate-Kole M, Affram K, Lee SJ et al. Hypertension and end-Stage renal failure in tropical Africa. J. Hum. Hypertens. 1993; 7: 443-6.

Odenigbo C.U. The prevalence and radiological markers of ROD in patients with chronic renal failure in Enugu FMCP, National Postgraduate Medical College of Nigeria May 2003.

Ojogwu L.I. The Pathological Basis of end-stage renal disease in Nigerians: experience from Benin City. West Afr.J. Med.1990;9: 193-6.

Ojogwu L.I. The clinical assessment of heamodialysis machine in the management of kidney failure. Nig. J.Biomedical Engineering 2001;(1):19-26.

Sanchez OP. Prevention and treatment of renal osteodystrophy in children with chronic renal insufficiency and end stage renal diaseses; Semin Nepphrol 2001; 21 (5): 441-50.

# 5

# Relationships Among Renal Function, Bone Turnover and Periodontal Disease

Akihiro Yoshihara and Lisdrianto Hanindriyo
*Division of Preventive Dentistry,*
*Department of Oral Health Science,*
*Graduate School of Medical and Dental Sciences,*
*Niigata University,*
*Japan*

## 1. Introduction

Chronic renal failure (CRF) is defined as a progressive decline in renal function associated with a reduced glomerular filtration rate. The most common causes are diabetes mellitus, glomerulonephritis and chronic hypertension (Proctor et al., 2004).

The clinical signs and symptoms of renal failure are collectively termed 'uremia'. CRF affects most body systems, and the clinical features are dependent upon the stage of renal failure and the systems involved.

Oral manifestations of CRF and related therapies:

a. Gingival enlargement
Gingival enlargement secondary to drug therapy is the most commonly reported oral manifestation of renal disease. It can be induced by cyclosporine and/or calcium channel blockers (Somacarrera et al., 1994; Kennedy and Linden 2000).
b. Oral hygiene and periodontal disease
The oral hygiene of individuals receiving hemodialysis can be poor. Deposits of calculus may be increased (Epstein et al., 1980; Gavalda et al., 1999). There is no good evidence of an increased risk of periodontitis (Brown et al., 1989; Thorstensson et al., 1996; Naugle et al., 1998), although premature bone loss has been reported (Locsey et al., 1986). Localized suppurative osteomyelitis, secondary to periodontitis, was observed in individuals receiving hemodialysis (Tomaselli et al., 1993).
c. Xerostomia
Symptoms of xerostomia can arise in many individuals receiving hemodialysis (Kho et al., 1999; Klassen and Krasko, 2002). Possible causes include restricted fluid intake, side-effects of drug therapy and/or mouth breathing (Porter et al., 2004).
d. Oral malodor/bad taste/halitosis
Uremic patients may have an ammonia-like oral odor (Kho et al., 1999), which also occurs in about one third of individuals receiving hemodialysis. CRF can give rise to altered taste sensation, and some patients complain of an unpleasant and/or metallic taste or a sensation of an enlarged tongue (Kho et al., 1999).

e. Mucosal lesions
   A wide range of oral mucosal lesions, particularly white patches and/or ulceration, have been described in individuals receiving dialysis and allografts (Proctor et al., 2004).
f. Oral malignancy
   Kaposi's sarcoma (KS) can occur in the mouths of immunosuppresed renal transplant recipients (Farge, 1993). Any increased risk of oral malignancy in CRF probably reflects the effects of iatrogenic immunosupression, which increases the risk of virally-associated tumors, such as KS or non-Hodgkin's lymphoma (Proctor et al., 2004).
g. Oral infections
   *Candidosis*, angular cheilitis has been described in up to 4% of hemodialysis and renal allograft recipients (King et al., 1994; Klassen and Krasko, 2002). Other oral candidal lesions—such as pseudomembranous (1.9%), erythematous (3.8%), and chronic atrophic candidosis (3.8%)—have been reported in allograft recipients (King et al., 1994).
   *Viral infection*, prior to the availability of appropriate anti-viral drugs (*e.g.*, acyclovir, gancyclovir, and valacyclovir), about 50% of renal allograft recipients, who were seropositive for herpes simplex, experienced recurrent, severe, and prolonged HSV infections (Armstrong et al., 1976). However, in recent years, the use of effective anti-herpetic regimes has significantly reduced the frequency of such infection (Kletzmayr et al., 2000; Squifflet and Legendre 2002).
h. Dental anomalies
   Delayed eruption of permanent teeth has been reported in children with CRF (Wolff et al., 1985; Jaffe et al., 1990). Enamel hypoplasia of the primary and permanent teeth (Kho et al., 1999; Koch et al., 1999; Al Nowaiser et al., 2003) with or without brown discoloration can also occur (Wolff et al., 1985).
i. Bone lesions
   A wide range of bone anomalies can arise in CRF. These reflect a variety of defects of calcium metabolism including, loss of hydroxylation of 1-hydroxycholecalciferol to active vitamin D (1,25-dihydroxycholecalciferol), decreased hydrogen ion excretion (and resultant acidosis); hyperphosphatemia, hypocalcemia and resultant secondary hyperparathyroidism and interference with phosphate metabolism by dialysis (Nadimi et al., 1993).
   Orofacial features of renal osteodystrophy due to hyperparathyroidism include bone demineralization, decreased trabeculation, decreased thickness of cortical bone, ground-glass appearance of bone, metastatic soft-tissue calcifications, radiolucent fibrocystic lesions, radiolucent giant cell lesions, lytic areas of bone, jaw fracture (due to trauma or during surgery) and abnormal bone healing after extraction. Orofacial features of renal osteodystrophy related to tooth and periodontium include delayed eruption, enamel hypoplasia, loss of the lamina dura, widening of the periodontal ligament, severe periodontal destruction, tooth mobility, drifting, pulp calcification and pulp narrowing (Damm et al., 1997; Okada et al., 2000; Klassen and Krasko, 2002).

## 2. The relationships among osteoporosis, renal function and periodontal disease

Osteoporosis is the most common metabolic bone disease among the elderly, and the incidence of osteoporotic fractures obviously increases with age (Honig, 2010). In addition, elderly people often experience periodontal destruction. Because bone loss is a common feature of periodontitis and osteoporosis, both diseases may share some common etiologic factors (Offenbacher, 1996). The final expression of periodontitis is governed by complex interactions among host, microbial and environmental factors occurring within an intricate cellular mosaic (Offenbacher, 1996).

In addition, CRF is associated with marked disturbances of bone structure and metabolism, and there is a slowly progressive loss of renal function over months or years (Ruggeneti, 1998). A significant decrease in bone mineral density after transplantation is a serious finding (Huang & Sprague, 2009). It is well known that impaired renal function increases osteoclast activity leading to bone turnover, and this may influence bone metabolic parameters (Couttenye et al., 1999; Cirillo et al., 1998). There is a growing body of evidence indicating that impaired renal function is associated with disrupted regulation of vitamin D (Rix et al., 1999; Hamdy et al., 1995). Whereas some systemic factors that contribute to loss of bone mass and periodontal progression have been identified, we hypothesized that renal function is associated with bone metabolism, and thus is also associated with periodontal disease. To test this hypothesis, it is essential to evaluate the relationships among bone turnover, renal function and periodontal disease.

We initiated a longitudinal interdisciplinary study on aging (the Niigata Study) in 1998 to examine the many links between oral health and general health and well being. In the present report, we reviewed the relationship between bone metabolism and periodontal disease, taking renal function into consideration, in elderly Japanese subjects from the Niigata Study.

## 3. Principal findings from the Niigata Study

### 3.1 Outline of the Niigata Study

According to a registry of residents, questionnaires were sent to all 70-year-olds among the 4,542 inhabitants of Niigata City in Japan. Participants were informed of the purpose of the survey, and the overall response rate was 81.4%. After dividing the residents into groups of males and females, 600 individuals (the screened population) were randomly selected in order to have approximately the same number of male and female participants in the study. Follow-up surveys were carried out every year in June from1998 to 2008 (11 times in 10 years), using the same methods that were used at baseline. All subjects were Japanese and did not require special care for their daily activities. Since age influences bone metabolism, renal function and periodontal disease, subjects were restricted to 70 years old at baseline (Ando et al., 2000).

### 3.2 Osteoporosis and periodontal disease

In addition to a strict age requirement, other study inclusion criteria included the following: blood sugar < 140 mg/dL with no history of diabetes, more than 20 teeth remaining, non-smokers, and no history of medication use for osteoporosis. There were 184 subjects among the screened population that met all the inclusion criteria.

We utilized data on bone mineral density (BMD) of the heel, which we measured using an ultrasound bone densitometer (Fig. 1, Achilles Bone Densitometer™, Luner Corporation,

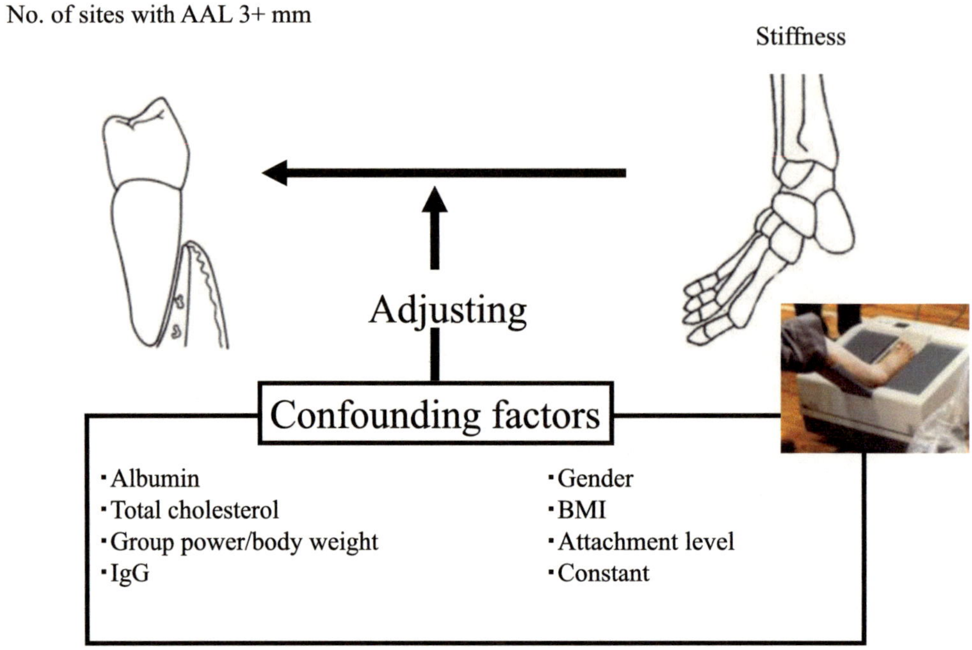


Fig. 1. Outline of the analysis between Osteoporosis and periodontal progression.
AAL: Additional attachment loss.

USA) (Lunar Corporation, 1991). Ultrasound densitometry enables the measurement of the physical properties of bone, specifically BMD. The ultrasound measurement contains two criteria, the velocity (speed of sound, SOS) and frequency attenuation (broadband ultrasound attenuation, BUA) of a sound wave as it travels through a bone. Stiffness is a clinical index combining SOS and BUA, and is calculated by the following formula: $(BUA - 50) \times 0.67 + (SOS - 1380) \times 0.28$.

Stiffness is indicated in the bone densitometer monitoring device as the percentage of the value for a normal younger population. Osteopenia was defined as a stiffness that was $\leq$ 85% for males and $\leq$ 69% for females. Follow-up clinical surveys were done by measuring the clinical attachment level after 3 years. Clinical attachment level is the amount of space between attached periodontal tissues and a fixed point, usually the cementoenamel junction. A measurement used to assess the stability of attachment as part of a periodontal maintenance program (Fig. 2). There were 179 subjects included in the final analysis, and all of these subjects participated in both the baseline and the follow-up examinations.

We measured the number of progressive sites that had $\geq$ 3 mm of additional attachment loss over 3 years (Fig. 2). After dividing the subjects into an osteopenia group (OG) and a no-osteopenia group (NOG), we evaluated the number of progressive sites that had $\geq$ 3 mm of additional attachment loss over 3 years by two-way analysis of variance (ANOVA).

The respective mean number of progressive sites for the OG and NOG were $4.7\pm5.5$ and $3.3\pm3.0$ in females, and $6.9\pm9.4$ and $3.4\pm2.8$ in males. The difference in the mean number of progressive sites between the OG and NOG was statistically significant by ANOVA after controlling for gender (Fig. 3, $p = 0.043$) (Yoshihara et al., 2004).

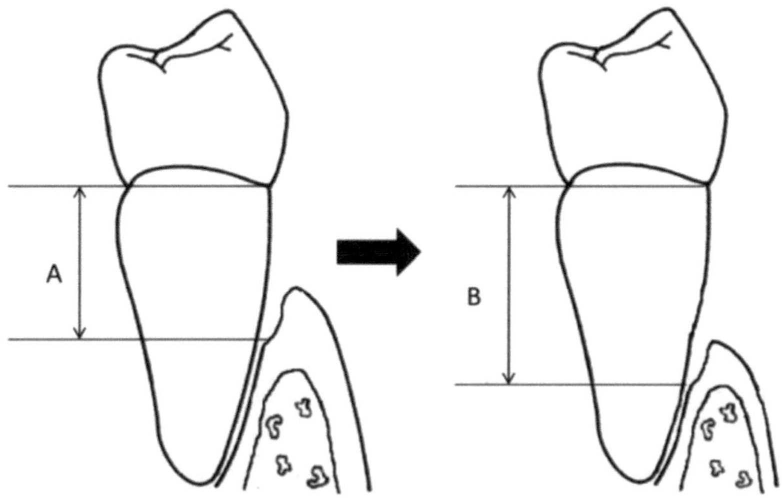


Fig. 2. Clinical attachment level and periodontal disease progression.
A, B = Clinical attachment level
B-A = Additional attachment loss

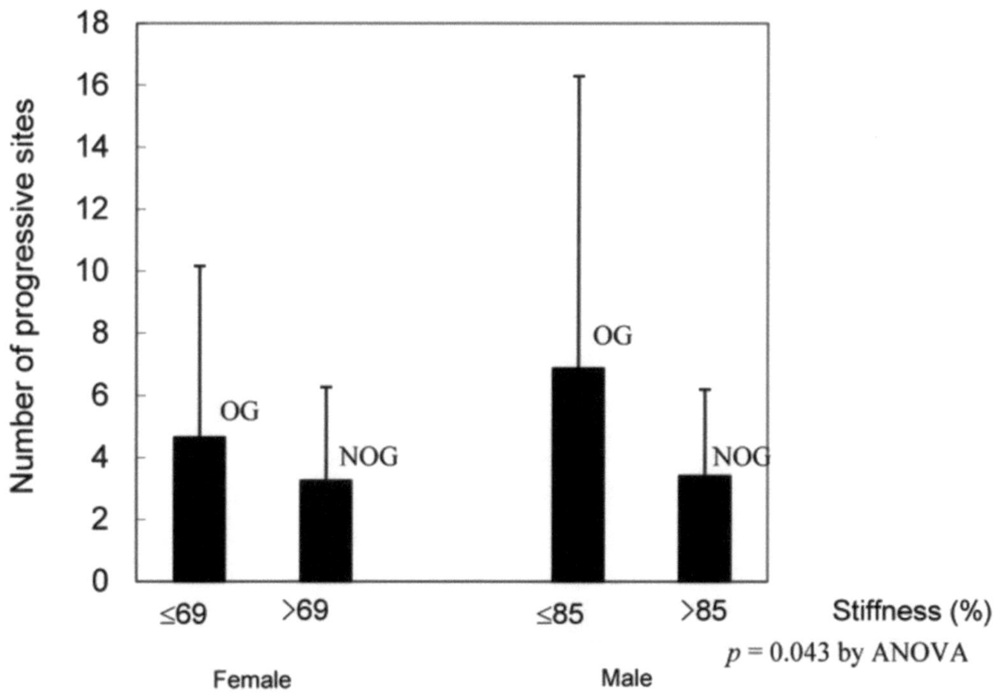


Fig. 3. Relationship between number of progressive sites with ≥3mm additional attachment loss and stiffness by gender.
The number of subjects: stiffness ≤69 (n=74) and >69 (n=19) for female, ≤85 (n=65) and >85 (n=22) for male.
OG: Osteopenia group, NOG: No-osteopenia group.

### 3.3 Bone metabolism and periodontal disease

A total of 398 subjects who turned 70 in 1998 had annual dental examinations. We selected 148 of these 398 subjects (79 males and 69 females) for participation in the study because they had one or more teeth, were not taking any medicine or supplements for bone disorders (tamoxifen, anabolic steroids, bisphosphonate, or estrogen), and did not have a diagnosis of fracture based on an X-ray assessment by a physician. The subject's blood was taken in the morning of the dental examination. Urine was collected over 24 hours (07:00 to 07:00 AM the day after the dental examination). During the day that urine was collected, usual food and fluid intake were ingested. Biochemical parameters of bone turnover were measured, including urinary deoxypyridinoline (U-DPD) (nM/nM*Cr) as a bone resorption marker, and serum osteocalcine (S-OC) (ng/mL) and serum bone alkaline phosphatase (S-BAP) (U/L) as bone formation markers. U-DPD data were corrected by the urinary creatinine concentration measured by a standard colorimetric method.

We categorized subjects by tertiles according to the percentage of sites with ≥6 mm clinical attachment level (6+ mm CAL). S-OC, S-BAP, and U-DPD were evaluated by analysis of covariance (ANCOVA) adjusted for smoking habit (0: none, 1: past or current). Differences in the distribution of bone turnover markers according to the percentage of sites with 6+ mm CAL per person are shown in Table 1. S-OC was significantly lower in the third tertile than in the first and second tertiles after adjusting for smoking habit (males: $p = 0.007$, females: $p = 0.042$, ANCOVA) (Yoshihara et al., 2009).

| | % of sites with 6mm attachment level | | | | | | | |
|---|---|---|---|---|---|---|---|---|
| | Males | | | | Females | | | |
| | 1st | 2nd | 3rd | *p* value* | 1st | 2nd | 3rd | *p* value* |
| Serum osteocalcin (ng/ml) | 8.5 ± 4.5 | 6.8 ± 2.7 | 5.7 ± 1.8 | 0.007 | 9.9 ±2.8 | 9.3 ± 2.4 | 9.1 ± 3.5 | 0.042 |
| Serum bone alkaline phosphatase (U/L) | 22.2 ± 5.9 | 23.3 ± 7.4 | 21.1 ± 6.2 | 0.212 | 29.3 ± 10.8 | 28.9 ± 8.1 | 27.4 ± 11.2 | 0.752 |
| Urinary deoxypyridinoline (nM/nM*Cr) | 4.8 ± 1.0 | 4.4 ± 1.2 | 4.0 ± 1.0 | 0.055 | 6.6 ± 1.4 | 6.8 ± 1.4 | 6.3 ± 1.7 | 0.664 |

* ANOCOVA adjusted for smoking habits.

Table 1. Relationship between % of sites with ≥ 6mm attachment level and bone metabolism markers controlling for confounding factors by multiple regression analysis.

### 3.4 Renal function and periodontal disease

We randomly selected 145 subjects among 398 healthy elderly subjects. All subjects were aged 77 years at the time of the renal function study in 2005. We evaluated the relationship between bone turnover markers and periodontal disease, taking renal function into consideration. Correlations among renal function and bone metabolism markers for periodontal disease, including the number of remaining teeth and smoking habit, were evaluated using multiple regression analysis.

To evaluate the relationship between periodontal disease and renal function markers (volume of urine per 24 hours [mL/day], creatinine clearance per 24 hours [L/day]) or bone metabolism markers (U-DPD [nM/nM*Cr] and S-OC [ng/mL]), multiple linear regression analysis was performed. For the final model, the confounding independent variables that had *p*-values less than 0.05 according to the statistical association with the percentage of sites with 6+ mm CAL by Pearson correlation coefficients, ANOVA, or chi-square test, were selected. Results of multiple linear regression analysis between the percentage of sites with 6+ mm CAL and renal function markers after controlling for confounding factors are shown in Table 2. Creatinine clearance for 24 hours was positively associated with the percentage of sites with 6+mm CAL (sta. coef. = 0.26, $p$ = 0.015). Furthermore, S-OC showed a negatively independent association with the percentage of sites with 6+vmm CAL after adjustment for the confounding factors (sta. coef. = -0.27, $p$ = 0.006, Table 3) (Yoshihara et al, 2007).

| | Dependent variable<br>% of sites with ≥6mm attachment level | |
|---|---|---|
| Independent variables | Sta. Coef (β).* | *p* value |
| Number of remaining teeth | -0.46 | <0.001 |
| Creatinine clearance for 24 h (L/day)† | 0.26 | 0.015 |
| Volume of urine for 24 h (ml/day) | 0.01 | 0.956 |
| Smoking habit | 0.08 | 0.500 |
| Gender | -0.17 | 0.121 |
| Use of interdental brushes or dental floss | -0.01 | 0.893 |
| Constant | | 0.074 |

†Creatinine (g/day) in urine per 24h/creatinine (g/L) in serum.
* Standardized coefficient.

Table 2. Relationship between % of sites with ≥6mm attachment level and renal function markers controlling for confounding factors by multiple regression analysis.

| | Dependent variable<br>% of sites with ≥6mm attachment level | |
|---|---|---|
| Independent variables | Sta. Coef (β).* | *p* value |
| Number of remaining teeth | -0.47 | <0.001 |
| Serum osteocalcin (ng/ml) | -0.27 | 0.006 |
| Urinary deoxypyridinoline (nM/nM*Cr) | -0.04 | 0.688 |
| Smoking habit | -0.10 | 0.406 |
| Gender | 0.10 | 0.481 |
| Use of interdental brushes or dental floss | -0.01 | 0.861 |
| Constant | | <0.001 |

* Standardized coefficient.

Table 3. Relationship between % of sites with ≥ 6mm attachment level and bone metabolism markers controlling for confounding factors by multiple regression analysis.

The results showed that the subjects in the OG had a higher number of progressive sites for additional attachment loss than the subjects in the NOG. This three-year longitudinal study clearly demonstrated that BMD is a risk factor for periodontal disease progression in an elderly population. In addition, according to our findings on linkage with BMD, there are some systemic factors that contribute to both loss of bone mass and periodontal disease progression (Kshirsagar, 2005). Systemic factors of bone remodeling may also modify the local tissue response to periodontal disease. The BMD of the mandible is affected by the mineral status of the skeleton and also by diseases that cause generalized bone loss (Davidovich, 2005). The mouth and face are highly accessible parts of the body, and reflect changes that occur internally. For the clinician, the mouth and face provide physical signs and symptoms of local and generalized disease. During routine oral examinations, periodontal disease including maxillary/mandibular general bone loss may be diagnostic of early osteoporotic changes in the skeleton. Some systemic factors of bone remodeling also modify the local tissue response to periodontal disease.

Osteoporosis and low renal function contribute to loss of bone mass. We were able to identify a weak but clear relationship between CAL and S-OC. There was a significant association between CAL and 24-hour creatinine clearance, which is a renal function marker. These findings suggest that S-OC is a valid marker of bone turnover when evaluating periodontal disease. It has been assumed that S-OC is associated with not only bone turnover but also low renal function. Periodontal conditions, including bone metabolism, may be affected by low renal function. The systemic bone metabolism, which might be affected by low renal function, is associated with periodontal disease.

## 4. Association between chronic renal failure and periodontal disease

Based on several studies, CRF and periodontal disease can have reciprocal effects (Fig. 3). CRF and renal therapy can greatly influence the dental management of renal patient. Moreover, chronic adult periodontitis can contribute to the overall systematic inflammatory burden and may therefore influence the management of the end-stage renal disease (ESRD) patient on hemodialysis maintenance therapy (Craig, 2008).

### 4.1 Possible association of chronic renal failure with periodontal disease

CRF can cause several changes that influence oral conditions such as decreased salivary flow rate, increase salivary urea level and calculus accumulation (Torres et al., 2010). CRF may have an effect on the periodontal status of an individual through several possible mechanisms.

a. A major clinical consequence of CRF is uremic syndrome (uremia). This condition leads to an immune dysfunction possibly caused by defects in lymphocyte and monocyte function, which in turn may increase the rate of gingival inflammation (Craig, 2008).
b. Several studies have found an increasing level of plaque formation, calculus, gingival inflammation and also decreasing saliva excretion, which can be considered together as reduced oral hygiene (Yoshihara et al., 2007). The intense psychological and time demands that are associated with hemodialysis in patients with ESRD may account for reduced oral hygiene (Craig, 2008).

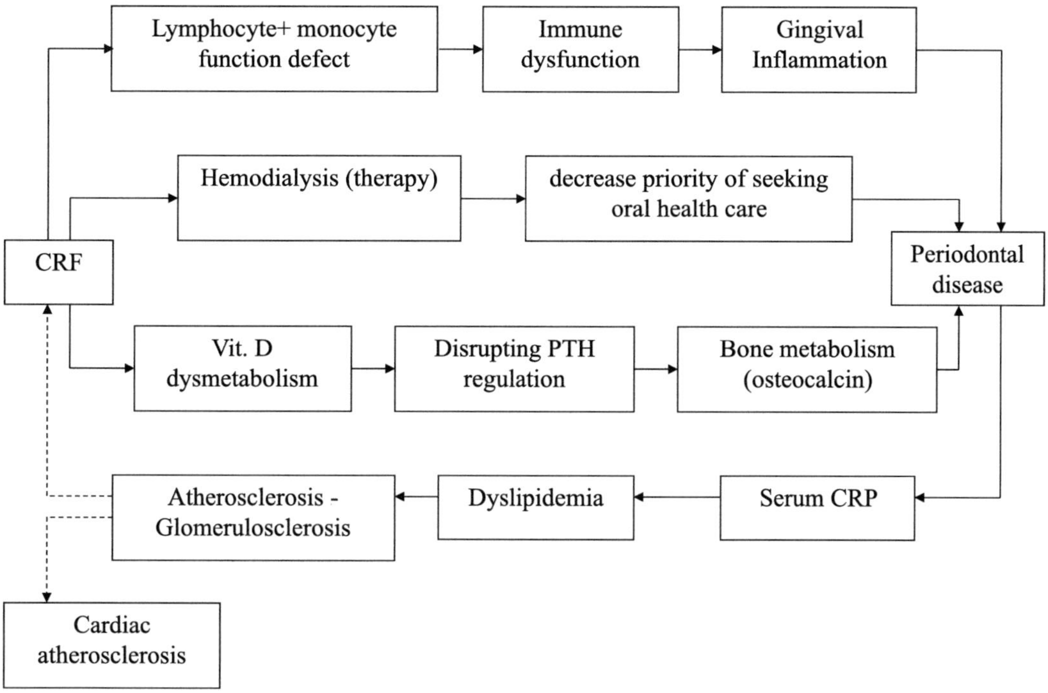


Fig. 4. The mechanism between low renal function and periodontal disease.

c. CRF has an important effect on vitamin D metabolism (Yoshihara et al., 2007). Since vitamin D is metabolized in the liver and kidney, the presence of CRF will automatically disturb vitamin D metabolism. Vitamin D is metabolized by kidney to its active metabolite, 1,25-dihydroxyvitamin D3. This substance subsequently interacts with vitamin D nuclear receptor in the intestine, bone and kidney. The functions of this substance are to regulate bone metabolism, immune response and also cell proliferation and differentiation. Regarding bone metabolism, vitamin D controls the availability of calcium phosphate by regulating the excretions of hormones such as the parathyroid hormone (PTH) (Souza et al., 2007). CRF may disrupt the regulation of PTH which may leads to hyperparathyroidism condition and increased rate of bone disease (Yoshihara et al., 2007). Vitamin D also contributes in the synthesis of bone matrix proteins such as type-I collagen, alkaline phosphatase, osteocalcin and osteopontin (Souza et al., 2007). Osteocalcin may exist in the circulating blood and undergo local accumulation in some parts of the body. Osteocalcin has been postulated to have a role in both bone resorption and mineralization and is currently considered the most specific marker of osteoblast function. The serum level of this protein is considered to be a marker of bone formation. Serum osteocalcin is presently considered a valid marker of bone turnover when resorption and formation are coupled and a specific marker of bone formation when formation and resorption are uncoupled (Bullon et al., 2005). Osteocalcin has also been found in the gingival crevicular fluid (GCF). Several studies found an increased level of serum osteocalcin in subjects with CRF. Moreover, the level of GCF osteocalcin was found to be significantly associated with periodontal disease, since there was an association with pocket depth, clinical attachment level and bleeding on probing (Bullon et al., 2005). Therefore, it might be reasonable to explain an effect of CRF on periodontal disease by its effect on bone metabolism (especially alveolar bone) which is specifically marked by the level of serum osteocalcin and/or GCF osteocalcin.

### 4.2 Possible association of periodontal disease with chronic renal failure

Periodontal disease may have an effect on CRF and also the treatment of CRF. Periodontal disease may have an effect on CRF through several possible mechanisms.

a. Moderate to severe periodontal disease may increase the serum level of C-reactive protein (CRP). CRP is an acute phase protein and systemic marker of inflammation which is also a major risk predictor for cardiac disorder and all other mortality cause of CRF persons (Craig, 2008). Several studies have reported periodontal disease to be associated with elevated CRP as well as other serum components of the acute phase response including decreased high density lipoprotein cholesterol, low density lipoprotein cholesterol, blood glucose and decreased peripheral blood neutrophil function and count (Muntner et al., 2000). Since all these factors are also risk factors for CRF, it might be justifiable to assume that periodontal disease may be considered as a predisposing factor and/or marker of CRF. Moreover, periodontal disease in a person with CRF has a strong tendency to increase the possibility of the complication of coronary atherosclerosis.
b. Several reports found that periodontitis may also contribute to the systemic inflammatory burden in ESRD. The level of IgG antibody particularly to *Porphyromonas gingivalis* correlated with elevated serum CRP (Muntner et al., 2000). Therefore, it is also important to consider an effective periodontal therapy in order to reduce the level of serum CRP which might eventually decrease the inflammatory burden of ESRD or CRF.

On the other hand, there are also some studies which failed to find the type of correlations mentioned above (Kitsou et al., 2000; Marakoglu et al., 2003; Duran et al., 2004; Bots et al., 2006). It is acknowledged that differences in research design, measurement methods instruments used, and other factors may have resulted in different findings. Therefore, it is still relevant and reasonable to execute further research using a more sophisticated and well-designed method to elucidate the relationship between CRF and periodontal disease.

## 5. References

Al Nowaiser A.; Roberts GJ.; Trompeter RS.; Wilson M.; Lucas VS. (2003). Oral health in children with chronic renal failure. *Pediatr Nephrol*, 18, pp. 39-45.

Ando, Y.; Yoshihara, A.; Seida, Y; et al. (2000). The study of sampling bias in an oral health survey of elderly. Comparison of oral and general health condition between respondents and non-respondents to a questionnaire and between participants and non-participants in an examination. *J Dent Hlth,* 50, pp. 322-333.

Armstrong JA.; Evans AS.; Rao N.; Ho M. (1976). Viral infections in renal transplant recipients. *Infect Immun,* 14, pp. 970-975.

Bots CP.; Poorterman JH.; Brand HS.; et al. (2006). The oral health status of dentate patients with chronic renal failure undergoing dialysis therapy. *Oral Dis,* 12, pp. 176-180.

Brown LJ.; Oliver RC.; Löe H. (1989). Periodontal diseases in the US in 1981: prevalence, severity, extent and role in tooth mortality. *J Periodontol,* 60, pp. 353-370.

Bullon, P.; Goberna, B.; Guerrero, J; et al. (2005). Serum, saliva, and gingival crevicular fluid osteocalcin: their relation to periodontal status and bone mineral density in postmenopausal women. *J Periodontol,* 76(4), pp. 513-519.

Cirillo, M.; Senigalliesi, L.; Laurenzi, M; et al. (1998). Microalbuminuria in nondiabetic adults: relation of blood pressure, body mass index, plasma cholesterol levels, and smoking: The Gubbio Population Study. *Arch Intern Med,* 158, pp. 1933-1939.

Couttenye, MM.; D'Haese, PC.; Verschoren, WJ; et al. (1999). Low bone turnover in patients with renal failure. *Kidney Int Suppl,* 73, pp. S70-S76.

Craig, RG. (2008). Interactions between chronic renal disease and periodontal disease. *Oral Dis,* 14, pp. 1-7.

Damm DD.; Neville BW.; McKenna S.; Jones AC.; Freedman PD.; Anderson WR.; et al. (1997). Macrognathia of renal osteodystrophy in dialysis patients. *Oral Surg Oral Med Oral Pathol,* 83, pp. 489-495.

Davidovich, E.; Schwarz, Z.; Davidovitch, M; et al. (2005). Oral findings and periodontal status in children, adolescents and young adults suffering from renal failure. *J Clin Periodontol,* 32, pp. 1076-1082.

Duran I. & Erdemir EO. (2004) Periodontal treatment needs of patients with renal disease receiving haemodialysis. *Int Dent J,* 54, pp. 274-278.

Epstein SR.; Mandell L.; Scopp IW. (1980). Salivary composition and calculus formation in patients undergoing hemodialysis. *J Periodontol,* 51, pp. 336-338.

Farge D. (1993). Kaposi's sarcoma in organ transplant recipients. *Eur J Med,* 2, pp. 339-343.

Gavalda C.; Bagan JV.; Scully C.; Silvestre F.; Milian M.; Jimenez V. (1999). Renal haemodialysis patients: oral, salivary, dental and periodontal findings in 105 adult cases. *Oral Dis,* 5, pp. 299-302.

Hamdy, NA.; Kanis, JA.; Beneton, MN; et al. (1995). Effect of alfacalcidol on natural course of renal bone disease in mild to moderate renal failure. *BMJ,* 310, pp. 358-363.

Honig, S. (2010). Osteoporosis - new treatments and updates. *Bulletin of the NYU Hospital for Joint Diseases,* 68, pp. 166-170.

Huang, M. & Sprague, SM. (2009). Bone disease in kidney transplant patients. *Semin Nephrol,* 29, pp. 166-173.

Jaffe EC.; Roberts J.; Chantler C.; Carter JE. (1990). Dental maturity in children with chronic renal failure assessed from dental panoramic tomographs. *J Int Assoc Dent Child*, 20, pp. 54-58.

Kao CH.; Hsieh JF.; Tsai SC.; Ho YJ.; Chang HR. (2000). Decreased salivary function in patients with end-stage renal disease requiring haemodialysis. *Am J Kidney Dis*, 36, pp. 1110-1114.

Kennedy DS. & Linden GJ. (2000). Resolution of gingival overgrowth following change from ciclosporin to tacrolimus therapy in a renal transplant patient. *J Ir Dent Assoc*, 46, pp. 3-4.

Kho H.; Lee S.; Chung SC.; Kim YK. (1999). Oral manifestations and salivary flow rate, pH, and buffer capacity in patients with end-stage renal disease undergoing haemodialysis. *Oral Surg Oral Med Oral Pathol*, 88, pp. 316-319.

King GN.; Healy CM.; Glover MT.; Kwan JT.; Williams DM.; Leigh IM.; et al. (1994). Prevalence and risk factors associated with leukoplakia, hairy leukoplakia, erythematous candidosis, and gingival hyperplasia in renal transplant recipients. *Oral Surg Oral Med Oral Pathol*, 78, pp. 718-726.

Kitsou VK.; Konstantinidis A.; Siamopoulos KC. (2000). Chronic renal failure and periodontal disease. *Ren Fail*, 22, pp. 307-318.

Klassen JT. & Krasko BM. (2002). The dental health status of dialysis patients. *J Can Dent Assoc*, 68, pp. 34-38.

Kletzmayr J.; Kreuzwieser E.; Watkins-Riedel T.; Berlakovich G.; Kovarik J.; Klauser R. (2000). Long-term oral ganciclovir prophylaxis for prevention of cytomegalovirus infection and disease in cytomegalovirus high-risk renal transplant recipients. *Transplantation*, 70, pp. 1174-1180.

Koch MJ.; Buhrer R.; Pioch T.; Scharer K. (1999). Enamel hypoplasia of primary teeth in chronic renal failure. *Pediatr Nephrol*, 13, pp. 68-72.

Kshirsagar, AV.; Moss, KL.; Elter, JR; et al. (2005). Periodontal disease is associated with renal insufficiency in the Atherosclerosis Risk In Communities (ARIC) study. *Am J Kidney Dis*, 45, pp. 650-657.

Locsey L.; Alberth M.; Mauks G. (1986). Dental management of chronic haemodialysis patients. *Int Urol Nephrol*, 18, pp. 211-213.

Lunar Corporation. Theory of ultrasound densitometry. In: Lunar Corporation, editors. Manual of Achilles ultrasound bone densitometer, B1–B7. Madison, Wis.: Lunar Corporation, 1991.

Marakoglu I.; Gursoy UK.; Demirer S.; Sezer H. (2003). Periodontal status of chronic renal failure patients receiving hemodialysis. *Yonsei Med J*, 44, pp. 648-652.

Muntner, P.; Coresh, J.; Smith, C; et al. (2000). Plasma lipids and risk of developing renal dysfunction: The Atherosclerosis Risk in Communities Study. *Kidney Int*, 58, pp. 293-301.

Nadimi H.; Bergamini J.; Lilien B. (1993). Uremic mixed bone disease. A case report. *Int J Maxillofac Surg*, 22, pp. 268-270.

Naugle K.; Darby ML.; Bauman DB.; Lineberger LT.; Powers R. (1998). The oral health status of individuals on renal dialysis. *Ann Periodontol*, 3, pp. 197-205.

Offenbacher, S. (1996). Periodontal diseases: pathogenesis. *Ann Periodontol*, 1, pp. 821-828.

Okada H.; Davies JE.; Yamamoto H. (2000). Brown tumour of the maxilla in a patient with secondary hyperparathyroidism: a case study involving immunohistochemistry and electron microscopy. *J Oral Maxillofac Surg*, 58, pp. 233-238.

Porter SR.; Hegarty A.; Scully C. (2004). An update of the etiology and management of xerostomia. *Oral Surg Oral Med Oral Pathol Oral Radiol Endod*, 97, pp. 28-46.

Proctor, R.; Kumar, N.; Stein, A; et al. (2005). Oral and Dental Aspects of Chronic Renal Failure. *J Dent Res*, 84, pp. 199-208.

Rix, M.; Andreassen, H.; Eskildsen, P; et al. (1999). Bone mineral density and biochemical markers of bone turnover in patients with predialysis chronic renal failure. *Kidney Int*, 56, pp. 1084-1093.

Ruggeneti, P.; Perna, A.; Gherardi, G; et al. (1998). Renal function and requirement for dialysis in chronic nephropathy patients on long-term ramipril: REIN follow-up trial. Gruppo Italiano di Studi Epidemiologici in Nefrologia (GISEN). Ramipril Efficacy in Nephropathy. *Lancet*, 352, pp. 1252-1256.

Scannapieco, FA. & Panesar, M. (2008). Periodontitis and chronic kidney disease. *J Periodontol*, 79, pp. 1617-1619.

Somacarrera ML.; Hernandez G.; Acero J.; Moskow BS. (1994). Factors related to the incidence and severity of ciclosporin-induced gingival overgrowth in transplant patients. A longitudinal study. *J Periodontol*, 65, pp. 671-675.

Souza, CM.; Braosi, APR.; Luczyszyn, SM; et al. (2007). Association between vitamin D receptor gene polimorphisms and susceptibility to chronic kidney disease and periodontitis. *Blood Purif*, 25, pp. 411-419.

Squifflet JP. & Legendre C. (2002). The economic value of valacyclovir prophylaxis in transplantation. *J Infect Dis*, 186(Suppl 1), pp. S116-S122.

Thorstensson H.; Kuylenstierna J.; Hugoson A. (1996). Medical status and complications in relation to periodontal disease experience in insulindependent diabetics. *J Clin Periodontol*, 23, pp. 194-202.

Tomaselli DL Jr.; Feldman RS.; Krochtengel AL.; Fernandez P. (1993). Osteomyelitis associated with chronic periodontitis in a patient with end-stage renal disease: a case report. *Periodontal Clin Investig*, 15, pp. 8-12.

Torres, SA.; Rosa, OP.; Hayacibara, MF; et al. (2010). Periodontal parameters and BANA test in patients with chronic renal failure undergoing hemodialysis. *J Appl Oral Sci*, 18, pp. 297-302.

Wolff A.; Stark H.; Sarnat H.; Binderman I.; Eisenstein B.; Drukker A. (1985). The dental status of children with chronic renal failure. *Int J Pediatr Nephrol*, 6, pp. 127-132

Yoshihara, A.; Deguchi, T.; Hanada, N; et al. (2007). Renal function and periodontal disease in elderly Japanese. *J Periodontol*, 78, pp. 1241-1248.

Yoshihara, A.; Deguchi, T.; Hanada, N; et al. (2009). Relation of bone turnover markers to periodontal disease and jaw bone morphology in elderly Japanese subjects. *Oral Dis*, 15, pp. 176-181.

Yoshihara, A.; Seida, Y.; Hanada, N; et al. (2004). A longitudinal study of the relationship between periodontal disease and bone mineral density in community-dwelling older adults. *J Clin Periodontol*, 31, pp. 680-684.

# 6

# Sarcoidosis and Kidney Disease

Tulsi Mehta, Anirban Ganguli and Mehrnaz Haji-Momenian
*Department of Medicine, Washington Hospital Center,*
*Washington DC,*
*USA*

## 1. Introduction

Sarcoidosis is an illness of granulomatous inflammation with multi-organ association. While most individuals exhibit pulmonary pathology, renal involvement is not without prevalence or significance. This chapter will review the current epidemiology of the disease and explore the two major pathways in the pathogenesis of renal sarcoidosis, mainly granulomatous deposition and deranged calcium management. With these concepts addressed, further inquiries into intrinsic renal disease will be provided along with explanations of renovascular complications, obstructive nephropathy, and transplant pathology. Each ailment will be accompanied by common presentation, more detailed pathophysiology, appropriate diagnostics, and current treatment recommendations. This chapter will seek to purvey a comprehensive but concise exploration of renal sarcoidosis.

## 2. Epidemiology & susceptibility

Sarcoidosis can affect a wide range of racial and ethnic groups but it has high prevalence in northern European countries, Japan, and the United States[1]. Certain countries have skewed incidences, for example: black Americans are three times more likely than white Americans to develop the disease (Iannuzzi et al. 2007). However, across the racial and ethnic groups, females are more prone to the illness than males (Iannuzzi et al. 2007). The disease manifests itself typically in patients less than 50 years of age and mainly in the third of fourth decade of life (Iannuzzi et al. 2011). A patient with a first degree relative with the disease has a five-fold increase of developing sarcoidosis. Nevertheless, this risk still does not exceed 1% (Iannuzzi et al. 2011). Patient susceptibility also increases with certain associations of genetics and environmental factors. Discoveries into HLA gene products and the butyrophilin-like2 (BTNL2) gene are the latest areas of genetic interests (Iannuzzi et al. 2007). A variety of environmental triggers including wood-burning stoves, tree pollen, inorganic particles, insecticides, and mold have also been scrutinized in addition to mycobacteria and propionibacteria antigens (Iannuzzi et al. 2007, 2011)· In fact, combinations of genetic and environmental activators have also been examined, for example: HLA-DQB1 and water damage or high humanity in the workplace (Iannuzzi et al. 2007). However, it seems that a ubiquitous number of agents may initiate a similar immunologic pathway that is pathognomonic for sarcoidosis.

## 3. Manifestations & pathogenesis

Sarcoidosis mainly affects the pulmonary system, with an over 90% occurrence rate in the afflicted, presenting as mostly hilar lymphadenopathy but also including pulmonary hyperternsion and obstructive and restrictive airway disease (Iannuzzi et al. 2011). Other major organ systems disturbed include the skin, the eye, the heart, and the nervous system with approximately 25 to 30% involvement (Iannuzzi et al 2011). Renal sarcoidosis is in fact rare with exact number relating prevalence difficult to come by. Unfortunately, the etiology for nephron-related disease is quite vast and it has been hard to delineate pure renal manifestations from simple metabolic disturbances (Berliner et al 2006). In order to understand the extent and pathogenesis of renal involvement, two central pathways for nephron insult has been validated including granulomatous deposition and deranged calcium management. While these pathways are by no means the only two routes of renal involvement, they are the most significant and the overriding themes for renal insult.

### 3.1 Granuloma formation

Many aspects of this process still require elucidation yet strong evidence reveals that granuloma formation centers on T cells reacting with unclear triggers and certain gene products to illicit cascades that either lead to complete resolution of inflammation or to irreversible fibrosis (Iannuzzi et al. 2007). Specifically, antigen presenting cells including macrophages with susceptible HLA or BTNL2 gene products present triggers including organic, inorganic, and infectious agents to the CD4 T cell. Once initiated, numerous peripheral cytokines, interleukins, and immune modulators steer T cells into a T Helper 1 or T Helper 2 response; where with the former, resolution of inflammation is more probable but with the later, fibrosis and irreversible damage is more probable (Iannuzzi et al. 2007, 2011). This deposition of macrophages, giant cells, and T helper cells form the pathognomonic, non-caseating granulomas that defines sarcoidosis (Casella and Allon 1983) See Figure 1. In renal disease, these granulomas are primarily in the cortex but may also be found in the medulla or capsule (Casella and Allon 1983). This process is the basis for granulomatous interstitial nephritis, which will be further discussed subsequently.

### 3.2 Deranged calcium management

Despite the granulomatous inflammation that marks sarcoidosis, deranged calcium homeostasis has a greater effect on the kidneys than the invasive granulomas themselves. Activated pulmonary macrophages express 1-α hydroxylase, which has important implications in maintaining appropriate levels of calcium in the body. In normal physiology, calcium balance is attained through the intricate interactions of parathyroid hormone (PTH), calcium, phosphorus, and Vitamin D. PTH upregulates renal 1-α hydroxylase, a cytochrome P450 enzyme located in the proximal tubule, to metabolize 25-hydroxy vitamin D to 1, 25-dihydroxy vitamin D, the bioactive form of Vitamin D, also known as calcitriol. Calcitriol, in turn, promotes calcium absorption in the intestines, kidneys, and bones. When calcium levels are adequate, normal physiological negative feedback mechanisms halt the PTH and calcitriol cycle. However, in sarcoidosis, extra-renal production of 1-α hydroxylase inappropriately increases calcitriol levels thereby increasing serum calcium and decreasing PTH. Unlike its renal equivalent, the granulomatous 1-α hydroxylase is immuned from the normal negative feedback mechanisms of hypercalcemia and is therefore unregulated,

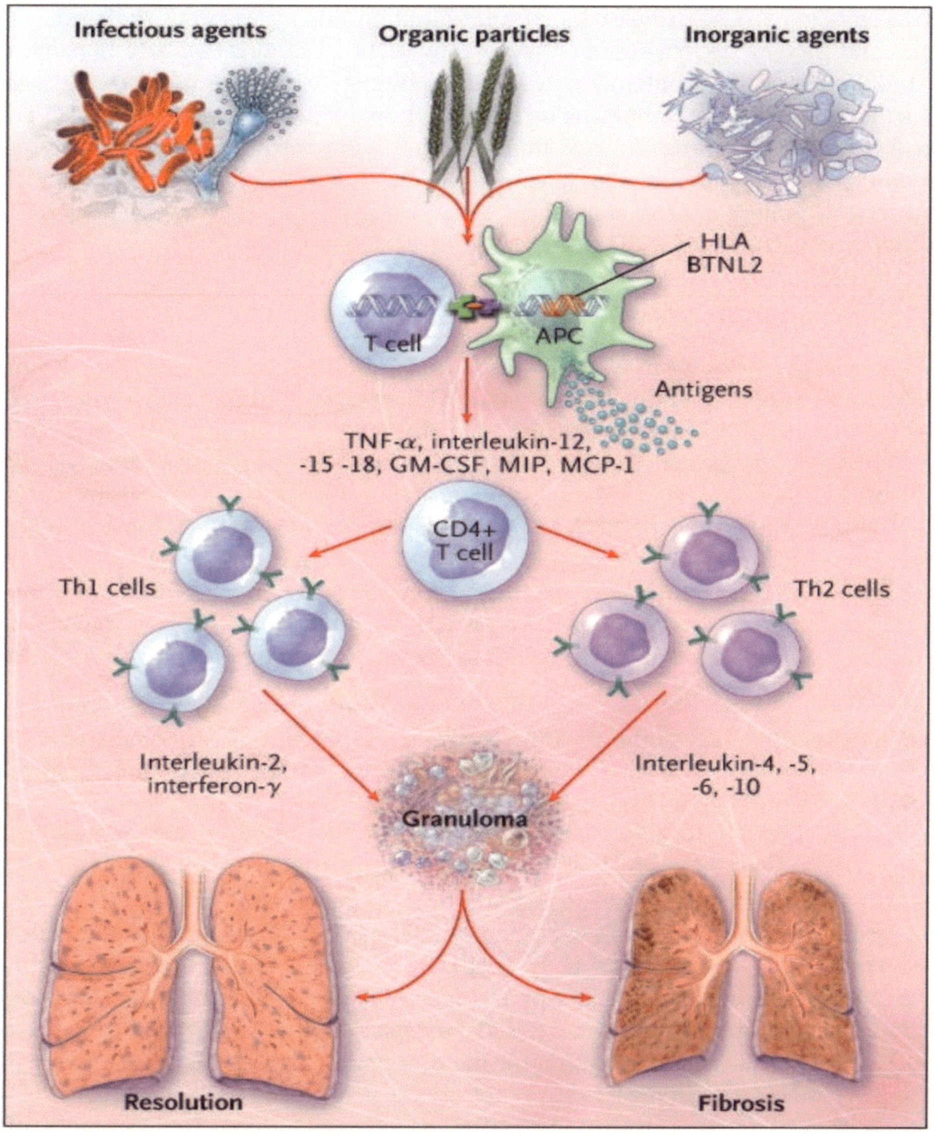


(Iannuzzi MC et al. N Engl J Med 2007;357:2153-2165.)

Fig. 1. Hypothesized Immunopathogenesis of Granuloma Formation.

causing disturbed calcium homeostasis. This not only causes hypercalcemia, hypercalciuria and possibly subsequent nephrolithiasis and nephrocalcinosis, which itself is the most common cause of progressive renal failure. The clinical consequences of each imbalance range from trivial presentation to overt pathology including dehydration, renal colic, and end-stage renal disease. Diagnosis may be established by laboratory findings, ultrasonography, and computed tomography. General treatments incorporate adequate oral hydration, minimization of dietary calcium and vitamin D, avoidance of UV light exposure, and possibly corticosteroid therapy (Sharma 1996).

Hypercalcemia may cause decrease glomerular filtration rate by vasoconstricting the afferent arterioles and thereby decreasing renal blood flow (Berliner et al 2006). Additionally, it may cause tubular necrosis, tubulointerstitial non-granulomatous inflammation with calcium deposits ultimately causing nephrocalcinosis and chronic kidney disease (Berliner et al 2006). Hypercalciuria, which is three times as more common as hypercalcemia, predisposes patients to calcium oxalate nephrolithiasis, which may ultimately lead to obstruction or chronic pyelonephritis (Berliner et al 2006 and Sharma 1996). Renovascular complications as well as obstructive nephropathy will also be further discussed subsequently.

## 4. Obstructive nephropathy

Abnormal calcium metabolism is a well known feature of sarcoidosis. Hypercalcemia and hypercalcuria is related to endogenous vitamin D. It is suggested that excess vitamin D may result in increased intestinal calcium absorption and consequent hypercalcemia, hypercalcuria and renal calculi. Hypercalcuria is defined as using excretion of 300 mg/day in men or 250 mg/day in women, about 2-5% healthy adults exhibit hypercalcuria. Hypercalcuria is the most common renal manifestation. It is caused by glomerular filtration of excess blood calcium and suppression by high calcitriol levels on PTH activity. It affects 50% of patients with sarcoidosis, often with an insidious onset because most patients remain normocalcemic. Sharma suggests that 10% of patients with sarcoidosis are diagnosed with hypercalcemia whereas 30% of patients with sarcoidosis show an increase in serum calcium. (Sharma, 1996)

In 1988, Foster described eight patients where he described extra uveitis may be the presenting sign of sarcoidosis. It was the first study that suggested that there may be unexpected presenting signs of sarcoidosis. (Foster, 1988) One of these symptoms may be nephrolithiasis. In a study from Italy, the charts 618 patients with histologically proven sarcoidosis was reviewed in 1978-92 in order to identify nephrolithiasis as a presenting feature of sarcoidosis. (Rizzato et al 1995) The authors concluded that calculi were the presenting feature of sarcoidosis in 6 out of 618 patients (1%) and was the first manifestation of disease in 14 (2. 2%) of the patients. In another 9 patients who presented with pulmonary involvement, persistent hematuria or pyuria led to discovery of stones via ultrasound or intravenous pyelography. Given that this is an uncommon disease, there is a very small chance that a physician seeing a patient for the first time with a new kidney stone will later prove to be is sarcoidosis. In the literature, the overall prevalence of nephrolithiasis is 10% in patients with sarcoidosis. (Muther et al 1981 and Rizzato 1995) The incidence of 2.2% exceeds more than 20 times the expected yearly rate of renal calculi in the general population (36 per 100, 000 in women and 123 in men in Rochester (Johnson et al 1979), 122 in California (Hiatt et al 1982) and 68 in Kyoto –Osaka. (Yoshida and Okada, 1990) In course of chronic sarcoidosis, approximately 10-13.8% of patients have at least 1 asymptomatic stone. (Lebacq, 1970)

Treatment of hypercalcuria involves minimization of dietary calcium and Vitamin D, avoidance of UV exposure, and dietary oxalate restriction. This is because an increase in intestinal calcium absorption caused by excess in 1, 25 dihydroxyvitamin D may result in an increase in urinary oxalate excretion especially if diet is low in calcium. Overabsorption of calcium leaves less of this divalent cation to complex with oxalate in the proximal intestine so more oxalate is delivered to the colon in which anion is hyperabsorbed. Corticosteriods are usually necessary to normalize these parameters as they can decrease inflammatory activity and reduce calcitriol syntheses.

Retroperitoneal lymph nodes can enlarge sufficiently to cause urethral obstruction.

(Frailly et al 1990). Sarcoidosis has also been shown to be responsible for bilateral hydronephrosis on the basis of retroperitoneal lymph node enlargement, with resolution after corticosteroid treatment. (Miyazaki 1995).

## 5. Glomerular diseases associated with sarcoidosis

Glomerular involvement in sarcoidosis is not very common. The spectrum of commonly reported glomerular diseases include focal segmental sclerosis, membranous glomerulonephritis (GN), mesangioproliferative glomerulonephritis, mesangiocapillary glomerulonephritis, IgA nephropathy and crescentric glomerulonephritis. (Sheffield 1997) The exact mechanisms of glomerular disease in sarcoidosis are not known. Due to the absence of a consistent glomerular pathology and a well described etiological pathway, most cases are believed to be coincidental associations. Broadly speaking, abnormalities in both the humoral and cellular immune system in sarcoidosis contribute to the development of immune complex -type glomerulonephritis which also explains why immunoglobulin and complement deposition are commonly observed in renal biopsies in sarcoidosis. (Gobel et al 2001).

### 5.1 Membranous glomerulonephritis

Overall, membranous glomerulonephritis (MGN) is the most commonly reported glomerular pathology. Amongst 39 cases of glomerular diseases reported in sarcoidosis, Vanhille et al found that 13 were MGN, largely occurring late in the course of overt disease. (Vanhille et al 1986) Khan et al. described a 56-yr-old woman with pulmonary sarcoidosis who developed heavy proteinuria. A renal biopsy revealed both interstitial granulomas and membranous glomerulonephritis. (Khan et al 1999) Rarely patients may be diagnosed to have sarcoidosis during the work up for secondary causes of nephrotic syndrome. Dimitriades et al. described a 13-yr-old girl who presented with the nephrotic syndrome and renal biopsy showed membranous nephropathy. (Dimitriades 1999) Typical subepithelial deposits were found with electron microscopy. Bilateral hilar adenopathy was present, which suggested sarcoidosis. The diagnosis was confirmed by a bone marrow biopsy, which disclosed noncaseating granulomas. The patient was treated with corticosteroids and cyclophosphamide, and her condition stabilized. In an experimental study, Maruyama et al, induced subepithelial deposits in pigs injected with heterologous antibodies to angiotensin converting enzyme (ACE). Confocal microscopy showed co localization of the granular deposits of ACE and anti ACE goat IgG on the outer aspect of glomerular basement. The authors conjectured that a similar autoimmune process may cause membranous GN in sarcoidosis. While traditionally idiopathic MGN is steroid resistant, most cases of MGN associated with sarcoidosis seem to respond to high dose steroid therapy especially if there is coexistent granulomatous interstitial nephritis (GIN) (Khan et al 1999). Others used pulse methylprednisolone plus oral cyclophosphamide to show remission of the nephrotic state. (Dimitriades et al 1999) See Figure 2. for histology of membranous nephropathy in sarcoidosis.

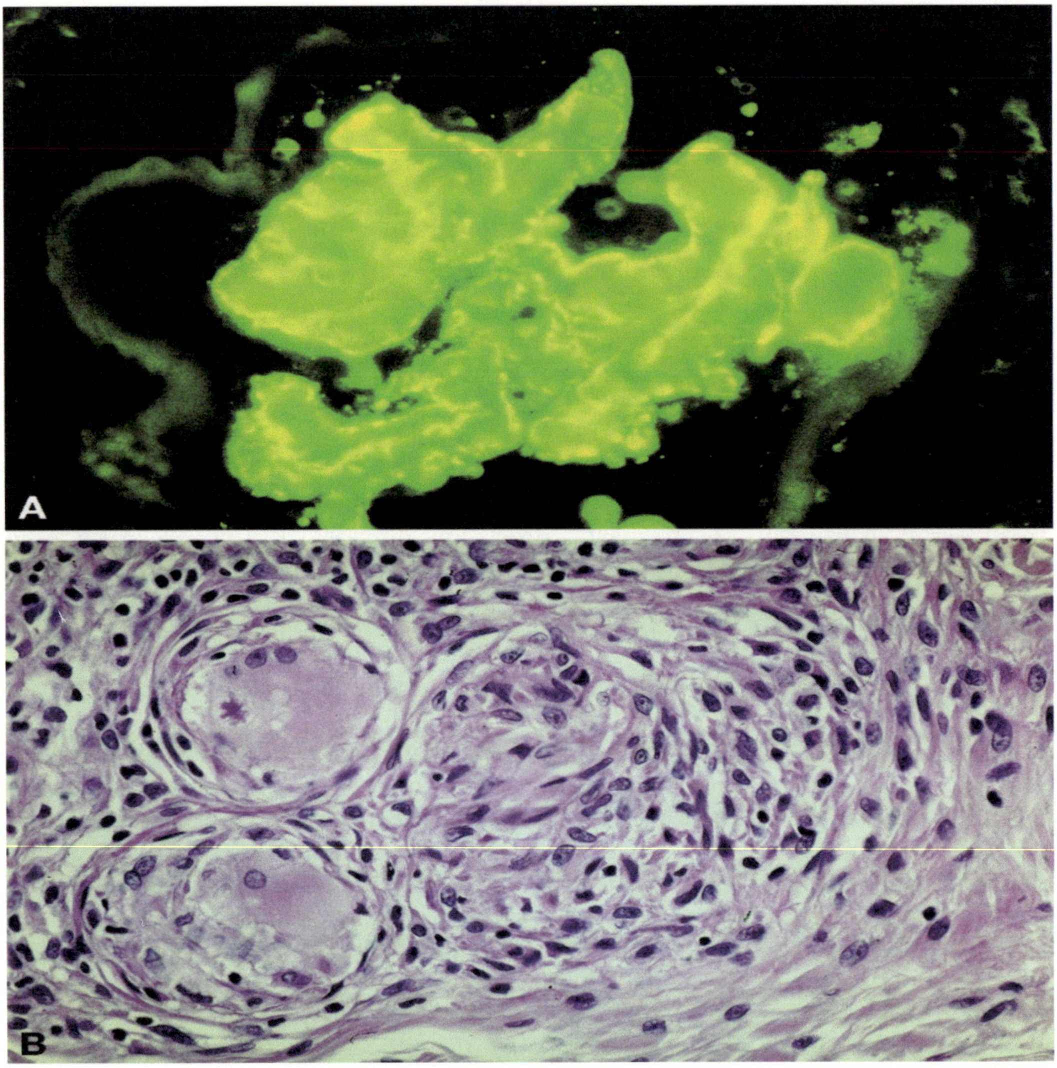

Fig. 2. (A) Immunofluorescence shows granular IgG deposits along the glomerular basement membrane consistent with membranous glomerulonephritis. (B) Left forearm biopsy with epithelioid granulomas. A star-shaped asteroid body is visible within a giant cell. Magnifications: x800 in A (IgG); x500 in B (hematoxylin and eosin). Gobel U et al. JASN 2001;12:616-623

### 5.2 Minimal change disease

Nephrotic syndrome due to minimal change disease (MCD) also has been described in patients with sarcoidosis. Mundlein et al, described a patient with Grave's disease with steroid dependent MCD who achieved complete remission with cyclophosphamide. (Mundlein et al 1996) Patient was subsequently diagnosed to have typical chest findings of pulmonary sarcoidosis. In contrast, Parry and Falk described a case of longstanding pulmonary sarcoidosis that later went on to develop steroid resistant MCD not responding to high dose steroids or cyclophosphamide. (Parry et al 1997) The patient had to be started on cyclosporine which was given for a year and a sustained remission was attained. Spontaneous occurrence and remission of heavy proteinuria coinciding with the relapse of the disease is also well described. (Mery 2005) The authors postulated that there is a functional and transient increase of glomerular permeability to proteins secondary to release of vascular permeability factor like lymphokines by activated T cells.

### 5.3 Crescentic glomerulonephritis

Crescent Glomerulonephrits (GN) has also been frequently reported in patients with sarcoidosis and co-existing ANCA associated vasculitis. ANCA are autoantibodies found in some autoimmune diseases, recognized by their reactivity with cytoplasmic antigens in neutrophils; two groups are recognized: c-ANCA, reacting with proteinase 3, is found in polyangiitis and Churg-Strauss syndrome; p-ANCA, reacting with myeloperoxidase is found in Wegener granulomatosis. Auinger et al described a patient with rapidly progressive glomerulonephritis and hepatosplenomegaly with no prior diagnosis of sarcoidosis whose renal biopsy showed crescentic GN. (Auinger et al 1997) Diagnosis of sarcoidosis was made with raised angiotensin converting enzyme (ACE) levels and both liver and kidney biopsies showing interstitial noncaseating granulomas. Patient was started on high dose steroids with which renal function improved. Subsequently, the patient developed anti- myeloperoxidase (MPO) antibodies. In contrast, Ahuja et al reported a patient with crescentic GN in the setting of Wegener's granulomatosis (WG). (Ahuja et al 1996). Patient responded well to long term oral cyclophosphamide treatment. Subsequently, the patient developed biopsy-confirmed pulmonary sarcoidosis months later. Given such close associations, it is believed that these sarcoidosis and granulomatous vasculitis like WG may have some common mechanisms. See Figure 3.

### 5.4 Other glomerular diseases

Rare associations of sarcoidosis with post-infectious GN have also been noted. Michaels et al. described two patients with sarcoidosis : one with recent history of pneumonia and other with elevated antistreptolysin O titres who developed acute renal failure with active urinary sediments and nephrotic range proteinuria (Michaels et al 2000). Biopsies disclosed diffuse endocapillary proliferative GN with hump-like epithelial deposits. Both patients responded well to corticosteroids with resolution of proteinuria and azotemia. Similarly IgA nephropathy (IgAN), coexisting with sarcoidosis is not unusual given the wide prevalence of IgAN. Taylor and Nishiki described a case of IgAN in sarcoidosis typically presenting as nephritic syndrome that responded well to steroids. (Taylor at el 1996 and Nishiki et al 2010) Renal amyloidosis (AA type) has also noted in patients with long standing sarcoidosis with the classical presentation of steroid resistant nephrotic syndrome with slow progression to end stage renal disease. (Tchenio et al. 1996 and Rainfray et al 1988).

## 6. Tubulointerstitial diseases

After excluding abnormalities affecting calcium homeostasis, tubulointerstitial diseases are the most commonly encountered renal abnormalities in sarcoidosis. They are

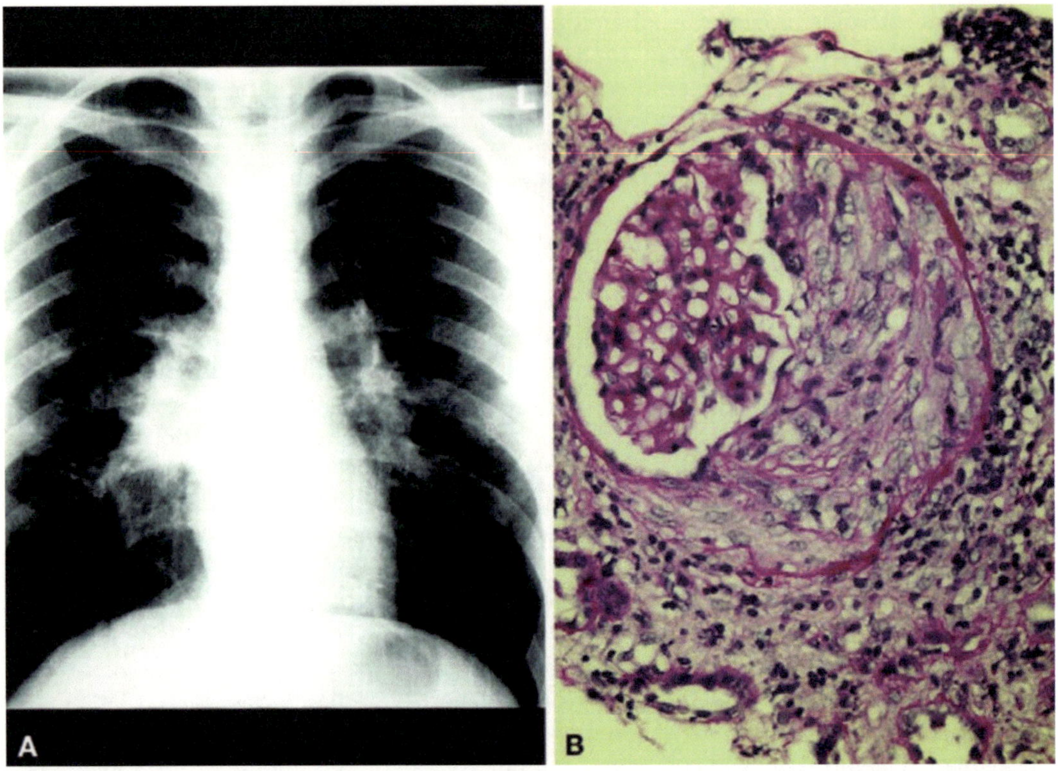


Fig. 3. (A) Roentgenogram showing bilateral hilar adenopathy in a patient with sarcoidosis. (B) Extracapillary glomerulonephritis with crescent formation. Magnification, x500 (periodic acid-Schiff). Gobel U et al. JASN 2001; 12:616-623

histopathologically described as granulomatous interstitial nephritis (GIN). Approximately 20% of patients with sarcoidosis show granulomatous inflammation in the kidney (Sheffield 1997) although values range from 15 to 40% (Mery 2005) reflecting differences in the indication for renal biopsies. In many instances, patients may be clinically silent and GIN may present with concomitant findings with well known clinicopathological syndromes. The variability in incidence of GIN also reflects sampling error in detecting scarce granulomas especially in inadequate biopsy specimens.

Overall GIN is a rare histologic diagnosis seen in 0. 5 and 0. 9% of native renal biopsies and 0. 6% of renal transplant biopsies (Joss et al 2007). Possible etiologies include medications, infections, sarcoidosis, Sjogren's syndrome, crystal deposits, paraproteinemia, Wegener's granulomatosis and idiopathic causes. Drugs implicated include anticonvulsants, antibiotics, nonsteroidal anti-inflammatory drugs, allopurinol, and diuretics. Mycobacteria and fungi are the main infective causes and seem to be the main causative factor in cases in renal transplants or in countries with high prevalence of tuberculosis. In the largest collection of data so far on this disease, Joss et al noted 18 cases of GIN from of etiologies such as sarcoidosis (n=5), drug induced (n=2), idiopathic (n=9) and tubulointerstitial nephritis with uveitis (n=2). The most common presentation of GIN was advanced renal failure with minimal proteinuria. (Joss 2007)

Despite great clinical variability, the most common clinical syndrome associated with sarcoidosis and GIN is chronic kidney disease with decline in renal function usually over weeks to months (Jean-Philllipe 2005). Acute renal failure as an initial presentation is also well known (O'Riordan et al 2001). Renal dysfunction may progress at variable rates but can irreversibly progress to end stage renal disease despite high dose glucocorticoid treatment. (Tsiouris et al 1999) Consistent with a pattern of tubulointerstitial disease, proteinuria is either absent or mild. Urine analysis shows leucocytes and granular casts. Rarely, patient may present as frank hematuria lasting several weeks. (Mills et al 1994) Functional tubular abnormalities can occur in as much as 50% of cases of sarcoidosis when aggressively investigated which include renal glycosuria, urinary sodium and potassium wasting, Fanconi's Syndrome, decreased urinary concentration ability, proximal or distal tubular acidosis. (Muther et al 1981) It is uncertain whether the presence of interstitial lesions solely contributes to these abnormalities but hypercalcemia and hypergammaglobulinemia also play a pathogenic role. (Mery, 2005)

GIN is usually associated with enlarged kidneys mimicking polycystic kidney disease or renal carcinoma. (Mery, 2005) Renal sonogram shows bilateral renal masses which are either hyper- or hypoechoic in comparison to adjacent renal parenchyma. Computer tomogram shows the renal masses to be low intensity. A Gallium-76 citrate scan commonly reveals increased uptake suggesting active granulomatous inflammation. (Mery and Kenouch, 1988) Serum ACE concentration is a poor marker of active renal lesion and may even be normal in active GIN with severe renal failure. (Hannedouche et al 1990)

In most cases, a diagnosis of GIN is made in the context of typical extra-renal manifestations of sarcoidosis and/or hyperkalemia. Rarely renal involvement may be isolated and preceding other sites of the disease for months to years. Some have even considered isolated GIN as a localized form of sarcoidosis. In such isolated cases, it is important to rule out drug induced interstitial nephritis which is far more easily treatable cause of GIN that sarcoidosis itself. (Muther et al 1981) Another syndrome commonly associated with Sjogren's Syndrome but also reported with sarcoidosis is the "TINU syndrome or the Dobrin Syndrome (Sinnamon et al 2008) which is characterized by acute interstitial nephritis, anterior uveitis and epitheliod granulomas in bone marrow and lymph nodes. The renal lesion consists of interstitial infiltrates mainly composed of mononuclear cells and few eosinophils. Although no interstitial granulomas are seen in TINU, the interstitial cell infiltrate is the same as a sarcoid granuloma. Therefore it is possible that some cases described as Dobrin syndrome may be atypical forms of sarcoidosis.

Analyzing all cases of GIN, Joss et al, noted that the background diagnosis of sarcoidosis was known in only 1 of 5 patients of GIN who eventually were categorized as sarcoid GIN. Mean age of presentation was 56. 8 years. ACE levels were elevated in a minority of patients (1 out of 5) and hypercalcemia was seen in only 2 patients. Pulmonary findings of hilar lymphadenopathy was seen in only 1 patient and one had the TINU syndrome.

(Joss et al 2007)

Renal pathology of GIN consists of the typical non-caseating granuloma widely distributed throughout the cortex and the medulla, although the density of these lesions may differ from patient to patient. (Mery 2005) The sarcoid granuloma consists of lymphocytes, mononuclear, cells and plasma cells. The center of the granuloma consists of epitheliod and multinucleate giant cells both of which are derived from activated macrophages. Multinucleate giant cells are formed by the coalescence of epitheliod cells. Lymphocytes largely consist of T-helper cells (CD $4^{+}$) in the center and CD $8^{+}$ lymphocytes in the periphery. Some granulomas have small arteries in their center. Although granulomas may also form in drug induced interstitial nephritis it is less well formed than in sarcoidosis. Varying degrees of fibrosis may also be present. The severity of fibrosis correlates with tubular atrophy and degeneration. In the absence of any predominant glomerular pathology, the glomeruli are either normal or show mesangial hypertrophy and thickening of the basement membrane. Electron microscopy may show fusion of epithelial foot processes (Farge et al 1986). However, there are no significant immune deposits in either the glomeruli or tubules as seen by immunoflourescent microscopy. In a significant number of cases, immunoflourescence with anti-ACE serum showed localization in the sarcoid granuloma in addition to normal staining of the brush border of the proximal tubules. (Mery et al 1988) See Figure 4.

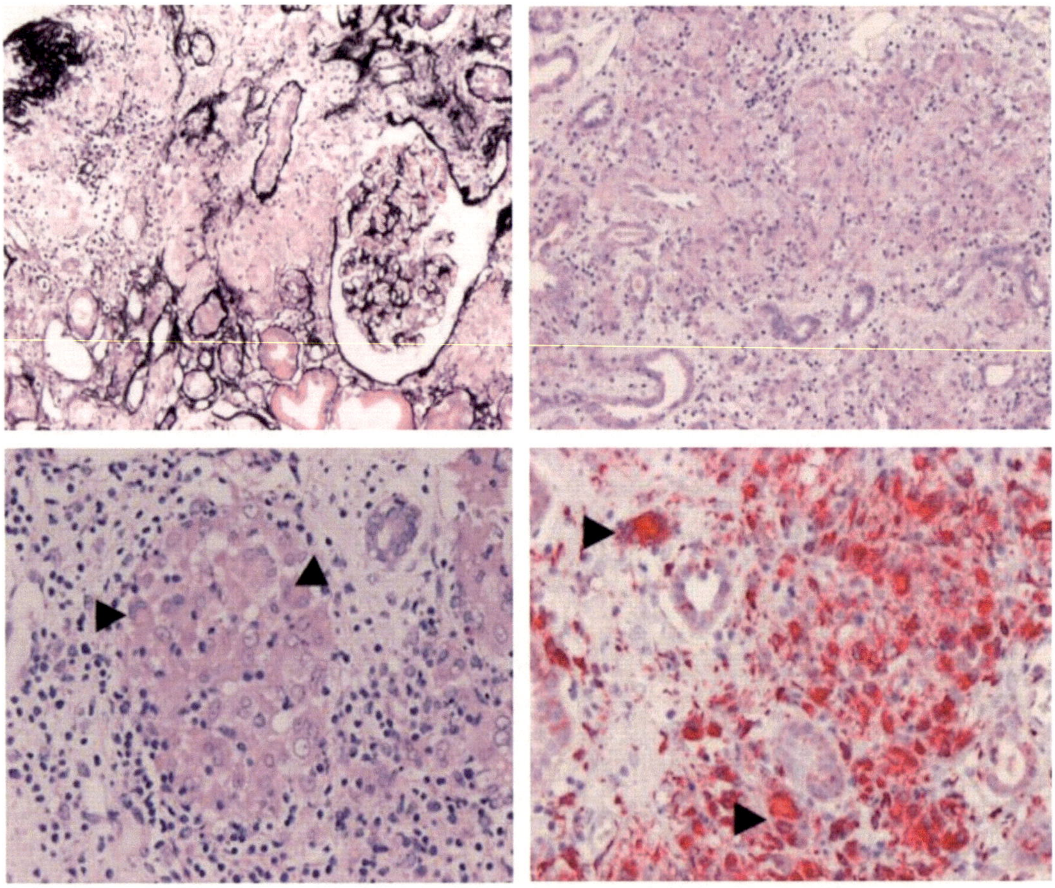

Fig. 4. Renal biopsy showed a granulomatous interstitial nephritis with a broadened interstitial, cellular infiltrates and granuloma with typical multinucleated giant cells (arrowheads). Kettritz R et al. Nephrol. Dial. Transplant. 2006; 21:2690-2694

In contrast to conventional pathological dogma, Joss et al showed that asteroid bodies and calcification were not common in sarcoid GIN. (Joss et al 2007) Interestingly, asteroid bodies were seen in 1 case of drug induced AIN. However, lymphocyte cuffing and giant cell infiltration were prominent in sarcoid granulomas in the kidney. Necrosis and eosinophil infiltration of the interstitum was more common in drug induced GIN as compared to sarcoidosis. It is now believed that idiopathic GIN, TINU and sarcoidosis represents a clinicopathological spectrum and that idiopathic GIN or TINU may subsequently develop typical extra-renal manifestations of sarcoidosis.

### 6.1 Treatment

The mainstay of treatment of sarcoid GIN is glucocorticoids. Initial treatment requires a daily dose of prednisone or prednisolone preferably 1-1. 5 mg/kg. Response to treatment can often be dramatic in terms of improvement of renal insufficiency. The best response to glucocorticoids was noted in a study by Mahevas et al. in which 47 patients with renal sarcoid received prednisolone while 10 also received pulse methylprednisolone. (Mahevas et al 2009) The authors concluded that at 24 months, a complete and partial remission occurred in 30 and 5 patients respectively. But no response was noted in patients with severe interstitial fibrosis of greater than 50%. Underlying functional tubular dysfunction improves with progressive drop in serum creatinine. An important point to realize here is that steroid treatment has to be prolonged and must exceed at least 6 months as nephropathy relapses very frequently with short term therapy (Gene and Cheviot 1988). A commonly followed strategy is to give the initial dose for 2 months followed by progressive taper and switching to an alternate -day therapy. A maintenance therapy period for 1 year at least is recommended. Serial renal biopsies have shown a regression of granuloma in conjunction with improvement of renal function (Farge et al 1986) although given the variability in results (Gene and Cheviot 1988) routine biopsies after starting steroids is not recommended. Treatment in advanced disease is often associated with interstitial fibrosis along with focal segmental glomerulosclerosis and vascular lesions. However, vascular lesions are more common with long term corticosteroid therapy and are associated with delayed development of hypertension which is a major contributor to progression of renal failure. (Mery and Kenouch 1988)

While analyzing outcomes of steroid treatment in a heterogeneous population of GIN, Joss et al, presented data of 16 patients of which 5 were labeled as sarcoidosis. Patients were treated with prednisolone (starting dose of 0. 55mg/kg) (Joss et al 2007) for a mean period of 25 months and then followed up for a period of 45 months. Overall, renal function stabilized or improved at the end of the study with mean GFR improving from 21 to 56 ml/min. One patient who was on dialysis at the beginning of therapy was able to discontinue dialysis within 3 months. Six patients relapsed on dose reduction of which 4 were sarcoid GIN who required azathioprine to break steroid dependence. Sarcoid patients required longer treatment (36 months) as compared to idiopathic or TINU patients. The greatest renal recovery occurred in the first year of treatment. There was no difference in renal outcome when analyzing the degree of interstitial fibrosis. Age less than 60 years was associated with a better outcome. Table 1 summarizes data on treatment of GIN in some important studies so far.

Long term results with steroid therapy in sarcoid GIN have not been rigorously tested in randomized controlled trials. In a large case series of 39 patients with sarcoid renal disease,

| Parameter | Joss et al | | Robson *et al.* | O'Riordan *et al.* | Hannedouche *et al.* | Brause *et al.* |
|---|---|---|---|---|---|---|
| *n* | 18 | 16[1] | 7 | 5 | 6 | 5 |
| Cause | Mixed | Idiopathic/ TINU/sarcoid | Idiopathic | Isolated sarcoid | Sarcoid | Sarcoid |
| Age (yr) | 55 | 56 | 69 | 48 to 71 | 62 | 61 |
| Male gender (%) | 61 | 56 | 71 | 60 | 50 | 60 |
| Renal function at baseline | | | | | | |
| BaselineCC (ml/min) | 21 | 24 | 14 | 6 | NA | NA |
| Baseline creatinine (μmol/L) | 373 | 357 | 420 | NA | 566 | 396 |
| Hypercalcemia | 3/18 | 3/16 | 2/7 | 0/5 | 2/6 | 1/5 |
| Raised serum ACE | 4/17 | 4/15 | 3/7 | 1/5 | 4/4 | 1/5 |
| Improved renal function | 17/18 | 15/16 | 5/7 | 4/5 | 6/6 | 5/5 |
| Long-term RRT | 0/18 | 0/16 | 2/7 | 0/5 | 0/6 | 0/5 |
| Prednisolone (%) | 89 | 88 | 100 | 100 | 100 | 100 |
| Mean follow-up (mo) | 45 | 48 | 25 | 35 | 75 | NA |
| Renal function at last visit | | | | | | |
| ECC (ml/min) at end of therapy | 56 | 53 | 22 | 20 | NA | NA |
| Creatinine (μmol/L) at end of study | 159 | 159 | 296 | NA | 192 | 225 |

[1] Data excluding the two cases of drug-induced GIN.

Table 1. Comparison on treatment of GIN in literature.

17 patients with biopsy-proven tubulo-interstitial nephritis with significant renal impairment were analyzed over a one year period of corticosteroid therapy. (Robson et al 2003). All patients were initially started on prednisolone at 0. 5 mg/kg body weight at a daily dose of 30–60 mg which was tapered by 5 mg each week once the renal function has improved and/or stabilized. Thereafter, patients were maintained on 5–7. 5 mg daily indefinitely. Mean duration of study was 84 months. Estimated glomerular filtration rate (eGFR) at baseline was 26. 814 ml/min which improved to 49. 65. 2 ml/min (P<0. 01) at 1 year, and 47. 96. 8 ml/min (P<0. 05) at last review. Interestingly, the response to treatment was similar regardless of the degree of renal impairment at baseline, race and the degree of tubulo-interstitial scarring on renal biopsy. Three patients developed side effects that could

be attributed to steroids which included acute psychosis and type 2 diabetes. Long term use of corticosteroids, especially in adolescents, can cause substantial side effects including diabetes, growth retardation and cataract. Alternative agents that have been attempted in treating sarcoid GIN include mycophenolate (Moudgil 2002) and mizoribine (Rajakariar et al 2006 and Ito et al 2009) which are limited to case reports and have been primarily used in pediatric patients to break steroid dependence or ameliorate significant side effects. Other agents which have been tried in systemic extra-renal sarcoidosis include mycophenolate mofetil, methotrexate, azathioprine, antimalarials, and phosphodiesterase inhibitors such as pentoxifylline and thalidomide although no data on treating renal sarcoidosis exists. (Baughman 2003) There has been great interest in the use of TNF-antagonists as another modality to treat sarcoid GIN in order to avoid use of steroids. TNF-alpha, which is expressed by monocytes, is critical in the development of these noncaseating granulomas. TNF-alpha receptor antagonists have also been shown to prevent the initiation and perpetuation of inflammation and subsequent interstitial fibrosis. Etanercept is a soluble TNF-alpha receptor fusion protein that binds TNF-alpha. Infliximab and adalimumab are monoclonal antibodies that bind specifically to and neutralize TNF-alpha. While etanercept is an ineffective agent in the treatment of systemic sarcoidosis, (Ulz et al 2003) infliximab has been shown to be effective in a case of renal sarcoid. Thumfart et al, described the case of a boy presenting with severe arterial hypertension and acute renal failure caused by an isolated sarcoid granulomatous interstitial nephritis. Renal function improved initially with prednisone treatment but later, the patient showed signs of severe steroid toxicity and progressive renal failure. Monthly treatment with infliximab was initiated resulting in a steady improvement in renal function and resolution of renal granulomata, as well as reduction in antihypertensive medication. (Thumfart 2005) Ahmed et al presented a patient with acute renal failure due to isolated granulomatous infiltration of the renal parenchyma. (Ahmed et al 2007) Renal biopsy showed granulomatous interstitial nephritis with noncaseating granulomas. There was no evidence of extrarenal sarcoid involvement. Prednisone 60mg daily resulted in significant improvement in renal function. Due to recurrent flares while tapering the prednisone and steroid toxicity, treatment with infliximab was instituted and resulted in stabilization of renal function. This case demonstrated that steroid-dependant or refractory renal sarcoidosis cases may respond to infliximab. We recently reported the case of a 46-year-old woman with multi-organ sarcoidosis, type 2 diabetes, subnephrotic-range proteinuria, hypertension and recurrent episodes of hypercalcemia-induced acute kidney injury who was referred for evaluation of worsening renal function and nephrotic range proteinuria. (Gupta et al 2008) A kidney biopsy showed sarcoid GIN with moderate-to-severe chronic tubulointerstitial disease, hypertensive vasculopathy, and diabetic glomerulosclerosis. Because steroids had caused multiple side effects including diabetes, hypertension and obesity and attempts to wean steroids had caused hypercalcemia and acute renal failure, Adalimumab (Humira™) 40 mg/0. 8 cc weekly for 6 months was initiated. After 6 months of treatment with adalimumab, serum creatinine improved from 345 µmol/L (3. 9 mg/dL) to 1. 8 mg/dl (her baseline for years) and proteinuria improved from 10 g/day to 3. 5 g in 24 hours respectively. A repeat biopsy showed persistent diabetic glomerulosclerosis, moderate chronic tubulointerstitial inflammation with complete resolution of interstitial epitheliod granulomas. Although adalimumab and infliximab are generally safe, some side effects include risk of lymphoma and reactivation of latent tuberculosis (Denys et al 2007). These agents may hold promise for the future once large scale randomized studies are available to show consistent benefits with minimal side effects.

## 7. Renovascular diseases associated with sarcoidosis

Renovascular diseases secondary to sarcoidosis are distinctly rare and attributed to a form of secondary vasculitides. Systemic vasculitis associated with sarcoidosis has been reported as an isolated entity in the literature after excluding other common causes of vasculitis. It is predominantly large vessel vasculitis although few instances of small vessel vasculitis have been reported. In a large case series and review of literature on sarcoid vasculitis, Fernandes et al, noted that most cases were children and clinical presentation resembled hypersensitivity vasculitis, Takayasu's arteritis, polyarteritis nodosa or microscopic polyangitis. (Fernandes 2000) Clinical features included fever, peripheral adenopathy, hilar adenopathy, rash, pulmonary parenchymal disease, musculoskeletal symptoms, and scleritis or iridocyclitis with biopsy showing necrotizing sarcoid granulomata. Interestingly, no renal involvement was noted. Notably the authors found large vessel vasculitis largely in the African American population while small vessel vasculitis predominantly affected white races. Godin et al described a known case of pulmonary sarcoidosis with persistent hypertension. (Godin et al 1980) Diagnostic evaluation for renovascular hypertension included aortography which showed severe stenosis of right renal artery. Surgical exploration showed extensive periaortic and perirenal fibrosis with extrinsic compression of renal artery. Pathological examination of the kidney revealed epitheloid infiltration of the adventia of renal artery suggestive of sarcoid angitis. Surgical biopsy was performed on both kidneys. The right kidney, protected by arterial stenosis, was slightly altered, while the left kidney showed extensive interstitial, tubular, and glomerular lesions which included focal and segmental hyalinosis. Marcussen et al, reported an autopsy case of a middle aged man who died of myocardial infarction secondary to fulminent vasculitis. (Marcussen and Lund 1989) Pathology showed widespread giant cell vasculitis with simultaneous involvement of the renal arteries, veins, and arterioles along with typical interstitial sarcoid granuloma. Shintaku et al, showed granulomatous inflammation of small renal vessels and crescentric GN on the autopsy of a patient with pulmonary hemorrhage and rapidly progressive renal failure. (Shintaku et al 1989) Thus, sarcoid angitis, especially causing small vessel vasculitis in the kidney may represent a very severe form of sarcoidosis. In their review, Fernandes et al, noted that four out of six patients responded well to steroid treatment alone but had relapses when attempts were made to taper or withdraw steroids. (Fernandes 2000) Frequently, there is an overlap between sarcoidosis and well known causes of granulomatous vasculitis. For instance, Watson et al described a case of longstanding pulmonary sarcoidosis presenting with rapidly progressive renal failure with p-ANCA positivity. (Watson 1996) Renal biopsy demonstrated focal and segmental fibrinoid necrosis with crescentric GN and focal fibrinoid necrosis in arterial wall, but no granulomata and pauci-immune deposits on immunofluorescence. Unlike patients with ANCA positive vasculitis, the index case responded poorly to pulse steroids and cyclophosphamide and progressed rapidly to end stage renal disease.

## 8. Kidney transplantation in patients with sarcoidosis

The usual cause of end stage renal disease in sarcoidosis requiring renal replacement therapy is usually due to hypercalcemic nephropathy rather than granulomatous interstitial nephritis or a glomerular disease. The outcome in renal transplantation in patients with sarcoidosis has been described in the literature. The first recurrence of sarcoid GIN in renal allograft was diagnosed 6 years after deceased donor kidney transplantation in a patient that was diagnosed with GIN before transplantation (Shen et al 1986). A recent French study aimed to describe a multicenter experience with kidney transplantation in patients with sarcoidosis. (Aouizerate et al 2010) In this study, the authors retrospectively identified 18 patients who underwent renal transplantation. Patient medical charts, demographics were reviewed. The median time between the last sarcoidosis episode and renal transplantation was 78 (8 to 900) months. Only 3 out of 18 patients had been on immunosuppression prior to transplantation. Vast majority of the patients had in the past received steroids and other immunosuppression for their sarcoid before transplantation. Renal disease was attributable to biopsy proven renal sarcoid in 10 out of the 18 patients and was attributed to other causes in 8 patients. Mean age of transplantation was 43. 5 +/- 11 years. 17 out of 18 patients had a deceased donor transplant. Mean donor age was 36. 5 +/ 15 years. Mean cold ischemia time was 16. 6 +/- 8 hours. 11 patients received induction therapy with anti-thymocyte globulin or Il-2 receptor antagonists. Maintenance immunosuppression included calcineurin inhibitor (CNI) for all patients, mycophenolate mofetil or azathiporine, sirolimus and corticosteroids for 16 out of the 18 patients. At the end of the 42 month follow up period, patient and death censored graft survival was 94. 4% and mean GFR was 60 cc/min per 1. 73 m2. Recurrence of sarcoidosis after renal transplantation was observed in 5 (27%) of patients. The median period between renal transplantation and recurrence was 13 months and four of five patients exhibited recurrence in the first 18 months after renal transplantation. Recurrences involved in the same organ in four of five patients and included renal involvement in three patients and lung and liver involvement in one patient. Mean GFR at end of follow-up was significantly lower in the three patients with recurrence than that for the entire cohort. (31 versus 60 cc/min per 1. 73 m2). Analysis of the recurrences showed that they occur in the first 18 months after transplantation. Primary disease related to sarcoidosis was strongly associated with recurrence (40% in the group with renal sarcoidosis versus 12. 5% in a group with a primary nephropathy, and median period between last episode of sarcoidosis and renal transplantation was shorter in the case of sarcoidosis recurrence (42 versus 78 months respectively). This study showed that patients with initial renal involvement display sensitivity to disease recurrence in allograft. The incidence of recurrence was significant as all patients were maintained on triple immunosuppressive therapy including steroids and mycophenolate mofetil. This study showed that renal transplant can be conducted safely in transplant patients with sarcoidosis, but recurrences do occur and affect overall graft outcome.

Kukura reported a case of recurrence of sarcoidosis in the renal allograft during pregnancy. (Kukura et al 2004) This was a 27 yr old female diagnosed with sarcoidosis at age 14 by lacrimal and parotid gland biopsy. 4 years after presentation, she developed hypertension and renal insufficiency. Kidney biopsy showed interstitial nephritis and nephrosclerosis, but no granulomas. Patient was eventually started in hemodialysis and underwent kidney transplantation with excellent graft function with a creatinine of 1. 32 mg/dl and a negative urinalysis. Patient was maintained on cyclosporine, azathioprine and prednisone 25 mg by mouth daily. 2 years after transplantation once the steroids were withdrawn, patient continued to have good kidney function with an allograft biopsy showing mild chronic allograft nephropathy only. Immunosuppression consisted of azathioprine and cyclosporine. At 3 years after kidney transplantation, patient became pregnant. 29 weeks into pregnancy, renal function worsened. Biopsy showed numerous noncaseating granulomas bound to the arteries, initial arteritis in one artery, mild interstitial mononuclear inflammation and tubulitis. Graft function improved with pulse methylprednisolone and tapered steroids were used. After delivery, renal allograft biopsy was performed 6 months which showed baseline disease of mild chronic allograft nephropathy and sporadic granulomas. This case demonstrates that steroid withdrawal after kidney transplantation may lead to sarcoidosis recurrence.

The implication that sarcoid reflects a disease phenomena related to the immunologic stimulus makes sarcoidosis an unlikely diagnosis to be made in an immunosuppressed patient such as an organ transplant recipient. However, Schmidt et al showed that after kidney transplantation, sarcoidosis can occur in the lung and pleura. (Schmidt et al 1999) In this case, a 41 yr old with history of IgA nephropathy and no past medical history received a living related kidney transplant and had been receiving tacrolimus therapy. He was found to have a large pleural effusion 17 months after kidney transplant. Diagnosis of sarcoidosis was established by identifying noncaseating granulomas, some with multinucleated giant cells in the pleural and lung tissue. All viral and bacterial workup was negative. The effusion resolved after initiating corticosteroid therapy. One month into therapy, the effusion resolved and patient continued to be asymptomatic twenty months after therapy. The authors did not speculate on the pathogenesis of granuloma formation since both tacrolimus and corticosteroids interfere with T lymphocyte function and granuloma formation. They speculated that activation of tissue chemokines of the IP-10 type during the posttransplant period, along with subsequent recruitment of lymphocytes and macrophages may have resulted in the sarcoidosis.

## 9. Conclusion

Sarcoidosis is a disease that primarily affects the reticuloendothelial system but can affect all tissues and organ systems. In this chapter, we described the effects of sarcoidosis on the kidneys. This disease affects patients worldwide and is defined pathologically by the presence of noncaseating granulomas in the involved tissue. The etiology of sarcoidosis has yet to be determined but some have proposed a possible infectious etiology. Commonly sarcoid patients present with hypercalcemia, hypercalcuria, and nephrolithiasis due to the overproduction of calcitriol from the epitheliod granulomas. We also described the rare glomerular and renovascular manifestations of sarcoidosis. Granulomatous interstitial nephritis is most commonly associated with sarcoidosis. It is a histological diagnosis and can be treated with both steroids and TNF-alpha antagonists. Kidney transplantation is safe in patients with sarcoidosis but we must keep in mind the disease can recur in the allograft. In conclusion, sarcoidosis is a complex disease and presents both a diagnostic and management challenge to the physician.

## 10. References


Ahmed MM, Mubashir E, Dossabhoy NR. Isolated renal sarcoidosis: a rare presentation of a rare disease treated with infliximab. Clin Rheumatol. 2007; 26(8):1346-9.

Ahuja TS, Mattana J, Valderrama E, Sankaran R, Singhal PC, Wagner JD: Wegener's granulomatosis followed by development of sarcoidosis. Am J Kidney Dis. 1996; 28:893 -898. 47.

Aouizerate, Jessie, Matignon, Marie et al: Renal Transplantation in Patients with Sarcoidosis: A French Multicenter Study. Clinical Journal of American Society of Nephrology 2010 5: 2101-2108.

Auinger M, Irsigler K, Breiteneder S, Ulrich W: Normocalcemic hepatorenal sarcoidosis with crescentic glomerulonephritis. Nephrol Dial Transplant. 1997; 12:1474 -1477.

Baughman, R. P, Lynch, J. Difficult treatment issues in sarcoidosis. J Intern Med. 2003 Jan; 253(1):41-5.

Berliner AR, Haas M, Choi MJ. Sarcoidosis: The Nephrologist's Perspective. Am J Kid Dis 2006; 48(5):856-870.

Brause M, Magnusson K, Degenhardt S, Helmchen U, Grabensee B: Renal involvement in sarcoidosis: A report of 6 cases. Clin Nephrol. 2002; 57 :142– 148.

Casella FJ, Allon M. The Kidney in Sarcoidosis. J Am Soc Nephrol 1993; 3: 1555-1562.

Denys, B. Bogaerts, Y. Coenegrachts, K. Et al. Steroid-resistant sarcoidosis: is antagonism of TNF-α the answer? Clinical Science. 2007; 11: 281–289.

Dimitriades C, Shetty AK, Vehaskari M, Craver RD, Gedalia A: Membranous nephropathy associated with childhood sarcoidosis. Pediatr Nephrol. 1999;13:444 -447.

Farge D, Loite F, Turner M. Granulomatous nephritis and chronic renal failure in sarcoidosis. Long term follow up studies in two patients. American J Nephrol. 1986; 6:22-27.

Fernandes SR, Singsen BH, Hoffman GS. Sarcoidosis and systemic vasculitis. Semin Arthritis Rheum. 2000 Aug; 30(1):33-46.

Foster S. Ocular manifestations of sarcoidosis preceding systemic manifestations. In: Grassi C. Rizzato G, Pzzi E, eds. *Sarcoidosis and other granuloamtous disorders.* Amsterdam: Elsevier; 1988: 1977-81.

Fraioli P, Montemurro L, Castrignano L, Rizzato G. Retroperitoneal involvement in sarcoidosis. Sarcoidosis. 1990;7(2):101.

Gobel U, Kettritz R, Schneider W, Luft F. The protean face of renal sarcoidosis. J Am Soc Nephrol. 2001; 12:616–623.

Godin M et al. Sarcoidosis, retroperitoneal fibrosis, renal artery involvement and unilateral focal glomerulosclerosis. Archives of Internal Medicine. 1980;140:1240-1242

Guenel J and Chevet D. Interstitial nephropathies in sarcoidosis. Effect of corticosteroid therapy and long-term evolution. Retrospective study of 22 cases. Nephrologie. 1988;9(6):253-7.

Gupta, R. Beaudet, Lisa and Mehta, Tulsi. Treatment of sarcoid granulomatous interstitial nephritis with adalimumab. NDT Plus. 2008;2(2): 139-142.

Hannedouche, T., Grateau, G., Noël, et al. Renal Granulomatous Sarcoidosis: Report of Six Cases. Nephrolo Dial Transplant. 1990;5(1):18-24.

Hiatt R, Dales L. Friedman G. Frequency of urolithiasis in a prepaid medical care program. Americal Journal Epidemiol 1982: 115: 255-65.

Iannuzzi MC, Rybicki BA, Teirstein AS. Medical Progress: Sarcoidosis. N Engl J Med 2007: 357(21). 2153-2165.

Iannuzzi MC, Fontana JR. Sarcoidosis: Clinical Presentation, Immunopathogenesis, and Therapeutics. JAMA 2011; 305(4):391-399.

Ito, Shuichi, Harada, Tomonori, Nakamura, Tomoko et al. Mizoribine for renal sarcoidosis: effective steroid tapering and prevention of recurrence. Pediatr Nephrol 2009; 24:411-414.

Johnson C, Wilson D, O'Fallon W et al. Renal stone epidemiology: a 25 year study in Rochester, Minnesota. Kidney International 1979: 16: 624-31.

Joss, Nicola, Morris, Scott and Young, B et al. Granulomatous Interstitial Nephritis. CJASN 2007; 2(2); 222-230.

Kettritz, R, Goebel U, Fiebeler, A, et al. The protean face of sarcoidosis revisited. Nephrol Dial Transplant 2006; 21:2690-2694.

Khan IH, Simpson JG, Catto GR, MacLeod AM: Membranous nephropathy and granulomatous interstitial nephritis in sarcoidosis. Nephron. 1999 66: 459 -461.

Kukura S, Viklicky o, Lacha J, et al: Recurrence of sarcoidosis in renal allograft during pregnancy. Nephrology Dialysis Transplant 2004; 19: 1640-1642.

Lebacq E, Desmet V, Verhaegen H. Renal involvement in sarcoidosis. Postgrad Med J 1970; 46: 526.

Mahévas M, Lescure FX, Boffa J et al. Renal sarcoidosis: clinical, laboratory, and histologic presentation and outcome in 47 patients. Medicine (Baltimore). 2009;88(2):98.

Marcussen N and Lund C. Combined sarcoidosis and disseminated visceral giant cell vasculitis. Pathology, Research and Practice. 1989;184:325-330.

Maruyama S, Cantu E 3rd, Demartino C, Vladutiu A, Caldwell PR, Wang CY, D'Agati V, Godman G, Stern DM, Andres G. Membranous glomerulonephritis induced in the pig by antibody to angiotensin-converting enzyme: considerations on its relevance to the pathogenesis of human idiopathic membranous glomerulonephritis. J Am Soc Nephrol. 1999 Oct;10(10):2102-8.

Mery, Jean-Phillippe. The patient with sarcoidosis. Oxford textbook of Clinical Nephrology, 3rd Edition (2005), Volume 1, Oxford University Press:733-740.

Mery J. P., Kenouch S. Les atteintes de l'interstitium rénal au cours des maladies systémiques. Seminares d'uro-nephrologie Pitie-Salpetriere, 1988; 57-89

Moudgil, A., Przygodzki, R. and Kher. K. Successful steroid-sparing treatment of renal limited sarcoidosis with mycophenolate mofetil. Pediatric Nephrol 2006;21(2):281-285.

Michaels S, Sabnis SG, Oliver JD, Guccion JG: Renal sarcoidosis with superimposed glomerulonephritis presenting as acute renal failure. Am J Kidney Dis. 2000; 36:1 -6.

Mills, PR, Burns AP, Dorman AM, Sweny PJ, Moorhead JF. Granulomatous sarcoid nephritis presenting as frank haematuria. Nephrol Dial Transplant. 1994;9(11):1649-51.

Miyazaki E, Tsuda T, et al. : Sarcoidosis presenting as bilateral hydronephrosis. Intern Med 35: 579-582, 1996

Mundlein E, Greten T, Ritz E: Graves' disease and sarcoidosis in a patient with minimal-change glomerulonephritis. Nephrol Dial Transplant. 1996; 11:860 -862.

Muther, R., Mc Carron D et al. Renal manifestations of sarcoidosis. Arch Intern Medicine 1981;141 :643-645.

Nishiki M, Murakami Y, Yamane Y, Kato Y: Steroid-sensitive nephrotic syndrome, sarcoidosis, and thyroiditis: A new syndrome? Nephrol Dial Transplant. 1999; 14:2008 -2010.

O'Riordan E, Willert RP, Reeve R et al. Isolated sarcoid granulomatous interstitial nephritis: review of five cases at one center. Clin Nephrol. 2001 Apr;55(4):297-302.

Parry RG, Falk C: Minimal change disease in association with sarcoidosis. Nephrol Dial Transplant. 1997;12 : 2159-2160.

Rainfray M. Renal amyloidosis complicating sarcoidosis. Thorax. 1988;43:422-423.

Rajakariar, E., Sharples, J et al. Sarcoid tubulo-interstitial nephritis: Long-term outcome and response to corticosteroid therapy. Kid Int. 2006; 70: 165–169.

Rizzato G, Fraioli P, Montemurro L. Nephrolithiasis as a presenting feature of chronic sarcoidosis. Thorax 1995; 50:555.

Rizzato G: Sarcoidosis in Italy. Sarcoidosis 9(supl): 145-147. 1995

Robson MG, Banerjee D, Hopster D, Cairns HS: Seven cases of granulomatous interstitial nephritis in the absence of extrarenal sarcoid. Nephrol Dial Transplant. 2003 ;18 :280- 284.

Schmidt, R., Bender, f. Change, W: Sarcoidosis After renal Transplantation. Transplantation 68(9) 1420-1423, 1999.

Sharma OP. Vitamin D, Calcium, and Sarcoidosis. Chest 1996; 109(2): 535-539.

Sheffield EA: Pathology of sarcoidosis. Clin Chest Med. 1997;18: 741-753.

Shen S, Hall-Craggs, M. et al : Recurrent sarcoid granulomatous nephritis and reactive tuberculin skin test in a renal transplant recipient. American Journal of Medicine 80:699-702, 1986.

Shintaku M, Mase K, Ohtsuki H, Yasumizu R, Yasunaga K, Ikehara S: Generalized sarcoidlike granulomas with systemic angiitis, crescentic glomerulonephritis, and pulmonary hemorrhage. Report of an autopsy case. Arch Pathol Lab Med. 1989; 113:1295 -129.

Sinnamon, T. Courtney, Harron, C et al. Tubulointerstitial nephritis and uveitis (TINU) syndrome: epidemiology, diagnosis and management. Nephrol Dial Transpl Plus. 2008; 2(1): 112-116.

Taylor JE, Ansell ID: Steroid sensitive nephrotic syndrome and renal impairment in a patient with sarcoidosis. Nephrol Dial Transplant. 1996; 11:355 -356.

Tchenio X et al. Amylose renale AA au cours d'une sarcoidose. Revue des Maladies Respiratoires. 1996; 13. 601-602.

Thumfart J. Isolated sarcoid granulomatous interstitial nephritis responding to infliximab therapy. Am J Kidney Dis 2005;45:411-414.

Tsiouris N, Kovacs B, Daskal I I, Brent LH, Samuels A. End stage renal disease in sarcoidosis of the kidney. 1999. Am J Kidney Disease. 1999;34: E21

Ulz JP, Limper AH, Kalra S, et al. Etanercept for the treatment of stage II and III progressive pulmonary sarcoidosis. Chest 2003;124:177.

Vanhille, Ph et al. Glomerulonephrite rapidement progressive a depots mesangiuax d'IgA au cours d'une sarcoidose. Nephrologie. 1986;5: 207-209.

Watson G, Hill C M, Biggart J D et al. Sarcoidosis and primary systemic vasculitis. Nephrol Dial Transplant. 1996;11: 1631-1633. 54.

Yoshida O, Okada Y. Epidemiology of urolithiasis in Japan: a chronological and geographical study. Urol Int 1990: 45: 104-11.

# 7

# Origins of Cardiorenal Syndrome and the Cardiorenal Connection

L. G. Bongartz[1,2], M. J. Cramer[1] and J. A. Joles[2]
[1]*Dept. of Cardiology, University Medical Center Utrecht, Utrecht*
[2]*Dept. of Nephrology, University Medical Center Utrecht, Utrecht*
*The Netherlands*

## 1. Introduction

In recent years, the relationship between the heart and the kidneys in disease has received increasing attention from the clinical and scientific medical community. This was initiated by epidemiological observations in the late 1990's of increasing patient numbers with concurrent heart and kidney problems, and the association with a significantly higher mortality ratio. This has led to intense discussions about the value of the recognition of cardiorenal disease on the one hand, and the existence of a specific "cardiorenal syndrome" on the other hand.[1-10]

The idea of specific interaction between heart and kidneys is not new. There are numerous examples and anecdotes that show that people in the past from various societies considered the heart and the kidneys to have a special relationship.

### 1.1 Heart and kidneys in ancient times

The Egyptian "Book of the Dead" (1600-1240 B.C.), which served as a reference work to assist the deceased in the afterlife, is one of the first known texts that mentions the heart and kidneys in parallel:

"*Homage to thee, O my heart! Homage to you, O my kidneys!*".[11]

The heart and the kidneys were the only organs left inside the body during the process of mummification. The heart was weighed against the feather of truth by the jackal-headed Anubis (Figure 1), but the exact role of the kidneys for the passage into afterlife is uncertain. Blood vessels are well preserved in mummies, and there is evidence that cardiovascular disease affecting both the heart and the kidneys were not uncommon.[12]

Eknoyan[13] researched the Bible and found that:

> "[T]he kidneys are mentioned five times in the Bible as the organs examined by God to pass judgment on a person. They are mentioned either before or after but always in parallel with the heart, as for example, "*I, the Lord, search the heart, I try the reins, even to give every man according to his ways, and according to the fruit of his doings*" (Jer. 17:10), and, "*Examine me, O Lord, and prove me; try my reins and my heart*" (Psalms 26:2)."

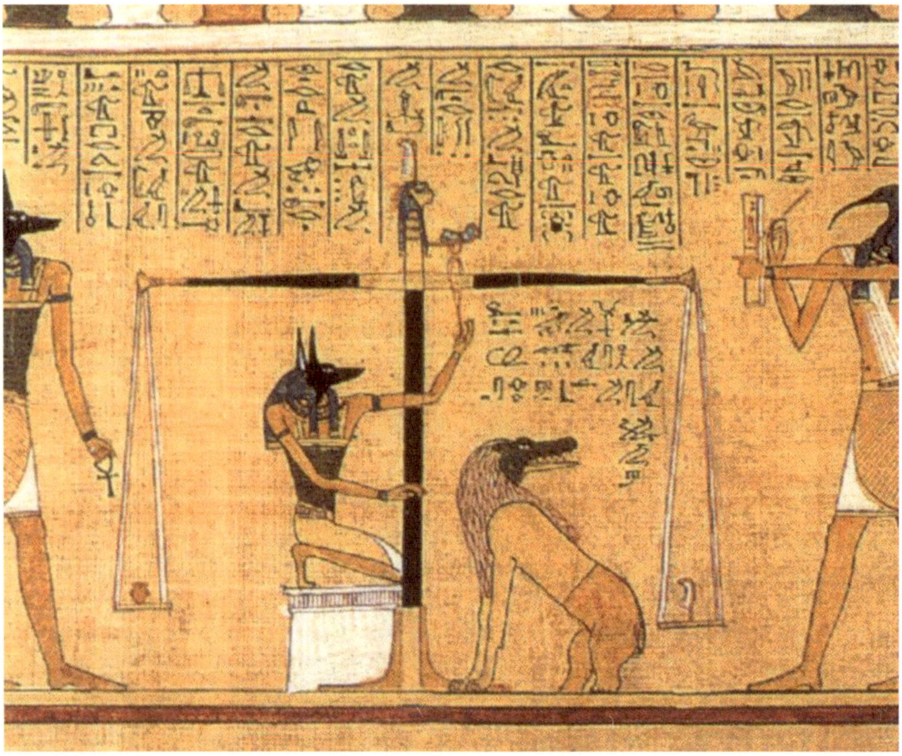

Fig. 1. The weighing of the heart against the feather of truth. This papyrus was found in the tomb of the scribe Hunefer in Thebes. It dates from the 19th Dynasty, about 1285 BC. It can be seen in the British Museum.

In Hebrew lore the kidneys owned the status as the organs which give the heart advice and counsel, and which symbolize the innermost sources of thought and desire, those hardly accessible to man but tested by God.[14]

## 1.2 Heart and kidneys in Traditional Chinese Medicine

No less lyrical, albeit more clinical descriptions are found in China, where the heart and the kidneys are described in various medical texts. In Traditional Chinese Medicine (TCM), the kidney represents water and is considered a 'yin' organ whereas the heart represents fire and is a 'yang' organ.[15] In TCM, the kidney not only regulates the urinary system, but also controls the reproductive, endocrine and nervous system. It stores Jing, which is considered a vital life force responsible for development and reproduction. The heart rules the blood vessels and blood supply to the organs, but also stores the "spirit", reflected in a person's mental, cognitive and intellectual abilities.

Dr. Shen Jin'ao writes in his book "Dr. Shen's Compendium of Honoring Life (*Shen Shi Zunsheng Shu*)" from 1773:

> "The heart resides in the vessels. It rules the kidney network, not via a controlling position in the restraining circle of relationship between the organ networks [where the kidney actually restrains the heart], but simply because it is the general master of all

organ networks. Before the heart fire can harmoniously blend with the kidney water, however, the kidney water must be sufficient. Otherwise the heart fire will flare out of control, and all kinds of heart and kidney ailments will arise."

In the 5 Elements network of Chinese medicine (Figure 2) a disorder called "heart and kidney failing to link" (*xin shen bu jiao*) is presented, resulting in a variety of symptoms ranging from restlessness and palpitations to dizziness, and dark, scanty urination or nocturia.[16] If both kidneys and heart are weakened, there may be palpitations, shortness of breath, dizziness, darken complexion, purple lips and nails, sensitivity to low temperatures, urinary difficulty, edema that is more apparent in the lower limbs, and a bulky tongue. If the kidneys and heart are in disharmony, there may be palpitations, dream-disturbed sleep, forgetfulness, dizziness, thirst, red cheeks, night sweats, lumbar and knee soreness, nocturnal emission, and a red tongue.

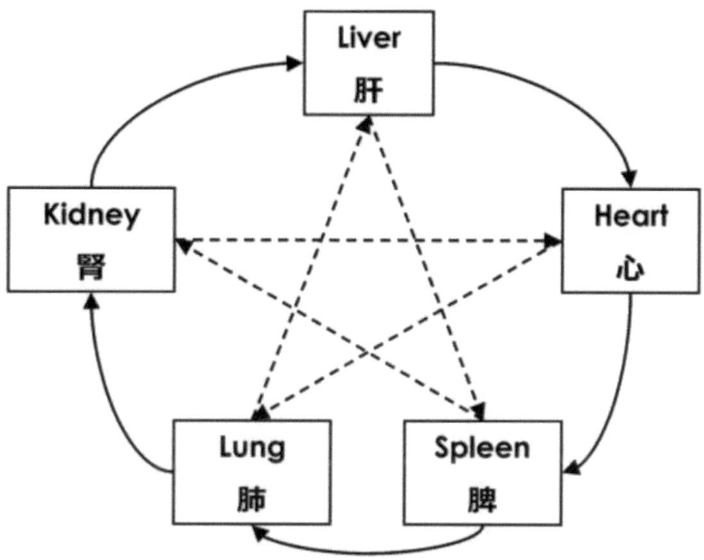


Fig. 2. The Five Elements theory of TCM and the relationships between the organs, with generation (solid arrows) and restriction cycles (dashed arrows).

Another piece of traditional Chinese Medicine text gives a pretty accurate description of the symptoms of cardiorenal failure:

> "When the kidney fails to evaporate fluid which then floods and ascends to depress the function of heart 'yang' there may be clinical manifestations such as oedema, chills and cold limbs, accompanied by palpitations, shortness of breath and stuffiness in the chest, indicating retained water affecting the heart."[17]

### 1.3 Cardiorenal disease in the European Middle Ages

In Western society, during the Middle Ages, heart disease per sé was not very well described in medical doctrines, although the heart was considered the source of the *spiritus vitalis*. Medieval doctors viewed the outward appearance and excretions of the whole body or body parts as a reflection of one's state of health, and as such the symptoms of congestive heart failure were approached as separate clinical entities.[18] The examination of urine was however a widely used diagnostic tool. As one of the first Western "cardio-nephrologists", Gentile da Foligno (Gentilis de Fulgineo; 1272? - 1348) considered heart disease as one of the major inflictions modulating the color and output of urine in his commentary on *De pulsibus* (About Pulses) composed by Aegidius Corboliensis (Figure 3).[19]

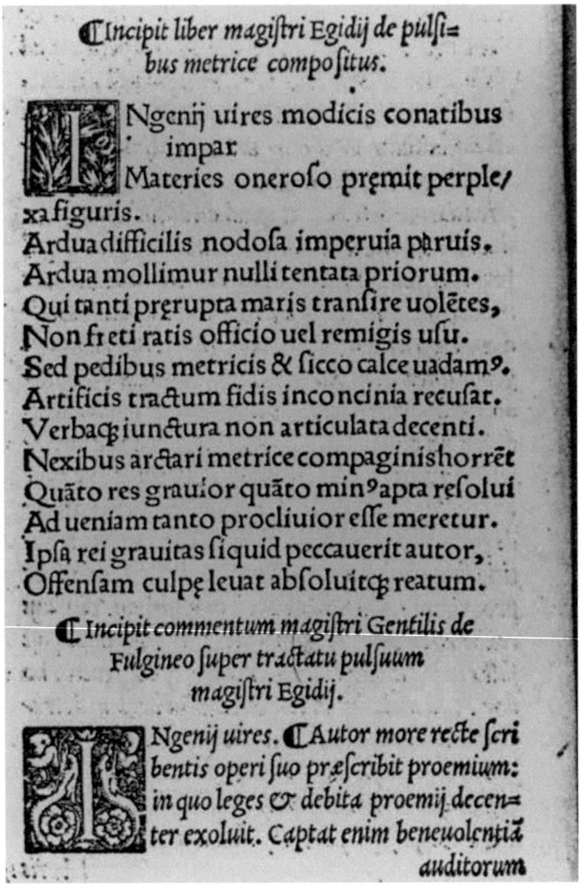

Incipit liber magistri Egidij de pulsibus metrice compositus.

Ingenij uires modicis conatibus impar
Materies oneroso premit perplexa figuris.
Ardua difficilis nodosa impervia paruis.
Ardua mollimur nulli tentata priorum.
Qui tanti prerupta maris transire uoletes,
Non freti ratis officio uel remigis usu.
Sed pedibus metricis & sicco calce uadamus.
Artificis tractum fidis inconcinia recusat.
Verbaqz iunctura non articulata decenti.
Nexibus arctari metrice compaginis horret
Quato res grauior quato min9 apta resolui
Ad ueniam tanto procliuior esse meretur.
Ipsa rei grauitas siquid peccauerit autor,
Offensam culpe leuat absoluitqz reatum.

Incipit commentum magistri Gentilis de Fulgineo super tractatu pulsuum magistri Egidij.

Ngenij uires. Autor more recte scribentis operi suo prescribit proemium: in quo leges & debita proemij decenter exoluit. Captat enim beneuolentiã auditorum

Fig. 3. First page of *De pulsibus*. Town Library, Foligno. Reproduced from ref. [19].

### 1.4 Heart-kidney interactions in the late 19$^{th}$ and early 20$^{th}$ century

During the Industrial Revolution the medical sciences expanded and scientific methods became more and more reliant on experiments and observation. Richard Bright (1789–1858) and Ludwig Traube (1818–1876) both documented that cardiac hypertrophy was a common anomaly resulting from chronic renal disease.[20, 21] Traube refers in his writings to William Senhouse Kirkes (1822 - 1864) who reviewed 14 autopsy cases of with apoplexy and diseased kidneys, of which only one did not have an enlarged heart (Figure 4).[22] He concludes that:

> "... I believe that the affection of the kidneys is the primary disease... [it] has among its most frequent and permanent accompaniments an hypertrophied condition of the left

ventricle ... of the various explanations of this pathological fact the most probable perhaps is that which regards the blood as so far altered from its normal constitution ... as to move with less facility through the systemic capillaries, and thus to require increased pressure, and consequently increased growth of the left ventricle, to effect its transmission."

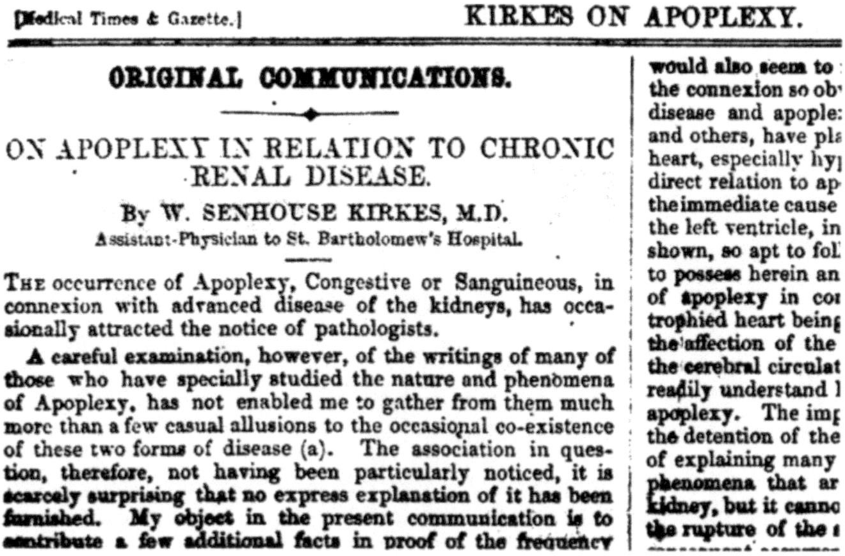

[Medical Times & Gazette.] KIRKES ON APOPLEXY.

ORIGINAL COMMUNICATIONS.

ON APOPLEXY IN RELATION TO CHRONIC RENAL DISEASE.

By W. SENHOUSE KIRKES, M.D.
Assistant-Physician to St. Bartholomew's Hospital.

The occurrence of Apoplexy, Congestive or Sanguineous, in connexion with advanced disease of the kidneys, has occasionally attracted the notice of pathologists.

A careful examination, however, of the writings of many of those who have specially studied the nature and phenomena of Apoplexy, has not enabled me to gather from them much more than a few casual allusions to the occasional co-existence of these two forms of disease (a). The association in question, therefore, not having been particularly noticed, it is scarcely surprising that no express explanation of it has been furnished. My object in the present communication is to contribute a few additional facts in proof of the frequency

would also seem to the connexion so ob disease and apople and others, have pl heart, especially hy direct relation to ap the immediate cause the left ventricle, in shown, so apt to fol to possess herein an of apoplexy in co trophied heart being the affection of the the cerebral circulat readily understand apoplexy. The im the detention of the of explaining many phenomena that ar kidney, but it canno the rupture of the

Fig. 4. Beginning of Kirkes' publication in the Medical Times & Gazette, 1855.

In a lecture delivered at the University College in London in 1913, Thomas Lewis[23] speaks about "paroxysmal dyspnoea in cardio-renal patients" and after a very interesting review of the clinical and pathological findings of multiple cases, he concludes:

> "We come to this standpoint-that the clinical or anatomical distinction between cardiac and renal asthma, is no certain one. Asthma occurring, in patients who show on the one hand prominent cardiac lesions, on the other hand prominent renal lesions, may or may not be due to a single cause."

Alfred Stengel[24] proposed a definition of "cardio-renal disease" (Figure 5) when he wrote in 1914:

> "The clinician encounters many cases, mainly in persons of middle age or older, in which evidences of cardiac weakness and other circulatory disturbances, such as high pressure, are associated with signs of failure of renal function or urinary indications of renal disease. When this combination of symptoms is of such character that the observer cannot readily assign to either the cardiovascular system or to the kidneys the preponderance of responsibility, the term "cardio-renal disease" is often employed. The term, therefore, comprises cases of combined cardiovascular and renal disease without such manifest predominance of either as to justify a prompt determination of the one element as primary and important and the other as secondary and unimportant."

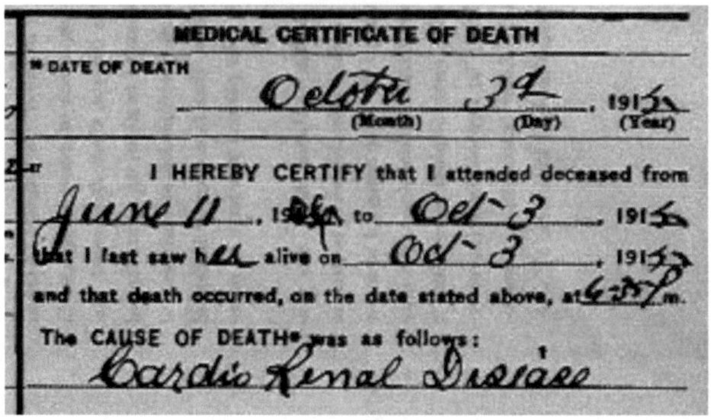
MEDICAL CERTIFICATE OF DEATH

DATE OF DEATH October 3, 1915 (Month) (Day) (Year)

I HEREBY CERTIFY that I attended deceased from June 11, 19 to Oct 3 1915

that I last saw her alive on Oct 3, 1915

and that death occurred, on the date stated above, at m.

The CAUSE OF DEATH was as follows:

Cardio Renal Disease

Fig. 5. Example from a 1915 Death Certificate from Massachusetts. From Rudy's List of Archaic Medical Terms at http://www.antiquusmorbus.com/English/Heart Stroke.htm

The observations on the cardiac consequences of chronic kidney disease were later expanded, and Gouley[25] was coined the term "uremic myocardiopathy" in 1940 and in 1944 Raab[26] proposed that cardiotoxic substances accumulate in uremia. Rössle,[27] and Langendorf and Pirani[28] later showed that interstitial widening and fibrosis were common in hearts of patients dying from uremia.

### 1.5 The Cardiorenal Syndrome in modern times

The advent of the Cimino-shunt and the development of hemodialysis (HD) as the mainstay treatment for end-stage renal disease (ESRD) resulted in further increasing interest in the structural and functional cardiac status of HD patients.[29-32] The full extent of the problem of cardiovascular disease in chronic kidney disease (CKD) and ESRD patients was then charted in the 1990's, showing that a large proportion of patients starting dialysis already suffers from cardiac abnormalities and dysfunction and that survival of these patients after a myocardial infarction (MI) was dismal.[33-35] In 2003, a statement from several councils from the American Heart Association (AHA) was published in Hypertension and Circulation underscoring the problem of increased cardiovascular risk in CKD, and the lack of knowledge on pathophysiology.[36] This was followed by two seminal papers published in the New England Journal of Medicine showing the exponentially increased risk for adverse outcome with decreasing kidney function, in "normal" patients but even more so after they had experienced a myocardial infarction.[37, 38] At the same time, the scientific and clinical community became increasingly aware of the effect of decreased kidney function or kidney damage on the prognosis of patients with heart failure.[39-41] Interestingly, in a study on the predictive value of 10 different biomarkers in over 3000 patients from the Framingham Heart Study, levels of brain natriuretic peptide and urinary albumin-to-creatinine ratio most strongly predicted major cardiovascular events.[42] One patient study even suggested that the decline of renal function is accelerated after an acute MI.[43] These epidemiological associations resulted in a strong clinical suspicion that the combination of heart and kidney disease is associated with accelerated disease progression and adverse outcome.

## 2. The Severe Cardiorenal Syndrome and the Cardiorenal Connection

The epidemiological data, the AHA statement, and our own clinical observations of cardiorenal failure in patients led us to propose the "Severe Cardiorenal Syndrome" (SCRS)

as a separate disease entity with the "Cardiorenal Connection" (CRC) as the putative pathophysiological model.[44] We defined the SCRS as a condition in which combined cardiac and renal dysfunction amplifies progression of failure of the individual organ, leading to grossly increased cardiovascular morbidity and mortality. The CRC works in conjunction with the hemodynamic control model of heart-kidney interactions as stipulated by the late professor Guyton (Figure 6).

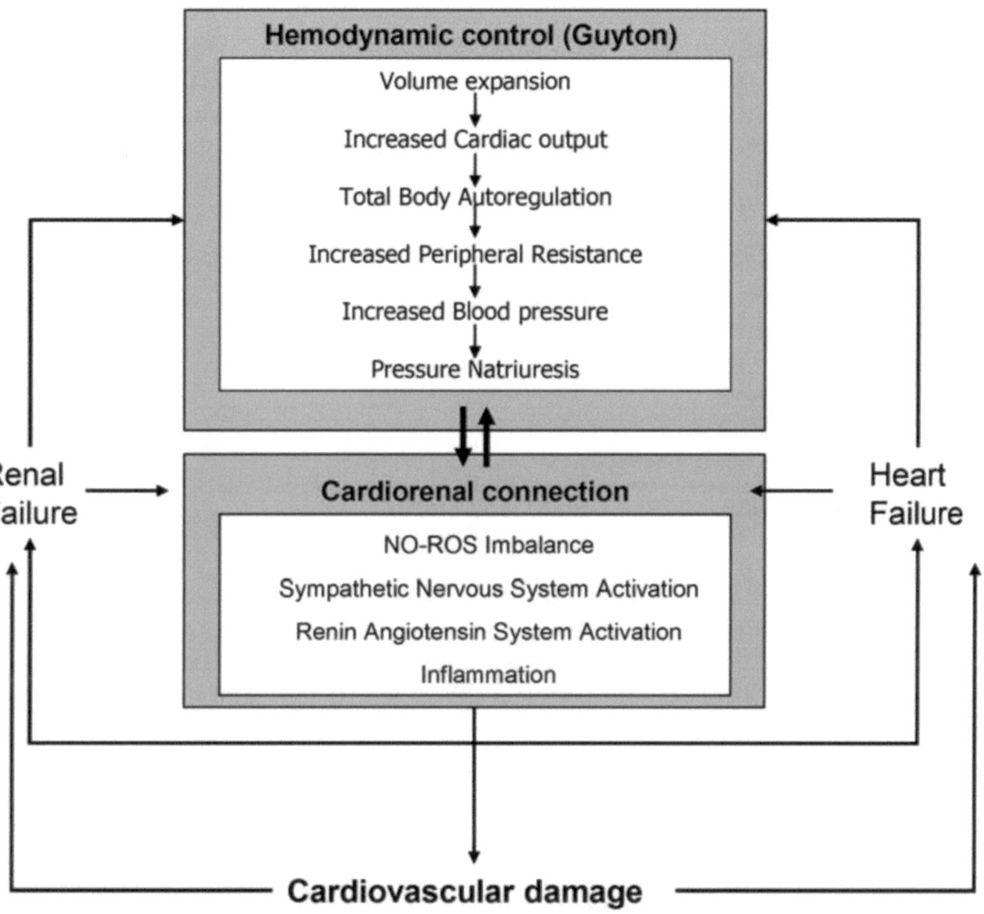


Fig. 6. The cardiorenal connection works extensive to Guyton's model to drive accelerated cardiovascular damage in combined renal and heart failure.

The "cardiorenal connectors" that we put forward were:

- the balance between nitric oxide (NO) and reactive oxygen species (ROS),
- the sympathetic nervous system (SNS)
- the renin-angiotensin system (RAS), and
- inflammation.

We envisioned that both heart and renal failure lead to derangement of the Guytonian model of hemodynamic control, but also results in activation/disturbance of the connectors of the CRC. The connectors have a modulating effect on hemodynamic control but can also induce cardiovascular damage, thereby mediating further functional deterioration.[44] We proposed that activation of the CRC leads to a vicious cycle in which all the connectors become disturbed, synergize and further activate each other. This ultimately results in worsening of both cardiac and renal damage and failure.

### 2.1 Summary of the Cardiorenal Connection

A shift in the balance between NO and ROS towards ROS is a central event in many cardiovascular diseases.[45] In the SCRS, the balance between NO and the ROS is skewed towards the latter by increased production of ROS, a low anti-oxidant status, and lower availability of NO.[46] In the cardiorenal connection, this imbalance may influence sympathetic nervous activity,[47] release of renin and angiotensin,[48] and promote inflammation by oxidative modification of substances.[49]

Sympathetic nervous activity is also increased in both renal and heart failure. By affecting the other cardiorenal connectors it can play a significant role in the SCRS. It stimulates renin release from the kidneys,[50] generates ROS which induces vascular wall growth,[51] and induces inflammation.[52]

The RAS is activated in both renal and heart failure [53, 54] and angiotensin II affects the other cardiorenal connectors in different ways. It activates the SNS in both heart and kidney failure,[55, 56] it generates ROS via nicotinamide adenine dinucleotide phosphate (NADPH)-oxidase,[57] and activates pro-inflammatory gene expression via nuclear factor-κB.[58]

Persistent inflammation has been found in both renal and heart failure. By altering the functioning of the RAS,[59] and promoting ROS[60] and noradrenaline formation,[61] inflammation can contribute to the positive feedback loops in the cardiorenal connection. The Severe Cardiorenal Syndrome is thus not a syndrome in which cardiac and renal failure simply co-exist side-by-side. Cardiac and renal failure are intimately linked by the cardiorenal connectors, because failure of either organ can excite the cardiorenal connectors, but the connectors themselves also affect the structure and function of both organs. Logically, the cardiorenal connectors become more pronounced in combined failure.[6]

## 3. Previous research on the cardiorenal interactions

In a recent comprehensive review in *Circulation,* Bock and Gottlieb[10] state that:

> "...each dysfunctional organ has the ability to initiate and perpetuate disease in the other organ through common hemodynamic, neurohormonal, and immunological/ biochemical pathways." They also write: "...our understanding of the complex physiological, biochemical, and hormonal derangements that encompass the CRS is woefully deficient...".

Despite general acknowledgement of the adverse prognosis of concurrent cardiac and renal disease, many clinicians and researchers are skeptical about the true existence of a specific heart-kidney interaction that goes beyond known physiological interactions. Thus the question was raised whether kidney disease and heart disease simply co-exist or that they indeed worsen each others progression. Clinical studies can not provide the answer to this question because they are observational, lack histological end-points, and are confounded by selection bias, inconsistent definition of end-points, and medication use. Therefore, further exploration of the mechanisms of cardiorenal interactions must rely on animal studies, in which timing and severity of the disease are controlled, progression of disease can be followed, and histological end-points are assessed.

Much of what we know today on the structural cardiac consequences of chronic kidney disease results from the extensive research in rats with CKD by the group of Kerstin Amann and Eberhard Ritz in the late 80's and early 90's.[62] Despite numerous cardiac changes, in the rat CKD model of subtotal (5/6$^{th}$) nephrectomy (SNX) cardiac systolic function is generally maintained.[63, 64] Conversely, after MI by ligation of the left coronary artery in rats, renal histological damage or proteinuria is absent although glomerular filtration rate (GFR) may be decreased.[65, 66] Thus, it appears that both organs need to be affected to cause acceleration of damage and failure typical for the CRS. Only two animal studies investigated the effect of 'dual damage' to heart and kidneys, with MI following shortly after a renal insult in rats, with conflicting results.[65, 67] Different models of nephrectomy exist in mice, but these are not as robust as those in rats, with variable changes in renal function and cardiac abnormalities.[68-72]

The renal hemodynamic response to heart failure (HF) induced by pacing in dogs has also been investigated,[73-75] but whether there is histological damage is unknown. Furthermore, there is no proven model of CKD in dogs. Taken together, there is still a paucity of models that investigate the interaction between kidney and heart failure in a chronic set-up with integrated physiological and histological assessment. From the available data, combining the SNX model of CKD and the coronary ligation model of HF appears to be the most robust option to investigate the SCRS.

### 3.1 The role of nitric oxide in the Severe Cardiorenal Syndrome

We developed a model of the SCRS based on CKD and depletion of NO availability. The rationale for these investigations was that the pathogenesis of CKD (in the presence of hypertension, diabetes or aging) is associated with low NO availability,[76,77] while experimental SNX induces nephron number reduction in a healthy animal. Furthermore, in SNX, cardiac systolic function generally remains preserved, while in patients left ventricular dysfunction (LVSD) develops during the course of CKD progression.[78]

Reduced NO availability is considered a hallmark of CKD.[46, 79] NO can function as an effector of the CRC by way of its vasodilatory action. It also modulates GFR and tubulo-glomerular feedback.[80] Reduced NO availability will result in tissue damage by oxidative stress. In extension to our proposal of the Cardiorenal Connection,[44] we postulated that the balance between NO and ROS is a key modulator of the other cardiorenal connectors.[81] Many effects of the other CRCs may be mediated by changes in the redox-balance and NO availability.[82, 83]

Also, it has been shown that constitutive NO production supports basal cardiac function.[84] Apart from its role in endothelial dysfunction, NO availability also modulates cardiac contractility, as NO synthase (NOS) inhibition reduces cardiac output, and causes cardiac damage in high doses.[85, 86]

We thus hypothesized that a reduction in NO availability would accelerate the development of cardiac dysfunction. Indeed, treatment with an oral NO synthase (NOS) inhibitor (L-NNA), at a very low dose, induced NO depletion and severe cardiac dysfunction.[87] Furthermore, proteinuria, severe glomerulosclerosis and cardiac interstitial fibrosis were worsened compared to rats with CKD without NOS inhibition. Another remarkable finding was that the effects on cardiorenal dysfunction but also on systemic NO production were irreversible after cessation of the NOS inhibitor, during a 7 week follow-up. A five times higher dose of NOS inhibition in control rats, which caused a similar level of hypertension and NO depletion, induced LVSD that was not as severe as in the CRS rats. Furthermore, all effects on blood pressure, cardiac function and NO availability were completely reversible, and had no effect on kidney structure and function. Combining NOS inhibition with SNX also, worsened kidney injury. The more severe hypertension and direct effects of NOS inhibition may have played a role in this.

We concluded that during CKD development the heart is very sensitive to depression of systemic NO availability. Compared to the normal kidney, the damaged kidney is more sensitive to alterations of NO availability as well, possibly because of a loss of autoregulation.[88] Thus, maintaining adequate NO availability appears to be very important for progression of cardiorenal failure during progression of CKD, and the combination of CKD and NO depletion appears to produce a functional model of the SCRS in which cardiac function is further compromised.

That supplementation of NO is useful as a rescue therapy was shown in a subsequent study, where treatment with the oral tolerance-free NO donor molsidomine (MOLS) significantly improved cardiac diastolic and systolic function, abrogated mortality, and also slightly improved kidney function and injury.[89] The cardiac effect of MOLS appeared to be a combination of reduced cardiac loading and improved contractility and relaxation. Systolic blood pressure was only mildly reduced and GFR was even slightly improved. Thus, MOLS appears to be an attractive and safe therapeutic option for CKD patients suffering from cardiac dysfunction of non-ischemic origin. The pathophysiology of the continuing low NO production in this model is likely very complex and may include low NOS expression or activity, substrate deficiency, high oxidative stress levels, and increased amounts of endogenous NOS inhibitors.[79]

In conclusion, the cardiorenal connection has intrigued scientists and physicians for centuries. The existence of a specific cardiorenal syndrome has been suggested since the start of the 20$^{th}$ century, but has recently gained widespread attention in the scientific literature. We proposed the Severe Cardiorenal Syndrome, in which CKD and HF induce derangements to cause a vicious cycle of cardiovascular damage and progression of failure of both organs. Understanding of pathophysiological mechanisms is expanding and animal models provide an invaluable tool to investigate the bidirectional nature of cardiorenal interactions.

## 4. References

[1] Parfrey PS, Harnett JD, Barre PE. The natural history of myocardial disease in dialysis patients. *J Am Soc Nephrol* 1991;2:2-12.

[2] Parfrey PS, Foley RN, Harnett JD, Kent GM, Murray DC, Barre PE. Outcome and risk factors for left ventricular disorders in chronic uraemia. *Nephrol Dial Transplant* 1996;11:1277-1285.
[3] Isles C. Cardiorenal failure: pathophysiology, recognition and treatment. *Clin Med* 2002;2:195-200.
[4] Zoccali C. Cardiorenal risk as a new frontier of nephrology: research needs and areas for intervention. *Nephrol Dial Transplant* 2002;17 Suppl 11:50-54.
[5] Shlipak MG, Massie BM. The clinical challenge of cardiorenal syndrome. *Circulation* 2004;110:1514-1517.
[6] Bongartz LG, Cramer MJ, Doevendans PA, Joles JA, Braam B. The severe cardiorenal syndrome: 'Guyton revisited'. *Eur Heart J* 2005;26:11-17.
[7] Schrier RW. Cardiorenal versus renocardiac syndrome: is there a difference? *Nat Clin Pract Nephrol* 2007;3:637.
[8] Ronco C. Cardiorenal and renocardiac syndromes: clinical disorders in search of a systematic definition. *Int J Artif Organs* 2008;31:1-2.
[9] van der Putten K, Bongartz LG, Braam B, Gaillard CA. The cardiorenal syndrome a classification into 4 groups? *J Am Coll Cardiol* 2009;53:1340; author reply 1340-1341.
[10] Bock JS, Gottlieb SS. Cardiorenal syndrome: new perspectives. *Circulation* 2010;121:2592-2600.
[11] Wallis Budge EA. The Egyptian Book of the Dead. The Papyrus of Ani. New York: Dover Publications Inc., 1967.
[12] Salem ME, Eknoyan G. The kidney in ancient Egyptian medicine: where does it stand? *Am J Nephrol* 1999;19:140-147.
[13] Eknoyan G. The kidneys in the Bible: what happened? *J Am Soc Nephrol* 2005;16:3464-3471.
[14] Kottek SS. "The kidneys give advice": some thoughts on nephrology in the Talmud and Midrash. *Korot* 1993;10:44-53.
[15] http://www.shen-nong.com/eng/front/index.html
[16] http://www.itmonline.org/5organs/heart.htm
[17] Lajoie G, Laszik Z, Nadasdy T, Silva FG. The renal-cardiac connection: renal parenchymal alterations in patients with heart disease. *Semin Nephrol* 1994;14:441-463.
[18] Jarcho S. The Concept of Heart Failure from Avicenna to Albertini. Cambridge: Harvard University Press, 1980.
[19] Timio M. Gentile da Foligno, a pioneer of cardionephrology: commentary on Carmina de urinarum iudiciis and De pulsibus. *Am J Nephrol* 1999;19:189-192.
[20] Traube L. Über den Zusammenhang von Herz- und Nierenkrankheiten. Berlin: August Hirschwald, 1856.
[21] Bright R. Cases and observations, illustrative of renal disease accompanied with the secretion of albuminous urine. *Guy's Hospital Reports* 1836;1:338-379.
[22] Kirkes WS. On apoplexy in relation to chronic renal disease. *Med Times Gaz* 1855;24:515-517.
[23] Lewis T. A Clinical Lecture ON PAROXYSMAL DYSPNOEA IN CARDIORENAL PATIENTS: WITH SPECIAL REFERENCE TO "CARDIAC" AND "URAEMIC"

ASTHMA: Delivered at University College Hospital, London, November 12th, 1913. *Br Med J* 1913;2:1417-1420.
[24] Stengel A. Cardiorenal disease: The clinical determination of cardiovascular and renal responsibility, respectively, in its disturbances. *J Am Med Assoc* 1914;LXIII:1463-1469.
[25] Gouley BA. The Myocadial Degeneration Associated With Uremia in Advanced Hypertensive Disease and Chrinic Glomerular Nephritis. *Am J Med Sci* 1940;200:39-49.
[26] Raab W. Cardiotoxic substances in the blood and heart muscle in uremia (their nature and action). *J Lab Clin Med* 1944;29:715-734.
[27] Rössle H. Über die seröse Entzündung der Organe. *Virchows Archiv* 1943; 311:252-284.
[28] Langendorf R, Pirani CL. The heart in uremia , , : An electrocardiographic and pathologic study. *American Heart Journal* 1947;33:282-307.
[29] Lindner A, Charra B, Sherrard DJ, Scribner BH. Accelerated atherosclerosis in prolonged maintenance hemodialysis. *N Engl J Med* 1974;290:697-701.
[30] Drueke T, Le Pailleur C, Meilhac B, Koutoudis C, Zingraff J, Di Matteo J, *et al.* Congestive cardiomyopathy in uraemic patients on long term haemodialysis. *Br Med J* 1977;1:350-353.
[31] Mir MA, Hearn DC. Cardiac function in renal failure. *Ann Intern Med* 1977;87:495.
[32] Hung J, Harris PJ, Uren RF, Tiller DJ, Kelly DT. Uremic Cardiomyopathy — Effect of Hemodialysis on Left Ventricular Function in End-Stage Renal Failure. *New England Journal of Medicine* 1980;302:547-551.
[33] Foley RN, Parfrey PS, Harnett JD, Kent GM, Martin CJ, Murray DC, *et al.* Clinical and echocardiographic disease in patients starting end-stage renal disease therapy. *Kidney Int* 1995;47:186-192.
[34] Harnett JD, Foley RN, Kent GM, Barre PE, Murray D, Parfrey PS. Congestive heart failure in dialysis patients: prevalence, incidence, prognosis and risk factors. *Kidney Int* 1995;47:884-890.
[35] Herzog CA, Ma JZ, Collins AJ. Poor long-term survival after acute myocardial infarction among patients on long-term dialysis. *N Engl J Med* 1998;339:799-805.
[36] Sarnak MJ, Levey AS, Schoolwerth AC, Coresh J, Culleton B, Hamm LL, *et al.* Kidney disease as a risk factor for development of cardiovascular disease: a statement from the American Heart Association Councils on Kidney in Cardiovascular Disease, High Blood Pressure Research, Clinical Cardiology, and Epidemiology and Prevention. *Circulation* 2003;108:2154-2169.
[37] Anavekar NS, McMurray JJ, Velazquez EJ, Solomon SD, Kober L, Rouleau JL, *et al.* Relation between renal dysfunction and cardiovascular outcomes after myocardial infarction. *N Engl J Med* 2004;351:1285-1295.
[38] Go AS, Chertow GM, Fan D, McCulloch CE, Hsu CY. Chronic kidney disease and the risks of death, cardiovascular events, and hospitalization. *N Engl J Med* 2004;351:1296-1305.
[39] Dries DL, Exner DV, Domanski MJ, Greenberg B, Stevenson LW. The prognostic implications of renal insufficiency in asymptomatic and symptomatic patients with left ventricular systolic dysfunction. *J Am Coll Cardiol* 2000;35:681-689.

[40] Hillege HL, Girbes AR, de Kam PJ, Boomsma F, de Zeeuw D, Charlesworth A, *et al.* Renal function, neurohormonal activation, and survival in patients with chronic heart failure. *Circulation* 2000;102:203-210.

[41] McAlister FA, Ezekowitz J, Tonelli M, Armstrong PW. Renal insufficiency and heart failure: prognostic and therapeutic implications from a prospective cohort study. *Circulation* 2004;109:1004-1009.

[42] Wang TJ, Gona P, Larson MG, Tofler GH, Levy D, Newton-Cheh C, *et al.* Multiple biomarkers for the prediction of first major cardiovascular events and death. *N Engl J Med* 2006;355:2631-2639.

[43] Hillege HL, van Gilst WH, van Veldhuisen DJ, Navis G, Grobbee DE, de Graeff PA, *et al.* Accelerated decline and prognostic impact of renal function after myocardial infarction and the benefits of ACE inhibition: the CATS randomized trial. *Eur Heart J* 2003;24:412-420.

[44] Bongartz LG, Cramer MJ, Braam B. The cardiorenal connection. *Hypertension* 2004;43:e14.

[45] Cai H, Harrison DG. Endothelial dysfunction in cardiovascular diseases: the role of oxidant stress. *Circ Res* 2000;87:840-844.

[46] Himmelfarb J, Stenvinkel P, Ikizler TA, Hakim RM. The elephant in uremia: oxidant stress as a unifying concept of cardiovascular disease in uremia. *Kidney Int* 2002;62:1524-1538.

[47] Lin HH, Chen CH, Hsieh WK, Chiu TH, Lai CC. Hydrogen peroxide increases the activity of rat sympathetic preganglionic neurons in vivo and in vitro. *Neuroscience* 2003;121:641-647.

[48] Katoh M, Egashira K, Usui M, Ichiki T, Tomita H, Shimokawa H, *et al.* Cardiac angiotensin II receptors are upregulated by long-term inhibition of nitric oxide synthesis in rats. *Circ Res* 1998;83:743-751.

[49] Witko-Sarsat V, Friedlander M, Nguyen Khoa T, Capeillere-Blandin C, Nguyen AT, Canteloup S, *et al.* Advanced oxidation protein products as novel mediators of inflammation and monocyte activation in chronic renal failure. *J Immunol* 1998;161:2524-2532.

[50] Reid IA. Interactions between ANG II, sympathetic nervous system, and baroreceptor reflexes in regulation of blood pressure. *Am J Physiol* 1992;262:E763-778.

[51] Bleeke T, Zhang H, Madamanchi N, Patterson C, Faber JE. Catecholamine-induced vascular wall growth is dependent on generation of reactive oxygen species. *Circ Res* 2004;94:37-45.

[52] Prabhu SD, Chandrasekar B, Murray DR, Freeman GL. beta-adrenergic blockade in developing heart failure: effects on myocardial inflammatory cytokines, nitric oxide, and remodeling. *Circulation* 2000;101:2103-2109.

[53] Brewster UC, Perazella MA. The renin-angiotensin-aldosterone system and the kidney: effects on kidney disease. *Am J Med* 2004;116:263-272.

[54] Schrier RW, Abraham WT. Hormones and hemodynamics in heart failure. *N Engl J Med* 1999;341:577-585.

[55] Ligtenberg G, Blankestijn PJ, Oey PL, Klein IH, Dijkhorst-Oei LT, Boomsma F, *et al.* Reduction of sympathetic hyperactivity by enalapril in patients with chronic renal failure. *N Engl J Med* 1999;340:1321-1328.

[56] Zhang W, Huang BS, Leenen FH. Brain renin-angiotensin system and sympathetic hyperactivity in rats after myocardial infarction. *Am J Physiol* 1999;276:H1608-1615.

[57] Griendling KK, Minieri CA, Ollerenshaw JD, Alexander RW. Angiotensin II stimulates NADH and NADPH oxidase activity in cultured vascular smooth muscle cells. *Circ Res* 1994;74:1141-1148.

[58] Pueyo ME, Gonzalez W, Nicoletti A, Savoie F, Arnal JF, Michel JB. Angiotensin II stimulates endothelial vascular cell adhesion molecule-1 via nuclear factor-kappaB activation induced by intracellular oxidative stress. *Arterioscler Thromb Vasc Biol* 2000;20:645-651.

[59] Wassmann S, Stumpf M, Strehlow K, Schmid A, Schieffer B, Bohm M, *et al.* Interleukin-6 induces oxidative stress and endothelial dysfunction by overexpression of the angiotensin II type 1 receptor. *Circ Res* 2004;94:534-541.

[60] Ward RA, McLeish KR. Polymorphonuclear leukocyte oxidative burst is enhanced in patients with chronic renal insufficiency. *J Am Soc Nephrol* 1995;5:1697-1702.

[61] Niijima A, Hori T, Aou S, Oomura Y. The effects of interleukin-1 beta on the activity of adrenal, splenic and renal sympathetic nerves in the rat. *J Auton Nerv Syst* 1991;36:183-192.

[62] Amann K, Ritz E. Structural basis of cardiovascular dysfunction in uremia. In: Loscalzo J, London GM, eds. Cardiovascular disease in end-stage renal failure, Oxford clinical nephrology series. Oxford ; New York: Oxford University Press, 2000:xiii, 495 p.

[63] Reddy V, Bhandari S, Seymour AM. Myocardial function, energy provision, and carnitine deficiency in experimental uremia. *J Am Soc Nephrol* 2007;18:84-92.

[64] Tian J, Shidyak A, Periyasamy SM, Haller S, Taleb M, El-Okdi N, *et al.* Spironolactone attenuates experimental uremic cardiomyopathy by antagonizing marinobufagenin. *Hypertension* 2009;54:1313-1320.

[65] van Dokkum RP, Eijkelkamp WB, Kluppel AC, Henning RH, van Goor H, Citgez M, *et al.* Myocardial infarction enhances progressive renal damage in an experimental model for cardio-renal interaction. *J Am Soc Nephrol* 2004;15:3103-3110.

[66] Bauersachs J, Braun C, Fraccarollo D, Widder J, Ertl G, Schilling L, *et al.* Improvement of renal dysfunction in rats with chronic heart failure after myocardial infarction by treatment with the endothelin A receptor antagonist, LU 135252. *J Hypertens* 2000;18:1507-1514.

[67] Windt WA, Henning RH, Kluppel AC, Xu Y, de Zeeuw D, van Dokkum RP. Myocardial infarction does not further impair renal damage in 5/6 nephrectomized rats. *Nephrol Dial Transplant* 2008;23:3103-3110.

[68] Kennedy DJ, Elkareh J, Shidyak A, Shapiro AP, Smaili S, Mutgi K, *et al.* Partial nephrectomy as a model for uremic cardiomyopathy in the mouse. *Am J Physiol Renal Physiol* 2008;294:F450-454.

[69] Siedlecki AM, Jin X, Muslin AJ. Uremic cardiac hypertrophy is reversed by rapamycin but not by lowering of blood pressure. *Kidney Int* 2009;75:800-808.

[70] Li Y, Takemura G, Okada H, Miyata S, Maruyama R, Esaki M, *et al.* Molecular signaling mediated by angiotensin II type 1A receptor blockade leading to attenuation of renal dysfunction-associated heart failure. *J Card Fail* 2007;13:155-162.

[71] Baumann M, Leineweber K, Tewiele M, Wu K, Turk TR, Su S, *et al.* Imatinib ameliorates fibrosis in uraemic cardiac disease in BALB/c without improving cardiac function. *Nephrol Dial Transplant* 2010;25:1817-1824.

[72] Bro S, Bollano E, Bruel A, Olgaard K, Nielsen LB. Cardiac structure and function in a mouse model of uraemia without hypertension. *Scand J Clin Lab Invest* 2008;68:660-666.

[73] Chen HH, Schirger JA, Chau WL, Jougasaki M, Lisy O, Redfield MM, *et al.* Renal response to acute neutral endopeptidase inhibition in mild and severe experimental heart failure. *Circulation* 1999;100:2443-2448.

[74] Martin FL, Stevens TL, Cataliotti A, Schirger JA, Borgeson DD, Redfield MM, *et al.* Natriuretic and antialdosterone actions of chronic oral NEP inhibition during progressive congestive heart failure. *Kidney Int* 2005;67:1723-1730.

[75] Martin FL, Supaporn T, Chen HH, Sandberg SM, Matsuda Y, Jougasaki M, *et al.* Distinct roles for renal particulate and soluble guanylyl cyclases in preserving renal function in experimental acute heart failure. *Am J Physiol Regul Integr Comp Physiol* 2007;293:R1580-1585.

[76] Blum M, Yachnin T, Wollman Y, Chernihovsky T, Peer G, Grosskopf I, *et al.* Low nitric oxide production in patients with chronic renal failure. *Nephron* 1998;79:265-268.

[77] Wever R, Boer P, Hijmering M, Stroes E, Verhaar M, Kastelein J, *et al.* Nitric oxide production is reduced in patients with chronic renal failure. *Arterioscler Thromb Vasc Biol* 1999;19:1168-1172.

[78] Kennedy DJ, Vetteth S, Periyasamy SM, Kanj M, Fedorova L, Khouri S, *et al.* Central role for the cardiotonic steroid marinobufagenin in the pathogenesis of experimental uremic cardiomyopathy. *Hypertension* 2006;47:488-495.

[79] Baylis C. Nitric oxide deficiency in chronic kidney disease. *Am J Physiol Renal Physiol* 2008;294:F1-9.

[80] Braam B. Renal endothelial and macula densa NOS: integrated response to changes in extracellular fluid volume. *Am J Physiol* 1999;276:R1551-1561.

[81] Jie KE, Verhaar MC, Cramer MJ, van der Putten K, Gaillard CA, Doevendans PA, *et al.* Erythropoietin and the cardiorenal syndrome: cellular mechanisms on the cardiorenal connectors. *Am J Physiol Renal Physiol* 2006;291:F932-944.

[82] Toledano MB, Leonard WJ. Modulation of transcription factor NF-kappa B binding activity by oxidation-reduction in vitro. *Proc Natl Acad Sci U S A* 1991;88:4328-4332.

[83] Cappola TP, Cope L, Cernetich A, Barouch LA, Minhas K, Irizarry RA, *et al.* Deficiency of different nitric oxide synthase isoforms activates divergent transcriptional programs in cardiac hypertrophy. *Physiol Genomics* 2003;14:25-34.

[84] Kojda G, Kottenberg K. Regulation of basal myocardial function by NO. *Cardiovasc Res* 1999;41:514-523.

[85] Klabunde RE, Ritger RC, Helgren MC. Cardiovascular actions of inhibitors of endothelium-derived relaxing factor (nitric oxide) formation/release in anesthetized dogs. *Eur J Pharmacol* 1991;199:51-59.

[86] Matsubara BB, Matsubara LS, Zornoff LA, Franco M, Janicki JS. Left ventricular adaptation to chronic pressure overload induced by inhibition of nitric oxide synthase in rats. *Basic Res Cardiol* 1998;93:173-181.

[87] Bongartz LG, Braam B, Verhaar MC, Cramer MJ, Goldschmeding R, Gaillard CA,Doevendans PA, Joles JA. Transient nitric oxide reduction induces permanent cardiac systolic dysfunction and worsens kidney damage in rats with chronic kidney disease. *Am J Physiol Regul Integr Comp Physiol* 2010;298:R815-R823.

[88] Bidani AK, Schwartz MM, Lewis EJ. Renal autoregulation and vulnerability to hypertensive injury in remnant kidney. *Am J Physiol* 1987;252:F1003-1010.

[89] Bongartz LG, Braam B, Verhaar MC, Cramer MJ, Goldschmeding R, Gaillard CA, *et al.* The Nitric Oxide Donor Molsidomine Rescues Cardiac Function In Rats with Chronic Kidney Disease and Cardiac Dysfunction. *Am J Physiol Heart Circ Physiol* 2010; 299:H2037-H2045.

# 8

# Sub-Types and Therapeutic Management of the Cardiorenal Syndrome

Margot Davis and Sean A. Virani
*University of British Columbia*
*Canada*

## 1. Introduction

Cardiorenal syndrome (CRS) describes the inter-relationship and complex pathophysiological processes by which dysfunction of either the heart or the kidneys is related to dysfunction in the other organ system. Historical definitions may have been overly simplistic; newer definitions have tried to capture the complex interactions and feedback processes which exist between the two organs. These definitions classify the CRS into five discrete categories, based on both the organ system in which the primary dysfunction occurs and the time course of disease development/progression.

The CRS is more common than many clinicians realize. Over one third of patients in heart failure (HF) registries have evidence of renal dysfunction, and a similar proportion of dialysis patients have symptoms of congestive HF or clinical evidence of left ventricular dysfunction (Adams et al., 2005; Stack & Bloembergen, 2001). Importantly, the presence of the CRS is a strong adverse prognostic marker in patients with either primary cardiac disease or primary renal disease.

While originally thought to reflect renal hypoperfusion secondary to low cardiac output, it is now understood that the CRS is underpinned by far more complex processes. From a hemodynamic standpoint, it seems likely that venous congestion is at least as important to the pathophysiology of disease progression as is low forward flow. Other contributing factors include activation of neurohormonal axes, including the sympathetic nervous system and the renin-angiotensin-aldosterone system, as well as oxidative injury and endothelial dysfunction (Bock & Gottlieb, 2010). More recently, it has become recognized that anemia may also be intimately involved in the process, both as a consequence and as a causative agent of the CRS. Finally, it is well recognized that many common risk factors for cardiovascular disease and for chronic kidney disease (CKD) co-exist in these patient cohorts.

Management of the CRS is challenging. Therapies for HF often cause worsening of renal function, while treatment of renal failure commonly involves fluid administration, which may precipitate disease decompensation among those with HF. Unfortunately, most large randomized trials in the HF population have excluded patients with elevated serum creatinine levels, and there is little evidence to guide therapy in this group of patients. Observational studies suggest that there may be a mortality benefit associated with the use of standard HF medications, such as angiotensin converting enzyme inhibitors, angiotensin receptor blockers and beta blockers in patients with HF and CKD, regardless of glomerular filtration rate (GFR) (Berger et al., 2007; Cice et al., 2003).

Many novel therapies for HF have been introduced over recent years, several of which were appealing for treatment of the CRS, given the pathophysiological processes towards which they were directed. Unfortunately, natriuretic peptides, vasopressin antagonists, and adenosine antagonists have all failed to show meaningful clinical benefits in patients with HF (Hernandez, 2010; Konstam et al., 2007; Massie et al., 2010). Other approaches, particularly peripheral ultrafiltration, have shown more promise in this patient population (Costanzo et al., 2005).

## 2. Definitions and sub-types of the cardiorenal syndrome

Historically, the CRS is thought to have been due to impaired renal perfusion secondary to low cardiac output states or the result of HF therapies negatively impacting renal function. In 2004, the National Heart, Lung and Blood Institute defined CRS as a "state in which therapy to relieve heart failure symptoms is limited by further worsening in renal function" (National Heart, Lung and Blood Institute, 2004). By this paradigm, the heart was considered to be the central driving force behind impaired renal function in patients with HF.

Our understanding of the pathophysiology behind the CRS has evolved in the last number of years and there is increasing recognition of the complexity of interactions which exist between the heart and the kidneys, particularly when either or both organs are diseased. This organ cross talk is bidirectional in nature and the resultant dialogue is dependent on whether the heart or the kidney is the primary affected organ as well as the time course over which the associated pathophysiological changes may occur.

It is within this context, that newer definitions for the CRS have been proposed which recognize that either the heart or kidney may be the primary site of organ injury. A more comprehensive definition and classification schema for the CRS has the advantage of allowing clinicians to make a more accurate diagnosis which in turn informs our understanding of a given patient's natural history, prognosis and optimal treatment strategy.

The definition and classification system for CRS introduced by Ronco and colleagues in 2008 (Ronco et al., 2008) is now widely considered to be the preferred mechanism for describing patients and the pathophysiological processes associated with CRS. Ronco and colleagues broadly define CRS as "a pathophysiological disorder of the heart and kidneys whereby acute or chronic dysfunction of one organ may induce acute or chronic dysfunction of the other." Additionally, they characterize five sub-types of the CRS based on this definition. These are described and discussed below. It should be noted that CRS types 1-5 may frequently co-exist in a given patient, underscoring the complexity of interaction between the heart and kidney and the importance of appointing chronology to these processes.

### 2.1 Cardiorenal syndrome type 1 (acute cardiorenal syndrome)

Type 1 CRS is distinguished by an acute deterioration in cardiac function or acute cardiac injury, from any cause, that secondarily results in acute kidney injury (AKI).

Pathophysiologically, Type 1 CRS is characterized by decreased cardiac output with impaired renal perfusion as well as elevated central venous pressures and acute renal edema. Renal ischemia may be mediated by decreased oxygen delivery due to impaired myocardial contractile performance, elevated interstitial pressures in the renal medulla and by peripheral/systemic vasoconstriction which occurs as a compensatory mechanism in the face of low cardiac output.

Historically, decreased forward cardiac flow was thought to be the primary determinant for AKI in this context, however recent clinical trials have suggested this mechanism may not be as important in the development of CRS Type I as previously hypothesized. Specifically, data from ADHERE (Acute Decompensated Heart Failure National Registry) which included over 100,000 patients admitted to hospital in the United States with acute decompensated heart failure (ADHF) showed that <2% of patients had systemic hypotension, a surrogate for low cardiac output, while the vast majority of patients had symptoms/signs of volume overload (Adams et al., 2005). This is corroborated by the findings of the ESCAPE (Evaluation Study of Congestive Heart Failure and Pulmonary Artery Catheterization Effectiveness) Trial in which 433 patients admitted to hospital with ADHF were randomized to pulmonary artery catheterization versus standard care to assess the efficacy of tailored haemodynamic therapy (Binanay et al., 2005). In the ESCAPE Trial, cardiac index was not associated with baseline renal function or deterioration in renal function, however right atrial pressure was weakly correlated with baseline creatinine and GFR (Nohria et al., 2008).

The impact of central venous pressures (CVP) on worsening renal function in the setting of ADHF has been receiving greater attention in recent years. Elevated CVP is more predictive of a decline in renal function than other relevant haemodynamic variables such as cardiac index, blood pressure and pulmonary capillary wedge pressure (Mullens et al., 2009). Moreover, elevated CVP predicts risk of re-hospitalization for HF and death suggesting that it is a potent prognosticator for poor outcomes and a potential target for therapy (Uthoff et al., 2011). Elevated intra-abdominal venous pressures have also been shown to have a similar relationship with GFR at baseline and changes in GFR with therapy (Bock & Gottlieb, 2010; S. E. Bradley & G. P. Bradley). This may be the result of a direct mechanical effect on renal blood flow or simply a reflection of elevated CVP.

Among patients with ADHF, activation of the sympathetic nervous system (SNS) and the renin-angiotensin-aldosterone system (RAAS) is a homeostatic mechanism intended to maintain intraglomerular perfusion pressures and preserve GFR. Paradoxically however, systemic vasoconstriction by these mechanisms increases cardiac afterload leading to further decline in cardiac output and renal blood flow. Additionally, these neurohormones have a maladaptive effect on the myocardium resulting in fibrosis and ventricular remodeling. Treatment with β-blockers is relatively contra-indicated in the face of an acute decompensation due to their negative inotropic effects and the relative dependence of cardiac output on heart rate in this patient population; therefore, SNS activation in CRS Type 1 may remain unchecked leading to ischemia of both renal and cardiac tissue beds.

Acute administration of RAAS inhibition may exacerbate renal injury in CRS Type 1 by reducing pressure in Bowman's capsule; this effect may be magnified in the presence of volume shifts associated with diuretics, which remains the mainstay of therapy. Moreover, diuretics may directly result in additional neurohormonal activation and there is now an increasing body of literature suggesting that diuretics, in and of themselves, may be associated with worse outcomes in patients with ADHF independent of other relevant clinical variables. In a single centre retrospective analysis of 1354 patients admitted with ADHF, Eshaghian and colleagues (Eshaghian et al., 2006) demonstrated that patients requiring the highest doses of diuretics, stratified by quartiles, had higher rates of sudden death, death due to progressive pump failure and all cause mortality compared to patients in the lowest quartile of diuretic dose. This type of observation has fueled a growing interest in identifying alternate strategies for fluid management in the acute setting, independent of diuretic administration (see section 3.8).

Of particular concern among patients who present with the features of CRS Type 1 is the impact of diagnostic imaging and invasive cardiac procedures which may have an additional and direct toxic effect on the kidneys through a variety of mechanisms. Individuals who present with an acute deterioration in cardiac function will frequently require imaging or investigation to identify a precipitant or cause for their symptoms. Independently, percutaneous interventions and cardiac surgery impart a risk of AKI which is higher in patients who have pre-existing or concomitant acute renal insufficiency (Anderson et al., 1999; Best et al., 2002).

Upwards of 70% of patients admitted to hospital with ADHF will experience a rise in serum creatinine over the course of their admission (Gottleib et al., 2002); this may be the result of therapies administered, either medical or invasive, or a consequence of the various pathophysiological processes which characterize CRS Type 1. Regardless of mechanism, worsening renal function portends a poor prognosis and is associated with higher mortality rates. (Gottleib et al., 2002; Damman et al., 2007).

### 2.2 Cardiorenal syndrome type 2 (chronic cardiorenal syndrome)

Chronic HF leading to chronic kidney disease is the hallmark of CRS Type 2. The prevalence of CKD in HF cohorts has been variably reported depending on the patient population examined – e.g. hospitalized versus ambulatory patients. Further complicating our understanding of disease prevalence is the fact that early clinical trials of chronic HF excluded patients with established renal insufficiency and most did not determine glomerular filtration rate (GFR) which is of particular clinical importance given that HF is a disease of the elderly.

For example, the SOLVD (Studies of Left Ventricular Dysfunction) trials examined the impact of the angiotensin converting enzyme (ACE) inhibitor Enalapril on mortality and symptom development in patients with left ventricular dysfunction (The SOLVD Investigators, 1991; The SOLVD Investigators, 1992). While those with serum creatinine levels >2.0 mg/dL were excluded from the original trial, a retrospective analysis of study patients revealed at least moderate renal impairment (GFR < 60 ml/min) was present in 26% and 56% of participants in the prevention and treatment arms of the trial, respectively (Dries et al., 2000). Across the series of trials which composed the CHARM (The Candesartan in Heart Failure: Assessment of Reduction in Mortality and Morbidity) Program, moderate renal impairment was detected in 36% of the 2680 study participants at baseline (Hillege et al., 2006).

Determining the prevalence of pre-existing CKD is particularly challenging among hospitalized HF patients. Some clinicians may attribute AKI at the time of HF hospitalization solely to CRS Type 1 thereby underestimating the presence of concomitant CRS Type 2 in this cohort of patients. Novel biomarkers of AKI may help clinicians to decipher the relative contributions of CRS Type 1 versus CRS Type 2 in patients hospitalized for HF who have poor renal function upon presentation (Siew et al., 2011; Coca et al., 2008).

Regardless of cause, renal insufficiency in hospitalized HF patients appears to be relatively common; among those enrolled in ADHERE, the prevalence of at least moderate renal impairment, as determined by GFR, was greater than 60% at baseline (Heywood et al., 2007). This is in sharp contrast to initial reports from the same registry which suggested a prevalence rate of only 20% when a serum creatinine of 2.0 mg/dL was employed as a cut off (Adams et al., 2005). Calculation of GFR, therefore, is paramount to accurately identifying the burden of renal disease in all forms of CRS.

The true burden of pre-existing renal dysfunction among patients with HF was best characterized in a meta-analysis performed by Smith and colleagues. In their systematic review of the literature, approximately 80,000 hospitalized and non-hospitalized patients with HF were identified across 16 clinical trials. While 29% of patients were found to have moderate to severe renal impairment (GFR <53 mL/min or cystatin C of >1.56 mg/dL), 63% were found to have at least some degree of impaired kidney function. Moreover, these findings are likely to underestimate the true prevalence of renal insufficiency in HF populations given that 8 of the clinical trials included in the meta-analysis excluded patients on the basis of age or an elevated serum creatinine at baseline (Smith et al., 2006).

In the meta-analysis performed by Smith and colleagues, renal impairment at baseline conferred an increased risk of mortality at one year follow-up compared to patients with normal kidney function (Smith et al., 2006). The adjusted hazard ratio for patients with any renal impairment or moderate to severe renal impairment was 1.56 and 2.31 respectively. Excess risk was conferred in an incremental fashion with each 10 mL/min reduction in GFR correlating to a 7% increase in the risk of death. This observation is strengthened by similar findings across a spectrum of clinical trials in both hospitalized and ambulatory HF populations (Adams et al., 2005; Dries et al., 2000; Fonarow et al., 2005; Heywood et al., 2007; Hillege et al., 2006).

Many of the pathophysiological mechanisms which characterize CRS Type 1 are also implicated in the development of CRS Type 2, although many of these processes may occur slowly and over longer periods of time. For example, elevated central venous pressure is strongly associated with a decline in eGFR among patients with chronic HF (Damman et al., 2009; Firth et al., 1988); as described above, the same is true for patients with ADHF and CRS Type 1. Elevated CVP and secondarily an elevation in renal venous pressure may trigger a number of downstream events, including interstitial ischemia, neurohormonal activation and decreased responsiveness to natriuretic peptides which all combine to reduce GFR directly or indirectly (Damman et al., 2007; Bock & Gottlieb, 2010) in the setting of chronic HF. Chronically low cardiac output, particularly in combination with micro and macrovascular renal disease, may also contribute to fibrosis and structural changes in the kidney which result in impaired renal function.

RAAS activation occurs in both HF and CKD with an associated increase in Angiotensin II levels (AII). AII mediates oxidative injury and endothelial dysfunction through both the formation of reactive oxygen species and a decrease in nitric oxide bioavailability. Each of these processes, in turn, can result in haemodynamic abnormalities at the level of the heart and kidney contributing to a decline in GFR (Bock & Gottlieb, 2010).

While neurohormonal inhibition and diuretic therapy are the mainstay of pharmacological HF management, these agents are also implicated in the worsening of GFR associated with CRS Type 2. ACE inhibitors and angiotensin receptor blockers (ARBs) result in systemic hypotension as well as efferent arteriolar vasodilatation with an associated decline in intraglomerular pressure and GFR. These effects may be magnified in the presence of concomitant diuretic use and relative intra-vascular volume depletion. The treatment of CRS is discussed in detail below.

The presence of anemia is common in patients with HF, an observation which is consistent across a number of clinical trials in the HF arena. A review of the literature suggests a prevalence rate of between 9-25% depending on the HF patient population studied and the cut-off criteria used to diagnose anemia (Virani et al., 2008; Al-Ahmad et al., 2001; Sharma et al., 2004; Anand et al., 2005; Horwich et al., 2002). Regrettably, many of these studies excluded patients based on renal function and therefore the relative contribution of low GFR to the development of anemia in these patient cohorts is lacking. Anemia in the presence of HF portends a poor prognosis with absolute haemoglobin (Hgb) levels correlating with 1 year survival; a precipitous increase in mortality is observed when Hgb drops below 120 g/L (Horwich et al., 2002; Ezekowitz et al., 2003).

The development of anemia in CRS Type 2 is likely multifactorial and underpinned by a number of processes occurring simultaneously; malnutrition, the formation of reactive oxygen species, cytokine release and erythropoietin (EPO) deficiency/resistance have all been implicated. When present, anemia may lead to further cardiac and renal dysfunction through impaired oxygen delivery and tissue hypoxia, neurohormonal activation, decreased renal blood flow and expansion of plasma volume with resultant cardiac remodeling (McCullough & Lepor, 2005). These mechanisms establish and propagate a vicious cycle of maladaptive processes which lead to worsening anemia, HF and kidney function as a net result.

### 2.3 Cardiorenal syndrome type 3 (acute renocardiac syndrome)

The RIFLE Criteria define acute kidney injury as a twofold increase in serum creatinine or a GFR decrease by 50 percent or urine output of <0.5 mL/kg per hour for 12 hours (Bellomo et al., 2004). By this definition, AKI is prevalent in nearly 9% of hospitalized patients (Uchino et al., 2006) with an associated 4-fold increased risk of mortality compared to patients without evidence of renal injury (Ricci et al., 2008). Much of that excess risk may be attributable to cardiac sequelae of AKI. CRS Type 3 characterizes this interaction and may be defined broadly as primary acute kidney injury, due to any number of causes, which secondarily leads to acute cardiac dysfunction.

A number of pathophysiological processes may be initiated as a consequence of AKI which have significant downstream cardiac effects. Biochemical abnormalities including hyperkalemia may pre-dispose to malignant cardiac arrhythmias and an increased risk of sudden cardiac death. Acidemia and uremia have direct myocardial depressant effects and may precipitate acute biventricular cardiomyopathy; these effects are exacerbated in the face of volume expansion.

Volume overload due to impaired solute and fluid clearance may also result in hypertension and pulmonary edema. Moreover, the resultant elevations in intra-cardiac filling pressures reduce the transmyocardial perfusion gradient during diastole leading to sub-endocardial ischemia and overall worsening of ventricular function. Release of pro-inflammatory cytokines and reactive oxygen species in response to renal injury may result in endothelial dysfunction in addition to having direct toxic effects on the myocardium with resultant apoptosis and myocardial fibrosis.

Activation of the SNS and RAAS as a result of AKI may also lead to deleterious haemodynamic consequences including increased systemic vascular resistance and increased myocardial oxygen consumption, both of which lead to decreased cardiac output. While AII also causes left ventricular hypertrophy, ventricular remodeling and accelerates the development of atherosclerosis, these effects are likely of greater relevance in the setting of Chronic Renocardiac Syndrome (CRS Type 4).

### 2.4 Cardiorenal syndrome type 4 (chronic renocardiac syndrome)

CRS Type 4 describes a clinical scenario where primary CKD leads to structural and/or functional cardiac abnormalities which may be associated with clinically significant adverse cardiac events. Indeed, the presence of CKD portends a poor cardiac prognosis with the attributable risk of adverse events correlating in a step-wise manner to reduction in GFR (Go et al., 2004). Moreover, individuals with CKD have an accelerated natural history of their cardiac disease and are more likely to die from cardiac causes rather than progress to renal replacement therapy (Collins et al., 2008; Foley et al., 2005; Keith et al., 2004).

For example, in ALLHAT (The Antihypertensive and Lipid-Lowering Treatment to Prevent Heart Attack Trial) the risk of myocardial infarction (MI)/stroke, revascularization, death due to coronary disease and all forms of atherosclerotic vascular disease was increased as GFR decreased (Wali & Henrich, 2005). Among patients with CKD who experience an acute coronary syndrome, prognosis may also be stratified according to GFR. Shlipak and colleagues reviewed approximately 130,000 elderly patients hospitalized with an acute coronary syndrome and found a 2.5 fold increased risk of death between patients in the highest (CrCl > 0.92 mL/sec) and lowest (CrCl 0.17-0.54 mL/sec) tertile of creatinine clearance (Shlipak et al., 2002). Moreover, an analysis of nearly 120,000 patients from the Cooperative Cardiovascular Project suggested that renal function was a more accurate predictor of long term mortality post-MI than left ventricular systolic function, the presence of heart failure or prior MI (Smith et al., 2008). This relationship has been demonstrated in a multitude of clinical trials across a variety of cardiac cohorts and the observation between CKD and poor cardiac outcomes remains robust (Ronco et al., 2008).

There are many postulates as to the mechanisms underlying poor cardiac outcomes in patients with chronic renal dysfunction. It would appear that the burden of coronary artery disease and myocardial ischemia is greater in patients with CKD than those without (Ix et al., 2003). This may be due to a higher preponderance of traditional risk factors for coronary artery disease in this patient population (Muntner et al., 2005; Parikh et al., 2006) or simply that CKD, in and of itself, imparts increased risk of adverse cardiac events (Levey et al., 2003). In the Framingham Offspring Cohort, two or more traditional cardiovascular risk factors were identified in 73% of patients with CKD (GFR <60 mL/min) compared to 51.4 %

of participants without CKD. A statistically significant increase in hypertension and diabetes along with a trend towards increased dyslipidemia were more prevalent in the CKD cohort (Parikh et al., 2006). Existing data would suggest that CKD is independently associated with a higher risk for cardiovascular endpoints in affected patients; the magnitude of this excess risk, however, does not support elevating CKD to the level of a cardiovascular disease equivalent as is the case with diabetes or prior MI (Wattanakit et al., 2006).

Other potential pathophysiological processes involved in the development and acceleration of coronary atherosclerosis in patients with CKD include abnormalities of mineral metabolism leading to vascular calcification and endothelial dysfunction secondary to both chronic inflammation and EPO deficiency. Uremia, hypertension and increased vascular stiffness contribute to progressive left ventricular hypertrophy and diastolic dysfunction, which in time may progress to systolic dysfunction. Neurohormonal activation results in myocardial fibrosis and maladaptive ventricular remodelling which may hasten this process. In the presence of volume expansion, patients with either systolic or diastolic dysfunction remain at high risk for developing decompensated heart failure.

Observational trials very clearly demonstrate that those with CKD, as a result of actual or perceived contraindications, are less likely to receive efficacious and evidence based therapies compared to cohorts of patients with normal renal function (Al-Suwaidi et al., 2002; Parikh et al., 2006). An even more important observation is that those patients with CKD who do receive appropriate guideline based interventions have better outcomes (Shlipak et al., 2002); therapeutic prejudice of healthcare teams and providers in relation to patients with renal dysfunction is most certainly misplaced, particularly since this group of patients have a high burden of disease and therefore may receive the greatest degree of benefit from aggressive intervention.

### 2.5 Cardiorenal syndrome type 5 (secondary cardiorenal syndrome)

Secondary cardiorenal syndrome is the result of a systemic disorder leading to simultaneous cardiac and renal injury; each of these processes may be acute or chronic in nature and CRS Type 5 does not preclude involvement of other organs and tissue beds. Moreover, other sub-types of the CRS may exist concomitantly due to pre-existing co-morbidities.

The prevalence of CRS Type 5 overall has not been well described, primarily due to a paucity of data in this arena, however the frequency of cardiac and renal involvement for specific systemic disease states may be described in the literature. For example, myocardial injury in the absence of an acute coronary syndrome, as manifested by a positive troponin assay, is present in up to one-half of patients with sepsis admitted to a critical care unit (Amman et al., 2003). Similarly, AKI may occur in 70% of this patient population (Kim et al., 2011). Dysfunction of either or both organ systems portends a poor prognosis.

Connective tissue disease, sarcoidosis, amyloidosis, diabetes and sepsis are the most commonly referred to systemic process that may predispose to secondary CRS (Ronco et al., 2008). While a discussion of cardiac and renal involvement in each of these disease states is beyond the scope of this chapter, it is clear that definitive treatment must be focused at correcting the underlying pathophysiological process while providing supportive care for the heart and kidneys in the interim.

## 3. Management of the cardiorenal syndrome

Management of the CRS presents a challenge to the clinician. Treatment of HF with standard therapies often results in worsening of renal function. Moreover, most randomized clinical trials of HF therapies, including β-blockers, ACE inhibitors, ARBs and aldosterone antagonists, have excluded patients with significant renal dysfunction. Therefore, the results of these trials, most showing significant reductions in morbidity and mortality in the general HF population, may not be applicable to the CRS population. Observational studies and small randomized studies, however, have suggested that many of these drug classes may have similar benefit in patients with renal dysfunction (Berger et al., 2007; Cice et al., 2003). A number of novel strategies have been described that may offer specific benefit in the CRS population, although data from clinical trials have not always been encouraging.

Management of chronic CRS is overall similar to the management of HF in general, employing a combination of diuretics, inhibitors of the RAAS, and β-blockers. In the hospitalized patient with CRS and ADHF, diuretics remain a mainstay of therapy, but may be supplemented by additional therapies including novel pharmacologic agents, inotropic support, and ultrafiltration.

### 3.1 Diuretics

While fluid removal with diuretics is a cornerstone of HF management, diuretic resistance is highly prevalent in patients with decreased renal function, making this aspect of care for the patient with CRS particularly challenging. Furthermore, effective diuresis can result in further deterioration in renal function, particularly when the rate of fluid removal exceeds the rate of fluid movement from the extravascular space to the intravascular space, resulting in low effective circulating volume. Thus, two of the greatest obstacles in treating patients with CRS are overcoming diuretic resistance and effectively removing fluid without compromising renal function.

Loop diuretics (LD) such as furosemide act at the thick ascending limb of the loop of Henle, inhibiting the $Na^+/K^+/2Cl^-$ cotransporter. LD are protein bound, preventing filtration at the glomerulus, but are actively secreted in the proximal tubule. Effective delivery to the loop of Henle requires effective delivery to the bloodstream (through intestinal absorption or direct intravenous administration), adequate renal blood flow, intact proximal tubule secretion, and delivery of tubular contents to the more distal nephron. There are therefore a number of mechanisms by which diuretic resistance may occur (Jentzer et al., 2010).

Delayed intestinal absorption is common in patients with HF, owing to intestinal wall edema. This can be most effectively overcome by using intravenous LD in patients who are markedly volume overloaded, and transitioning to oral administration once signs of congestion elsewhere (i.e. peripheral edema, venous congestion on chest X-ray) have resolved. Reduced renal blood flow (RBF) and GFR are also prevalent in patients with HF and CRS as a result of intrinsic renal dysfunction, decreased cardiac output, and alteration in glomerular haemodynamics by agents such as non-steroidal anti-inflammatory drugs (NSAIDs), ACE inhibitors, and ARBs. Avoiding agents such as NSAIDs, optimizing systemic hemodynamics, and increasing LD dose can help to overcome this aspect of resistance to LD. Similarly, proximal tubular secretion of LD is reduced in patients with CRS because organic acids that accumulate in the uremic state compete for the same transporters; increased doses of LD may be required to overcome this problem.

Through intravascular volume depletion, LD may result in activation of the RAAS. This leads to increased sodium absorption by the proximal and distal tubule. This issue is compounded by the fact that post-diuretic rebound sodium avidity occurs between bolus doses of LD, negating much of the natriuretic benefit achieved. Strict dietary sodium restriction and administration of RAAS antagonists (i.e. ACE inhibitors and ARBs) may help to prevent this. Historically, it has been believed that continuous infusions of diuretics may also be effective in minimizing rebound sodium absorption; the recent DOSE (Diuretic Strategies in Patients with Acute Decompensated Heart Failure) trial suggests that there may be no difference in diuretic efficacy between intermittent intravenous bolus dosing and continuous infusions (Felker et al., 2011).

The "braking phenomenon" is a short-term effect, whereby the nephron becomes less sensitive to LD after an initial dose. This is thought to result from upregulation of the $Na^+/K^+/2Cl^-$ cotransporter in the thick ascending loop of Henle. Higher doses of LD may be necessary to overcome this. With chronic LD administration, distal tubule hypertrophy occurs. This allows increased distal sodium reabsorption, tending to negate the inhibition of sodium reabsorption that has occurred in the loop of Henle.

A strategy of combination diuretic administration, with the addition of a thiazide diuretic such as metolazone 5-10 mg 30 minutes prior to LD administration can help to prevent sodium retention by this mechanism. Thiazides inhibit the NaCl cotransporter in the distal convoluted tubule. Caution is needed, however, as combination diuretic therapy can result in profound electrolyte abnormalities. Serum levels of potassium and magnesium must be closely monitored and infrequent metolazone dosing (i.e. three times per week) or co-administration of a potassium-sparing diuretic may be necessary to prevent life-threatening hypokalemia.

Finally, sodium and water retention may be upregulated in the distal nephron in patients with CRS, mediated by elevated levels of aldosterone and vasopressin, respectively. Administration of aldosterone antagonists or other potassium-sparing diuretics will minimize sodium retention in this situation; the new vasopressin antagonists have a role in preventing excessive absorption of free water (see section 3.6). Free water restriction may also be necessary in patients with refractory fluid overload or significant hyponatremia. An important caveat to the use of aldosterone antagonists in CRS is the risk of hyperkalemia in patients with renal impairment; these agents should generally be avoided in patients with GFR <30 mL/min.

Major drawbacks to the use of LD include neurohormonal activation, ototoxicity, electrolyte abnormalities (particularly hypokalemia and hypomagnesemia), dysrhythmias, and intravascular volume depletion with resultant worsening renal function and/or hypotension in patients who are preload-dependent or receiving concomitant vasodilator therapy.

A novel approach to diuretic use involves the co-administration of loop diuretics and hypertonic saline solution (HSS). Small studies in patients with ADHF have demonstrated that, compared to intravenous bolus loop diuretics with a low sodium diet, administration of intermittent boluses of HSS with loop diuretics and moderate dietary sodium restriction resulted in more rapid diuresis, normalization of neurohormonal activity, shorter hospitalizations, and less renal dysfunction (Licata et al., 2003; Paterna et al., 2000). After discharge, these results were maintained by continuing moderate sodium restriction (<2.8 g/day) with strict fluid restriction (<1 L/day), resulting in fewer readmissions and improved survival compared to continued strict sodium (<2 g/day) and similar fluid restriction. The mechanism by which HSS provides these benefits is unclear, but may be related to the osmotic load drawing interstitial fluid into the intravascular space, leading to neurohormonal blockade, reduced vascular resistance, improved cardiac output, and reduced interstitial edema. In addition, the sodium load in the kidney may induce a sort of transient diabetes insipidus, resulting in rapid diuresis (Di Pasquale et al., 2007). Further research and larger scale studies are required to confirm the benefits of HSS in patients with CRS.

### 3.2 Renin-angiotensin-aldosterone system antagonists

Inhibitors of the renin-angiotensin system, including ACE inhibitors and ARBs have proven survival benefit in patients with left ventricular dysfunction (The SOLVD Investigators, 1991; The SOLVD Investigators, 1992), and have also been shown to slow the rate of decline of renal function in patients with diabetic chronic kidney disease (Lewis et al., 1993). It stands to reason, therefore, that these agents would be beneficial in the CRS, although large-scale clinical trials in the HF population have typically excluded patients with significant renal dysfunction.

The CHARM studies investigated the effects of candesartan compared with placebo in a broad population of patients with HF. Patients with serum creatinine >3.0 mg/dL were excluded, but among the study population, there was no statistically significant interaction between eGFR and treatment effect, suggesting a mortality benefit of ARBs in patients with HF and mild-to-moderate renal dysfunction that is equivalent to that seen in patients with HF and preserved renal function (Hillege et al., 2006). An analysis of CONSENSUS (Cooperative North Scandinavian Enalapril Survival Study) which demonstrated a mortality benefit of enalapril compared to placebo in patients with HF, found a greater benefit in patients with baseline serum creatinine above the median (123 umol/L) than in those with serum creatinine below the median (Swedberg et al., 1990). A retrospective analysis of the Minnesota Heart Survey stratified 4573 patients hospitalized with HF by GFR, and revealed that patients at all stages of CKD had reduced in-hospital mortality when an ACE inhibitor or ARB was used in hospital, and reduced one-year mortality when discharged on an ACE inhibitor or ARB (Berger et al., 2007). This same analysis, however, demonstrated that patients with severe renal dysfunction were far less likely to receive either agent than those with normal renal function.

In HF, elevated angiotensin II levels cause efferent arteriolar vasoconstriction, elevating glomerular filtration pressure and preserving GFR. Inhibition of this process with ACE inhibitors or ARBs may result in an initial decline in GFR, but in the long term protects the glomerulus from high filtration pressures and may help to preserve long-term renal function (Heywood, 2004). Although there appear to be benefits of using these agents in the CRS population, caution must be taken when initiating ACE inhibitors and ARBs in patients with renal dysfunction, particularly with regard to volume status and avoidance of NSAIDs.

Volume depletion increases the risk of significant renal dysfunction associated with ACE inhibitors and ARBs. Increases in creatinine of up to 30% are acceptable, and may identify a group of patients most likely to benefit from angiotensin inhibition (Koniari et al., 2010). HF patients who are unable to tolerate ACE inhibitor therapy because of hypotension, renal dysfunction, or hyperkalemia have a particularly high one-year mortality rate, in excess of 50% (Kittleson et al., 2003).

### 3.3 β-adrenergic receptor blockers

β-blockers are considered standard therapy in patients with HF and systolic dysfunction. They exert a number of beneficial effects, including prevention of ventricular arrhythmias, prevention of ventricular remodeling, reduction in myocardial oxygen demand, increased myocardial oxygen supply, and inhibition of other deleterious neurohormonal pathways. Their significant mortality benefit in patients with HF is well established through large clinical trials. Unfortunately, the majority of these studies excluded patients with significant renal dysfunction, but retrospective analyses of trials data have offered insight into the benefits in patients with mild-to-moderate renal impairment. COPERNICUS (Carvedilol Prospective Randomized Cumulative Survival Study), for example, demonstrated a 35% reduction in the risk of death in patients with severe HF treated with carvedilol compared to placebo, but excluded patients with a serum creatinine greater than 2.8 mg/dL. Similarly, the CAPRICORN (Carvedilol Post-Infarct Survival Control in Left Ventricular Dysfunction) trial showed a 23% reduction in all-cause mortality in patients with EF ≤40% after myocardial infarction treated with carvedilol compared with placebo, but excluded patients with significant renal impairment (Dargie, 2001). A post-hoc analysis of individual patient data from these two trials, however, demonstrated that in patients with HF and mild-to-moderate CKD, carvedilol was safe and efficacious, associated with reductions in all-cause mortality, cardiovascular mortality, and HF hospitalization (Wali et al., 2011). CIBIS-II (The Cardiac Insufficiency Bisoprolol Study II) demonstrated a 34% reduction in mortality in patients with HF treated with bisoprolol compared to placebo, and excluded patients with serum creatinine ≥300 umol/L (3.4 mg/dL) (CIBIS-II Investigators and Committees, 1999). A post-hoc analysis of this trial showed that although patients with GFR <60 mL/min had higher overall mortality than those with GFR ≥60 mL/min, the benefit of bisoprolol was similar in both groups (Erdmann et al., 2001). The relative risk of mortality in the group with GFR <60 mL/min treated with bisoprolol compared to placebo was 0.66, and there was a non-significant trend towards an even greater benefit in the small number of patients with GFR <30 mL/min.

An analysis of MADIT-II (Multicenter Automatic Defibrillator Implantation Trial II), which demonstrated a 31% reduction in the risk of all-cause mortality with the addition of an implantable cardioverter-defibrillator to medical therapy in patients with ischemic cardiomyopathy and EF ≤30%, examined the predictors of sudden cardiac death (SCD) in the subset of patients in the medical arm of the study with impaired renal function, defined as GFR ≤75 mL/min. β-blocker therapy was a negative predictor of SCD, with a hazard ratio of 0.61 (Chonchol et al., 2007).

Smaller studies have examined the benefits of β-blocker therapy in patients with end-stage renal failure. In a non-randomized study of 134 patients with HF and either chronic renal impairment, anemia, or both, treatment with β-blockers for 12 months was associated with improvement in both creatinine clearance and hemoglobin levels, while those patients who did not receive β-blockers had worsening renal function and anemia over the same time period (Khan et al., 2006). In patients with HF and normal renal function at baseline, lack of treatment with a β-blocker was associated with increased risk of developing renal failure over 20 years of follow-up (Tanaka et al., 2007). In hemodialysis patients with dilated left ventricles, treatment with metoprolol resulted in reduced ventricular dimensions, increased fractional shortening, and reduced levels of natriuretic peptides (Hara et al., 2001). A randomized trial of 114 hemodialysis patients with dilated cardiomyopathy showed that carvedilol, compared to placebo, was associated with improved ejection fraction, improved survival, and fewer HF hospitalizations (Cice et al., 2003). Although large-scale clinical trials in this population are lacking, the weight of evidence suggests that treatment with β-blockers in the CRS population is likely to be associated with reductions in mortality and morbidity.

### 3.4 Inotropic agents

Inotropic medications such as dobutamine and milrinone are frequently used in patients with ADHF, particularly in the setting of the CRS where low cardiac output is felt to be a major contributor to rapidly declining renal function. Both agents are vasodilating inotropes, but they have different mechanisms of action. Dobutamine is an adrenergic agonist that affects inotropy and chronotropy via β-1 activity and peripheral vasodilation via β-2 activity. Milrinone is an inhibitor of type III phosphodiesterase and results in increased intracellular cyclic adenosine monophosphate (cAMP). This, in turn, results in increased inotropy (without chronotropy) as well as peripheral vasodilation. Although both agents have attractive hemodynamic profiles in the treatment of CRS, evidence suggests that they should not be part of standard therapy in this condition. OPTIME-CHF (Outcomes of a Prospective Trial of Intravenous Milrinone for Exacerbations of Chronic Heart Failure) compared intravenous milrinone to placebo in patients with ADHF not requiring inotropic therapy for shock or other indications. There was no difference between the two groups in the primary endpoint of total number of days in hospital by 60 days after randomization. There was also no difference in the rate of progression of HF, but the patients treated with milrinone had higher rates of treatment failure, largely driven by higher rates of hypotension and atrial arrhythmias.

The ADHERE registry compared outcomes of patients with ADHF treated with vasodilating medications (nitroglycerin, nesiritide) and inotropic agents (dobutamine, milrinone). Even after adjustment for baseline variables including age, gender, blood pressure, BUN, creatinine, sodium, heart rate, and symptom severity, odds ratios for mortality between individual inotropes and individual vasodilators ranged from 1.45 to 2.17. Inotropic agents, therefore, are recommended by major society guidelines only for short-term use in patients with cardiogenic shock or refractory volume overload with diuretic resistance, and not recommended for routine use in hospitalized patients with ADHF. In addition, patients receiving these agents must be carefully monitored for hypotension and arrhythmias, and it should be recognized that the use of these agents is associated with a worse prognosis.

Dopamine is an endogenous catecholamine that binds dopamine receptors (D1-D5) as well as α and β adrenergic receptors with varying affinity depending on the dose administered. At low doses (2-5 mcg/kg/min), it primarily binds dopaminergic receptors and causes vasodilation of renal, splanchnic, cerebral, and coronary vessels. At higher doses, β adrenergic effects dominate, resulting in positive inotropy and chronotropy as well as β adrenergic-mediated vasodilation, with progressively increasing α adrenergic activity at still higher doses resulting in vasoconstriction.

For many years the use of "renal-dose" dopamine was advocated in acute renal failure, the rationale being that dopamine in doses up to 5 mcg/kg/min in animals and healthy volunteers resulted in increased renal blood flow and natriuresis via selective dopamine receptor binding. In recent years this approach has fallen out of favor, as multiple retrospective and small prospective studies failed to convincingly demonstrate any benefit in terms of renal function or survival. A meta-analysis of 61 trials comparing low-dose dopamine to placebo or no treatment found that dopamine was associated with a 24% increase in urine output on day 1 but was not associated with reductions in mortality, need for renal replacement therapy, or adverse events (Friedrich et al., 2005). Only one of the 61 studies included patients with HF, and this study did not assess mortality; only three of the studies included patients who were receiving diuretics. More recently, data from the DAD-HF (Dopamine in Acute Decompensated Heart Failure) trial has been presented, comparing low-dose dopamine plus low-dose furosemide to high-dose furosemide alone in patients with ADHF. The two regimens were not associated with statistically significant rates of diuresis, but the patients receiving dopamine plus low-dose furosemide were less likely to develop worsening renal function (36% and 4% of patients in dopamine/furosemide and furosemide only groups, respectively, had >25% increase in serum creatinine). As more data become available regarding outcomes with low-dose dopamine in this specific population, "renal-dose" dopamine may turn out to be useful after all.

### 3.5 Vasodilators

Nesiritide, a synthetic B-type natriuretic peptide (BNP), has been used in the management of ADHF, particularly in patients at risk for worsening renal function with standard therapies. Like naturally occurring BNP, released from ventricular myocardium under conditions of increased wall stress, nesiritide is a vasodilator, causing both arterial and venous dilatation as well as mild diuresis. Its rapid onset of action, apparent neurohormonal benefits, and lack of need for invasive hemodynamic monitoring led to much initial enthusiasm for its use in ADHF, as well as FDA approval for this indication (Publication Committee for the VMAC Investigators, 2002). Use of this agent took a sharp decline, however, after meta-analyses suggested increased 30-day mortality and increased risk of renal failure with nesiritide (Hauptman et al., 2006; Sackner-Bernstein et al., 2005a; 2005b). The definitive randomized clinical trial, ASCEND-HF (Acute Study of Clinical Effectiveness of Nesiritide in Decompensated Heart Failure), recently demonstrated that while nesiritide is safe with no increased risk of 30-day death or hospitalization or increased risk of renal failure, it offers no significant clinical benefit when added to standard therapy in patients with ADHF (Hernandez, 2010).

### 3.6 Vasopressin antagonists

Arginine vasopressin (AVP), a nonapeptide synthesized by the hypothalamus and released by the posterior pituitary gland in response to increased plasma osmolality or decreased plasma volume, binds to 3 distinct receptor subtypes (V1a, V1b, and V2). V1 receptors mediate cardiac myocyte hypertrophy, vasoconstriction, and platelet aggregation. When AVP binds V2 receptors expressed in the renal collecting duct, the short-term result is increased translocation of vesicles containing aquaporin-2 (AQP2) water channels to the apical membrane of principal cells; in the long-term, AVP-V2 receptor binding results in the up-regulation of AQP2 protein expression. AQP2 mediates water transport across the apical membrane of the principal cell, resulting in urinary concentration and increased solute-free water retention (Schrier et al., 2009). AVP also stimulates urea reabsorption, resulting in an augmented medullary concentrating gradient and increased levels of blood urea nitrogen (Sands, 2003).

In HF and CRS, low cardiac output causes nonosmotic AVP release, leading to inappropriate water retention. Low serum sodium and elevated blood urea nitrogen are strong predictors of mortality in HF, and both are mediated, at least in part, by AVP activity in the kidney. Augmentation of cardiac output with vasodilator medications is associated with reductions in plasma AVP (Bichet et al., 1986). Early studies demonstrated effective water removal without worsening renal function (Gheorghiade et al., 2007). Thus, the use of agents that interfere with AVP-mediated water retention has been an attractive concept in CRS. The SALT-1 and SALT-2 trials showed that tolvaptan, a selective oral V2 receptor antagonist, caused increases in serum sodium levels in patients with HF, cirrhosis, and the syndrome of inappropriate antidiuretic hormone (Schrier et al., 2006). Unfortunately, the randomized EVEREST (Efficacy of Vasopressin Antagonism in Heart Failure Outcome Study with Tolvaptan) trial subsequently failed to demonstrate a mortality benefit or reduction in HF morbidity in patients hospitalized with HF treated with tolvaptan, despite sustained reductions in body weight with preserved renal function (Konstam et al., 2007). It seems, therefore, that vasopressin antagonists have little role in influencing clinical outcomes in patients hospitalized with HF and the CRS, although they may be useful in patients with hyponatremia that is difficult to manage with standard therapies. Additional studies are needed to further define the role of tolvaptan and other vasopressin antagonists in the outpatient setting.

### 3.7 Adenosine antagonists

Adenosine is a purine nucleoside breakdown product of adenosine triphosphate. It interacts with four main receptor subtypes: A1, A2a, A2b, and A3. With the exception of coronary vasodilatation and increased renal medullary blood flow, its cardiovascular and renal effects are largely mediated via the A1 receptor. Binding of adenosine to A1 receptors in the heart results in slowing of the heart rate and decreased atrial contraction. In the kidney, adenosine is released from the macula densa in response to sodium delivery to the distal nephron via tubuloglomerular feedback (TGF). Adenosine released through TGF acts on local A1 receptors, causing afferent arteriolar vasoconstriction and reduction in GFR as well as increased proximal tubular sodium reabsorption. Blockade of these receptors should, therefore, result in improved renal blood flow and GFR and decreased sodium and water reabsorption.

In the setting of CRS, loop diuretics cause increased sodium delivery to the distal tubule, making the role of adenosine particularly relevant in this population. Animal studies showed that rolofylline, a selective A1 receptor antagonist, caused increased urine flow and urinary sodium excretion without increasing potassium excretion and without affecting either blood pressure or renal function, and protected against nephrotoxic medication-induced acute renal failure (Nagashima & Karasawa, 1996; Yao et al., 1994). A small clinical study supported this, demonstrating that the addition of rolofylline to diuretics in patients with volume overload and renal impairment resulted in an improvement in renal function and increased diuresis with reduced diuretic requirements (Givertz et al., 2007). Unfortunately, the PROTECT (Placebo-Controlled Randomized Study of the Selective $A_1$ Adenosine Receptor Antagonist Rolofylline for Patients Hospitalized With Acute Decompensated Heart Failure and Volume Overload to Assess Treatment Effect on Congestion and Renal Function) study, which randomized 2033 patients with ADHF to intravenous rolofylline or placebo, failed to demonstrated any difference between groups in the primary endpoint of treatment success (moderate or marked improvement in dyspnea at 24 and 48 hours without treatment failure), treatment failure (death or readmission for HF by 7 days, persistent worsening renal failure, or worsening HF), or no change (Massie et al., 2010). There were no differences in the number of patients who developed renal impairment or in the secondary endpoint of death or rehospitalization for cardiac or renal causes at 60 days. The overall adverse event rates were similar between groups, although more patients in the rolofylline group had seizures, a known side effect of A1 antagonists mediated via central nervous system A1 receptors that regulate electrical excitability. Based on the lack of clinical efficacy, coupled with the increased risk of seizures, rolofylline is not recommended for the treatment of CRS.

Another intravenous selective A1 antagonist, tonapofylline, was also investigated in Phase II clinical trials after preclinical studies and small human studies suggested effective natriuresis. The TRIDENT-1 (Safety and Tolerability of IV Tonapofylline in Subjects With Acute Decompensated Heart Failure and Renal Insufficiency) and POSEIDON (Oral BG9928 in Patients with Heart Failure and Renal Insufficiency) trials were both terminated early after review of interim safety data from TRIDENT-1 revealed that two patients in the tonapofylline group had had seizures (Ensor & Russell, 2010). Of note, seizures were not reported in studies of oral tonapofylline, and in rat studies, tonapofylline did not cross the blood-brain barrier (Ensor & Russell, 2010). There is insufficient data to determine whether oral formulations of A1 antagonists are safe or clinically useful.

### 3.8 Ultrafiltration

Extracorporeal fluid removal has been used for decades in ADHF, typically reserved for patients with fluid overload states that are refractory to diuretics and other medical therapies. Small studies of ultrafiltration in HF have previously demonstrated effective fluid removal, rapid symptom improvement, attenuated neurohormonal activity, and hemodynamic improvements including reduced LV filling pressures and reduced pulmonary arterial pressures without reductions in systemic blood pressure or cardiac index (Marenzi et al., 1993; Rimondini et al., 1987). The landmark UNLOAD (Ultrafiltration versus intravenous diuretics for patients hospitalized for acute decompensated heart failure) trial randomized 200 patients with ADHF and volume overload to veno-venous ultrafiltration or intravenous diuretics (Costanzo et al., 2005). Patients in both groups had similar improvements in dyspnea scores, but the patients in the ultrafiltration group had greater weight loss and net fluid loss at 48 hours. Importantly, there were fewer rehospitalizations, rehospitalization days, and unscheduled clinic visits at 90 days in the ultrafiltration group than in the IV diuretic group. No differences in renal outcomes were seen.

Ultrafiltration can be performed via peripheral or central veins, with rates of fluid removal regulated by a hematocrit sensor and ranging from 10 to 500 mL per hour. Blood flow rates range from 10 to 40 mL per minute, and total extracorporeal blood volume can be as low as 33 mL. Maintenance of a constant hematocrit ensures that the rate of fluid removal from the intravascular compartment is equivalent to the rate of fluid shift from the extravascular to intravascular compartments. Low extracorporeal blood volume and slow fluid removal minimize neurohormonal activation and prevent hypotension. In contrast to the hypotonic fluid removal that occurs with diuresis, ultrafiltration removes isotonic fluid, potentially resulting in greater total sodium removal. The mechanism of the sustained benefit seen in the UNLOAD trial is thought to be related to the attenuation of neurohormonal activity and to the removal of isotonic fluid.

The major limitation to the widespread use of ultrafiltration in HF and the CRS is likely to be the cost of the filters used. In addition, questions remain about patient selection, optimal timing of initiation of therapy, and determination of total fluid volume to be removed. The specific role of ultrafiltration in patients who develop worsening renal function with diuretic therapy is being investigated in CARESS-HF (Cardiorenal Rescue Study in Acute Decompensated Heart Failure), and will help to define the role of this therapy specifically in the CRS population.

### 3.9 Erythropoietin and correction of anemia

Anemia is common in both HF and CKD, and the term "cardiorenal-anemia syndrome" refers to the coexistence of anemia and the CRS. EPO is widely used in the CKD population to correct anemia to a moderate degree. Studies in this population have shown improved parameters of cardiac performance with EPO therapy, including reduction of left ventricular hypertrophy and dilatation, improved left ventricular ejection fraction, and increased cardiac output (Linde et al., 1996; Low et al., 1989; Low-Friedrich et al., 1991). Studies of EPO and iron administration to patients with HF with or without CKD have shown inconsistent results, but some studies have demonstrated modest improvements in symptoms and functional capacity as well as renal function, ejection fraction, and left ventricular dimensions (Bolger et al., 2006; Palazzuoli et al., 2006; Silverberg et al., 2000; Toblli et al., 2007). The FAIR-HF (Ferric Carboxymaltose in Patients with Heart Failure and Iron Deficiency) study demonstrated improved symptoms and functional capacity in patients with HF and iron deficiency, even in the absence of overt anemia, treated with intravenous iron as compared to placebo (Anker et al., 2009). The ongoing IRON-HF (Iron Supplementation in Heart Failure Patients With Anemia) and RED-HF (Reduction of Events With Darbepoetin Alfa in Heart Failure ) studies will likely further clarify the role of iron and EPO therapies in patients with HF and provide additional insights into the management of the CRS.

## 4. Conclusions and future directions

The Cardiorenal Syndrome is a pathophysiologic state involving complex feedback processes between the failing heart and failing kidneys, and is associated with a significantly increased risk of morbidity and mortality compared to either disease process alone. New classification schemes add to our understanding of the processes involved, and help to guide therapy. As the pathophysiology of the CRS becomes better understood, there is potential for the development of novel and rational treatment strategies. Although many promising agents introduced in recent years have produced disappointing results in clinical trials, other strategies, including HSS, ultrafiltration, and low-dose dopamine still hold potential. Larger scale trials of these and other agents are required before their use can be widely adopted. Fortunately, such trials are already underway for ultrafiltration, EPO, and dopamine and the results of these studies are eagerly anticipated. Similarly, established therapies such as β-blockers, ACE inhibitors, and ARBs must be rigorously tested in patients with concomitant cardiac and renal dysfunction to ensure they provide clinical benefit across the spectrum of disease states which characterize the cardiorenal syndrome.

## 5. References

Adams, K. F., Fonarow, G. C., Emerman, C. L., LeJemtel, T. H., Costanzo, M. R., Abraham, W. T., Berkowitz, R. L., Galvao, M., Horton, D. P. ; ADHERE Scientific Advisory Committee and Investigators. (2005). Characteristics and outcomes of patients hospitalized for heart failure in the United States: rationale, design, and preliminary observations from the first 100,000 cases in the Acute Decompensated Heart Failure National Registry (ADHERE). *Am Heart J*, 149(2), 209–16.

Al-Ahmad, A., Rand, W. M., Manjunath, G., Konstam, M. A., Salem, D. N., Levey, A. S. & Sarnak, M. J. (2001). Reduced kidney function and anemia as risk factors for mortality in patients with left ventricular dysfunction. *J Am Coll Cardiol*, 38(4), 955-62.

Al-Suwaidi, J., Reddan, D. N., Williams, K., Pieper, K. S., Harrington, R. A., Califf, R. M., Granger, C. B., Ohman, E. M., Holmes, D. R.; GUSTO-IIb, GUSTO-III, PURSUIT. Global Use of Strategies to Open Occluded Coronary Arteries. Platelet Glycoprotein IIb/IIIa in Unstable Angina: Receptor Suppression Using Integrilin Therapy; PARAGON-A Investigators. Platelet IIb/IIIa Antagonism for the Reduction of Acute coronary syndrome events in a Global Organization Network. (2002) Prognostic implications of abnormalities in renal function in patients with acute coronary syndromes. *Circ*, 106(8), 974-80.

Ammann, P., Maggiorini, M., Bertel, O., Haenseler, E., Joller-Jemelka, H. I., Oechslin, E., Minder, E. I., Rickli, H. & Fehr, T. (2003). Troponin as a risk factor for mortality in critically ill patients without acute coronary syndromes. *J Am Coll Cardiol*, 41(11), 2004-9.

Anand, I. S., Kuskowski, M. A., Rector, T. S., Florea, V. G., Glazer, R. D., Hester, A., Chiang, Y. T., Aknay, N., Maggioni, A. P., Opasich, C., Latini, R. & Cohn, J. N. (2005). Anemia and change in hemoglobin over time related to mortality and morbidity in patients with chronic heart failure: results from Val-HeFT. *Circ*, 112(8), 1121-7.

Anderson, R. J., O'brien, M., MaWhinney, S., VillaNueva, C. B., Moritz, T. E., Sethi, G. K., Henderson, W. G., Hammermeister, K. E., Grover, F. L. & Shroyer, A. L. (1999). Renal failure predisposes patients to adverse outcome after coronary artery bypass surgery. VA Cooperative Study #5. *Kidney Int*, 55(3), 1057-62.

Anker, S. D., Comin Colet, J., Filippatos, G., Willenheimer, R., Dickstein, K., Drexler, H., Luscher, T. F., Bart, B., Banasiak, W., Niegowska, J., Kirwan, B. A., Mori, C., von Eisenhart Rothe, B., Pocock, S. J., Poole-Wilson, P. A., & Ponikowski, P. (2009). Ferric carboxymaltose in patients with heart failure and iron deficiency. *N Engl J Med*, 361(25), 2436-48.

Bellomo, R., Ronco, C., Kellum, J. A., Mehta, R. L., Palevsky, P.; Acute Dialysis Quality Initiative Workgroup (2004). Acute renal failure - definition, outcome measures, animal models, fluid therapy and information technology needs: the Second International Consensus Conference of the Acute Dialysis Quality Initiative (ADQI) Group. *Crit Care*, 8(4), R204-12.

Berger, A. K., Duval, S., Manske, C., Vazquez, G., Barber, C., Miller, L., & Luepker, R. V. (2007). Angiotensin-converting enzyme inhibitors and angiotensin receptor blockers in patients with congestive heart failure and chronic kidney disease. *American Heart Journal*, 153(6), 1064-73.

Best, P. J., Lennon, R., Ting, H. H., Bell, M. R., Rihal, C. S., Holmes, D. R. & Berger, P. B. (2002). The impact of renal insufficiency on clinical outcomes in patients undergoing percutaneous coronary interventions. *J Am Coll Cardiol*, 39(7), 1113-9.

Bichet, D. G., Kortas, C., Mettauer, B., Manzini, C., Marc-Aurele, J., Rouleau, J. L. & Schrier, R. W. (1986). Modulation of plasma and platelet vasopressin by cardiac function in patients with heart failure. *Kidney Int*, 29(6), 1188-96.

Binanay, C., Califf, R. M., Hasselblad, V., O'Connor, C. M., Shah, M. R., Sopko, G., Stevenson, L. W., Francis, G. S., Leier, C. V. & Miller, L. W.; ESCAPE Investigators and ESCAPE Study Coordinators. (2005). Evaluation study of congestive heart failure and pulmonary artery catheterization effectiveness: the ESCAPE trial. *JAMA*, 294(13), 1625-33.

Bolger, A. P., Bartlett, F. R., Penston, H. S., O'Leary, J., Pollock, N., Kaprielian, R., & Chapman, C. M. (2006). Intravenous iron alone for the treatment of anemia in patients with chronic heart failure. *J Am Coll Cardiol*, 48(6), 1225-7.

Bock, J. S. and Gottlieb, S. S. (2010). Cardiorenal syndrome: new perspectives. *Circ*, 121(23), 2592-600.

Bradley, S.E. and Bradley, G.P. (1947). The effect of increased intra-abdominal pressure on renal function. *Am J Physiol*, 26(5), 1010-22.

Chonchol, M., Goldenberg, I., Moss, A. J., McNitt, S., & Cheung, A. K. (2007). Risk factors for sudden cardiac death in patients with chronic renal insufficiency and left ventricular dysfunction. *Am J Nephrol*, 27(1), 7-14.

Cice, G., Ferrara, L., D'Andrea, A., D'Isa, S., Di Benedetto, A., Cittadini, A., Russo, P. E., Golino, P., & Calabro, R. (2003). Carvedilol increases two-year survivalin dialysis patients with dilated cardiomyopathy: a prospective, placebo-controlled trial. *J Am Coll Cardiol*, 41(9), 1438-44.

Collins, A. J., Li, S., Gilbertson, D. T., Liu, J., Chen, S. C. & Herzog, C. A. (2008). Chronic kidney disease and cardiovascular disease in the Medicare population. *Kidney Int Suppl*, 87, S24-31.

Coca, S. G., Yalavarthy, R., Concato, J. & Parikh, C. R. (2008). Biomarkers for the diagnosis and risk stratification of acute kidney injury: a systematic review. *Kidney Int*, 73(9), 1008-16.

Committees, C.-I. I. a. (1999). The Cardiac Insufficiency Bisoprolol Study II (CIBIS-II): a randomised trial. *Lancet*, 353(9146), 9-13.

Costanzo, M. R., Saltzberg, M., O'Sullivan, J., & Sobotka, P. (2005). Early ultrafiltration in patients with decompensated heart failure and diuretic resistance. *J Am Coll Cardiol*, 46(11), 2047-51.

Damman, K., Navis, G., Smilde, T. D., Voors, A. A., van der Bij, W., van Veldhuisen, D. J. & Hillege H. L. (2007). Decreased cardiac output, venous congestion and the association with renal impairment in patients with cardiac dysfunction. Eur J Heart Fail, 9(9), 872-8.

Damman, K., Navis, G., Voors, A. A., Asselbergs, F. W., Smilde, T. D., Cleland, J. G., van Veldhuisen, D. J. & Hillege, H. L. (2007). Worsening renal function and prognosis in heart failure: systematic review and meta-analysis. *J Card Fail*, 13(8), 599-608.

Damman, K., van Deursen, V. M., Navis, G., Voors, A. A., van Veldhuisen, D. J. & Hillege, H. L. (2009). Increased central venous pressure is associated with impaired renal function and mortality in a broad spectrum of patients with cardiovascular disease. *J Am Coll Cardiol*, 53(7), 582-8.

Dargie, H. J. (2001). Effect of carvedilol on outcome after myocardial infarction in patients with left-ventricular dysfunction: the CAPRICORN randomised trial. *Lancet*, 357(9266), 1385-90.

Di Pasquale, P., Sarullo, F. M., & Paterna, S. (2007). Novel strategies: challenge loop diuretics and sodium management in heart failure--part II. *Congest Heart Fail*, 13(3), 170-6.

Dries, D. L., Exner, D. V., Domanski, M. J., Greenberg, B. & Stevenson, L. W. (2000). The prognostic implications of renal insufficiency in asymptomatic and symptomatic patients with left ventricular systolic dysfunction. *J Am Coll Cardiol*, 35(3), 681-9.

Ensor, C. R., & Russell, S. D. (2010). Tonapofylline: a selective adenosine-1 receptor antagonist for the treatment of heart failure. *Expert Opin Pharmacother*, 11(14), 2405-15.

Erdmann, E., Lechat, P., Verkenne, P., & Wiemann, H. (2001). Results from post-hoc analyses of the CIBIS II trial: effect of bisoprolol in high-risk patient groups with chronic heart failure. *Eur J Heart Fail*, 3(4), 469-79.

Eshaghian S., Howrich, T. B. & Fonarow, G. C. (2006). Relation of loop diuretic dose to mortality in advanced heart failure. *Am J Cardiol*, 97(12), 1759-64.

Ezekowitz, J. A., McAlister, F. A. & Armstrong, P. W. (2003) Anemia is common in heart failure and is associated with poor outcomes: insights from a cohort of 12, 065 patients with new-onset heart failure. *Circ*, 107(2), 223-5.

Felker, G. M., Lee, K. L., Bull, D. A., Redfield, M. M., Stevenson, L. W., Goldsmith, S. R., LeWinter, M. M., Deswal, A., Rouleau, J. L., Ofili, E. O., Anstrom, K. J., Hernandez, A. F., McNulty, S. E., Velazquez, E. J., Kfoury, A. G., Chen, H. H., Givertz, M. M., Semigran, M. J., Bart, B. A., Mascette, A. M., Braunwald, E., & O'Connor, C. M. (2011). Diuretic strategies in patients with acute decompensated heart failure. *N Engl J Med*, 364(9), 797-805.

Firth, J. D., Raine, A. E. & Ledingham, J. G. (1988). Raised venous pressure: a direct cause of renal sodium retention in oedema? *Lancet,* 1(8593), 1033-5.

Foley, R. N., Murray, A. M., Li, S., Herzog, C. A., McBean, A. M., Eggers, P. W. & Collins, A. J. (2005). Chronic kidney disease and the risk for cardiovascular disease, renal replacement, and death in the United States Medicare population, 1998 to 1999. *J Am Soc Nephrol,* (16)2, 489-95.

Fonarow, G. C., Adams, K. F., Abraham, W. T., Yancy, C. W. & Boscardin, W.J.; ADHERE Scientific Advisory Committee, Study Group, and Investigators. (2005) Risk Stratification for in-hospital mortality in acutely decompensated heart failure: classification and regression tree analysis. *JAMA,* 293(5), 572-80.

Friedrich, J. O., Adhikari, N., Herridge, M. S., & Beyene, J. (2005). Meta-analysis: low-dose dopamine increases urine output but does not prevent renal dysfunction or death. *Ann Intern Med,* 142(7), 510-24.

Gheorghiade, M., Konstam, M. A., Burnett, J. C., Jr., Grinfeld, L., Maggioni, A. P., Swedberg, K., Udelson, J. E., Zannad, F., Cook, T., Ouyang, J., Zimmer, C., & Orlandi, C. (2007). Short-term clinical effects of tolvaptan, an oral vasopressin antagonist, in patients hospitalized for heart failure: the EVEREST Clinical Status Trials. *JAMA,* 297(12), 1332-43.

Givertz, M. M., Massie, B. M., Fields, T. K., Pearson, L. L., & Dittrich, H. C. (2007). The effects of KW-3902, an adenosine A1-receptor antagonist,on diuresis and renal function in patients with acute decompensated heart failure and renal impairment or diuretic resistance. *J Am Coll Cardiol,* 50(16), 1551-60.

Go, A. S., Chertow, G. M., Fan, D., McCulloch, C. E. & Hsu, C. Y. (2004). Chronic kidney disease and the risks of death, cardiovascular events, and hospitalization. *NEJM,* 351(13), 1296-305.

Gottlieb, S. S., Abraham, W., Butler, J., Forman, D. E., Loh, E., Massie, B. M., O'connor, C. M., Rich, M. W. , Stevenson, L. W. , Young, J. & Krumholz, H. M. (2002). The prognostic importance of different definitions of worsening renal function in congestive heart failure. *J Card Fail,* 8(3), 136-41.

Hara, Y., Hamada, M., Shigematsu, Y., Murakami, B., & Hiwada, K. (2001). Beneficial effect of beta-adrenergic blockade on left ventricular function in haemodialysis patients. *Clin Sci (Lond),* 101(3), 219-25.

Hauptman, P. J., Schnitzler, M. A., Swindle, J., & Burroughs, T. E. (2006). Use of nesiritide before and after publications suggesting drug-related risks in patients with acute decompensated heart failure. *JAMA,* 296(15), 1877-84.

Hernandez, A. F. (2010). *Acute Study of Clinical Effectiveness of Nesiritide in Decompensated Heart Failure Trial (ASCEND-HF) – Nesiritide or placebo for improved symptoms and outcomes in acute decompensated HF.* Paper presented at the American Heart Association 2010 Scientific Sessions.

Heywood, J. T. (2004). The cardiorenal syndrome: lessons from the ADHERE database and treatment options. *Heart Failure Reviews,* 9(3), 195-201.

Heywood, J. T., Fonarow, G. C., Costanzo, M. R., Mathur, V. S., Wigneswaran, J. R., Wynne, J.; ADHERE Scientific Advisory Committee and Investigators. (2007). High prevalence of renal dysfunction and its impact on outcome in 118, 465 patients hospitalized with acute decompensated heart failure: a report from the ADHERE database. *J Card Fail,* 13(6), 422-30.

Hillege, H. L., Nitsch, D., Pfeffer, M. A., Swedberg, K., McMurray, J. J., Yusuf, S., Granger, C. B., Michelson, E. L., Ostergren, J., Cornel, J. H., de Zeeuw, D., Pocock, S., & van Veldhuisen, D. J. (2006). Renal function as a predictor of outcome in a broad spectrum of patients with heart failure. *Circulation,* 113(5), 671-8.

Horwich, T. B., Fonarow, G. C., Hamilton, M. A., MacLellan, W. R. & Borenstein J. (2002). Anemia is associated with worse symptoms, greater impairment in functional capacity and a significant increase in mortality in patients with advanced heart failure. *J Am Coll Cardiol,* 39(11), 1780-6.

Ix, J. H., Shlipak, M. G., Liu, H. H., Schiller, N. B. & Whooley, M. A. (2003). Association between renal insufficiency and inducible ischemia in patients with coronary artery disease: the heart and soul study. *J Am Soc Nephrol,* 14(12), 3233-8.

Jentzer, J. C., DeWald, T. A., & Hernandez, A. F. (2010). Combination of loop diuretics with thiazide-type diuretics in heart failure. *J Am Coll Cardiol,* 56(19), 1527-34.

Khan, W., Deepak, S. M., Coppinger, T., Waywell, C., Borg, A., Harper, L., Williams, S. G., & Brooks, N. H. (2006). Beta blocker treatment is associated with improvement in renal function and anaemia in patients with heart failure. *Heart,* 92(12), 1856-7.

Keith, D. S., Nichols, G. A., Gullion, C. M., Brown, J. B. & Smith, D. H. (2004). Longitudinal follow-up and outcomes among a population with chronic kidney disease in a large managed care organization. *Arch Int Med,* 164(6), 659-63

Kim, W.Y., Huh, J. W., Lim, C. M., Koh, Y. & Hong, S.B. (2011). Analysis of progression in risk, injury, failure, loss, and end-stage renal disease classification on outcome in patients with severe sepsis and septic shock. *J Crit Care,* doi:10.1016/j.physletb.2003.10.071

Kittleson, M., Hurwitz, S., Shah, M. R., Nohria, A., Lewis, E., Givertz, M., Fang, J., Jarcho, J., Mudge, G., & Stevenson, L. W. (2003). Development of circulatory-renal limitations to angiotensin-converting enzyme inhibitors identifies patients with severe heart failure and early mortality. *J Am Coll Cardiol,* 41(11), 2029-35.

Koniari, K., Nikolaou, M., Paraskevaidis, I., & Parissis, J. (2010). Therapeutic options for the management of the cardiorenal syndrome. *Int J Nephrol,* 2011, 194910.

Konstam, M. A., Gheorghiade, M., Burnett, J. C., Jr., Grinfeld, L., Maggioni, A. P., Swedberg, K., Udelson, J. E., Zannad, F., Cook, T., Ouyang, J., Zimmer, C., & Orlandi, C. (2007). Effects of oral tolvaptan in patients hospitalized for worsening heart failure: the EVEREST Outcome Trial. *JAMA,* 297(12), 1319-31.

Levey, A. S., Coresh, J., Balk, E., Kausz, A. T., Levin, A., Steffes, M. W., Hogg, R. J., Perrone, R. D., Lau, J., Eknoyan, G.; National Kidney Foundation. (2003). National Kidney Foundation practice guidelines for chronic kidney disease: evaluation, classification, and stratification. *Ann Intern Med,* 139(2), 137-47.

Lewis, E. J., Hunsicker, L. G., Bain, R. P., & Rohde, R. D. (1993). The effect of angiotensin-converting-enzyme inhibition on diabetic nephropathy. The Collaborative Study Group. *N Engl J Med,* 329(20), 1456-62.

Licata, G., Di Pasquale, P., Parrinello, G., Cardinale, A., Scandurra, A., Follone, G., Argano, C., Tuttolomondo, A., & Paterna, S. (2003). Effects of high-dose furosemide and small-volume hypertonic saline solution infusion in comparison with a high dose of furosemide as bolus in refractory congestive heart failure: long-term effects. *Am Heart J*, 145(3), 459-66.

Linde, T., Wikstrom, B., Andersson, L. G., & Danielson, B. G. (1996). Renal anaemia treatment with recombinant human erythropoietin increases cardiac output in patients with ischaemic heart disease. *Scand J Urol Nephrol*, 30(2), 115-20.

Low, I., Grutzmacher, P., Bergmann, M., & Schoeppe, W. (1989). Echocardiographic findings in patients on maintenance hemodialysis substituted with recombinant human erythropoietin. *Clin Nephrol*, 31(1), 26-30.

Low-Friedrich, I., Grutzmacher, P., Marz, W., Bergmann, M., & Schoeppe, W. (1991). Therapy with recombinant human erythropoietin reduces cardiac size and improves heart function in chronic hemodialysis patients. *Am J Nephrol*, 11(1), 54-60.

Marenzi, G., Grazi, S., Giraldi, F., Lauri, G., Perego, G., Guazzi, M., Salvioni, A., & Guazzi, M. D. (1993). Interrelation of humoral factors, hemodynamics, and fluid and salt metabolism in congestive heart failure: effects of extracorporeal ultrafiltration. *Am J Med*, 94(1), 49-56.

Massie, B. M., O'Connor, C. M., Metra, M., Ponikowski, P., Teerlink, J. R., Cotter, G., Weatherley, B. D., Cleland, J. G., Givertz, M. M., Voors, A., DeLucca, P., Mansoor, G. A., Salerno, C. M., Bloomfield, D. M., & Dittrich, H. C. (2010). Rolofylline, an adenosine A1-receptor antagonist, in acute heart failure. *N Engl J Med*, 363(15), 1419-28.

McCullough, P. A. & Lepor, N. E. (2005). Piecing together the evidence on anemia: the link between chronic kidney disease and cardiovascular disease. *Rev Cardiovasc Med*, 6(Suppl 3), S4-12.

Mullens, W., Abrahams, Z., Francis, G. S., Sokos, G., Taylor, D. O., Starling, R. C., Young, J. B. & Tang, W. H. (2009). Importance of venous congestion for worsening of renal function in advanced decompensated heart failure. *J Am Coll Cardiol* 53(7), 589-96.

Muntner, P., He, J., Astor, B. C., Folsom, A.R. & Coresh, J. (2005). Traditional and nontraditional risk factors predict coronary heart disease in chronic kidney disease: results from the atherosclerosis risk in communities study. *J Am Soc Nephrol*, 16(2), 529-38.

Nagashima, K., & Karasawa, A. (1996). Effects of KW-3902 (8-(noradamantan-3-yl)-1,3-dipropylxanthine), an adenosine A1-receptor antagonist, on urinary excretions of various electrolytes in rats. *Biol Pharm Bull*, 19(7), 940-3.

Nohria, A., Hasselblad, V., Stebbins, A., Pauly, D. F., Fonarow, G. C., Shah, M., Yancy, C. W., Califf, R. M. , Stevenson, L. W. & Hill, J. A. (2008). Cardiorenal interactions: Insights from the ESCAPE trial. *J Am Coll Cardiol*, 51(13), 1268-74.

Palazzuoli, A., Silverberg, D., Iovine, F., Capobianco, S., Giannotti, G., Calabro, A., Campagna, S. M., & Nuti, R. (2006). Erythropoietin improves anemia exercise tolerance and renal function and reduces B-type natriuretic peptide and hospitalization in patients with heart failure and anemia. *Am Heart J*, 152(6), 1096 e1099-1115.

Parikh, N. I., Hwang, S. J., Larson, M. G., Meigs, J. B., Levy, D. & Fox, C. S. (2006). Cardiovascular disease risk factors in chronic kidney disease: overall burden and rates of treatment and control. *Arch Intern Med,* 166(17), 1884-91.

Paterna, S., Di Pasquale, P., Parrinello, G., Amato, P., Cardinale, A., Follone, G., Giubilato, A., & Licata, G. (2000). Effects of high-dose furosemide and small-volume hypertonic saline solution infusion in comparison with a high dose of furosemide as a bolus, in refractory congestive heart failure. *Eur J Heart Fail,* 2(3), 305-13.

Publication Committeee for the VMAC Investigators (2002). Intravenous nesiritide vs nitroglycerin for treatment of decompensated congestive heart failure: a randomized controlled trial. *JAMA,* 287(12), 1531-40.

Ricci, Z., Cruz, D. & Ronco C. (2008). The RIFLE criteria and mortality in acute kidney injury: A systematic review. *Kidney Int,* 73(5), 538-46.

Rimondini, A., Cipolla, C. M., Della Bella, P., Grazi, S., Sisillo, E., Susini, G., & Guazzi, M. D. (1987). Hemofiltration as short-term treatment for refractory congestive heart failure. *Am J Med,* 83(1), 43-8.

Ronco, C., Haapio M., House, A. A., Anavekar N. & Bellomo, R. (2008). Cardiorenal Syndrome. *J Am Coll Cardiol,* 52(19), 1527-39.

Sackner-Bernstein, J. D., Kowalski, M., Fox, M., & Aaronson, K. (2005). Short-term risk of death after treatment with nesiritide for decompensated heart failure: a pooled analysis of randomized controlled trials. *JAMA,* 293(15), 1900-5.

Sackner-Bernstein, J. D., Skopicki, H. A., & Aaronson, K. D. (2005). Risk of worsening renal function with nesiritide in patients with acutely decompensated heart failure. *Circulation,* 111(12), 1487-91.

Sands, J. M. (2003). Mammalian urea transporters. *Annu Rev Physiol,* 65, 543-66.

Schrier, R. W., Gross, P., Gheorghiade, M., Berl, T., Verbalis, J. G., Czerwiec, F. S., & Orlandi, C. (2006). Tolvaptan, a selective oral vasopressin V2-receptor antagonist, for hyponatremia. *N Engl J Med,* 355(20), 2099-112.

Schrier, R. W., Masoumi, A., & Elhassan, E. (2009). Role of vasopressin and vasopressin receptor antagonists in type I cardiorenal syndrome. *Blood Purif,* 27(1), 28-32.

Sharma, R., Francis, D. P., Pitt, B., Poole-Wilson, P. A., Coats, A. J. & Anker, S. D. (2004). Haemoglobin predicts survival in patients with chronic heart failure: a substudy of the ELITE II trial. *Eur Heart J,* 25(12), 1021-8.

Shlipak, M. G., Heidenreich, P. A., Noguchi, H., Chertow, G. M., Browner, W. S. & McClellan, M. B. (2002). Association of renal insufficiency with treatment and outcomes after myocardial infarction in elderly patients. *Ann Intern Med,* 137(7), 555-62.

Siew, E. D., Ware, L. B. & Ikizler, T. A. (2011). Biological markers of acute kidney injury. *J Am Soc Nephrol,* 22(5), 810-20.

Silverberg, D. S., Wexler, D., Blum, M., Keren, G., Sheps, D., Leibovitch, E., Brosh, D., Laniado, S., Schwartz, D., Yachnin, T., Shapira, I., Gavish, D., Baruch, R., Koifman, B., Kaplan, C., Steinbruch, S., & Iaina, A. (2000). The use of subcutaneous erythropoietin and intravenous iron for the treatment of the anemia of severe, resistant congestive heart failure improves cardiac and renal function and functional cardiac class, and markedly reduces hospitalizations. *J Am Coll Cardiol,* 35(7), 1737-44.

Smith, G. L., Lichtman, J. H., Bracken, M. B., Shlipak, M. G., Phillips, C. O., DiCapua, P. & Krumholz, H. M. (2006). Renal impairment and outcomes in heart failure: systematic review and meta-analysis. *J Am Coll Cardiol*, 47(10), 1987-96.

Smith, G. L., Masoudi, F. A., Shlipak, M. G., Krumholz, H. M. & Parikh, C. R. (2008). Renal impairment predicts long-term mortality risk after acute myocardial infarction. *J Am Soc Nephrol*, 19(1), 141-50.

Swedberg, K., Eneroth, P., Kjekshus, J., & Snapinn, S. (1990). Effects of enalapril and neuroendocrine activation on prognosis in severe congestive heart failure (follow-up of the CONSENSUS trial). CONSENSUS Trial Study Group. *Am J Cardiol,* 66(11), 40D-44D; discussion 44D-45D.

Tanaka, K., Ito, M., Kodama, M., Maruyama, H., Hoyano, M., Mitsuma, W., Iino, N., Hirono, S., Okura, Y., Gejyo, F., Tanabe, N., & Aizawa, Y. (2007). Longitudinal change in renal function in patients with idiopathic dilated cardiomyopathy without renal insufficiency at initial diagnosis. *Circ J,* 71(12), 1927-31.

The National Heart, Lung and Blood Institute Working Group. (2004) Executive Summary, In: *Cardio-Renal Connections in Heart Failure and Cardiovascular Disease,* 06.23.2011, Available from: www.nhlbi.nih.gov/meetings/workshops/cardiorenal-hf-hd.htm

The SOLVD Investigators (1991). Effect of enalapril on survival in patients with reduced left ventricular ejection fractions and congestive heart failure. *New England Journal of Medicine,* 325(5), 293-302.

The SOLVD Investigators (1992). Effect of enalapril on mortality and the development of heart failure in asymptomatic patients with reduced left ventricular ejection fractions. *New England Journal of Medicine,* 327(10), 685-91.

Toblli, J. E., Lombrana, A., Duarte, P., & Di Gennaro, F. (2007). Intravenous iron reduces NT-pro-brain natriuretic peptide in anemic patients with chronic heart failure and renal insufficiency. *J Am Coll Cardiol,* 50(17), 1657-65.

Uchino, S., Bellomo, R., Goldsmith, D., Bates, S. & Ronco, C. (2006). An Assessment of the RIFLE criteria for acute renal failure in hospitalized patients. *Crit Care Med,* 34(7), 1913-17.

Uthoff, H., Breidthardt, T., Klima, T., Aschwanden, M., Arenja, N., Socrates, T., Heinisch, C., Noveanu, M., Frischknecht, B., Baumann, U., Jaeger, K. A. & Mueller, C. (2011) Central venous pressure and impaired renal function in patients with acute heart failure. *Eur J Heart Fail* 13(4), 432-9.

Virani, S. A., Khosla A. & Levin A. (2008). Chronic kidney disease, heart failure and anemia. *Can J Cardiol,* 24(Suppl B), 22B-24B.

Wali, R. K. & Henrich, W. L. (2005). Chronic kidney disease: a risk factor for cardiovascular disease. *Cardiol Clin,* 23(3), 343-62.

Wali, R. K., Iyengar, M., Beck, G. J., Chartyan, D. M., Chonchol, M., Lukas, M. A., Cooper, C., Himmelfarb, J., Weir, M. R., Berl, T., Henrich, W. L., & Cheung, A. K. (2011). Efficacy and safety of carvedilol in treatment of heart failure with chronic kidney disease: a meta-analysis of randomized trials. *Circ Heart Fail,* 4(1), 18-26.

Wattanakit, K., Coresh, J., Muntner, P., Marsh, J. & Folsom, A. R. (2006). Cardiovascular risk among adults with chronic kidney disease, with or without prior myocardial infarction. *J Am Coll Cardiol*, 48(6), 1183-9.

Yao, K., Kusaka, H., Sato, K., & Karasawa, A. (1994). Protective effects of KW-3902, a novel adenosine A1-receptor antagonist, against gentamicin-induced acute renal failure in rats. *Jpn J Pharmacol, 65*(2), 167-70.

# 9

# Atherosclerotic Renovascular Disease

Gen-Min Lin, Chih-Lu Han, Chung-Chi Yang
and Cheng-Chung Cheng
*National Defense Medical Center*
*Taiwan*

## 1. Introduction

Atherosclerotic renovascular disease (ARVD), also known as atherosclerotic renal artery stenosis is increasingly recognized to be a cause of chronic renal failure. According to a recent administrative data regarding general population of the elderly greater than 65 years of age in the United States, the prevalence and incidence rates of ARVD were estimated 0.5% and 3.7 per each 1000 person-years respectively (Kalra et al., 2005). In addition, some epidemiological researches demonstrated that the prevalence among those with end-stage renal disease beginning renal replacement therapy was estimated from 5% to 22% (Rimmer & Gennari, 1993; Mailloux et al., 1994; Appel et al., 1995; van Ampting et al., 2003). Of note, ARVD is not only responsible to impaired kidney function but also reflects a status of patients at risk for systemic cardiovascular diseases (Kalra et al., 2005). It has been well known that a variety of risk factors for atherosclerosis share common pathway underlying atherosclerotic renal artery stenosis, coronary artery disease, and peripheral vascular disease. On the contrary, significant high-grade bilateral or isolated renal artery stenosis may cause renovascular hypertension estimating over 50% of ARVD populations by activation of renin-angiotensin-aldosterone system and lipoxygenase pathway that further deteriorate the kidney function (Romero 1997). A previous report uncovered that ARVD was estimated from 1% to 6% in patients with hypertension (Simon et al., 1972). In this regard, a vicious cycle will be established in the progression of renal arterial atherosclerosis, which is characterized by refractory hypertension, acute cardiac events (ie, heart failure, cardiogenic pulmonary edema or acute coronary syndrome), and hence leads to acute or chronic renal failure due to hypertensive or ischemic nephropathy (Buller et al., 2004). Therefore, an early alert of patients at risk for ARVD is critical in slowing down the rate of kidney function loss and providing treatment for underlying cardiovascular disease as well. In this chapter, we will fuel the readers with the classic knowledge in this field and propose the latest evidence-based medicine to manage patients with this disease.

## 2. The pathogenesis of atherosclerosis

Atherosclerosis is affected by the traditional risk factors including hypertension, smoking, hyperlipidemia, diabetes mellitus and family history of premature coronary artery disease systemically. Regionally, blood flow disturbances near arterial branches, bifurcations and curvatures result in complex spatiotemporal shear stresses that are associated with atherosclerosis susceptibility (Davies, 2009). In these predisposed areas, hemodynamic shear stress, the frictional force acting on the endothelial cell surface is weaker than in protected regions. Studies have identified shear stress to be an important determinant of endothelial function and phenotype. High shear stress (>15 dyne/cm$^2$) induces endothelial quiescence and an atheroprotective gene expression profile, while low shear stress (<4 dyne/cm$^2$), which is prevalent at atherosclerosis-prone sites, stimulates an atherogenic phenotype (Malek et al, 1999). As we know, thrombosis formation in situ and distal embolic dislodge from great vessels, determined by the burden and the stability of atherosclerosis, are the two major mechanisms leading to target organ infarction. With recent substantial evidence, systemic inflammation caused by either external stimulus such as microbial infection or internal immunologic response may trigger acute vascular events via pathogenic athroma plaque rupture. Therefore, when and how to stablize and regress the process of atherosclerosis becomes a cirtical step to prevent target organ damage.

### 2.1 Systemic arterial atherosclerosis: the evidence from angiography and autopsy

Advanced atherosclerosis is highly prevalent among patients with ARVD characterized by coexistence with abdominal aortic aneurysm, severe coronary artery disease, ischemic stroke and peripheral vascular disease in post-mortem and angiographic studies (Table 1).

| | ANG (Patient: n) | Age (year) | CAD (%) | PAD (%) | ARVD (%) | Predictors |
|---|---|---|---|---|---|---|
| Crowley, 1998 | CAD: 14,152 | 61±12 | 63% | NA | 6.3% (bil: 1.3%) | Predictors for ARVD progression:<br>-Female gender, OR: 1.8<br>-PAD, OR: 1.8<br>-Hypertension, OR: 1.5<br>-significant CAD, OR: 1.2 |
| Conlon, 2001 | CAD: 3,987 | 61±9 | 100% | NA | 9.1% (4.8%)* | -CAD: 2VD vs.1VD, OR: 1.9<br>-CAD: 3VD vs 1VD, OR: 2.5 |
| Liu, 2004 | CAD: 141 | 59±10 | 31% | NA | 18.4% | -CAD vs. non-CAD, HR: 2.8 |
| Leandri, 2004 | CAD: 467 | 64±11 | 69% | NA | 9.0% | -CAD: 2VD vs.1VD, OR: 2.8<br>-CAD: 3VD vs 1VD, OR: 3.0 |
| Buller, 2004 | ARVD: 837 | 67±10 | 68% | -Carotid: 12%<br>-A.A.A or lower limb PAD: 12% | 14.4% (bil: 3.1%) | -Age per 10 year, OR:1.7<br>-Female gender. OR:1.9<br>-A.A.A or lower limb PAD, OR: 2.1<br>-Carotid, OR: 3.0 |
| Zhang, 2006 | CAD: 1,200 | 62±10 | 51% | NA | 9.7% (bil: 1.7%) | Age, hypertension, renal insufficiency, CAD |
| Ozkan, 2009 | PAD: 629 | 62±11 | 43% | Aortoiliac, crural, femoropopliteal: 83% | 9.6%§ | Age, hypertension and aortoiliac stenosis |

| | ANG (Patient: n) | Age (year) | CAD (%) | PAD (%) | ARVD (%) | Predictors |
|---|---|---|---|---|---|---|
| Kuroda, 2000 | Stroke: 346 | 69±11 | 33% | -Carotid: 29.2%<br>-A.A.A: 13.3% | 10.4%* | -Renal insufficiency, OR: 6.6<br>-Hypertension:, OR: 4.1<br>-Carotid >50%, OR: 4.8<br>-Female gender, OR: 3.4 |
| Fujii, 2006 | Stroke: 346 | 71±11 | 39% | NA | 26.1%*<br>(bil: 19%) | Hypertension, renal insufficiency, PAD |

Table 1. Associations between systemic atherosclerosis and ARVD: n: number; ANG: renal angiography; CAD: coronary artery stenosis>50%; ARVD: renal artery stenosis>50%; PAD: peripheral artery stenosis>50%; NA: not available; A.A.A: abdominal aortic aneurysm;; carotid: carotid artery stenosis>50%; HR: hazard ratio; OR: odds ratio; VD: number of diseased coronary artery; § renal artery stenosis>60%; * renal artery stenosis>75%.

### 2.1.1 The nature course of ARVD

According to the shear stress rule, ostial and proximal lesions are mostly encountered and 20%-50% of cases are bilateral sites in ARVD (Safian & Textor, 2001). A significant progression of ARVD was observed in 11.1% of 14,152 subjects with high cardiovascular risks within a 2.6-year period in an angiographic study (Crowley et al, 1995) and in 35%-51% from 3 to 5 years in a doplex unltrasonography study (Caps et al, 1998). From these reports, the predictors to disease progression include old age, female gender, hypertension, diabetes and the presence of significant coronary artery disease or peripheral vascular disease in which the odds ratios range from 1.2 to 2.1. On the other hand, patients with ARVD are associated with approximately 2-times risk of the occurrence of adverse coronary events and mortality as compared to those without ARVD in a long-term follow-up (Conlon et al, 2001; Edwards et al, 2005).

### 2.2 How to select patients at risk for prompt screening

As prescribed previously, patients at higher risk for atherosclerosis should receive an advanced step for screening the presence of ARVD (table 2)

Among these clinical features, the only statistically significant predictor to ARVD is the presence of abdominal bruit. The prevalence ranges from 6.5% to 31% in the healthy population (Watson & William, 1973), and 28% in hypertensive patients (Julius and Steward, 1967). However, in patients with angiographically proven ARVD, the prevalence increases up to 80% (Turnbull, 1995). Besides, the sensitivity of a systolic-diastolic abdominal bruit in the diagnosis of RAS has been reported from 39% to 63% and the specificity of 90% to 99% ((Turnbull, 1995). Thus, the presence of a systolic-diastolic bruit is highly suggestive of RAS and should be screened for, while the absence of a bruit does not exclude RAS (Rosener 2001).

### 2.2.1 Differential diagnosis

Some clinical situations have to been addressed in the diffential diagnosis of ARVD (table 3).

| Categories | Criteria |
|---|---|
| Physical findings | -Abdominal or flank bruit |
| Metabolic syndorme | *International Diabetes Federation*:<br>- Central obesity is defined as waist circumference with ethnicity specific values or if BMI is >30 $kg/m^2$, central obesity can be assumed and waist circumference does not need to be measured.<br>**And and any two of the following**:<br>-Triglycerides: > 150 mg/dl, or specific treatment for this lipid abnormality.<br>- HDL cholesterol: < 40 mg/dl in males, < 50 mg/dl in females, or specific treatment for this lipid abnormality<br>- BP: systolic BP > 130 mmHg or diastolic BP >85 mm Hg, or treatment of previously diagnosed hypertension.<br>- FPG >100 mg/dl, or previously diagnosed type 2 diabetes. If FPG>100 mg/dl, OGTT glucose tolerance test is strongly recommanded but is not necessary to define presense of the syndrome |
| Hypertension | -Refractory hypertension (BP >160/95 mm Hg while receiving three or more antihypertensive agents) or associataed acute pulmonary edema<br>-Accelerated hypertension (increase in BP>15% in 6 months)<br>-Severe hypertension (DBP >115 mm Hg or Grade III or IV retinopathy)<br>-Recent-onset (within the last 2 years) hypertension<br>-Onset of hypertension after age 60 |
| Renal insufficiency | -Elevated serum blood urea nitrogen > 20mg/dl or creatinine > 1.4 mg/dl<br>-Cockcroft-Gault CrCl < 50 ml/min without clear etiology<br>-Acute renal failure attributable to ACEI or ARB therapy |
| Atheroscelrosis | -Abdominal aortic atherosclerosis or lower extremity artery stenosis<br>-Peripheral artery disease or carotid artery stenosis / ischemic stroke<br>-Coronary artery disease > 2 vessel disease |

Table 2. Patients at risk for further ARVD screening. BP: blood pressure; DBP: diastolic BP; FPG: Fasting plasma glucose; OGTT: oral glucose tolerance test; CrCl: creatinine clearance; ACEI: ACE inhibitors; ARB: angiotensin II receptor blockers.

| Clinical situations | Differential diagnosis |
|---|---|
| Abdominal bruit | Splenic arteriovenous fistula, hepatic cirrhosis, hepatoma, abdominal aortic aneurysm and coarctation, celiac artery compression syndrome, intestinal ischemia, and pancreatic carcinoma |
| Rrogressive renal insufficiency or renovascular hypertension | -Benign hypertensive nephrosclerosis<br>-Atheroembolic renal disease |
| Renal artery stenosis | -Renal artery dissection<br>-Fibromuscular dysplasia |

Table 3. Differential diagnosis of ARVD.

Most of these clinical situations could be differentiataed correctly by the image study such as computed tomography and renal angiography. They are not neccessry mutually exclusive and may be coexisted. For instance, benign hypertensive nephrosclerosis, a renal parenchymal disease can be present together with ARVD. Atheroembolic renal disease is associated with aortic manupulation or occurs spontaneously. The clinical features include abrupt decline of renal functions and evidence of atrial fibrillation with extrarenal embolism (Hazanov, 2004). Fibromuscular dysplasia (FMD) characterized by fibrous thickening in arterial wall usually involves 60%-75% of renal and 25%-30% of carotid artery stenosis (Luscher et al, 1981; Gray et al 1996) and is respoisble for 25 % cases of renovascular hypertension (Pickering, 1989). In angiographic findings, FMD demostrates classic images of " string-of-beads" appearance, aneurysm, and focal or tubular stenosis. In conrast to ARVD, FMD occurs predominantly in young women of childbearing age and involves the middle and distal portion of main renal artery (Das et al, 2007).

### 2.3 The screening and diagnostic modality

With the progression of the technology, a variety of modalities emerge for screening and diagnosis of ARVD (table 4). In addition to renogram and nuclear scintigraphic captopril renogram, doplex ultrasonography has been used successfully to detect the presence of renal artery stenosis due to the non-invasive and contrast-free characteristics. However, it is usually limited by a wide operator-dependent variation, obesity of patient and time consuming. Magnetic resonance (MR) angiography increases the comparability between examinations (Fig. 1A). Both of the sensitivity and specificity are estimated within 90-95%. Till now, multi-detector computed tomography (MDCT) angiography (Fig. 1B) almost replaces the role of catheter angiography as the first diagnostic tool for ARVD because of its high utility and detection rate in evaluation of other abdominal problems.

| Categories | Sensitivity/specificity | PPV/NPV | Limitations |
|---|---|---|---|
| Renogram | 75% /75% | 50-75% /60% | Almost for screening only |
| Captopril renogram | 83-90% / 80-93% | 70-92% /60-100% | Hypotension |
| Doplex ultrasonography | 75-90% /62-90% | 60% /95% | Wide operator-dependent variation, time consuming |
| MR angiography | 88-95% /90-95% | 60-75% /90-98% | Gadolinium-induced renopathy |
| MDCT angiography | 94-100% / 93-100% | 71-100% /95-100% | Contrast-induced renopathy |
| Catheter angiography | 100% | 100% | Contrast-induced renopathy, bleeding, arterial dissection, distal embolism |

Table 4. Diagnostic modalities for ARVD. PPV: positive predictive value; NPV: negative PV.

### 2.4 Therapeutic indications

As we know, ARVD is highly associated with systemic atherosclerosis and occurs after the occurrence of coronary artery disease and peripheral artery disease. Accordingly, an early medical intervention and risk factors reductions to prevent the development of ARVD in the

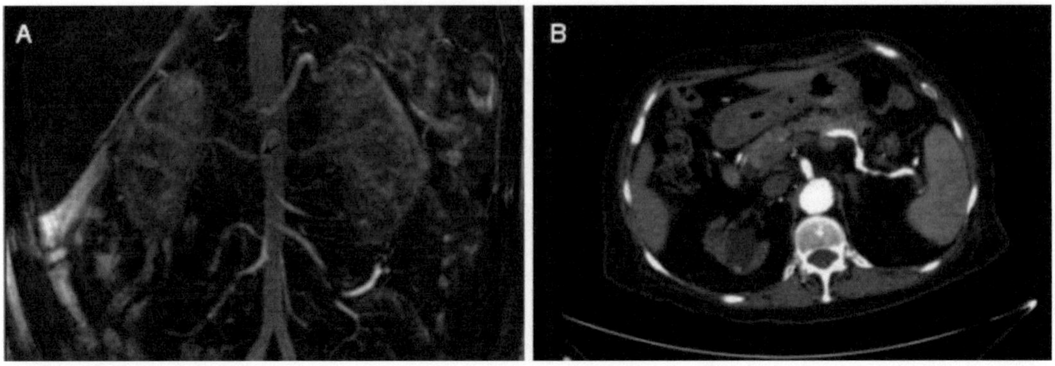


Fig. 1. A: MR angiography demonstrates a right ostial renal artery stenosis (an arrowhead); B: MDCT angiography demonstrates diffuse atherosclerosis of left renal artery (an arrowhead indicate the proximal lesion of left renal artery).

presence of systemic atherosclerosis and many risk factors is important. On the other hand, a critically unilateral or bilateral stenosis of renal artery disease may need further mechanical manipulations such as renal angioplasty, stenting and bypass surgery. We will describe the two parts of therapy in detail in the following paragraphs.

#### 2.4.1 Medical treatment

Life style modification and a control of established risk factors is the golden rule for most atherosclerotic vascular disease including diabetes, obesity, hypertension, low density lipoprotein cholesterol (LDL-C), inflammation and smoking. However, no reports prove the effect of medical control to reduce the occurrence of ARVD or prevent disease progression. It is reasonable that medical treatment should be started in middle-aged persons at risk to prevent ARVD. The choice of pharmacological agents and the goal aimed to achieve with or without vascular events will be listed in table 5.

Among the antihypertensive agents, ACE inhibitors or angiotensin II receptor blockers (ARBs) are observed with the most effectiveness in control of the blood pressure for patients with ARVD (Dworkin & Jamerson, 2007). Surgical intervention should be considered if refractory hypertension persisits. However, adequate control of blood pressure by chronic administration of antihypertensive drugs can not be guarantteed the prevention of stenotic lesions progression and post-stenotic renal.atrophy.

#### 2.4.2 Interventional treatment

Renal artery revascularization for bilateral or unilateral disease in a single viable kidney is indicated in the following situations (Greco & Breyer, 1997; Textor, 2004).

1. Severe or refractory hypertension
2. Recurrent episodes of acute pulmonary edema
3. Unexplained progressive renal insufficiency
4. Progressive renal function impairment with optimal blood pressure control.

Beyond these criteria mentioned above, the procedure of revascularization should be performed after weighing the benefits against the hazards. Therefore revascularization

| Risk factors | Medications | (non) CVD / Goal | Precautious |
|---|---|---|---|
| Diabetes mellitus | Insulin, secretagogues, sensitizers, α-glucosidase inhibitors, peptide analogs | Non-CVD/ HbA1c< 6.5 %<br>CVD/ LDL-C < 7.0 % | Adverse cadiovascualr effects and metabolic abnormalities of anti-diabetic agents |
| Hypertension | ACEI/ ARB, BB, CB, diuretics | Non-CVD/ BP< 120/85 mg/L<br>CVD/ BP< 140/90mg/dl | -A J-curve relationship between hypertension and cardiovascular mortality<br>-ACEI/ARB should be used carefully in bilateral ARVD |
| LDL-C | Statin, fibrates, resins, niacin, ezetimibe, | Non-CVD/ LDL-C< 100 mg/L<br>CVD/ LDL-C < 70mg/dl | Multi-drug interaction and dose effect related rhabdomyolysis |
| Inflammation | -Antiplatelet agents<br>-Statin<br>-Investagated drugs | Non-CVD/ hs-CRP< 2mg/L<br>CVD/ not established | According to the JUPITER trial only (Ridker et al, 2008) |

Table 5. Modifiable risk factors for ARVD. CVD: cardiovascular disease including myocardial infarction and ischemic stroke; ACEI: ACE inhibitors; ARB: angiotensin II receptor blockers; BP: blood pressure; BB: beta-blocker; CB: calcium receptor blocker; JUPITER: Justification for the Use of Statins in Primary Prevention: An Intervention Trial Evaluating Rosuvastatin trial; CRP: C-reactive protein.

should be aimed for patients with a reversible status of chronic renal insufficiency and resistant hypertension instead of reduing their mortality. A review literature has demonstrated that half of patients with ARVD have no change in renal function, while one fourth improve and one fifth deterioate their renal function after renal stenting (Fig.1A & B) (Leertouwer et al, 2000).

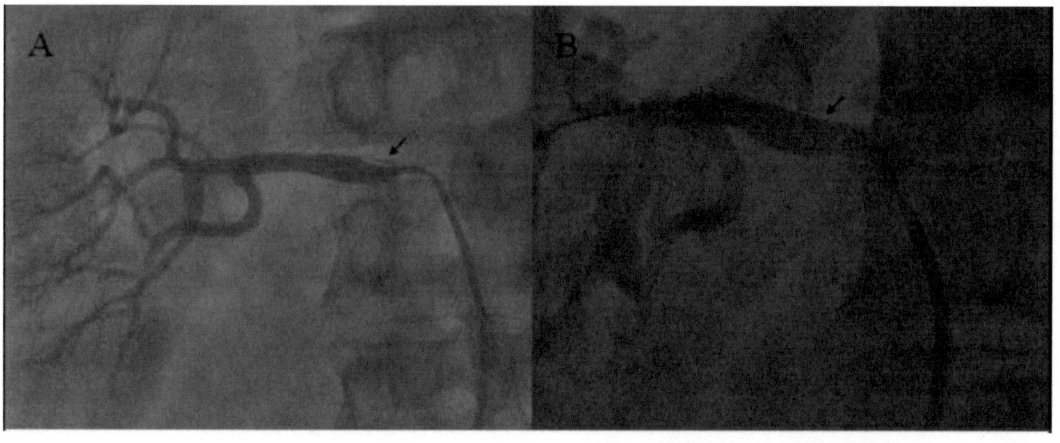


Fig. 2. An atherosclerotic ostial lesion at right renal artery. Panel A: catheter renal angiography (An arrowhead indicates a lesion from ostial to proximal right renal artery; Panel B: post-percutaneous transluminal angioplasty with stenting (An arrowhead indicates stenting site of right renal artery).

Accordingly, only 20-25% of patients may be eligible for elective renal revascularization. There have some image, histology and clinical evidence to select patients with ARVD having benefits to undergo renal artery revascularization which is described as follow (Novick et al, 1987; Muray et al, 2002).

1. Visualization of the collecting system either on an intravenous pyelogram or during the pyelogram phase after renal arteriography
2. Kidney length ≥9 cm.
3. The presence of intact glomeruli on frozen section biopsy at the time of surgery.
4. Rapid decline of renal functions after ACEI/ARB administrations.

There are three methods for renal artery revascularization (table 6).

| Revascularization | Indications | Comments |
|---|---|---|
| PTA without stenting (Connolly et al, 1994) | Non-ostial lesions | -65-70% success rate for lesions<br>-35-50% improvement of renal functions |
| PTA with stenting (ASTRAL investigators, 2009; Stone et al, 2011; White, 2010; Davies et al, 2009) | Ostial and non-ostial lesions | -Significantly lower restenosis rate than PTA alone<br>-98.8% success rate for lesions<br>-10.6-19% TVR rate within 5-10 years period<br>-Inconclusive results of the improvement of renal functions<br>-Complication rate: 9% in 24 hours; 20% in 1 month; mortality rate <1% |
| Bypass surgery (ACC/AHA 2005 guidelines; Hansen et al, 1992) | -Multiple small renal arteries<br>-Early primary branching of the main renal artery<br>-Aortic reconstruction near the renal arteries | -85-90% success rate for lesions<br>-55-65% improvement of lesions of renal functions<br>-In-hospital mortality rate: 3-10% |

Table 6. Comparison of three types of revascularization intervention. PTA: percutaneous transluminal angioplasty; TVR: target vessel revascularization; ASTRAL: Angioplasty and Stenting for Renal Artery Lesions; ACC/AHA: American College of Cardiology Foundation/American Heart Association.

## 3. Conclusion

ARVD reflecting a status of systemic atherosclerosis is associated with chronic renal disease. Life style modification and risk factors reduction are important for the primary prevention of ongoing renal dysfunction and secondary prevention of subsequent cardiovascular events. Some clinical features of patients at risk for ARVD should be highlighted and both medical treatment and mechanical procedures should be taken as early as possible if uncontrolled hypertension leading to end-organ damage or progressive renal insufficiency develops.

## 4. Acknowledgement

We thank Dr. Yu-Guang Chen, Tri-Service General Hospital for his kindly providing the image of MDCT angiography.

## 5. References

Appel, RG, Bleyer, AJ, Reavis, S, Hansen, KJ. (1995). Renovascular disease in older patients beginning renal replacement therapy. *Kidney Int*, Vol. 48, No.1, (May 2011), pp.171-176, ISSN 1523-1755

ASTRAL Investigators, Wheatley, K, Ives, N, Gray, R, Kalra, PA, Moss, JG, Baigent, C, Carr, S, Chalmers, N, Eadington, D, Hamilton, G, Lipkin, G, Nicholson, A, Scoble, J. (2009). Revascularization versus medical therapy for renal-artery stenosis. *N Engl J Med*, Vol. 361, No. 20, (May 2011), pp.1953-1962, ISSN1046-6673

Buller, CE, Nogareda, JG, Ramanathan, K, Ricci, DR, Djurdjev, O, Tinckam, KJ, Penn, IM, Fox, RS, Stevens, LA, Duncan, JA, Levin, A. (2004). The profile of cardiac patients with renal artery stenosis. *J Am coll cardiol*, Vol. 43, No.9, (May, 2011), pp.1614-1616, ISSN 0735-1097.

Caps, MT, Perissinotto, C, Zierler, RE, Polissar, NL, Bergelin, RO, Tullis, MJ, Cantwell-Gab, K, Davidson, RC, Strandness, DE Jr.(1998). Prospective study of atherosclerotic disease progression in the renal artery. *Circulation*, Vol.98, No.25, (May 2011), pp.2866-2872, ISSN 0009-7322

Conlon, PJ, Little, MA, Pieper, K, Mark, DB. (2001). Severity of renal vascular disease predicts mortality in patients undergoing coronary angiography. *Kidney Int*, Vol. 60, No.4, (May 2011), pp.1490-1497, ISSN 1523-1755

Connolly, JO, Higgins, RM, Walters, HL, Mackie, AD, Drury, PL, Hendry, BM, Scoble, JE. (1994). Presentation, clinical features and outcome in different patterns of atherosclerotic renovascular disease. *QJM*, Vol.87, No.7, (May 2011), pp.413-421, ISSN 1460-2725.

Crowley, JJ, Santos, RM, Peter, RH, Puma, JA, Schwab, SJ, Phillips, HR, Stack, RS, Conlon, PJ. (1998). Progression of renal artery stenosis in patients undergoing cardiac catheterization. *Am Heart J*, Vol.136, No.5, (May 2011), pp.913-918, ISSN 0002-8703

Davies, MG, Saad, WA, Bismuth, JX, Peden, EK, Naoum, JJ, Lumsden, AB. (2009). Outcomes of endoluminal reintervention for restenosis after percutaneous renal angioplasty and stenting. *J Vasc Surg*, Vol.49, No.4, (May 2011) pp.946-52, ISSN 1532-2165

Davies PF. (2009). Hemodynamic shear stress and the endothelium in cardiovascular pathophysiology. *Nat Clin Pract Cardiovasc Med*, Vol.6, No.1 (May, 2011), pp.16-26, ISSN 1743-4297

de Mast, Q, Beutler, JJ. (2009). The prevalence of atherosclerotic renal artery stenosis in risk groups: a systematic literature review. *J Hypertens.*, Vol.27, No.7, (May 2011), pp.1333-1340, ISSN 0263-6352

Dworkin, LD, Jamerson, KA. (2007). Is renal artery stenting the correct treatment of renal artery stenosis? Case against angioplasty and stenting of atherosclerotic renal artery stenosis. *Circulation.*, Vol. 115, No. 2, (May 2011), pp.271-276, ISSN 0009-7322

Edwards, MS, Craven, TE, Burke, GL, Dean, RH, Hansen, KJ. (2005). Renovascular disease and the risk of adverse coronary events in the elderly: a prospective, population-based study. *Arch Intern Med.*, Vol.165, No.2, (May 2011), pp.207-213., ISSN 0003-9926

Fraioli, F, Catalano, C, Bertoletti, L, Danti, M, Fanelli, F, Napoli, A, Cavacece, M, Passariello, R. (2006). Multidetector-row CT angiography of renal artery stenosis in 50 consecutive patients: prospective interobserver comparison with DSA. *Radiol Med.*, Vol.111, No.3, (May 2011), pp.459-468. ISSN 0033-8362

Fujii, H, Nakamura, S, Kuroda, S, Yoshihara, F, Nakahama, H, Inenaga, T, Ueda-Ishibashi, H, Yutani, C, Kawano, Y. (2006). Relationship between renal artery stenosis and intrarenal damage in autopsy subjects with stroke. *Nephrol Dial Transplant.*, Vol.21, No.1, (May 2011): pp.113-119. ISSN 0931-0509

Greco, BA, Breyer, JA. (1997). Atherosclerotic ischemic renal disease. *Am J Kidney Dis.*, Vol. 29, No.2, (May 2011), pp.167-187, ISSN 0272-2386

Gray, GH, Young, JR, Olin, JW. (1996). Miscellaneous arterial diseases. In: *Peripheral Vascular Diseases. 2nd ed.*, Young, JR, Olin, JW, Bartholomew, J, pp.425-440, Mosby ISBN, 0815187853-9780815197850, St Louis

Hazanov, N, Somin, M, Attali, M, Beilinson, N, Thaler, M, Mouallem, M, Maor, Y, Zaks, N, Malnick, S. (2004). Acute renal embolism. Forty-four cases of renal infarction in patients with atrial fibrillation. *Medicine* (Baltimore), Vol.83, No.5, (May 2011), pp.292-299, ISSN 0025-7974

Hansen, KJ, Starr, SM, Sands, RE, Burkart, JM, Plonk, GW Jr, Dean, RH. (1992). Contemporary surgical management of renovascular disease. *J Vasc Surg*, Vol.16, No.3, (May 2011), pp.319-330, ISSN 1078-5884

Kalra, PA, Guo, H, Kausz, AT, Gilbertson, DT, Liu, J, Chen, SC, Ishani, A, Collins, AJ, Foley, RN. (2005). Atherosclerotic renovascular disease in United States patients aged 67 years or older: risk factors, revascularization, and prognosis. *Kidney Int.*, Vol.68, No.1 (May 2011), pp.293-301, ISSN 1523-1755

Leandri, M, Lipiecki, J, Lipiecka, E, Hamzaoui, A, Amonchot, A, Mansour, M, Albuisson, E, Citron, B, Ponsonnaille, J, Boyer, L. (2004). Prevalence of renal artery stenosis in patients undergoing cardiac catheterization: when should abdominal aortography be performed? Results in 467 patients. *J Radiol*, Vol.85, No.5pt 1, (May 2011), pp.627-633, ISSN 0952-4746

Leertouwer, TC, Gussenhoven, EJ, Bosch, JL, van Jaarsveld, BC, van Dijk, LC, Deinum, J, Man In 't Veld, AJ. (2000). Stent placement for renal arterial stenosis: where do we stand? A meta-analysis. *Radiology.*, Vol. 216, No.1, (May 2011), pp.78-85, ISSN 0033-8419

Liu, BC, Tang, RN, Feng, Y, Wang, YL, Yin, LF, Ma, GS. (2004). A single Chinese center investigation of renal artery stenosis in 141 consecutive cases with coronary angiography. *Am J Nephrol*, Vol.24, No.6, (May 2011), pp.630-634. ISSN 0250-8095

Luscher, TF, Lie, JT, Stanson, AW, Houser, OW, Hollier, LH, Sheps, SG. (1987). Arterial fibromuscular dysplasia. *Mayo Clin Proc.*, Vol.62, No.10, (May 2011), pp.931-952, ISSN 0025-2196

Mailloux, LU, Napolitano, B, Bellucci, AG, Vernace, M, Wilkes, BM, Mossey, RT. (1994). Renal vascular disease causing end-stage renal disease, incidence, clinical correlates, and outcomes: a 20-year clinical experience. *Am J Kidney Dis.*, Vol.24, No.4, (May 2011), pp.622-629, ISSN 0272-2386

Malek, AM, Alper, SL, Izumo, S. (1999). Hemodynamic shear stress and its role in atherosclerosis. *JAMA.*, Vol.282, No.21, (May 2011), pp.2035-2042, ISSN 0098-7484.

Muray, S, Martín, M, Amoedo, ML, García, C, Jornet, AR, Vera, M, Oliveras, A, Gómez, X, Craver, L, Real, MI, García, L, Botey, A, Montanyà, X, Fernández, E. (2002) Rapid decline in renal function reflects reversibility and predicts the outcome after angioplasty in renal artery stenosis. *Am J Kidney Dis.*, Vol.39, No.1, (May 2011), pp.60-66, ISSN 0272-2386

Novick, AC, Ziegelbaum, M, Vidt, DG, Gifford, RW Jr, Pohl, MA, Goormastic, M. (1987) Trends in surgical revascularization for renal artery disease. Ten years' experience. *JAMA*, Vol.257, No.4, (May 2011), pp.498-501, ISSN 0098-7484

Ozkan, U, Oguzkurt, L, Tercan, F, Nursal, TZ. (2009) The prevalence and clinical predictors of i ncidental atherosclerotic renal artery stenosis. *Eur J Radiol.*, Vol.69, No.3 (May 2011), pp.550-554. ISSN 0720-048X

Pickering, TG (1989) Renovascular hypertension: etiology and pathophysiology. *Semin Nucl Med*,Vol.19, (May 2011), pp.79–88, ISSN 0001-2998

Ridker, PM, Danielson, E, Fonseca, FA, Genest, J, Gotto, AM Jr, Kastelein, JJ, Koenig, W, Libby, P, Lorenzatti, AJ, MacFadyen, JG, Nordestgaard, BG, Shepherd, J, Willerson, JT, Glynn, RJ; JUPITER Study Group. (2008). Rosuvastatin to prevent vascular events in men and women with elevated C-reactive protein. *N Engl J Med.*, Vol.359, No.21, (May 2011), pp.2195-2207, ISSN 0028-4793

Rimmer, JM, Gennari, FJ. (1993). Atherosclerotic renovascular disease and progressive renal failure. *Ann Intern Med.*, Vol.118, No.9, (May 2011), pp.712-719, ISSN 0003-4819.

Romero, JC, Feldstein, AE, Rodriguez-Porcel, MG, Cases-Amenos, A. (1997) New insights into the pathophysiology of renovascular hypertension. *Mayo Clin Proc.*,Vol. 72, No.3, (May 2011), pp.251-60, ISSN 0025-2196

Rountas, C, Vlychou, M, Vassiou, K, Liakopoulos, V, Kapsalaki, E, Koukoulis, G, Fezoulidis, IV, Stefanidis, I. (2007) Imaging modalities for renal artery stenosis in suspected renovascular hypertension: prospective intraindividual comparison of color Doppler US, CT angiography, GD-enhanced MR angiography, and digital substraction angiography. *Ren Fail.*, Vol.29, No.3, (May 2011), pp.295-302, ISSN 0886-022X

Safian, RD, Textor, SC. (2001) Renal-artery stenosis. *N Engl J Med*, Vol.344, No. (May 2011), pp.431–442, ISSN 0028-4793

Simon, N, Franklin, SS, Bleifer, KH, Maxwell, MH. (1972) Clinical characteristics of renovascular hypertension. *JAMA.*, Vol.220, No.9, (May 2011), pp.1209-18.

Soulez, G, Pasowicz, M, Benea, G, Grazioli, L, Niedmann, JP, Konopka, M, Douek, PC, Morana, G, Schaefer FK, Vanzulli A, Bluemke DA, Maki JH, Prince MR, Schneider, G, Ballarati, C, Coulden, R, Wasser, MN, McCauley, TR, Kirchin, MA, Pirovano, G. (2008) Renal artery stenosis evaluation: diagnostic performance of gadobenate dimeglumine-enhanced MR angiography--comparison with DSA. *Radiology*, Vol.247, No.1, (May 2011), pp.273-285, ISSN 0033-8419

Stone, PA, Campbell, JE, Aburahma, AF, Hamdan, M, Broce, M, Nanjundappa, A, Bates, MC. (2011). Ten-year experience with renal artery in-stent stenosis. *J Vasc Surg*, Vol.53, No.4, (May 2011), pp.1026-1031, ISSN 1532-2165

Textor, SC. (2004) Ischemic nephropathy: where are we now? *J Am Soc Nephrol.*, Vol.15, No.8 (May 2011), pp. 1974-1982, ISSN 1046-6673 van Ampting, JM, Penne, EL, Beek, FJ, Koomans, HA, Boer, WH, Beutler, JJ. (2003) Prevalence of atherosclerotic renal artery stenosis in patients starting dialysis. *Nephrol Dial Transplant*, Vol. 18, No.6, (May 2011), pp.1147-1151, ISSN 0931-0509

White, CJ. (2010). Optimizing outcomes for renal artery intervention. *Circ Cardiovasc Interv*, Vol.3, No.2 (May 2011), pp.184-192, ISSN 1941-7640

Zhang, Y, Ge, JB, Qian, JY, Ye, ZB. Prevalence and risk factors of atherosclerotic renal artery stenosis in 1,200 chinese patients undergoing coronary angiography. *Nephron Clin Pract.* 2006, Vol.104, No.4, (May 2011), pp.c185-192, ISSN 1660-2110.

# 10

# Pharmacologic Adjuvants to Reduce Erythropoietin Therapy Dose in Anemia of Chronic Kidney Disease and End Stage Renal Disease

Adeel Siddiqui, Aqeel Siddiqui and Robert Benz
*Lankenau Medical Center and Lankenau Institute for Medical Research*
*Wynnewood, Pennsylvania*
*USA*

## 1. Introduction

Anemia is one of the leading causes of morbidity in chronic renal failure.[1] Chronic kidney disease (CKD) associated anemia is largely due to reduced erythropoietin (EPO) release and, to a lesser degree, to shortened red cell survival.[2] To overcome EPO deficiency in this population, the development and administration of erythropoiesis-stimulating agents (ESAs) such as recombinant human EPO and darbepoetin alfa (DPO) has resulted in substantial health benefits, including improved quality of life, reduced blood transfusion requirements, decreased left ventricular mass, diminished sleep disturbance and enhanced exercise capacity.[1-7] Unfortunately in recent clinical trials, a proportion of patients exhibited complications such as fatal or nonfatal stroke, access thrombosis, increase in thrombotic events and exacerbation of malignancy associated with overly aggressive correction of anemia. [8-10] It is not established whether these complications are related to higher dose of EPO, underlying EPO resistance factors (i.e. inflammation) or achieving higher hematocrit (HCT). A multifactorial combination of predisposing circumstances is possible. A number of pharmacologic agents have been evaluated as adjuvant to ESAs therapy. These agents include iron, L-carnitine, ascorbic acid, androgens, statins, pentoxifylline and N-acetylcysteine. In this review article we will focus on the agents that have been used in conjunction with EPO to correct anemia in patient with chronic kidney disease and end-stage renal disease in an effort to reduce the dose requirement of EPO.

## 2. Iron

Iron is one of the most integral components of hematopoiesis in the anemia of kidney disease. "Trapped" iron storage or decreased availability of iron is the most common factor for the resistance to the effect of ESAs. Absolute iron deficiency is likely to be present in patients with CKD when: the percent transferrin saturation (plasma iron divided by total iron binding capacity x 100) falls below 20; the serum ferritin concentration is less than 100 ng/mL among advance CKD("predialysis") and peritoneal dialysis patients and less than

200 ng/mL among home hemodialysis patients.[11] However, functional iron deficiency is associated with transferrin saturation (TSAT) ≤20 percent and elevated ferritin levels (between approximately 200 to 800 ng/mL) or higher. An elevated ferritin level in this condition is likely secondary to the acute phase reaction of underlying inflammation. The 2006 K/DOQI guidelines recommend goals of iron therapy during administration of ESAs. For predialysis and peritoneal dialysis patients: TSAT >20 percent or content of hemoglobin (Hb) in reticulocytes >29 percent and serum ferritin concentration >100 ng/mL. For patients undergoing hemodialysis: transferrin saturation >20 percent or content of Hb in reticulocytes >29 percent and serum ferritin concentration >200 ng/mL.[12]

A number of clinical trials have compared which route of iron administration Intravenous (IV) vs Oral (PO) is superior in treating anemia of CKD. [13-22]

First we will discuss this issue in the Chronic Kidney Disease (CKD) population.

## 3. Anemia in chronic kidney disease

In a prospective trial by Stoves et.al, PO vs IV route of iron administration was studied. Forty five anemic patients with CKD, not on dialysis, were randomized to receive oral (ferrous sulfate 200 mg tid) or intravenous (300 mg iron sucrose monthly) iron therapy. EPO was started at the same time and the dose adjusted according to a pre-established protocol. After an average follow up of 5.2 months, there were no significant differences in Hb response and EPO dose between the two groups.[13] A prospective study by Charytan et. al. in 96 CKD anemic patients on EPO compared the efficacy of IV iron (5 doses of 200 mg iron sucrose weekly) to oral iron (ferrous sulfate 325 mg tid). They found an increase in Hb and ferritin following IV iron, whereas the oral iron group demonstrated an increase in Hb without increase in iron stores.[14] Both of the above studies failed to show IV iron superior to PO in either selected group of CKD patients. Van Wyck et.al. conducted a larger study of 182 non dialysis-dependent CKD (stages 3 to 5) patients to compare oral iron vs. IV iron. That randomized, controlled, multicenter trial tested IV iron as sucrose 1 g in divided doses over 14 days vs oral ferrous sulfate 325 mg three times a day for 56 days. Inclusion criteria for the group were Hb ≤11 g/dL, TSAT ≤25%, and ferritin ≤300ng/mL. EPO/DPO dose was not changed for eight weeks prior to or during the study. The proportion of patients achieving the primary outcome (Hb increase ≥1 g/dL) was greater in the IV iron treatment group than in the oral iron treatment group (44.3% vs. 28.0%, P = 0.0344), as was the mean increase in Hb by day 42 (0.7 vs. 0.4 g/dL, P = 0.0298).[15] Agarwal and colleagues conducted a randomized, multicenter, controlled trial in 75 adult, anemic, iron-deficient, non-dialysis CKD patients not receiving ESAs. The patients were randomly assigned to receive either IV ferric gluconate 250 mg weekly for 4 weeks or oral ferrous sulfate 325 mg three times a day for 42 days. Both oral and IV iron similarly increased Hb in anemic CKD patients not receiving ESAs.[16]

A new IV iron preparation, ferumoxytol has been approved in the United States. It appears to be safe and effective when given as a rapid infusion of up to 510 mg in patients with CKD and patients on dialysis. A Phase III trial randomly assigned 304 patients with CKD in a 3:1 ratio to two 510-mg doses of intravenous ferumoxytol within 5 ± 3 days or 200 mg of elemental oral iron daily for 21 days. Among patients who were not receiving ESAs, Hb increased 0.62 ± 1.02 g/dL with ferumoxytol vs. 0.13±0.93

g/dL with oral iron. Among patients who were receiving ESAs, Hb increased 1.16±1.49 g/dL with ferumoxytol vs. 0.19±1.14 g/dL with oral iron. The increase in Hb at day 35, the primary efficacy end point, was 0.82+/-1.24 g/dL with ferumoxytol and 0.16+/-1.02 g/dL with oral iron (P<0.0001).[17] The authors concluded that a regimen of two doses of 510 mg of intravenous ferumoxytol administered rapidly within 5±3 days was well tolerated and had the intended therapeutic effect. The side effects associated with IV iron in the above-mentioned studies were headache, myalgia, and hypotension (particularly in thin, older women<65 kg). Intravenous iron sucrose has shown better tolerability. Oral iron has more GI associated side effects including constipation, diarrhea, nausea and vomiting.[13-17]

As a result of these studies the K/DOQI guidelines have recommended that either oral iron therapy or intravenous iron therapy can be given in CKD patients.

## 4. Anemia in end stage renal disease

Among hemodialysis patients, studies show that transferrin saturation and serum ferritin levels usually continue to fall and anemia fails to correct despite ongoing oral iron therapy. MacDougall et.al. studied 37 iron-replete hemodialysis patients beginning EPO therapy randomized into three groups with different iron supplementation: Group1, IV iron dextran 5 ml (equivalent to 250 mg of elemental iron) every 2 weeks; Group 2, oral ferrous sulfate 200 mg tid; Group 3, no iron. Subjects were treated with 25 U/kg of EPO thrice weekly subcutaneously. After a period of 16 weeks, the Hb response in the group receiving IV iron (7.3+/-0.8 to 11.9+/-1.2 g/dL) was significantly greater than that for the other two groups (7.2 +/-1.1 to 10.2 +/-1.4 g/dL and 7.3+/-0.8 to 9.9+/-1.6 g/dL for Groups 2 and 3, respectively; p < 0.005 for both groups vs. Group 1 at 16 weeks). Serum ferritin levels remained constant in those receiving IV iron (345 +/-273 to 359+/-140 mcg/L) in contrast to the other two groups in which ferritin levels fell significantly (309+/-218 to 116+/- 87 mcg/L and 458+/-206 to 131+/- 121 mcg/L for Groups 2 and 3, respectively; p < 0.0005 for Group 1 vs. Group 2, and p < 0.005 for Group 1 vs. Group 3 at 16 weeks). Dosage requirements of EPO were also less in Group1.These results suggested that even in iron-replete patients, those supplemented with IV iron have an enhanced Hb response to EPO with better maintenance of iron stores and lower dosage requirements of EPO.[18]

Wingard et.al. conducted a prospective study on 46 EPO treated hemodialysis patients and randomized them into four different oral iron preparations. These four preparations included Chromagen (ferrous fumarate from Savage Laboratories), Feosol (ferrous sulphate from Smith Kline Beecham), Niferex (polysaccharide, Central Pharmaceutical) or Tabron (ferrous fumarate; Parke-Davis). All patients were prescribed approx 200 mg of elemental iron daily with at least 100 mg of ascorbic acid for six months. The study concluded that with emphasis on compliance, oral iron supplementation at the dose used for this study was able to maintain adequate iron status in the short term (less than 6 months) without the need for IV iron dextran. However, IV iron dextran eventually (after 6 months) would be necessary because of the downward trend in iron stores.[19]

Ferumoxytol was studied in a randomized, open-label, controlled, multicenter Phase 3 trial by Provenzano et.al. to evaluate the safety and efficacy of IV ferumoxytol compared with oral iron.[20] Anemic patients on HD and on a stable ESA regimen received either two injections of 510 mg of ferumoxytol within 7 days (n = 114) or 200 mg elemental oral iron daily for 21 days (n = 116). Ferumoxytol resulted in a mean increase in Hb of 1.02+/-1.13 g/dL at day 35 compared with 0.46+/-1.06 g/dL with oral iron (p = 0.0002). There was a greater mean increase in TSAT with ferumoxytol compared with oral iron at day 35 ($p < 0.0001$).

## 5. Conclusion

For patients with chronic kidney disease who are not on dialysis, oral iron or IV iron can be used for iron supplementation. This conclusion is consistent with the opinion of the Work Group from K DOQI guidelines.

The preferred route of administration of iron in patients with chronic kidney disease on hemodialysis is intravenous as supported by K DOQI guidelines as of 2006.

## 6. Ascorbic acid

Vitamin C or ascorbic acid has been studied in the metabolism of iron and anemia management. The first studies were performed in guinea-pigs. It was found that ascorbic acid deprivation increased the total non-haem iron concentration in the spleen and reduced it in the liver, and in both organs ferritin was diminished and haemosiderin increased. Repleting the ascorbic acid restored the normal distribution of iron between the two storage compounds, and in the spleen the total storage iron concentration returned to control levels within 24 hours.[21] Another important property of ascorbic acid is its ability to increase the availability of storage iron to chelators.[22] In hemodialysis patients this role of ascorbic acid was investigated by Deicher who conducted a cross-sectional, single-centre observational study. Pre-dialysis plasma Vitamin C concentrations were measured and response to EPO (Hb concentration/ international units EPO/kg/week) was recorded. Univariate analysis yielded a significant correlation between Vitamin C plasma levels and response to EPO. It was found that in unselected hemodialysis patients Vitamin C plasma levels account, at least partially for the response to EPO.[23] That work led to ascorbic acid investigations for use in EPO-treated hemodialysis patients, particularly those with EPO- hypo responsiveness, elevated serum ferritin levels, and functional iron deficiency (transferrin saturation ≤20 percent and elevated ferritin level between 200 to 800 ng/ml or higher). Studies evaluated the role of IV Vitamin C in hemodialysis patients and showed that in those patients who develop resistance to EPO with "functional iron deficiency", the resistance can be overcome by giving Vitamin C instead of iron,thus avoiding hemosiderosis.[24] In another comparative larger study, Tarng et.al. were able to show similar results in a prospective trial of dialysis patients. Sixty-five HD patients with serum ferritin levels greater than 500 mcg/L were recruited and divided into the control (N = 19) and intravenous ascorbic acid IVAA (N = 46) groups. IVAA patients with a hematocrit (HCT) of less than 30% received 300 mg of ascorbic acid three times per week for eight weeks. Controls had a HCT of more than 30% and did not receive the adjuvant therapy. Red blood cell and reticulocyte counts, iron metabolism indices, erythrocyte zinc protoporphyrin (E-ZPP), and the concentrations of plasma ascorbate and oxalate were examined before and following the therapy. Thirteen patients (four controls and nine IVAA patients) withdrew by the end of the study. Eighteen patients had a dramatic response to IVAA with a significant increase in Hb and reticulocyte index and a concomitant 24% reduction in EPO dose after eight weeks. This paralleled a significant rise in serum iron and TSAT and a fall in E-ZPP and serum ferritin (baselines vs. 8 weeks, serum iron 68+/-37 vs. 124 +/-64 mcg/dL, TSAT 27+/-10 vs. 48+/-19%, E-ZPP 123+/-44 vs. 70+/-13 micromol/mol heme, and serum ferritin 816+/-435 vs. 587+/-323 mcg/L, $p<0.05$). Compared with responders, mean values of Hb, EPO dose, iron metabolism parameters, and E-ZPP showed no significant changes in controls (N = 15) and in non-responders (N = 19).[25]

A single PO study by Benz et. al. was conducted in 21 EPO resistant anemic hemodialysis patients with ferritin levels greater than 350 ng/mL had received oral daily ascorbic acid at a dose of 500 mg/day and were retrospectively studied. Hemoglobin, HCT, EPO dose, ferritin, and transferrin saturation were recorded at baseline and after three months of treatment. EPO dose/HCT was calculated. Serum oxalate levels were also measured. In this study, daily oral ascorbic therapy decreased ferritin levels and EPO dose requirements while raising Hb and HCT level. Hb increased 9% from 11.4 to 12.2 gm/dl ($p$ = 0.05), HCT increased 10% from 33.3 to 36.7% ($p$ = 0.05), and EPO dose requirement decreased 33% from 26,229 to 17,559 U/week ($p$ = 0.03). Ferritin levels decreased 21% from 873 to 691 ng/mL ($p$ = 0.004) Patients with oxalate levels >27 micromol/L were instructed to stop ascorbic acid treatment, and mean levels decreased from 107 to 19 micromol/L ($p$ = 0.01) over a mean time of 71 days. This beneficial profile of the effects of ascorbic acid therapy is consistent with improvement of EPO resistance and cost savings in this population.[26]

The primary concern for using Vitamin C in dialysis patients is secondary oxalosis because of the impairment in renal excretion and inadequate removal by dialysis procedures.[27-28] Tarng et.al. showed that oxalate levels increase modestly after 8 weeks of IV Vitamin C but information on longer courses of treatment is limited.[25] Canavese prospectively studied the dose of Vitamin C and effect on oxalate levels in 30 dialysis patients. Eighteen patients were administered intravenous ascorbate during 18 months (250 mg/wk, subsequently increased to 500 mg), and 12 patients were taken as reference untreated cases. The study found that plasma oxalate levels progressively increased as the dose of IV Vitamin C was increased from 250 to 500 mg/week. After six months at a dose of 500 mg per week, 7 of 18 patients (40 percent) attained plasma oxalate levels that exceeded the range that would be associated with calcium oxalate super saturation at usual calcium concentrations.[29]

The 2006 K/DOQI guidelines for anemia in CKD stated that there was insufficient evidence to recommend Vitamin C as an adjuvant to EPO therapy.[30] However, several of the clinical studies were published subsequent to the development of those guidelines.

## 7. Pentoxifylline

Pentoxifylline (PTX) is a methyl xanthine derivative, which is approved for use in peripheral vascular disease and may also have anti-inflammatory effects according to studies. Benbernou et. al. studied pentoxifyline and examined its regulatory effect on T helper (TH1-and TH2) cell-derived cytokines in human whole blood and peripheral blood mononuclear cells stimulated with phytohemagglutinin and phorbol myristate acetate. The results showed that PTX at the appropriate concentrations ($5 \times 10^{(-4)}$M ) could induce selective suppression of interleukin (IL) -2 and interferon (INF) -gamma, whereas at high concentrations this drug could act as a suppressive agent of both TH1- and TH2-derived cytokines.[31] Bienvenu showed similar results that PTX possesses a much broader spectrum of activity on cytokine production than was initially described, and it appears to be a potential and promising immunotherapeutic agent.[32] These studies led to PTX's possible role in treating EPO resistant anemia. Navarro et. al. conducted a prospective small study of 7 anemic patients with CKD, who were treated with pentoxifylline (400 mg orally daily) for 6 months with the goal of defining the effects of pentoxifylline, as an agent with anti-tumor necrosis factor (TNF)-alpha properties. The results showed Hb significantly increased in the pentoxifylline-treated patients at the 6th month (9.9+/-0.5 g/dL at baseline;10.6+/-0.6 g/dL at the 6th month, respectively, $p < 0.01$), whereas no increase was seen in the control group. Serum EPO levels remained stable in all patients. However, the serum TNF-alpha concentration decreased significantly in patients receiving pentoxifylline. The study suggested that the inhibition of erythropoiesis by cytokines may play a significant role in renal anemia. The administration of agents with anti-cytokine properties, such as pentoxifylline, can improve the hematologic status in this population.[33] Another small study was conducted by Cooper and colleagues on 16 dialysis EPO resistant anemic patients. The patients were treated with oral pentoxifylline 400 mg daily for 4 months. Ex-vivo T cell generation of TNF-alpha and IFN-gamma from the patients was assessed before and 6 to 8 weeks after the therapy. A total of 12 of 16 patients completed the study. Before therapy, mean Hb concentration was 9.5+/-0.9 g/dL. After 4 months, the mean Hb concentration increased to 11.7+/-1.0 g/dL ($p = 0.0001$). Baseline ex vivo T cell expression of TNF-alpha decreased from 58% +/-11% to 31%+/-23% ($p= 0.0007$) after therapy. Likewise, IFN-gamma expression decreased from 31%+/-10% to 13%+/-10% ($p = 0.0002$). EPO doses remained unchanged in all but one patient in whom the dose was reduced in response to a higher Hb. One patient who was previously transfusion dependent was able to stop receiving monthly transfusions. Pentoxifylline therapy may significantly improve Hb response in patients with EPO–resistant anemia in renal failure.[34]

This small, open-label, uncontrolled study suggests the need for a larger, controlled trial with this agent. Until such a trial is conducted, pentoxifylline is not recommended as an EPO-adjuvant except in the experimental setting.

## 8. Statins

Statins (HMG-CoA reductase inhibitors) are a class of drugs used to lower cholesterol levels by inhibiting the enzyme HMG-CoA reductase, which plays a central role in the production of cholesterol in the liver. As mentioned above, cytokines play a role in inhibition of erythropoiesis. Statins have been evaluated as an adjuvant to EPO with the thought that they have anti-oxidant and anti-inflammatory properties. In one retrospective study, 70 HD patients were treated with statins for a period of 4.7 months and were found to have the mean Hb level rise from 10.6 to 12.5 g/dL ($p < 0.0005$) with an associated 25 percent decrease in EPO requirements.[35] Another study investigated whether the anti-inflammatory effect of statins improved EPO responsiveness in hemodialysis patients. It examined patients with Type 2 diabetes mellitus, who had been shown to have EPO resistance. One hundred and three patients were stratified into statin and non-statin groups.The outcome of interest was EPO dose. The mean EPO dose (units/kg per week) was significantly lower in the statin group (275.6 ± 273.2, vs. 449.5 ± 555.9, $p < 0.05$). Twenty percent of patients in the statin group required EPO dose in excess of an EPO equivalent of 500 units/kg per week, compared to 30.88% in the non-statin group. The two-way analysis of variance showed no interaction between the use of statins and the presence of Type 2 diabetes mellitus on EPO dose. This study demonstrated that hemodialysis patients who were on statins had a significantly lower EPO requirement. This association is possibly due to the pleiotropic effect of statins.[36]

A prospective study tested the effect of statin therapy on ESA hypo- responsiveness, and emphasized its anti-inflammatory benefits in maintenance hemodialysis patients. This study enrolled 30 patients with baseline cholesterol >220 mg/dL. Low-dose atorvastatin (10 mg/day) was prescribed for 12 weeks. They prospectively recorded biochemistry and hematological profiles, ESAs prescription and inflammatory markers at baseline, 4 weeks and 12 weeks. Statistically significant changes were noted after 4 and 12 weeks of statin therapy for cholesterol (272.5 to 184.4 and 196.4 mg/dL, $p < 0.05$) and ESA hypo-responsiveness, reported as EPO to HCT ratio (EHR) (129.3+/-58.2 to 122.3+/-53.5 and 121.0+/-53.3 EPO U/HCT/week, $p < 0.05$). Mean values for proinflammatory cytokines included interleukin-6 and TNF-alpha levels decreased by 30.8 and 10.6%, respectively. These data suggest that statin therapy may benefit patients with ESA hypo-responsiveness. This benefit in ESA hypo-responsiveness is associated with the effects of statins on inflammation.[37]

These preliminary studies may justify future studies to use statins as an EPO dose reducing adjuvant in patients with inflammation-mediated EPO resistant anemia of CKD.

## 9. Carnitine

L-carnitine is a small molecule (molecular weight: 161.2) that is derived from dietary products, mainly red meat and milk. Endogenous carnitine production takes place in the liver from lysine, methionine, ascorbate, niacin and pyridoxine. L-carnitine is required for the transport of long-chain fatty acids into the mitochondria and is an integral part of energy metabolism via ATP formation.

L-carnitine has been shown to improve anemia in uremic patients by stabilizing erythrocyte membrane function or erythropoiesis. End-stage renal disease patients are known to have carnitine deficiency.[38] This could be a contributing factor of anemia requiring higher dose of EPO. Thus, it has been used therapeutically in dialysis patients with and without concomitant EPO. Carnitine's role as an adjuvant to EPO in kidney disease is unclear. Most studies have involved HD patients with IV carnitine administration.

A 2002 meta-analysis evaluated the efficacy of IV carnitine supplementation in lowering the required dose of EPO using data from six randomized trials. The EPO dose was found to be significantly lower among those administered carnitine, with a beneficial response reported in four of the six studies.[38] Two studies showed improvement in Hb and HCT with PO carnitine but they were published before EPO was available.[39,40] In one study, 24 dialysis anemic patients were divided into two groups, controls (inert placebo), treated patients (L-carnitine 1.6 g PO daily) for one year. A significant increase in HCT, Hb, red cell count and mean corpuscular Hb concentration was observed. In comparison with the control group, an early improvement could be detected by the 3rd month, with further increases in the successive months of treatment in the L-carnitine cohort.

There is some evidence in the literature suggesting that accumulation of metabolites (trimethyleamine and trimethylamines-N-oxide)of oral carnitine, may have potential toxicity[41]. Marcus et.al. conducted a study using oral carnitine and showed that a small dose of L-carnitine is sufficient to increase the blood concentration of carnitine.[41] The concern remains about the accumulation of trimethylamines-N-oxide and its potential toxicologic effects include neurological toxicity and uremic breath.

The 2006 K/DOQI guidelines for anemia in CKD stated that there was insufficient evidence to recommend L-carnitine.[42]

## 10. Androgens

There is no literature available in CKD patients not on dialysis. Before EPO was available, androgens (which may increase endogenous EPO production, sensitivity of erythroid progenitors to the effects of EPO, and red blood cell survival) were used regularly in the treatment of anemia in dialysis patients.[43-46] Their use for anemia in dialysis patients has declined markedly since EPO was approved.

EPO and androgen's combination in hemodialysis patients has been studied:

Ballal et.al. performed a study in a group of 15 adult male hemodialysis patients.[47] Seven patients were treated with EPO alone at a dose of 2,000 U intravenously (IV) three times a week. An additional group of eight patients was treated with 2,000 U of EPO three times a week and also received 100 mg of nandrolone decanoate intramuscularly (IM) each week. After 12 weeks of therapy, HCT values increased slightly in the group receiving EPO alone, from 25.3+/-0.8 to 27.4+/-1.5. In contrast, EPO in combination with nandrolone decanoate resulted in a greater increase in HCT values, from 24.4+/-1.4 to 32.9 +/-1.8 ($p < 0.001$). The results showed that the groups receiving low-dose EPO alone had a poor erythropoietic response. In contrast, patients receiving androgen in addition to EPO had a significantly greater increase in HCT values with treatment. These data show that androgen therapy significantly augments the action of exogenous EPO such that lower doses of EPO may be sufficient for an adequate hematopoietic response.

In a prospective, randomized study by Berns et al. in a chronic hemodialysis population, patients received EPO 40 U/kg intravenously three times weekly either alone (Group 1, n = 6) or with weekly intramuscular injection of 2 mg/kg nandrolone decanoate (Group 2, n = 6) for up to 16 weeks. Baseline HCT, ferritin, N-terminal parathyroid hormone, and aluminum levels were similar. The mean weekly rate of rise in HCT was 0.32+/-0.13% in Group 1 and 0.37+/-0.11% in Group 2, (p = NS). Three of 6 patients in Group 1, but only 1 of 6 patients in Group 2, reached the target HCT of 30% within 16 weeks. Two patients in Group 2 requested that the nandrolone decanoate be stopped prior to reaching target HCT because of unacceptable side effects (acne). [48] Nandrolone decanoate did not enhance the response rate to this EPO dose and is associated with significant side effects.

In a longer open-label study with low-dose EPO therapy, 19 chronic hemodialysis patients were randomly assigned to receive EPO (1,500 units IV at each HD treatment) either alone or with nandrolone decanoate (100 mg intramuscularly weekly) for 26 weeks.[49] The mean increase in HCT and the final achieved HCT were greater in the nandrolone decanoate treated group (8.2 and 33.2 percent, respectively) than in the group treated with EPO alone (3.5 percent and 28.3 percent, respectively). No serious side effects were reported.

Thirty two hemodialysis patients were randomly assigned to receive low dose EPO therapy (1,000 units SC at each HD treatment) either alone or with nandrolone decanoate 50 mg intramuscularly twice weekly for six months.[50] The increase in Hb in the nandrolone decanoate treated group (from 7.5 to 10.4 g/dL) was not statistically different from the control group (7.3 to 10.0 g/dL). Side effects, including gynecomastia, hirsutism, menstrual irregularity, and increases in liver enzymes and triglyceride levels, were common.

The limiting factor in these studies was small size and relatively short follow ups, and none attempted to maintain currently recommended Hb levels. The 2006 K DOQI guidelines for anemia in CKD stated that androgens should not be used as an adjuvant to EPO.

## 11. N-acetylcysteine

N-acetylcysteine (NAC) is a drug and nutritional supplement used primarily as a mucolytic agent and also in the management of acetaminophen overdose. To explore the efficacy of oral NAC supplementation for anemia and oxidative stress in hemodialysis patients, Chien et al studied 325 dialysis patients. In this study, 49 pateints received NAC 200 mg orally three times a day during the first 3 months of dialysis, while the other 276 patients not receiving NAC were observed. During the 4-month study, 11 patients receiving NAC withdrew but had no severe adverse effects, while 49 patients not receiving NAC had negative confounding events. Thus only the data of the remaining patients, 38 taking NAC and 227 not taking NAC, were analyzed for efficacy.

When the EPO dosage was stable, only the NAC group had a significant increase in HCT, accompanied with a decrease in plasma levels of 8-isoprostane and oxidized low-density lipoprotein. Analyzed as a nested case-control study, NAC supplementation was also found to be a significant predictor of positive outcomes in uremic anemia. [51] To determine the contribution of injectable iron administered to hemodialysis patients in causing oxidative stress and the beneficial effect of NAC in reducing it, Swarnalatha et al conducted a prospective, double blinded, controlled, cross over trial on 14 adult hemodialysis patients who were randomized into two groups; one group received NAC in a dose of 600 mgs by mouth twice daily for 10 days prior to intravenous iron therapy and the other group received placebo. Both groups received intravenous iron therapy, 100 mg of iron sucrose in 100 mL of normal saline given over a period of one hour. Blood samples for the markers of oxidative stress were taken before and after the iron therapy. After a week of wash-out period for the effect of NAC, subjects crossed over to the opposite regimen. They measured the lipid peroxidation marker, malondiaaldehyde (MDA), to evaluate the oxidative stress and total anti-oxidant capacity (TAC) for the antioxidant level in addition to the highly sensitive C-reactive protein (HsCRP). Non-invasive assessment of endothelial dysfunction was measured by digital plethysmography before and after intravenous iron therapy. There was an increase of MDA (21.97 + 3.65% vs 7.06 + 3.65%) and highly sensitive C-reactive protein (HsCRP) (11.19 + 24.63% vs 13.19 + 7.7%) after iron administration both in the placebo and the NAC groups. NAC reduced the baseline acute systemic generation of oxidative stress when compared to placebo, which was statistically significant with MDA (12.76 +/- 4.4% vs 9.7 +/- 4.4%) but not with HsCRP. Pre-treatment with NAC reduced the endothelial dysfunction when compared to placebo, but it was not statistically significant.

The author concluded that in those HD patients, NAC reduced the oxidative stress before and after the administration of intravenous iron therapy in addition to the endothelial dysfunction induced by this treatment. [52]

Finnigan and Benz reported the results of treating 12 ESRD EPO resistant hemodialysis subjects with oral NAC 600 mg by mouth twice daily for 6 months. In that small pilot study, NAC therapy was associated with a 53% reduction in the EPO Resistance Index (weekly EPO dose/weight in Kg/Hb). [53]

These preliminary studies suggest the need for a larger, controlled trial with NAC. Until then, routine use of NAC as an EPO- adjuvant cannot be recommended.

## 12. Discussion

Anemia of CKD/ESRD has multiple etiologies, although the decrease in EPO production by the diseased kidneys is the major contributor. Recently, studies targeting higher Hb levels or using higher EPO dosing regimens in the correction of anemia have shown detrimental effects including increased all cause mortality, cardiac and cerebral vascular events and vascular access thrombosis[8-10,54] It is not clear whether this is due to higher HCT or EPO the molecule itself at higher concentration. This review article focused on adjuvant oral and parenteral agents that have been used along with EPO to reduce its dose and give foundation to research in randomized control trials. There may also be a potential benefit of these agents to use along with EPO in reducing cost and expenditures especially when the bundling method of dialysis payment is in effect.

## 13. References

[1] Valderrabano F. EPO in chronic renal failure. Kidney Int. 1996; 50:1373 – 91

[2] Benz RL, Pressman MR, Hovick ET, Peterson DD. A preliminary study of the effects of correction of anemia with recombinant human EPO therapy on sleep, sleep disorders, and daytime sleepiness in hemodialysis patients (The SLEEPO study). Am. J. Kidney Dis. 1999; 34: 1089–95

[3] Revicki DA , Brown RE, Feeney DH, Henry D, Teehan BP, Rudnick MR, Benz RL: Health - related quality of life associated with recombinant human EPO therapy for predialysis chronic renal disease patients . Am J Kidney Dis 25:548-554, 1995

[4] Evans RW, Rader B, Manninen DL, and the Cooperative Multicenter EPO Clinical Trial Group: The quality of life of hemodialysis recipients treated with recombinant human EPO. JAMA 263: 825-830, 1990

[5] Barany P, Petterson E, Bergstron J: EPO treatment improves quality of life in hemodialysis patients. Scand J Urol Neprol 131: 55 -60, 1990 (suppl)

[6] Auer J, Oliver DO, Winearls CG: The quality of life of dialysis patients treated with recombinant human EPO. Scand J Urol Nephrol 131: 61-65, 1990 ( suppl)

[7] Wolcott DL, Marsh jt, La Rue A, Carr C, Nissenson AR: Recombinant human EPO treatment may improve quality of life and cognitive function in chronic hemodialysis patients. Am J Kidney Dis 13: 478 – 485 , 1989

[8] Pfeffer MA, Burdmann EA, Chen CY, Cooper ME, de Zeeuw D, Eckardt KU, Feyzi JM, Ivanovich P, Kewalramani R, Levey AS, Lewis EF, McGill JB, McMurray JJ, Parfrey P, Parving HH, Remuzzi G, Singh AK, Solomon SD, Toto R, TREAT Investigators A trial of darbepoetin alfa in type 2 diabetes and chronic kidney disease. N Engl J Med. 2009;361(21):2019.

[9] Drüeke TB, Locatelli F, Clyne N, Eckardt KU, Macdougall IC, Tsakiris D, Burger HU, Scherhag A, CREATE Investigators Normalization of hemoglobin level in patients with chronic kidney disease and anemia. N Engl J Med. 2006;355(20):2071.

[10] Singh AK, Szczech L, Tang KL, Barnhart H, Sapp S, Wolfson M, Reddan D, CHOIR Investigators Correction of anemia with epoetin alfa in chronic kidney disease. N Engl J Med. 2006;355(20):2085.

[11] Fernandez-Rodriguez AM; Guindeo-Casasus MC; Molero-Labarta T; Dominguez-Cabrera C; Hortal-Casc n L; Perez-Borges P; Vega-Diaz N; Saavedra-Santana P; Palop-Cubillo L Diagnosis of iron deficiency in chronic renal failure Am J Kidney Dis 1999 Sep;34(3):508-13.

[12] K/DOQI Clinical Practice Guidelines and Clinical Practice Recommendations for anemia in Chronic Kidney Disease. Am J Kidney Dis 2006; 47(suppl 3):S1

[13] Stoves J; Inglis H; Newstead CG A randomized study of oral vs. intravenous iron supplementation in patients with progressive renal insufficiency treated with EPO. Nephrol Dial Transplant 2001 May; 16(5):967-74.

[14] Charytan, C, Ounibi, W, Bailie, GR. Comparison of intravenous iron sucrose to oral iron in the treatment of anemic patients with chronic kidney disease not on dialysis. Nephron Clin Pract 2005; 11:100.

[15] Van Wyck DB; Roppolo M; Martinez CO; Mazey RM; McMurray S A randomized, controlled trial comparing IV iron sucrose to oral iron in anemic patients with non dialysis-dependent CKD. Kidney Int. 2005 Dec; 68(6):2846-56.

[16] Agarwal R; Rizkala AR; Bastani B; Kaskas MO; Leehey DJ; Besarab A A randomized controlled trial of oral versus intravenous iron in chronic kidney disease Am J Nephrol. 2006; 26(5):445-54. Epub 2006 Oct 11

[17] Spinowitz BS, Kausz AT, Baptista J, Noble SD, Sothinathan R, Bernardo MV, Brenner L, Pereira BJ Ferumoxytol for treating iron deficiency anemia in CKD. Journal of the American Society of Nephrology 2008 Aug;19(8):1599-605

[18] MacDougall IC; Tucker B; Thompson J; Tomson CR; Baker LR; Raine AE A randomized controlled study of iron supplementation in patients treated with EPO. Kidney Int 1996 Nov;50(5):1694-9

[19] Wingard RL; Parker RA; Ismail N; Hakim RM Efficacy of oral iron therapy in patients receiving recombinant human EPO. Am J Kidney Dis 1995 Mar; 25(3):433-9.

[20] Provenzano R, Schiller B, Rao M, Coyne D, Brenner L, Pereira BJ Ferumoxytol as an intravenous iron replacement therapy in hemodialysis patients. Clinical Journal of the American Society of Nephrology 2009 Feb; 4(2):386-93.

[21] Lipschitz, DA, Bothwell, TH, Seftel, HC, et al. The role of ascorbic acid in the metabolism of storage iron. Br J Haematol 1971; 20:155.

[22] Bridges KR; Hoffman KE The effects of ascorbic acid on the intracellular metabolism of iron and ferritin. J Biol Chem 1986 Oct 25; 261(30):14273-7.

[23] Deicher R; Ziai F; Habicht A; Bieglmayer C; Schillinger M; Horl WH Vitamin C plasma level and response to EPO in patients on maintenance hemodialysis. Nephrol Dial Transplant 2004 Sep; 19(9):2319-24.

[24] Gastaldello K; Vereerstraeten A; Nzame-Nze T; Vanherweghem JL; Tielemans C Resistance to EPO in iron-overloaded hemodialysis patients can be overcome by ascorbic acid administration. Nephrol Dial Transplant 1995; 10 Suppl 6:44-7.

[25] Tarng DC; Wei YH; Huang TP; Kuo BI; Yang WC Intravenous ascorbic acid as an adjuvant therapy for recombinant EPO in hemodialysis patients with hyperferritinemia. Kidney Int 1999 Jun; 55(6):2477-86.

[26] Sirover WD; Siddiqui AA; Benz RL Beneficial hematologic effects of daily oral ascorbic acid therapy in ESRD patients with anemia and abnormal iron homeostasis: a preliminary study. Ren Fail. 2008; 30(9):884-9.

[27] Balcke, P, Schmidt, P, Zazgornik, J, et al. Ascorbic acid aggravates secondary hyperoxalemia in patients on chronic hemodialysis. Ann Intern Med 1984; 101:344.

[28] Pru C; Eaton J; Kjellstrand C Vitamin C intoxication and hyperoxalemia in chronic hemodialysis patients. Nephron 1985; 39(2):112-6.

[29] Canavese C; Petrarulo M; Massarenti P; Berutti S; Fenoglio R; Pauletto D; Lanfranco G; Bergamo D; Sandri L; Marangella M Long-term, low-dose, intravenous vitamin C leads to plasma calcium oxalate super saturation in hemodialysis patients. Am J Kidney Dis 2005 Mar;45(3):540-9

[30] K/DOQI Clinical Practice Guidelines and Clinical Practice Recommendations for anemia in Chronic Kidney Disease. Am J Kidney Dis 2006; 47(suppl 3):S1.

[31] Benbernou N; Esnault S; Potron G; Guenounou M Regulatory effects of pentoxifylline on T-helper cell-derived cytokine production in human blood cells. J Cardiovasc Pharmacol 1995;25 Suppl 2:S75-9.

[32] Bienvenu J; Doche C; Gutowski MC; Lenoble M; Lepape A; Perdrix JP Production of proinflammatory cytokines and cytokines involved in the TH1/TH2 balance is modulated by pentoxifylline J Cardiovasc Pharmacol 1995;25 Suppl 2:S80-4.

[33] Navarro JF; Mora C; Garcia J; Rivero A; Macia M; Gallego E; Mendez ML; Chahin J Scand Effects of pentoxifylline on the hematologic status in anemic patients with advanced renal failure. J Urol Nephrol 1999 Apr;33(2):121-5 .

[34] Cooper A; Mikhail A; Lethbridge MW; Kemeny DM; MacDougall IC Pentoxifylline improves Hb levels in patients with EPO-resistant anemia in renal failure. J Am Soc Nephrol 2004 Jul; 15(7):1877-82.

[35] Sirken G; Kung SC; Raja R ASAIO Decreased EPO requirements in maintenance hemodialysis patients with statin therapy. J 2003 Jul-Aug; 49(4):422-5.

[36] K. Tangdhanakanond and R. Raja Effect of statins on EPO responsiveness in Type 2-diabetic versus non-diabetic hemodialysis patients Clinical Nephrology, Vol. 73 – No. 1/2010 (1-6)

[37] Chiang CK, Yang SY, Peng YS, Hsu SP, Pai MF, Huang JW, Hung KY, Wu KD. Atorvastatin increases EPO-stimulating agent hypo responsiveness in maintenance hemodialysis patients: role of anti- inflammation effects. Am J Nephrol. 2009; 29(5):392-7. Epub 2008 Oct 31

[38] Hurot JM; Cucherat M; Haugh M; Fouque D Effects of L-carnitine supplementation in maintenance hemodialysis patients: a systematic review J Am Soc Nephrol 2002 Mar; 13(3):708-14.

[39] Trovato GM, Ginardi V, Di Marco V, Dell'Aira AE, Corsi M: Long term L-carnitine treatment of chronic anemia of patients with end stage renal failure. *Curr Ther Res* 31: 1042–1049, 1982.

[40] Bellinghieri G, Savica V, Mallamace A, Di Stefano C, Consolo F, Spagnoli LG, Villaschi S, Palmieri G, Corsi M, Maccari F: Correlation between increased serum and tissue L-carnitine levels and improved muscle symptoms in hemodialyzed patients. Am J Clin Nutr 38: 523–531, 1983

[41] Bain MA; Faull R; Milne RW; Evans AM Oral L-carnitine: metabolite formation and hemodialysis Curr Drug Metab. 2006 Oct; 7(7):811-6.

[42] K/DOQI Clinical Practice Guidelines and Clinical Practice Recommendations for anemia in Chronic Kidney Disease. Am J Kidney Dis 2006; 47(suppl 3):S1.

[43] Teruel JL, Marcen R, Navarro-Antolin J, Aguilera A, Fernandez-Juarez G, Ortuo J Androgen versus EPO for the treatment of anemia in hemodialyzed patients: a prospective study. J Am Soc Nephrol. 1996; 7(1):140-4.

[44] Gascn A, Belvis JJ, Berisa F, Iglesias E, Estopin V, Teruel JL Nandrolone decanoate is a good alternative for the treatment of anemia in elderly male patients on hemodialysis. Geriatr Nephrol Urol. 1999; 9(2):67-72.

[45] Navarro JF, Mora-Fernandez C, Rivero A, Macia M, Gallego E, Chahin J, Mendez ML, Garcia J Androgens for the treatment of anemia in peritoneal dialysis patients. Adv Perit Dial. 1998; 14:232-5.

[46] Navarro JF, Mora C, Macia M, Garcia J Randomized prospective comparison between EPO and androgens in CAPD patients. Kidney Int. 2002; 61(4):1537-44.

[47] Ballal SH, Domoto DT, Polack DC, Marciulonis P, Martin KJ Androgens potentiate the effects of EPO in the treatment of anemia of end-stage renal disease. Am J Kidney Dis. 1991; 17(1):29-33.

[48] Berns JS, Rudnick MR, Cohen RM A controlled trial of recombinant human EPO and nandrolone decanoate in the treatment of anemia in patients on chronic hemodialysis. Clin Nephrol. 1992; 37(5):264-7.

[49] Gaughan WJ, Liss KA, Dunn SR, Mangold AM, Buhsmer JP, Michael B, Burke JF A 6-month study of low-dose recombinant human EPO alone and in combination with androgens for the treatment of anemia in chronic hemodialysis patients Am J Kidney Dis. 1997;30(4):495-500.

[50] Sheashaa, H, Abdel-Razek, W, El-Husseini, A, et al. Use of nandrolone decanoate as an adjuvant for EPO dose reduction in treating anemia in patients on hemodialysis. Nephron Clin Pract 2005; 99c:102.

[51] Shih-Ping Hsu, Chih-Kang Chiang, Shao-Yu Yang, Chiang-Ting Chien N-Acetylcysteine for the Management of Anemia and Oxidative Stress in Hemodialysis Patients Nephron Clin Pract 2010;116:c207-c216

[52] Swarnalatha G, Ram R, Neela P, Naidu MU, Dakshina Murty KV. Oxidative stress in hemodialysis patients receiving intravenous iron therapy and the role of N-acetylcysteine in preventing oxidative stress Saudi J Kidney Dis Transpl. 2010 Sep;21(5):852-8.

[53] Finnigan N., Chernick M. and Benz R. Nephrology, N-Acetylcysteine (NAC) May Improve Erythropoietin Resistant Anemia ( ERA) in hemodialysis patients[SA-PO2587] ASN Renal week 2010 Abstracts
[54] Fishbane S, Besarab A.Mechanism of increased mortality risk with erythropoietin treatment to higher hemoglobin targets. Clin J Am Soc Nephrol 2007;2:1274-1282

# 11

# Molecular Mechanisms of Nephro-Protective Action of HE-86 Liquid Extract in Experimental Chronic Renal Failure

Li-qun He[1], Dong Feixia[2], Qiang Fu[3] and Jun Li[4]

[1]*Department of Nephrology, Shuguang Hospital Affiliated with Shanghai University of Traditional Chinese Medicine, Ministry of Education Key Laboratory of Liver and Kidney Disease Syndrome, E-Institutes of Shanghai Municipal Education Commission, Innovative Research Team in Universities of Shanghai Municipal Education Commission*

[2]*Department of Nephrology, Wenzhou TCM Hospital Affiliated to Zhejiang University of Traditional Chinese Medicine, Wenzhou*

[3]*Heilongjiang University of Traditional Chinese Medicine, HeiLongJiang*

[4]*Zhuhai City NO 5 Hospital, GuangDong*

*China*

## 1. Introduction

Chronic renal injury can be mediated by angiotensin II (Ang II) through hemodynamic and inflammatory mechanisms and attenuated by individual suppression of these mediators. Hypertension is usually associated with the development of vascular and renal fibrosis [3]. This pathophysiological process is characterized by structural changes in vasculature caused by increased synthesis and rearrangement of extracellular matrix proteins, such as the collagen type I [4]. Several studies support a major role for the renin-angiotensin system in the development of fibrosis [5, 6].

Hypertension injures blood vessels and thereby causes end-organ damage. The mechanisms are complicated and although they have been studied for decades in experimental animal models [7], they are only currently being elucidated. From the efforts of many investigators, we are now in the position of constructing a chain of events from the endothelium to the underlying matrix, to the vascular smooth muscle cells, and beyond to the adventitia, and surrounding tissues. The endothelial layer acts as a signal transduction interface for hemodynamic forces in the regulation of vascular tone and chronic structural remodeling of arteries [8]. Infiltration of the permeabilized endothelium by leukocytes sets the stage for an inflammatory cascade, involving cytokines, chemokines, growth factors, and matrix metalloproteinases. Altered integrin signaling, the production of tenacin, epidermal growth factor signaling, tyrosine phosphorylation, and activation of downstream pathways culminate in vascular smooth muscle cell proliferation [9]. Evidence is accumulating that matrix molecules provide an environment which decreases the rate of programmed cell death [10].

Hypertension is a major risk factor for renal and cardiac damage, however, the mechanisms are incompletely understood. Angiotensin (Ang) II, the key effector of the local and circulating renin-angiotensin system (RAS), plays a central role [11-12]. In addition to its vasoactive and growth-promoting action, Ang II stimulates circulating leukocytes and endothelial cells, thereby promoting inflammation and interstitial extracellular matrix accumulation [13-17]. Many inflammation-mediating genes are activated by the transcription nuclear factor-$\kappa$B (NF-$\kappa$B), which resides inactive and bound to the inhibitory protein I-$\kappa$B in the cytoplasm of T lymphocytes, monocytes, macrophages, endothelial cells, and smooth muscle cells [18-19]. Ang II stimulates NADPH oxidase, which generates reactive oxygen species (ROS) [20]. ROS may act as signal transduction messengers for several important transcription factors, including NF-$\kappa$B and AP-1 (activator protein-1) [21]. Recently, Ozes et al [22]showed that Akt/protein kinase B (Akt) is essential in tumor necrosis factor-$\alpha$ (TNF-$\alpha$)–induced activation of NF-$\kappa$B. Takahashi et al, [23] as well as Ushio-Fukai et al, [24] have demonstrated Akt activation by Ang II, which may involve ROS. Akt-induced activation of NF-kB upregulates numerous genes, including interleukin (IL)-1, IL-6, IL-8, interferon-$\gamma$, TNF-$\alpha$, intercellular adhesion molecule-1 (ICAM-1), vascular cell adhesion molecule-1 (VCAM-1), and the chemokine MCP-1 (monocyte chemoattractant protein-1). Several reports [25-27] indicated that angiotensin converting enzyme (ACE) inhibition decreased NF-$\kappa$B in renal disease.

We have previously demonstrated that traditional Chinese medicine prescription documented in the ancient Chinese pharmacopoeia or monographs promoted blood circulation, decreased blood stasis, and improved renal function. They decreased urinary protein excretion ,balanced lipid metabolism and enhanced the effects of antioxidant in the treatment of patients with early and middle stage chronic renal failure [28-32].

It has been showen broad foreground to postpone progression of chronic renal dysfunction. But it is unclear that effective composition and mechanism of renal protection. Therefore, the study presented here was designed to test the hypothesis that HE-86 liquid extract, which is effective unite refined from above Chinese prescription, would prevent chronic renal failure rats induced by nephrectomized, in association with decreased expression of angiotensin II and AT- II receptors, further to suppress high expression of inflammatory and growth factors. In an attempt to obtain more effective renal protection, research design consisted of a group of Nx rats receiving a HE-86 liquid extract treatment comparing with chronic renal failure rats induced by subtotal nephretomized without treatment. At same time, in the present study, we also assess the influence of renal mass reduction (RMR) caused by subtotal (5/6) nephrectomy on gene expression for NF-$\kappa$B, TNF-$\alpha$ and TGF-beta1 and evaluate the correlation between expression of these genes and activity of the intrarenal renin-angiotensin systems. The research result showed HE-86 played a critical role in improving renal disease and was a key mediator in delay process of vascular fibrosis, characterized by reduced lumen diameter and arterial wall thickening attributable to excessive deposition of extracellular matrix (ECM) through by the model study.

## 2. Materials and methods

### 2.1 Experimental design

Thirty-six of the normal kidney mass were removed from adult male Munich-Wistar rats (BiKai, Shanghai, China) weighing 200–210 g to make animal models of CRF. In a first session, two thirds of the left kidney were removed. One week after the first operation, the right kidney was removed. These procedures were performed under anaesthesia with sodium pentobarbital (The ShuGuang pharmaceutical factory in Shanghai). Two weeks after 5/6-nephrectomy, 24 rats were divided into pairs such that both rats in each pair exhibited almost the same levels of serum creatinine, blood urea nitrogen (BUN) (Table 1). One rat from each pair was assigned to (i) control uraemic group (n=12), the other to (ii) treatment uraemic group (n=12) which received HE-86, extract liquid which is effective composition isolated from Chinese medicine prescription, everyday at a dose of 0.75 g/100 g body weight for 8 weeks. For normal controls, rats underwent a sham operation consisting of laparotomy and manipulation of the renal pedicles but without damage to the kidney(n=12). The treatment group were administered by HE-86 infuse the stomach as pair-fed with the control uraemic rats, and the normal rats were fed ad libitum with standard solid chow (BiKai Animal Lab. Company, Shanghai, China) containing 24.5% protein.

| | N | BUN(mmol/L) | Scr(μmol/L) |
|---|---|---|---|
| sham | 12 | 7.51±0.75 | 19.00±4.00 |
| control | 12 | 16.17±0.99* | 49.50±6.53* |
| treatment | 12 | 16.18±2.42* | 49.23±9.36* |

Table 1. The variation of serum creatinine and blood urea nitrogen before treatment.

Blood pressure was measured before treatment and every two weeks after surgery. The levels of serum creatinine (Scr), Blood urea nitrogen (BUN), 24h urine protein excreation and urine TGF-β were determined at 4 or 8 weeks after starting the administration of HE-86, respectively. The remnant kidneys were removed after perfusion at the end of experiment for histopathological and gene expression studies.

## 2.2 Analytical procedures

**Renal Function Assessment and Blood Pressure Measurement**

Serum creatinine (Scr) and Blood urea nitrogen (BUN) were measured using a Beckman Cx4 analyser (Fullerton, CA, USA), respectively.

24h Urinary protein concentrations were determined by the Bradford method, adapted to a microtiter plate assay. Coomassie reagent (USB, Cleveland, OH) was added to the diluted urine samples. After 10 minutes, the absorbance at 595-nm wavelength was read on ELX800 microplate reader (Bio-Tek Instruments, VT). The protein concentrations were calculated by reference to bovine serum albumin (Sigma) standards.

Systolic blood pressure was recorded by tail plethysmography using the BP2000 blood pressure analysis system (Visitech Systems, Inc., Apex, NC) in conscious rats at baseline and every 2 weeks throughout the experimental time course.

### 2.3 Immunohistochemical analysis

Immunostaining of NF-κb (Sigma) in renal tissue sections was performed using the streptavidin–biotinylated peroxidase complex (SABC) method. The tissue specimens were divided into thin sections (4-μm thick) that were then deparaffinized. The sections were washed three times with distilled water for 5 min. The sections were treated with Protease K (Try box produced by BSD living creature technique company of Wuhan) in distilled water at 37°C for 15 min, and washed three times with PBS for 10 min. Endogenous peroxidase activity was blocked by incubating the sections with 0.3% H2O2 in methanol for 20 min at room temperature. The sections were washed three times with PBS for 5 min. The sections were incubated with 10% rabbit serum at 37°C for 60 min to reduce the non-specific background staining, and washed three times with PBS for 5 min. Then, the sections were incubated with a monoclonal anti- NF-κb antibody (7 μg/ml) dissolved in PBS containing 3% BSA and 0.1% NaN3 at 4°C overnight, and washed three times with PBS for 10 min; followed by incubation with a biotinylated rabbit antibody against mouse IgG+IgA+IgM (10 μg/ml) at 37°C for 40 min. The sections were washed three times with PBS for 5 min, and then incubated with peroxidase-labelled streptavidin at 37°C for 30 min. After washing three times with PBS for 10 min, the reaction was completed by the addition of diaminobenzidine–H2O2 solution for 15 min, and washed three times with distilled water for 5 min, then the slides were counter-stained with methylgreen.

The primary anti- NF-κb antibody (1 : 100) was incubated with NF-κb (10 mg/ml) at 4°C overnight. After centrifuging the mixture at 10,000xg for 30 min, the supernatant was used as negative control for the primary antibody solution followed by the usual SABC method. There was no positive staining in the renal cortex when the primary antibody was pre-incubated with NF-κb.

The immunostaining of NF-κb was quantified using an image analyser IMS (FUDAN university of medical science portrait examination center) by evaluating the positively stained area of the sections under the same light intensity for microscopy. The intensity of colour component for red, green or blue was graded from 0 to 256°. Areas which showed intense brown color were extracted from the microscopic fields (number of fields for each tissue sample, six fields; magnification on the display: x300) under the following conditions; red component ranging from 104 to 158°, green component from 81 to 129°, and blue component from 70 to 123°.

## 3. Real-time quantitative Polymerase Chain Reaction (PCR) for TNF－α, Ang II and AT1R

To investigate the expression of TNF–α mRNA, Ang II and AT1R real-time PCR (BC living creature technique company, Shanghai, China) was performed with the Opticon real-time PCR machine (FX scientific research Inc. Shanghai, China). Briefly, total RNA was extracted from renal tissues. All of the RNA samples were treated with the RNase-free DNase I (GIBCO BRC Inc, Shanghai, China) before the RT-PCR. Real-time quantitative one-step RT-PCR assay was performed to quantify mRNA using real-time PCR machine (FX scientific research Inc. Shanghai, China). The primers used for real-time RT-PCR were as follows: TNF-a: forward 5′-CTCATTCCCGCTCGTGG-3′ reverse 3′-CGTTTGGTGGTTCGTCTCC- 5′;

AT1R: forward 5′-CTTGTTCCCTTTCCTTATC -3′reverse 3′-ACTCCACCTCACTGTCCA -5′. Ang II : forward 5'- ACCTG CATGA GTGTT GATAGG-3' reverse 3'-ACTTCA ATATC GTCAGT AACTGGAC-5'.

Total RNA of osteoblasts was isolated by using TRIzol reagent (Invitrogen) and reverse transcription was performed follow manufacturer's manual(BioTNT, Shanghai, China). Quantitative real-time PCR, enabling the quantification of relative gene expression, was performed using SYBR green DNA binding fluorescent dye. 10 μL of QuantiTect TM SYBR Green PCR Master Mix, 4 μL of QuantiTect TM SYBR Green primer assay (osteocalcin, b-actin; all provided by BioTNT), 5 μL of RNase free water and 1 μL of cDNA (1 ng/μL) were used for one reaction. Quantitative real-time PCR was performed in triplicates with the following cycler program: 95°C 10 min, denaturation step: 95°C 15 s, annealing step: 60°C 15 s, elongation step: 72°C 30 s; dissociation: 95°C 15 s, 60°C 1min, 95°C 15 s, 40 cycles were performed in total. B-actin was taken as an endogenous standard and relative gene expression was determined using the ΔΔCt method. Gene expression was compared by setting control cultures to 1 (reference value) as indicated in the relevant figures.

Quantitative analyses of TNF, α, Ang II and AT1R expression were performed using a quantitative image analysis system (FR-2000,FR Science and technology Inc, Shanghai China). Because the pattern of expression of TNFα, Ang II and AT1R are diffuse in nature, the percentage of positive staining in the renal tissue was quantified under a ×20 power field of microscope. Briefly, up to 10 random areas of kidney with the early stage (media:intima ≥1) and advanced stage (media:intima <1) were chosen from each tissue section and examined. The examined area was outlined, the positive staining patterns were identified, and the percent positive area in the examined area was then measured. Data were expressed as the percentage of mean±SEM.

## 4. Characterization of monoclonal anti-TGF–β antibody

The reactivity of the produced monoclonal antibodies with Urine TGF–β was screened by enzyme-linked immunosorbent assay (ELISA) using kit produced by Section living creature technique limited company of Hangzhou, China (NO,13409007) The sample solution (40 μl) was incubated with the monoclonal anti- TGF–β antibody (40 μl) at room temperature for 1 h in an TGF–β–transferrin attached microplate. After washing with phosphate-buffered saline (PBS) containing 0.05% Tween 20, 0.1 ml of peroxidase-labelled goat F(ab')2 fragment to mouse IgG(Fc) was added into the microplate, followed by incubation at room temperature for 1 h. After washing with PBS containing 0.05% Tween 20, 0.2 ml of o-phenylenediamine hydrochloride (1 mg/ml) containing 0.0124% H2O2 was added to the microplate, and then incubated at room temperature for 30 min. The reaction was terminated with 1.3 M H2SO4. The absorption at 492 nm was measured.

### 4.1 Statistical analysis

Data obtained from this study are expressed as the means ± SEM. Statistical analyses were performed using GraphPad Prism 3.0 (GraphPad Software, Inc., San Diego, CA). Differences in blood pressure, serum creatinine, blood urea nitrogen, 24h urine protein and Urine TGF–β at different time points (weeks 0 to 8) within the groups, and differences of Ang II and

AT1R activation, TNF–α expression and NF-κb accumulation in sham, control and HE86-treated animals were assessed by one-way analysis of variance, followed by t-test. Results were considered statistically significant when the P value was <0.05.

## 5. Result

Renal and systemic parameters obtained at 0 (before treatment), 32and 64 days after Nx are given in Table 1-5, Figure 1-5. Nx groups exhibited limited growth compared with Sham. In all Nx groups except treatment group, body weights were statistically different from those observed before treatment. Average food intake was similar among groups.

## 6. Effects of HE-86 administration on biochemical parameters in uraemic rats

Table2-3 shows the summary of renal function and 24h urine protein level. There was significant change in body weight between the control uraemic (control) and HE-86 treated uraemic (treatment) rats, although they were pair-fed. body weight of treatment group was showed more than control uraemic. Even 4 weeks after 5/6-nephrectomy, the levels of serum creatinine and BUN were markedly increased as compared to sham rats. Not only at 4 week but also at 8 week, the uraemic rats treated with HE-86 were manifested significantly decreased levels of serum creatinine, BUN, respectively. Urinary protein excretion was also suppressed obviously at 8 week as comparing with control uraemic rats.

| | N | BUN(mmol/L) | Scr(μmol/L) |
|---|---|---|---|
| sham | 12 | 6.79±0.70 | 26.25±1.04 |
| control | 12 | 12.09±3.37 | 50.56±15.83 |
| treatment | 12 | 9.81±2.93 | 38.83±12.00# |

Table 2. Serum creatinine and blood urea nitrogen after 4 week treatment. #P<0.05, ##P<0.01,when compared against empty vector-treated controls

| | N | BUN(mmol/L) | Scr(μmol/L) | 24h urine protein(mg) |
|---|---|---|---|---|
| sham | 12 | 9.31±1.05 | 18.88±1.55 | 22.34±4.4 |
| control | 12 | 14.85±2.83 | 53.38±12.05 | 41.47±8.07 |
| treatment | 12 | 13.62±2.81 | 41.00±10.51## | 29.14±5.68## |

Table 3. Serum creatinine, blood urea nitrogen and twenty-four-hour urinary protein excretion after 8 week treatment. #P<0.05, ##P<0.01,when compared against empty vector-treated controls

## 7. Effects of HE-86 administration on mean arterial blood pressure in uraemic rats

After subtotal nephrectomy, hypertension developed in both HE-86 treatment and control uremic rats. Blood pressure was significantly elevated from second to eighth week after nephrectomy compared to sham-operated animals (P < 0.05-0.01), and the rise in blood pressure was equivalent (systolic blood pressure 180 to 200 mmHg) in control group. After using HE-86 liquid extract, hypertension was obviously suppressed in treatment group, showing average systolic blood pressure 140 to 160 mmHg (Table 4).

| | Before treatment | After treatment | | | |
|---|---|---|---|---|---|
| | | Second week | Forth week | Sixth week | Eighth week |
| sham | 137.31±14.72 | 139.13±14.06 | 125.50±7.15 | 150.56±13.97 | 129.63±29.16 |
| control | 140.50±23.55* | 212.46±43.26 | 199.92±23.55 | 156.33±20.72 | 202.44±15.09 |
| treatment | 141.77±26.45* | 148.50±38.82## | 152.46±29.54## | 141.00±14.73# | 176.00±30.70# |

Table 4. Systolic blood pressure. Data represent the means ± SEM for groups of twelve rats treated with either HE-86 or empty vector (#P<0.05,##P<0.01,when compared against empty vector-treated controls;*P<0.05,**P<0.01, when compared to normal sham-controls).

## 8. Effects of HE-86 administration on urine TGF−β1

High excreation of urine TGF−β1, which express both glomerular and tubulointerstitial injuries. To demonstrate further the anti-inflammatory effect of HE-86 on rat chronic renal failure, we determined the TGF−β1 levels within the urine by ELISA. Results demonstrated that compared with vehicle, He-86 treatment significantly reduced urinary TGF−β1 levels, corrected by decrease level of serum creatinine, throughout the entire disease course (P<0.05), indicating that HE-86 treatment may primarily suppress the local immune and inflammatory response within the diseased kidney. In contrast, overexpression of urine TGF−β1 was found in control uraemic rats as compared with normal rats (Table 5). The experimental result showed the administration of HE-86 significantly inversed high expression of urine TGF−β in uraemic rats, manifesting HE-86 to attenuate the development of glomerular sclerosis.

| | N | Urine TGF−β(ug/L) |
|---|---|---|
| sham | 12 | 1.83±0.64 |
| control | 12 | 1.90±0.56* |
| treatment | 12 | 1.77±0.43# |

Table 5. Effect of HE-86 liquid extract on urine TGF−β excretion in 5/6 nephrectomy in rats. (#P<0.05, ##P<0.01,when compared against empty vector-treated controls; *P<0.05, **P<0.01, when compared to normal sham-controls)

## 9. Effects of HE-86 administration on localization of NF-κB in renal tissue

Immunohistochemical analysis was performed to determine the localization of NF-κB in the renal cortex (Fig.1-2). NF-κB, a critical transcriptional factor for controlling inflammatory response, has been shown to play a central role in inflammatory diseases, including kidney diseases [33]. In normal rats, only tubular epithelial cells were weakly stained by the monoclonal anti-NF-κB antibody, while glomeruli were hardly stained. In control uraemic rats, however, proximal tubular epithelial cells, especially of dilated tubules, were intensively stained by the anti-NF-κB antibody. In contrast, in the HE-86-treated uraemic rats activation of the NF-κB in tubular epithelial cells was less prominent as compared with that in the control uraemic rats. The staining of NF-κB as shown in the control uraemic rats found increased NF-κB -positive (intensively stained) area in the renal cortex, whereas HE-86-treated rats showed markedly decreased NF-κB -positive area as compared to the control uraemic rats. These data demonstrate that HE-86 markedly reduces the overexpress of NF-κB on the remnant tubular cells.

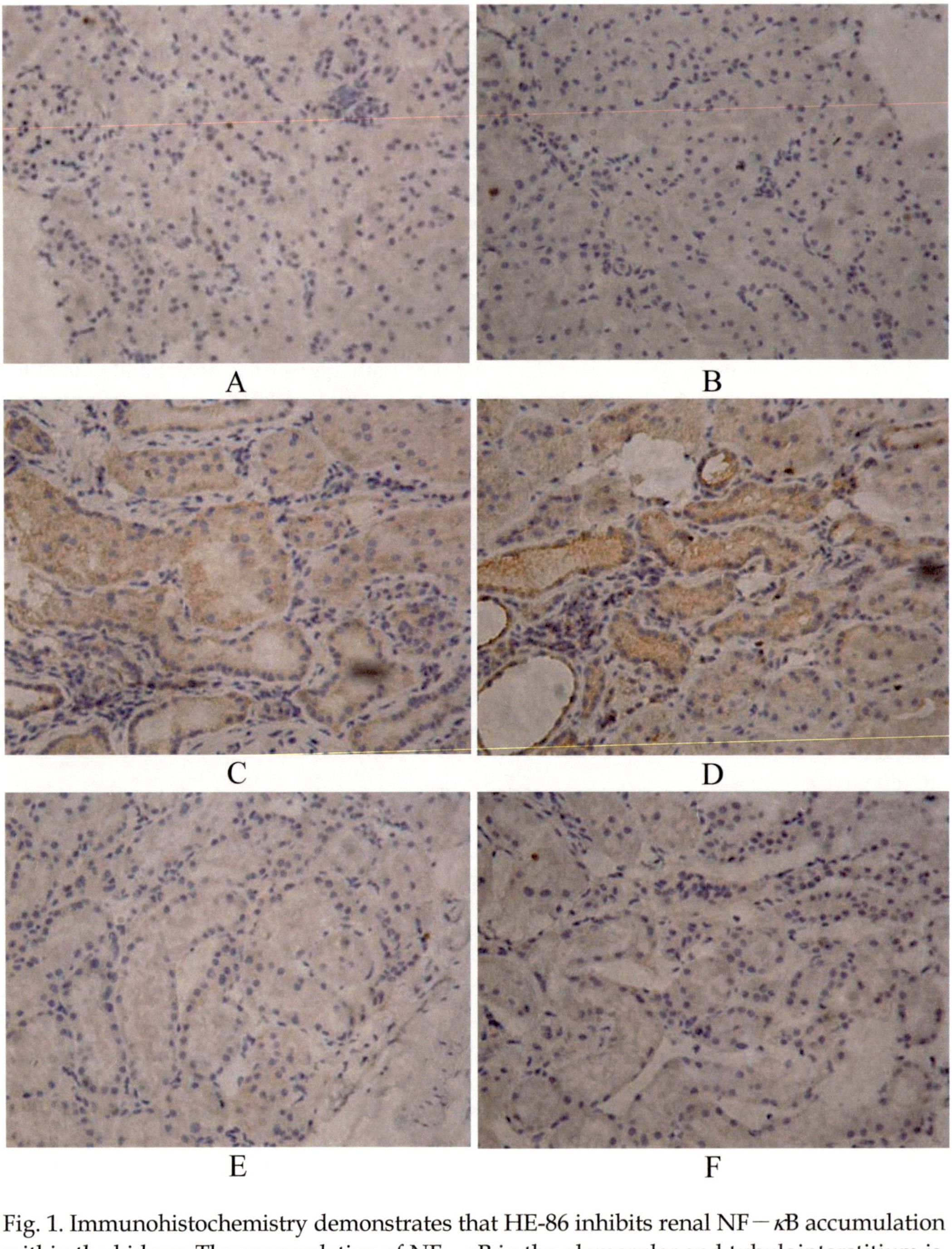

Fig. 1. Immunohistochemistry demonstrates that HE-86 inhibits renal NF$-\kappa$B accumulation within the kidney. The accumulation of NF$-\kappa$B in the glomerular and tubulointerstitium is markedly increased in empty vector-treated animals (C, D), compared to normal sham-controls (A,B), which is substantially inhibited in 5/6 nephrectomized rats treated with HE-86 (E, F). Original magnifications, x100.

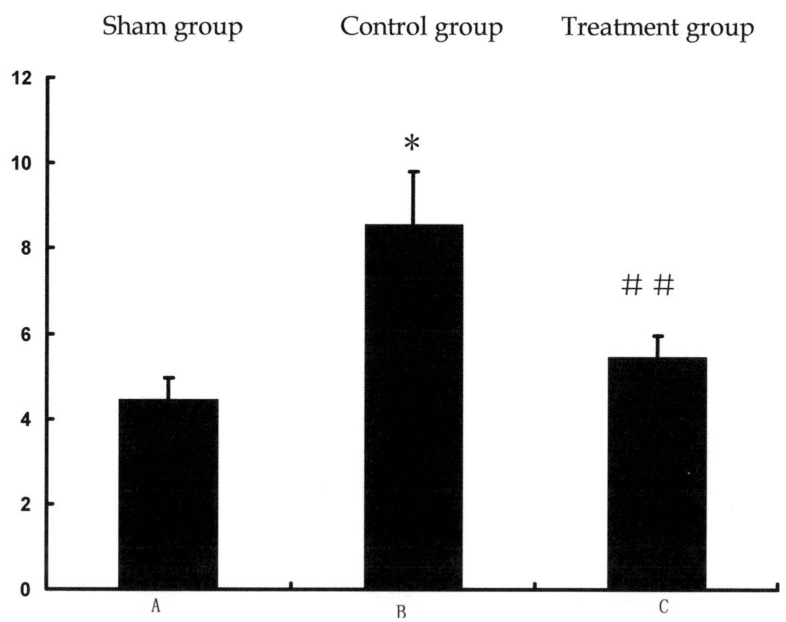


Fig. 2. Semiquantitative analysis of the therapeutic effect of HE-86 on NF-$\kappa$B localization in the glomerulus and tubulointerstitium using the Quantitative Image System. A: Percentage of glomerular and tubulointerstitial NF-$\kappa$B deposition in sham group. B: Percentage of NF-$\kappa$B localization in glomerular and tubulointerstitial without treatment C: Percentage of glomerular and tubulointerstitial NF-$\kappa$B accumulation in twelve rats treated with HE-86 was decreased significantly. Each bar represents data (mean ± SEM) #, $P < 0.05$ and ##, $P < 0.001$, when compared to empty vector-treated controls; *, $P < 0.05$ and **, $P < 0.01$, when compared to the normal sham-control.

## 10. Effects of HE-86 administration on mRNA levels of TNF-α, Ang II and AT II R in renal tissue

The effects of HE-86 on the gene expression of Ang II (Figure 3), AT1R (Figure 4) and TNF-$\alpha$ (Figure 5) in the renal cortex were examined. We investigated the potential mechanisms whereby HE-86 suppressed rat tubular interstitial fibrosis and glomerular cirrhosis. TNF-$\alpha$, being key proinflammatory cytokines in anti-GBM glomerulonephritis, and a group of chemotactic and adhesion molecules including ICAM-1, MCP-1, was examined. In vehicle-treated chronic renal failure rats, there was a substantial increase in renal mRNA expression of TNF-$\alpha$, Treatment with HE-86 significantly reduced upregulation of TNF-$\alpha$ inflammatory genes examined (P<0.05). Furthermore, HE-86 was capable of attenuating renal cortical mRNAs for Ang II and AT1R as compared with the control uraemic rats when they were administered after the establishment of nephrectomized. However, the renal mRNA levels of Ang II and AT1R were markedly increased in control uraemic rats as compared with normal rats. The variation in the mRNA levels of TNF–$\alpha$, Ang II and AT1R in both HE-86-treated and control uraemic rats are related to variation in the extent of CRF.

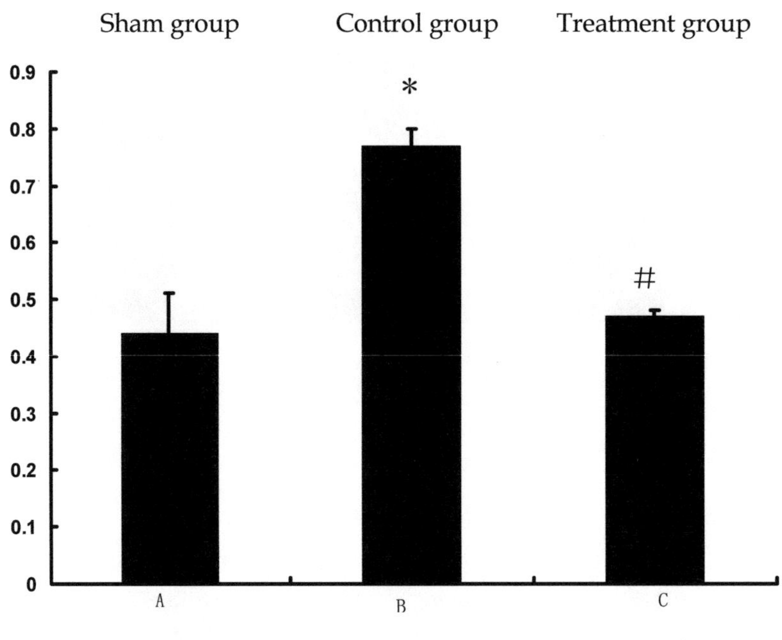


Fig. 3. Real-time PCR reveals the inhibitory effect of HE-86 liquid extract on renal Ang II mRNA expression(A). and Semiquantitative analysis of the therapeutic effect of HE-86 on Ang II mRNA localization in the glomerulus and tubulointerstitium using the FR-2000 Image Analyze System. A: Degree of glomerular and tubulointerstitial Ang II mRNA expression in sham group. B: Numbers of Ang II mRNA expression in glomerular and tubulointerstitial without treatment C: Numbers of glomerular and tubulointerstitial cells with nuclear localization of Ang II mRNA in twelve rats treated with HE-86 was decreased significantly. Each bar represents data (mean ± SEM) #, $P < 0.05$ and # #, $P < 0.01$, when compared to empty vector-treated controls; *, $P < 0.05$ and **, $P < 0.01$, when compared to the normal sham-control.

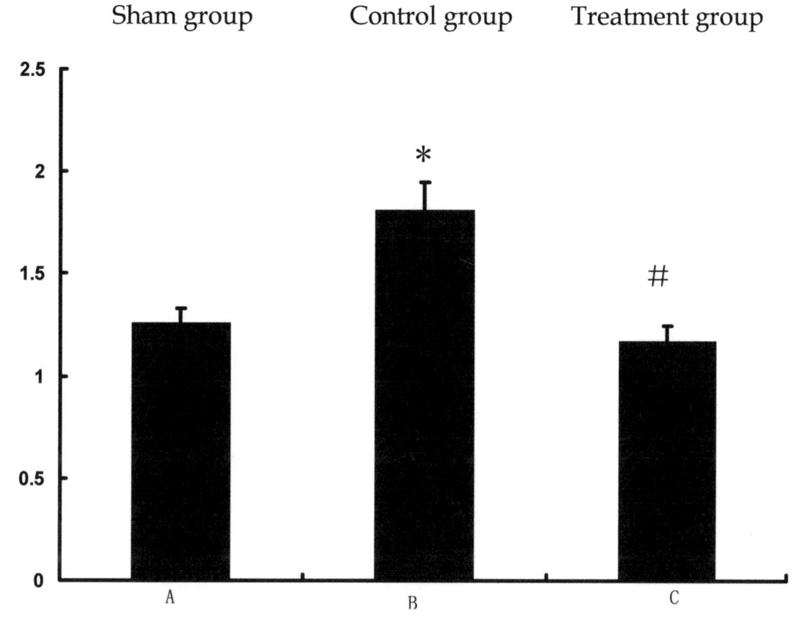


Fig. 4. Real-time PCR reveals the inhibitory effect of HE-86 liquid extract on renal AT1RmRNA expression(B). and Semiquantitative analysis of the therapeutic effect of HE-86 on AT1RmRNA localization in the glomerulus and tubulointerstitium using the FR-2000 Image Analyze System. A: Degree of glomerular and tubulointerstitial AT1RmRNA expression in sham group. B: Numbers of AT1RmRNA expression in glomerular and tubulointerstitial without treatment C : Numbers of glomerular and tubulointerstitial cells with nuclear localization of AT1RmRNA in nephrectomized rats treated with HE-86 was decreased significantly. Each bar represents data (mean ± SEM) #, P < 0.05 and # #, P < 0.01, when compared to empty vector-treated controls; *, P < 0.05 and **, P < 0.01, when compared to the normal sham-control

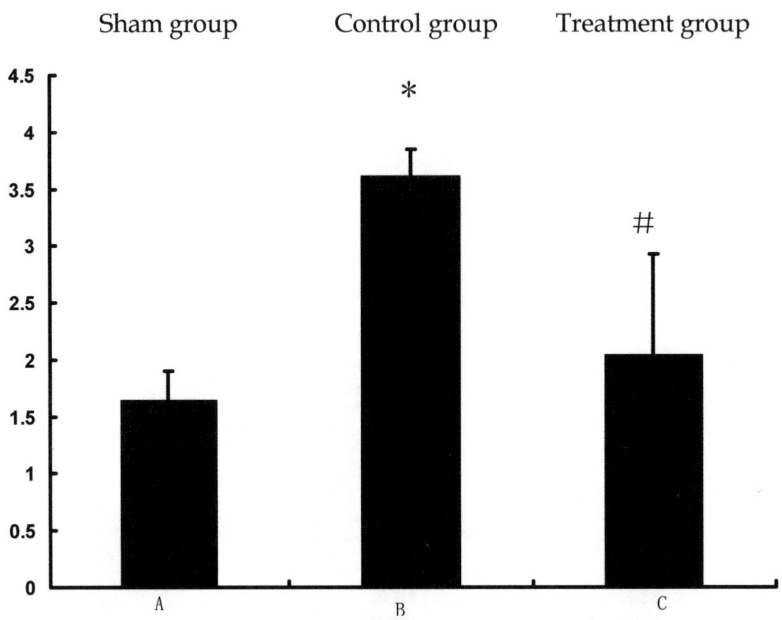


Fig. 5. Real-time PCR reveals the inhibitory effect of HE-86 liquid extract on renal TNF−αmRNA expression(C). and Semiquantitative analysis of the therapeutic effect of HE-86 on TNF−αmRNA within the glomerulus and tubulointerstitium using the FR-2000 Image Analyze System. A: Degree of glomerular and tubulointerstitial TNF−αmRNA expression in sham group. B: Numbers of TNF−αmRNA expression in glomerular and tubulointerstitial without treatment C: Numbers of glomerular and tubulointerstitial cells with nuclear localization of TNF−αmRNA in nephrectomized rats treated with HE-86 was decreased significantly. Each bar represents data (mean ± SEM) #, $P < 0.05$ and ##, $P < 0.01$, when compared to empty vector-treated controls; *, $P < 0.05$ and **, $P < 0.01$, when compared to the normal sham-control.

## 11. Discussion

Renal fibrosis is a final common pathway to end-stage renal disease. Recent studies have shown that hypertensive nephropathy is a major leading cause of end-stage renal disease and the renin-angiotensin system plays a pivotal role in the development of progressive renal injury [34-35]. Clinical trials have shown that blocking the effects of angiotensin II (Ang II) with angiotensin-converting enzyme inhibitors and angiotensin-receptor blockers can prevent or slow the progression of kidney damage in patients with diabetes and hypertension [34-36].

As expected, 5/6 renal ablation promoted growth retardation, systemic arterial hypertension, impaired renal function, and severe albuminuria. These functional changes were accompanied by severe glomerulosclerosis, as well as expansion and intense macrophage infiltration of the interstitial area. Mounting evidence indicates that these renal structural abnormalities, which are characteristic of the Nx and other models of progressive nephropathies, are a consequence of the concerted action of mechanical stress, caused by glomerular hypertension and hypertrophy [37-38], and inflammatory phenomena, comprising cell infiltration and/or proliferation and extracellular matrix accumulation [38-39]. Moreover, a causal relationship appears to exist between these phenomena, because the distension of the glomerular walls due to intracapillary hypertension may trigger the local release of cytokines, growth factors, and, particularly, Ang II and AT-1 receptors [40-41].

The beneficial effect of RAS suppressors was initially attributed to amelioration of the glomerular hemodynamic dysfunction associated with progressive nephropathies. However, recent observations suggest that the nonhemodynamic effects of RAS suppressors may be equally important, given the strong proinflammatory and profibrotic effects of Ang II [42]. A substantial fraction of this proinflammatory ANG II may originate in the renal parenchyma, rather than in renal vessels or in the systemic circulation [43]. Increased intrarenal production of ANG II was described in various models of renal fibrosis [44-46]. A preliminary report has suggested that, in the 5/6 renal ablation (Nx) model, ANG II is expressed in renal interstitial cells, paralleling the severity of renal injury [47].

Increasing evidence shows that angiotensin II (Ang II) plays a critical role in cardiovascular disease and is a key mediator in the process of vascular fibrosis, characterized by reduced lumen diameter and arterial wall thickening attributable to excessive deposition of extracellular matrix (ECM). Vascular fibrosis is a major complication of hypertension and diabetic mellitus. It has been shown that upregulated tissue rennin-angiotensin system is involved in development of vascular lesions in both human and experimental vascular diseases [48-49]. This observation is confirmed by the finding that infusion of Ang II is able to induce vascular fibrosis in rats [50]. The functional importance of Ang II in vascular fibrosis is further supported by the evidence that blockade of Ang II inhibits vascular fibrosis in diabetic and subtotal nephrectomy rats and NO-deficient mice [51-53].

Both the hemodynamic and proinflammatory effects of Ang II are mediated by AT-1 receptors (AT1R) [54], extensively expressed in renal tissue. In the normal rat kidney, AT1R are predominantly expressed in tubular cells and vessels [55]. Recent data obtained with the Nx model have suggested that AT1R expression is shifted from the glomerular to the tubulointerstitial compartment 4 wk after ablation [56]. However, the renal distribution of AT1R in this model and its temporal evolution have not been established.

Beyond its hemodynamic effects, Ang II is recognized as a cytokine with an active role in cardiovascular remodeling. It is well known that Ang II signals through its Ang II receptor 1 (AT1) receptor to exert most of its biological functions [57]. After binding to the AT1 receptor, Ang II activates multiple downstream intracellular signaling pathways, including tyrosine kinase, mitogen-activated protein kinase (MAPK), p38, and Janus family kinase

[58]. Activation of these pathways leads to numerous heterogeneous downstream events that play essential roles in the biological activities of Ang II, such as cell growth and migration, ECM production, and apoptosis [58].

Renal expression of AT1R in rats appeared mostly in tubular cells, and to a lesser extent, at the interstitial area, whereas weaker expression was seen in vessels and glomeruli. This pattern was completely disrupted after Nx, when dense AT1R expression could be demonstrated in interstitial cells, far exceeding in intensity the expression of AT1R in tubules. The exact meaning of this finding and the cell types involved are uncertain. Several inflammatory cells known to infiltrate the renal interstitium in the Nx model have the potential to express AT1R, such as lymphocytes [59] and macrophages [60]. In addition, AT1R may be expressed by myofibroblasts originating from tubular cell transdifferentiation [61]. This hypothesis is particularly attractive because it helps to explain the progressive shift in AT1R expression, from tubules to the interstitial area, observed in Nx rats, and also because tubular cells already express AT1R under normal conditions. The simultaneous presence at the interstitial area of large amounts of Ang II and of the AT1R may accelerate the progression of the nephropathy by a positive-feedback mechanism. Consistent with this view is the aggravation of the renal structural injury of Nx, which was paralleled by the intensity of the inflammatory infiltration and of the interstitial expression of Ang II.

It is well accepted that NF-$\kappa$B is a key transcriptional factor to regulate a variety of inflammatory responses [75]. NF-$\kappa$B is composed of p50 and p65 subunits, among which p65 is a potent transcriptional activator, strongly promoting inflammatory reaction in kidney diseases [76]. NF$\kappa$B total protein expression, and inflammation, which may have resulted from blockade of the oxidative stress pathway [77-78]. This was accompanied by a substantial attenuation in renal fibrosis, which might have resulted from the modulating actions of vitamins on lipid peroxidation and profibrotic activity involved in renal tissue damage [79-82]. In this study, marked activation of NF-$\kappa$B was closely correlated with the renal inflammation. In our study, using liquid extract isolated from clinical effective Chinese prescription, we were able to show that overexpression activation of NF-$\kappa$B was substantially suppressed as compared with control group. These findings are consistent with the improving renal function and correcting high blood pressure.

Tumour necrosis fator-α(TNF-α)is a potent pro-inflammatory cytokine which is produced by many cell types including monocytes/macrophages, and renal mesangial and epithelial cells. It induces the expression of major histocompatibility complex (MHC) class I and II molecules, endothelial adhesion molecules and procoagulant activity of endothelium. TNF-α stimulates the release of other pro-inflammatory cytokines, chemokines and growth factors, including interleukin-1β(IL-1β), monocyte chemoattractant protein-1 (MCP-1) and transforming growth factor-β(TFG-β) [83-84]. The biological effects of TNF-α are mediated by binding to specific receptors which are widely distributed. TNF-α binds to two types of receptor: TNF receptor type 1 and TNF receptor type 2, which have molecular weights of 55 kDa (p55) and 75 kDa (p75), respectively. Both receptors are necessary and act synergistically for cell proliferation and maturation, cytotoxicity and antiviral activity, but p55 is responsible for activation of NFκB and mediation of apoptosis [85].

TNF-$\alpha$ may contribute to renal damage by inciting an inflammatory response within the kidney via induction of a variety of chemokines and adhesion molecules [86-87]. There is a mounting evidence to implicate TNF-α in the pathogenesis of glomeruli of rodents with experimental nephritis, and is found in renal biopsies, sera and urine of patients with different types of glomerulonephritis [88-91]; In vitro and in vivo studies document that TNF-α is produced locally within inflamed glomeruli by mesangial and epithelial cells, as well as by infiltrating monocytes/macrophages [89,91]; Systemic administration of TNF-α results in glomerular damage in rabbits [92] and exacerbates the degree of glomerular injury in nephrotoxic nephritis in rats [93]; and blocking endogenous TNF-α in nephrotoxic nephritis in rats ameliorates acute glomerular inflammation [94], and down-regulates glomerular IL-1βmRNA and circulating TNF-α concentrations [95].

Treatment of Nx rats with the HE-86 promoted a significant regression of hypertension, high level of creatinine and blood urea nitrogen, albuminuria, and inflammatory signs such as urine TGF-ß and renal tissue TNF-α, NF-κB, Ang II and AT1R expression, whereas the parameters of renal structural tissue injury were strongly attenuated, compared with pretreatment levels. The protection achieved with effective unit from clinical prescription treatment was much greater than that obtained with traditional prescription alone. On the basis of the present study, we cannot exclude the hypothesis that the success of HE-86 was due to a particularly effective hemodynamic action, although previous observations from this laboratory [96] indicated that NOF, a new nonsteroidal anti-inflammatory, had no significant effect on glomerular hemodynamics. Because treatment with NOF alone had no effect on blood pressure, it seems unlikely that the hemodynamic effect of NOS was directly intensified by its association with NOF. Therefore, the efficacy of extract HE-86 was likely due to the simultaneous blockade of the hemodynamic and proinflammatory actions of Ang II, AT1R and its derivatives as TNF-*α*, NF-*κ*B, TGF-ß and by abrogation of the complex interplay between hypertension and inflammation. The present findings support other scholars' observations of the Nx model, which similarly indicated the superiority of the combination of a RAS suppressor with an anti-inflammatory agent [97-99]. It is noteworthy that HE-86 afforded partial regression of the nephropathy associated with Nx even though it was started 4 week after surgery, when renal injury was already established. This observation suggests that both continued stimulation of Ang II and AT1 receptors and production of inflammatory factors continue to play an important pathogenic role even during the late phases of the process, necessitating vigorous and persistent treatment to prevent further renal deterioration.

Taken together with our previous data and the present results, it is likely that HE-86-induced reduction of renal rennin-angentensin system is mediated, at least partly, by reducing the overload of inflammatory factors activity on remnant kidney unit. In summary, HE-86effective composition coming from clinical validly treating patients with chronic renal failure especially for early and middle stage, partially reversed the nephropathy and renal inflammation associated with the Nx model, showing much more effective protection than with traditional Chinese medicine prescription.

## 12. References

[1] Wolf G, Ziyadeh FN. Renal tubular hypertrophy induced by angiotensin II. Semin Nephrol. 1997;17:448–454

[2] Guijarro C, Egido J: Transcription factor-kappa B (NF-kappa B) and renal disease. Kidney Int 59: 415–424, 2001

[3] Weistuch JM, Dworkin LD. Does essential hypertension cause end-stage renal disease? Kidney Int. 1992;41:S33–S37.

[4] Yoshioka K, Tohda M, Takemura T, Akano N, Matsubara K, Ooshima A, Maki S. Distribution of the type I collagen in human kidney diseases in comparison with type III collagen. J Pathol. 1990;162:141–148.

[5] Albaladejo P, Bouaziz H, Duriez M, Gohlke P, Levy BI, Safar ME, Benetos A. Angiotensin-converting enzyme inhibition prevents the increase in aortic collagen in rats. Hypertension. 1994;23:74–82.

[6] Anderson S, Meyer TW, Renke HG, Brenner BM. Control of glomerular hypertension limits glomerular injury in rats with reduced renal mass. J Clin Invest. 1985;76:612–619.

[7] Wilson C, Byrom FB. Renal changes in malignant hypertension. Lancet. 1939;i:136–143.

[8] Davies PF, Barbee KA, Volin MV, Robotewskyj A, Chen J, Joseph L, Griem ML, Wernick MN, Jacobs E, Polacek DC, dePaola N, Barakat AI. Spatial relationships in early signaling events of flow-mediated endothelial mechanotransduction. Ann Rev Physiol. 1997;59:527–549.

[9] Jones PL, Crack J, Rabinovitch M. Regulation of tenacin-C, a vascular smooth muscle cell survival factor that interacts with the alpha v beta 3 integrin to promote epidermal growth factor receptor phosphorylation and growth. J Cell Biol. 1997;139:279–293.

[10] Isik FF, Gibran NS, Jang YC, Sandell L, Schwartz SM. Vitronectin decreases microvascular endothelial cell apoptosis. J Cell Physiol. 1998;175:149–155.

[11] Ingelfinger JR, Dzau VJ. Molecular biology of renal injury: emphasis on the role of the renin-angiotensin system. J Am Soc Nephrol. 1991;2:S9–S20.

[12] Lindpaintner K, Ganten D. The cardiac renin-angiotensin system: an appraisal of present experimental and clinical evidence. Circ Res. 1991;68:905–921.

[13] Haller H, Park JK, Dragun D, Lippoldt A, Luft FC. Leukocyte infiltration and ICAM-1 expression in two-kidney one-clip hypertension. Nephrol Dial Transplant. 1997;12:899–903.

[14] Hsueh WA, Law RE, Do YS. Integrins, adhesion, and cardiac remodeling. Hypertension. 1998;31:176–180.

[15] Roy-Chaudhury P, Hillis G, McDonald S, Simpson JG, Power DA. Importance of the tubulointerstitium in human glomerulonephritis, II: distribution of integrin chains beta 1, alpha 1 to 6 and alpha V. Kidney Int. 1997;52:103–110.

[16] Ridker PM, Hennekens CH, Roitman Johnson B, Stampfer MJ, Allen J. Plasma concentration of soluble intercellular adhesion molecule 1 and risks of future myocardial infarction in apparently healthy men. Lancet. 1998;351:88–92.

[17] Remuzzi G, Bertani T. Pathophysiology of progressive nephropathies. N Engl J Med. 1998;339:1448–1456.

[18] Lenardo MJ, Baltimore D. NF-kappa B: a pleiotropic mediator of inducible and tissue-specific gene control. Cell. 1989;58:227–229.

[19] Barnes PJ, Karin M. Nuclear factor-kappaB: a pivotal transcription factor in chronic inflammatory diseases. N Engl J Med. 1997;336:1066–1071.

[20] Marumo T, Schini Kerth VB, Brandes RP, Busse R. Glucocorticoids inhibit superoxide anion production and p22 phox mRNA expression in human aortic smooth muscle cells. Hypertension. 1998;32:1083–1088.

[21] Sen CK, Packer L. Antioxidant and redox regulation of gene transcription. FASEB J. 1996;10:709–720.

[22] Ozes O, Mayo L, Gustin J, Pfeffer S, Pfeffer L, Donner D. NF-kappaB activation by tumour necrosis factor requires the Akt serine-threonine kinase. Nature. 1999;401:82–85.

[23] Takahashi T, Taniguchi T, Konishi H, Kikkawa U, Ishikawa Y, Yokoyama M. Activation of Akt/protein kinase B after stimulation with angiotensin II in vascular smooth muscle cells. Am J Physiol. 1999;276:H1927–H1934.

[24] Ushio-Fukai M, Alexander R, Akers M, Yin Q, Fujio Y, Walsh K, Griendling K. Reactive oxygen species mediate the activation of Akt/protein kinase B by angiotensin II in vascular smooth muscle cells. J Biol Chem. 1999;274:22699–22704.

[25] Hernandez-Presa MA, Bustos C, Ortego M, Tunon J, Ortega L, Egido J. ACE inhibitor quinapril reduces the arterial expression of NF-kappaB-dependent proinflammatory factors but not of collagen I in a rabbit model of atherosclerosis. Am J Pathol. 1998;153:1825–1837.

[26] Morrissey JJ, Klahr S. Rapid communication: enalapril decreases nuclear factor kappa B activation in the kidney with ureteral obstruction. Kidney Int. 1997;52:926–933.

[27] Ruiz-Ortega M, Bustos C, Hernandez-Presa M, Lorenzo O, Plaza J, Edigo J. Angiotensin II participates in mononuclear cell recruitment in experimental immune complex nephritis through nuclear factor-kB activation and monocyte chemoattractant protein-1 synthesis. J Immunol. 1998;161:430–439.

[28] He Li qun, Wang yi, Cao he xin, Li jun. The effect of kangxianling decoction on PDGF-mRNA 、TNF $\alpha$-mRNA expression of CRF Rat renal tissue J. China experiments the square to learn 2003,9: （5）:29-32

[29] He liqun 、Li jun 、Li yi. The effect of "FUZHENGHUOXUE Decoction" on the expressions of fibronectin and transforming growth factor-$\beta$ mRNA in renal tissue of the CRF rats. J. Chinese medicine 2005. 46： （6） ：454-457

[30] LI Jun 、HE Li-Qun 、LI Yi 、HOU Wei-Guo：The Effect of kang xian ling 2 decoction on serum lipide metabolism of chronic renal fail rats. J. International medical science of China 2003, 3:(3）204-206

[31] Wang chen 、He liqun. Experimental Study on Effect of Renal Failure Granule in Treating Uremia CJIM, 2002;8(3):208-211

[32] HE Li-Qun Cai Gan The clinical observation of the JIAN-PI-QIN-HUI prescription on spleen deficiency and dampness heat style patients with chronic renal failure J.The combination with Chinese and western medicine 2005, 14： （4） ：270-274

[33] Muller DN, Dechend R, Mervaala EM, Park JK, Schmidt F, Fiebeler A, Theuer J, Breu V, Ganten D, Haller H, Luft FC. NF-$\kappa$B inhibition ameliorates angiotensin II–induced inflammatory damage in rats. Hypertension. 2000; 35:193–201.

[34] Flack JM, Peters R, Shafi T, Alrefai H, Nasser SA, Crook E: Prevention of hypertension and its complications: theoretical basis and guidelines for treatment. J Am Soc Nephrol 2003, 14(Suppl 2):S92-S98

[35] Klahr S, Morrissey J: Progression of chronic renal disease. Am J Kidney Dis 2003, 41(Suppl 1):S3-S7

[36] Taal MW, Brenner BM: Renoprotective benefits of RAS inhibition: from ACEI to angiotensin II antagonists. Kidney Int 2000, 57:1803-1817

[37] Brenner BM. Nephron adaptation to renal injury or ablation. Am J Physiol Renal Fluid Electrolyte Physiol 249: F324-F337, 1985.

[38] Fujihara CK, Antunes GR, Mattar AL, Andreoli N, Malheiros DM, Noronha IL, and Zatz R. Cyclooxygenase-2 (COX-2) inhibition limits abnormal COX-2 expression and progressive injury in the remnant kidney. Kidney Int 64: 2172-2181, 2003

[39] Floege J, Burns MW, Alpers CE, Yoshimura A, Pritzl P, Gordon K, Seifert RA, Bowen-Pope DF, Couser WG, and Johnson RJ. Glomerular cell proliferation and PDGF expression precede glomerulosclerosis in the remnant kidney model. Kidney Int 41: 297-309, 1992.

[40] Akai Y, Homma T, Burns KD, Yasuda T, Badr KF, and Harris RC. Mechanical stretch/relaxation of cultured rat mesangial cells induces protooncogenes and cyclooxygenase. Am J Physiol Cell Physiol 267: C482-C490, 1994.

[41] Lee LK, Meyer TW, Pollock AS, and Lovett DH. Endothelial cell injury initiates glomerular sclerosis in the rat remnant kidney. J Clin Invest 96: 953-964, 1995.

[42] Ruiz-Ortega M, Lorenzo O, Suzuki Y, Ruperez M, and Egido J. Proinflammatory actions of angiotensins. Curr Opin Nephrol Hypertens 10: 321-329, 2001.

[43] Van Kats JP, Schalekamp MA, Verdouw PD, Duncker DJ, and Danser AH. Intrarenal angiotensin II: interstitial and cellular levels and site of production. Kidney Int 60: 2311-2317, 2001

[44] Gilbert RE, Wu LL, Kelly DJ, Cox A, Wilkinson-Berka JL, Johnston CI, and Cooper ME. Pathological expression of renin and angiotensin II in the renal tubule after subtotal nephrectomy: implications for the pathogenesis of tubulointerstitial fibrosis. Am J Pathol 155: 429-440, 1999

[45] Pelayo JC, Quan AH, and Shanley PF. Angiotensin II control of the renal microcirculation in rats with reduced renal mass. Am J Physiol Renal Fluid Electrolyte Physiol 258: F414-F422, 1990

[46] Rodriguez-Iturbe B, Quiroz Y, Nava M, Bonet L, Chavez M, Herrera-Acosta J, Johnson RJ, and Pons HA. Reduction of renal immune cell infiltration results in blood pressure control in genetically hypertensive rats. Am J Physiol Renal Physiol 282: F191-F201, 2002

[47] Noronha IL, Fujihara CK, and Zatz R. The inflammatory component in progressive renal disease—are interventions possible (Abstract)? Nephrol Dial Transplant 17: 363, 2002

[48] Ford CM, Li S, Pickering JG, Itoh H, Mukoyama M, Pratt RE, Gibbons GH, Dzau VJ. Angiotensin II stimulates collagen synthesis in human vascular smooth muscle cells. Involvement of the AT(1) receptor, transforming growth factor-beta, and tyrosine phosphorylation. Arterioscler Thromb Vasc Biol. 1999;19:1843–1851.

[49] Miao CY, Tao X, Gong K, Zhang SH, Chu ZX, Su DF. Arterial remodeling in chronic sinoaortic-denervated rats. J Cardiovasc Pharmacol. 2001;37:6–15.

[50] Lombardi DM, Viswanathan M, Vio CP, Saavedra JM, Schwartz SM, Johnson RJ. Renal and vascular injury induced by exogenous angiotensin II is AT1 receptor-dependent. Nephron. 2001;87:66–74.
[51] Hayashi T, Sohmiya K, Ukimura A, Endoh S, Mori T, Shimomura H, Okabe M, Terasaki F, Kitaura Y. Angiotensin II receptor blockade prevents microangiopathy and preserves diastolic function in the diabetic rat heart. Heart. 2003;89:1236–1242.
[52] Kakinuma Y, Kawamura T, Bills T, Yoshioka T, Ichikawa I, Fogo A. Blood pressure-independent effect of angiotensin inhibition on vascular lesions of chronic renal failure. Kidney Int. 1992;42:46–55.
[53] Boffa JJ, Lu Y, Placier S, Stefanski A, Dussaule JC, Chatziantoniou C, Tharaux PL, Ardaillou R. Regression of renal vascular and glomerular fibrosis: role of angiotensin II receptor antagonism and matrix metallo-proteinases. J Am Soc Nephrol. 2003;14:1132–1144.
[54] Ruiz-Ortega M, Lorenzo O, Suzuki Y, Ruperez M, and Egido J. Proinflammatory actions of angiotensins. Curr Opin Nephrol Hypertens 10: 321-329, 2001
[55] Harrison-Bernard LM, Navar LG, Ho MM, Vinson GP, and el-Dahr SS. Immunohistochemical localization of ANG II AT1 receptor in adult rat kidney using a monoclonal antibody. Am J Physiol Renal Physiol 273: F170-F177, 1997
[56] Cao Z, Bonnet F, Candido R, Nesteroff SP, Burns WC, Kawachi H, Shimizu F, Carey RM, de Gasparo M, and Cooper ME. Angiotensin type 2 receptor antagonism confers renal protection in a rat model of progressive renal injury. J Am Soc Nephrol 13: 1773-1787, 2002.
[57] Zhuo J, Moeller I, Jenkins T, Chai SY, Allen AM, Ohishi M, Mendelsohn FA. Mapping tissue angiotensin-converting enzyme and angiotensin AT1, AT2 and AT4 receptors. J Hypertens. 1998;16:2027–2037.
[58] Touyz RM, Berry C. Recent advances in angiotensin II signaling. Braz J Med Biol Res. 2002;35:1001–1015.
[59] Nath KA, Chmielewski DH, and Hostetter TH. Regulatory role of prostanoids in glomerular microcirculation of remnant nephrons. Am J Physiol Renal Fluid Electrolyte Physiol 252: F829-F837, 1987
[60] Okamura A, Rakugi H, Ohishi M, Yanagitani Y, Takiuchi S, Moriguchi K, Fennessy PA, Higaki J, and Ogihara T. Upregulation of renin-angiotensin system during differentiation of monocytes to macrophages. J Hypertens 17: 537-545, 1999
[61] Ng YY, Huang TP, Yang WC, Chen ZP, Yang AH, Mu W, Nikolic-Paterson DJ, Atkins RC, and Lan HY. Tubular epithelial-myofibroblast transdifferentiation in progressive tubulointerstitial fibrosis in 5/6 nephrectomized rats. Kidney Int 54: 864-876, 1998.
[62] Border WA, Noble NA: Interactions of transforming growth factor-beta and angiotensin II in renal fibrosis. Hypertension 1998, 31:181-188
[63] Gaedeke J, Peters H, Noble NA, Border WA: Angiotensin II, TGF-beta and renal fibrosis. Contrib Nephrol 2001, 135:153-160
[64] Wolf G: Link between angiotensin II and TGF-beta in the kidney. Miner Electrolyte Metab 1998, 24:174-180

[65] Wolf G, Haberstroh U, Neilson EG: Angiotensin II stimulates the proliferation and biosynthesis of type I collagen in cultured murine mesangial cells. Am J Pathol 1992, 140:95-107
[66] Kagami S, Border WA, Miller DE, Noble NA: Angiotensin II stimulates extracellular matrix protein synthesis through induction of transforming growth factor-beta expression in rat glomerular mesangial cells. J Clin Invest 1994, 93:2431-2437
[67] Wolf G, Zahner G, Schroeder R, Stahl RA: Transforming growth factor beta mediates the angiotensin-II-induced stimulation of collagen type IV synthesis in cultured murine proximal tubular cells. Nephrol Dial Transplant 1996, 11:263-269
[68] Wolf G, Ziyadeh FN, Stahl RA: Angiotensin II stimulates expression of transforming growth factor beta receptor type II in cultured mouse proximal tubular cells. J Mol Med 1999, 77:556-564
[69] Gibbons GH, Pratt RE, Dzau VJ: Vascular smooth muscle cell hypertrophy vs hyperplasia: autocrine transforming growth factor-beta 1 expression determines growth response to angiotensin II. J Clin Invest 1992, 90:456-461
[70] Rumble JR, Gilbert RE, Cox A, Wu L, Cooper ME: Angiotensin converting enzyme inhibition reduces the expression of transforming growth factor-beta(1) and type IV collagen in diabetic vasculopathy. J Hypertens 1998, 16:1603-1609
[71] Peters H, Border WA, Noble NA: Targeting TGF-beta overexpression in renal disease: maximizing the antifibrotic action of angiotensin II blockade. Kidney Int 1998, 54:1570-1580
[72] Benigni A, Zoja C, Corna D, Zatelli C, Conti S, Campana M, Gagliardini E, Rottoli D, Zanchi C, Abbate M, Ledbetter S, Remuzzi G: Add-on anti-TGF-beta antibody to ACE inhibitor arrests progressive diabetic nephropathy in the rat. J Am Soc Nephrol 2003, 14:1816-1824
[73] Houlihan CA, Akdeniz A, Tsalamandris C, Cooper ME, Jerums G, Gilbert RE: Urinary transforming growth factor-beta excretion in patients with hypertension, type 2 diabetes, and elevated albumin excretion rate: effects of angiotensin receptor blockade and sodium restriction. Diabetes Care 2002, 25:1072-1077
[74] Agarwal R, Siva S, Dunn SR, Sharma K: Add-on angiotensin II receptor blockade lowers urinary transforming growth factor-beta levels. Am J Kidney Dis 2002, 39:486-492
[75] Barnes PJ, Karin M: Nuclear factor-kappaB: A pivotal transcription factor in chronic inflammatory diseases. N Engl J Med 336 : 1066 –1071, 1997
[76] Guijarro C, Egido J: Transcription factor-kappa B (NF-kappa B) and renal disease. Kidney Int 59 : 415 –424, 2001
[77] Nava M, Quiroz Y, Vaziri N, Rodriguez-Iturbe B: Melatonin reduces renal interstitial inflammation and improves hypertension in spontaneously hypertensive rats. Am J Physiol Renal Physiol 284: F447–454, 2003
[78] Rodriguez-Iturbe B, Zhan CD, Quiroz Y, Sindhu RK, Vaziri ND: Antioxidant-rich diet relieves hypertension and reduces renal immune infiltration in spontaneously hypertensive rats. Hypertension 41: 341–346, 2003
[79] Chade AR, Rodriguez-Porcel M, Herrmann J, Krier JD, Zhu X, Lerman A, Lerman LO: Beneficial effects of antioxidant vitamins on the stenotic kidney. Hypertension 42: 605–612, 2003

[80] Chade AR, Rodriguez-Porcel M, Herrmann J, Zhu X, Grande JP, Napoli C, Lerman A, Lerman LO: Antioxidant intervention blunts renal injury in experimental renovascular disease. J Am Soc Nephrol 15: 958–966, 2004
[81] Hahn S, Kuemmerle NB, Chan W, Hisano S, Saborio P, Krieg RJ Jr, Chan JC: Glomerulosclerosis in the remnant kidney rat is modulated by dietary alpha-tocopherol. J Am Soc Nephrol 9: 2089–2095, 1998
[82] Li D, Saldeen T, Romeo F, Mehta JL: Oxidized LDL upregulates angiotensin II type 1 receptor expression in cultured human coronary artery endothelial cells: The potential role of transcription factor NF-kappaB. Circulation 102: 1970–1976, 2000
[83] Vassalli P. The pathophysiology of tumor necrosis factor. Annu Rev Immunol 1992; 10: 411-452
[84] Feldmann M, Brennan FM, Maini R. Cytokines in autoimmune disorders. Int Rev Immunol 1998; 17: 217-228
[85] Tartaglia LA, Ayres TM, Wong GHW, Goeddel DV. A novel domain within the 55 kd TNF receptor signals cell death. Cell 1993; 74: 845-853
[86] Tipping PG, Kitching AR, Cunningham MA, Holdsworth SR. Immunopathogenesis of crescentic glomerulonephritis. Curr Opin Nephrol Hypertens 1999; 8: 281–286
[87] Couser WG. Sensitized cells come of age: a new era in renal immunology with important therapeutic implications. J Am Soc Nephrol 1999; 10: 664–665
[88] Ortiz A, Egidl J. Is there a fole for specific anti-TNF strategies in glomerular diseases. Nephrol Dial Transplant 1995; 10:309-311
[89] Takemura T, Yoshioka K, Murakami K, Akano N, Okada M, Aya N, Maki S. Cellular localization of inflammatory cytokines in human glomerulonephritis. Virchows Arch 1994; 424: 459-464
[90] Ozen S, Saatci U, Tinaztepe K, Bakkaloglu A, Barut A. Urinary tumor necrosis factor levels in primary glomerulopathies. Nephron 1994; 66:291-294
[91] Noronha IL, Kruger C, Andrassy K, Ritz E, Waldherr R. In situ production of TNF-alpha, IL-1 beta and IL-2R in ANCA-positive glomerulonephritis. Kidney Int 1993; 43: 682-692
[92] Bertani T, Abbate M, Zoja C et al. Tumor necrosis factor induces glomerular damage in the rabbit. Am J Pathol 1989; 134: 419-430
[93] Tomosugi NI, Cashman SJ, Hay H et al. Modulation of antibody-mediated glomerular injury in vivo by bacterial lipo-polysaccharide, tumor necrosis factor and IL-1. J Immunol 1989; 142: 3083-3090
[94] Karkar AM, Tam FWK, Steinkasserer A et al. Modulation of antibody-mediated glomerular injury in vivo by IL-1ra, soluble IL-1 receptor and soluble TNF receptor. Kidney Int 1995; 40: 1738-1746
[95] Karkar AM, Koshino Y, Cashman SJ et al. Passive immunization against TNF alpha and IL-1B protects from LPS enhancing glomerular injury in nephrotoxic nephritis in rats. Clin Exp Immunol 1992; 90: 312-318
[96] Fujihara CK, Malheiros DM, Donato JL, Poli A, De Nucci G, and Zatz R. Nitroflurbiprofen, a new nonsteroidal anti-inflammatory, ameliorates structural injury in the remnant kidney. Am J Physiol Renal Physiol 274: F573-F579, 1998.

[97] Fujihara CK, Noronha IL, Malheiros DM, Antunes GR, de Oliveira IB, and Zatz R. Combined mycophenolate mofetil and losartan therapy arrests established injury in the remnant kidney. J Am Soc Nephrol 11: 283-290, 2000.
[98] Hamar P, Peti-Peterdi J, Razga Z, Kovacs G, Heemann U, and Rosivall L. Coinhibition of immune and renin-angiotensin systems reduces the pace of glomerulosclerosis in the rat remnant kidney. J Am Soc Nephrol 10, Suppl 11: S234-S238, 1999
[99] Remuzzi G, Zoja C, Gagliardini E, Corna D, Abbate M, and Benigni A. Combining an antiproteinuric approach with mycophenolate mofetil fully suppresses progressive nephropathy of experimental animals. J Am Soc Nephrol 10: 1542-1549, 1999.

# 12

# The Effects of Asymmetric Dimethylarginine (ADMA), Nitric Oxide (NO) and Homocysteine (Hcy) on Progression of Mild Chronic Kidney Disease (CKD): Relationship Between Clinical and Biochemical Parameters

A. Atamer[1], S. Alisir Ecder[2], Y. Atamer[3], Y. Kocyigit[4], N. Bozkurt Yigit[5] and T. Ecder[6]

*[1]Haydarpasa Training and Research Hospital, Department of Internal Medicine, Division of Gastroenterology, Istanbul*
*[2]Goztepe Training and Research Hospital, Department of Internal Medicine, Division of Nephrology, Istanbul*
*[3]Dicle University Medical Faculty, Department of Clinical Biochemistry, Diyarbakir*
*[4]Dicle University Medical Faculty, Department of Physiology, Diyarbakir*
*[5]Yalova University, Termal Vocational School, Department of Physical Medicine and Rehabilitation, Yalova*
*[6]Istanbul University, Istanbul Medical Faculty, Department of Internal Medicine, Division of Nephrology, Istanbul, Turkey*

## 1. Introduction

Chronic kidney disease (CKD) is a syndrome characterized by the progressive and irrevocable loss of nephrons due to several diseases. Chronic kidney disease has a varying spectrum ranging from normal renal function to uremic syndrome. Actually, the stages of renal failure have interpenetrated each other and it is not possible to draw a clear line between them. The most important reason of mortality and morbidity of patients with CKD are cardiovascular diseases and atherosclerotic complications; cardiac insufficiency 15%, myocardial infarction 10%, pericarditis 3% (1, 2). Development of vascular injury in CKD is caused by both classic (Framingham) risk factors (hypertension, dyslipidemia, smoking, diabetes mellitus) and CKD specific factors (anaemia, secondary hyperparathyroidism etc). Besides, there are papers reporting that recently defined potential risk factors such as homocysteine (Hcy), C-reactive protein (CRP), interleukin-6 (IL-6), fibrinogen, soluble intracellular adhesion molecule (sICAM-1), asymmetric dimethyl arginine (ADMA), cardiac specific troponin-I (cTnI), advanced glycation endproducts have a role in the development of accelerated atherosclerosis seen in patients with CKD (2-13). Asymmetric dimethylarginine (ADMA) is an endogenous competitive inhibitor of nitric oxide (NO) synthase and it is a guanidine analogue of L-arginine aminoacid detectable in human urine and plasma synthesized from endothelial cells (Figure 1). It is shown that high ADMA level increases the cardiovascular incident risk by 34% and mortality risk by 52% (4-8). Increased ADMA concentration has a high prevalence in hyperhomocysteinemia, coronary artery diseases, hypercholesterolemia, diabetes mellitus, hypertension, preeclampsia, peripheral arterial occlusive disease, impaired renal function and other diseases (7,9,10). Reduced nitric oxide (NO)-dependent vasodilation is regarded as an early indicator of atherosclerotic diseases (7,14). It is documented that adult patients with renal failure have 2-6 times higher ADMA than healthy subjects due to reduced renal excretion and reduced enzymatic degradation (15). NO is synthesized from L-arginine via NO synthase enzyme. NO inhibition decreases endothelial derived vasodilation and increases vascular resistance. Reduced NO availability can occur in patients with CKD. Moreover CKD can contribute to the accelaration of hypertension and cardiovascular complications. It appears that the increase in endogenic NO inhibitors like ADMA plays a major role in this process (11, 15-17). It has been shown that Hcy stimulates ADMA formation and plasma ADMA levels elevate in humans and animals by hyperhomocysteinemia (18-20). Increased serum Hcy level in adult CKD patients is an independent risk factor for cardiovascular system mortality. Elevated ADMA and hyperhomocysteinemia may be due to decreased renal excretion (18-22). It is reported that ADMA formation may be related with Hcy metabolism (18,19). It was found that there is a significant interaction of serum fibrinogen and CKD with respect to risk of both fatal/nonfatal coronary events and death (20–24).

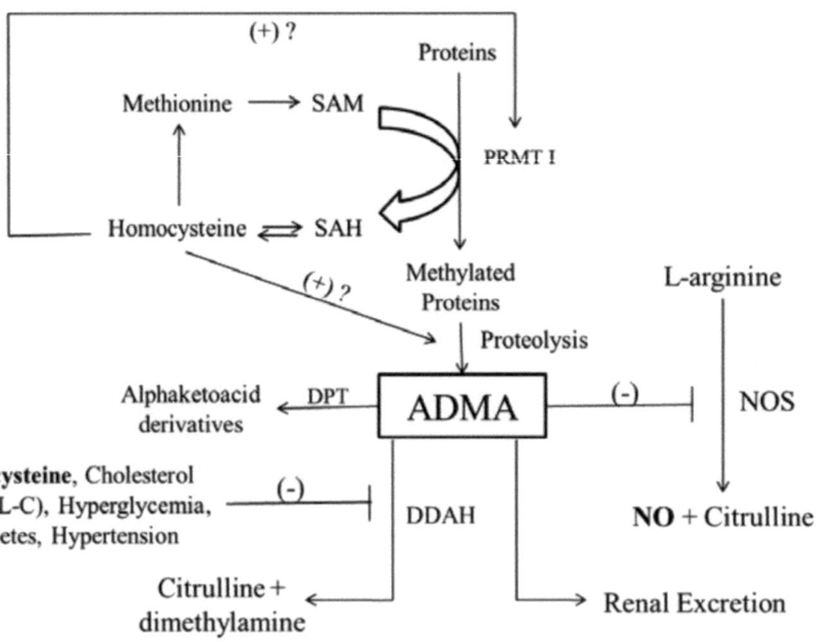


*PRMT I: Protein arginine methyltransferase type I; DDAH: Dimethylaminohydrolase; DPT: Dimethyl arginine piruvate aminotransferase; NOS: Nitric oxide synthase; SAM: S-Adenosylmethionine; SAH: S-Adenosylhomocysteine; Ox LDL-C: Oxidized low density lipoprotein cholesterol*

Fig. 1. Biochemical pathway for generation and degradation of ADMA and homocysteine.

The aim of this study was to investigate the role of uremia-related cardiovascular risk factors, such as ADMA, NO, Hcy and fibrinogen, in the pathogenesis and progression of early stage CKD and to evaluate the relation of these parameters with each other.

## 2. Material and methods

### 2.1 Subjects

This prospective study was carried out in 65 untreated mild chronic kidney disease (35 men and 30 women; mean age 55.2 ± 9.6 years) and 65 healthy control subjects with matched age, sex and body mass index (BMI). The creatinine clearance was calculated by the Cockcroft-Gault Formula (25). Patients having creatinine clearance less than 75 ml/min were considered to have mild CKD. Body mass index was determined as weight divided by the square of height ($kg/m^2$). The underlying causes of CKD were glomerulonephritis (n=17), interstitial nephropathy (n=12), autosomal dominant polycystic kidney disease (n=13), chronic pyelonephritis (n=7) and urological problems (n=5). No cause was identified in 11 cases. The exclusion criteria were diabetes mellitus, active hepatitis, malignancy, smoking and infectious disease. Patients using vitamin supplements were also excluded.

The study protocol was approved by the Ethics Committee of the Dicle University School of Medicine (Diyarbakir, Turkey) and written informed consent was obtained from each participant.

### 2.2 Methods

In all patients, venous blood samples were drawn between 7:00 AM after a 12-h fastened, and the serum was frozen at -70° C in aliquots until biochemical analysis were performed.

*ADMA Measurement:* ADMA was measured by HPLC according to the method described by Chen et al. (26). Mobile phases consisting of 50 mM sodium acetate (pH 6.8), methanol and tetrahydrofuran (THF) (A, 82:17:1; B, 22:77:1) were used. All separations were performed at 27$^0$C and at a flow-rate of 1.0 ml/min. The wavelengths of fluorescence detector were set at 338 nm and 425 nm for excitation and emission, respectively. 20 mg of 5-sulfosalicylic acid (5-SSA) was added to 1 ml plasma, and the mixture was left in an ice bath for 10 min. The precipitated protein was removed by centrifugation at 2000 g for 10 min. o-Phthaldialdehyde (OPA) (10 mg) was dissolved in 0.5 ml of methanol, and 2 ml of 0.4 M borate buffer (0.4 M boric acid adjusted to pH 10.0 with potassium hydroxide) and 30 µl of mercaptoethanol were added. The derivatization was performed by mixing 10 µl of sample or working standard solution and 100 µl of OPA reagent and reacting for 3 min before autoinjecting onto the column.

*NO Measurement:* The serum level of NO was measured using a colorimetric method based on the Griess reaction (27), in which nitrite is reacted with sulphanilamide and N-(1-naphthyl) ethylenediamine to produce an azo dye that can be detected at 540 nm. This was carried out after enzymatic reduction of nitrate to nitrite with nitrate reductase.

*Hcy Measurement:* Serum level of Hcy was measured using HPLC with fluorescence detection (Shimadzu RF-10A fluorescence detector; Shimadzu Co., Kyoto, Japan).

Urea, creatinine, calcium, phosphate, albumin, protein, high sensitive CRP (hsCRP), insulin, glucose, total cholesterol, high-density lipoprotein cholesterol (HDL-C), low-density lipoprotein cholesterol (LDL-C) and triglyceride assays were determined by standard laboratory methods according to the established methodology. The serum level of fibrinogen was measured by the Clauss method using a commercial kit. All routine laboratory measurements were carried out using certified assay methods.

Statistical analysis of the differences between groups of subjects was performed using the Kolmogorov-Smirnov and unpaired student's t-test or by the Mann-Whitney non-parametric test as appropriate. Pearson's correlation analyses were performed.

## 3. Results

Serum levels of ADMA, Hcy, creatinine, LDL-C and hsCRP were significantly ($p<0.001$) higher in patients with mild CKD than in healthy controls. Also, systolic and diastolic blood pressures were increased ($p<0.001$). There were no significant differences in levels of serum fasting blood glucose, insulin, total cholesterol, HDL-C, triglyceride, calcium and phosphate between the mild CKD and healthy controls ($P>0.05$). Serum NO and creatinine clearance levels were decreased in patients with mild CKD than in healthy controls ($p<0.001$). Clinical and laboratory data are reported in Table 1. In multiple linear regression analysis, ADMA level was negatively correlated with NO ($r = -0.861$; $p<0.001$) as shown in Figure 2A, and positively correlated with Hcy ($r = 0.547$; $p<0.001$, Figure 2B) and fibrinogen ($r = 0.704$; $p<0.01$, Figure 2C). ADMA level was positively correlated with creatinine ($r=0.510$;$p<0.001$), LDL-C ($r=0.420$;$p<0.01$), hsCRP ($r=0.525$;$p<0.001$), systolic ($r=0.375$; $p<0.001$) and diastolic blood pressure ($r=0.410$;$p<0.001$) levels. ADMA level was negatively correlated with GFR ($r=-0.720$;$p<0.001$). Also, serum NO level was negatively correlated with homocystein ($r = -0.390$; $p<0.001$, Figure 3). We found no association between ADMA and HDL-C or other parameters in either subjects with mild CKD.

## 4. Discussion

The findings of the present study are as follows: (1) Serum ADMA level is increased in patients with CKD compared with healthy subjects and is associated with decreased NO and GFR. (2) Elevation of circulating serum ADMA is associated with increased Hcy and fibrinogen in CKD patients. (3) Serum NO level as dependent variable was also negatively correlated with Hcy. Our findings suggested that the ADMA levels can reflect a possible independent role in CKD pathogenesis. Increased ADMA serum levels cause persistent renal vasoconstriction and sodium retention, and contributes to the development of high blood pressure (11). In addition, it might influence NO and GFR levels and affect atherosclerosis formation.

Several studies suggested that ADMA level can be an independent risk factor for progression of CKD (3-13). Elevated ADMA reduces bioavailability of NO and induces endothelial dysfunction and may be involved in the pathophysiology of cardiovascular disease in CKD (8). ADMA fulfils many of the characteristic features of an uremic toxin (14,15). Elevation of circulated ADMA, an endogenous inhibitor of nitric oxide synthase, is an independent risk factor for cardiovascular diseases in predialysis patients with CKD (5,14,15). High ADMA levels lead to NO depletion, impaired endothelium-dependent

| | Healthy Subjects (n=65) | Chronic Kidney Disease (n=65) |
|---|---|---|
| Age (years) | 54.9 ± 10.1 | 55.2 ± 9.6 |
| Number of patients (M/F) | 35/30 | 35/30 |
| Body mass index (kg/m2) | 24.90 ± 2.1 | 24.70 ± 2.6 |
| Systolic BP (mmHg) | 110.20 ± 10.4 | *128.40 ± 22.4 |
| Diastolic BP (mmHg) | 72.20 ± 11.6 | *84.40 ± 16.3 |
| Creatinine clearance (ml/min) | 90.20 ± 15.1 | *52.50 ± 15.3 |
| Urea (mg/dl) | 31.50 ± 6.2 | *61.30 ± 14.6 |
| Creatinine (mg/dl) | 1.20 ± 0.42 | *1.61 ± 0.73 |
| Calcium (mg/dl) | 8.73 ± 1.2 | 8.91 ±1.08 |
| Phosphate (mg/dl) | 4.10 ± 1.09 | 4.09 ± 1.2 |
| Albumin (g/dl) | 3.82 ± 0.9 | 3.94 ± 0.5 |
| Protein (g/dl) | 6.40 ± 1.1 | 6.01 ± 0.3 |
| Glucose (mg/dl) | 87.90 ± 16.2 | 90.10 ± 15.4 |
| Insulin (µu/ml) | 11.60 ± 2.9 | 12.04 ± 2.83 |
| Triglyceride(mg/dl) | 118.30 ± 20.2 | 120.10 ± 18.5 |
| Total cholesterol (mg/dl) | 184.20 ± 22.1 | 185.60 ± 19.4 |
| HDL-C (mg/dl) | 45.80 ± 12.4 | 42.02 ±14.3 |
| LDL-C (mg/dl) | 113.20 ± 12.8 | *142.12 ± 18.6 |
| hsCRP (mg/dl) | 1.914 ± 0.667 | *7.048 ±2.249 |
| Fibrinogen (g/L) | 2.835 ± 0.646 | *4.574±0.521 |
| ADMA (µmol/L) | 0.512 ± 0.116 | *0.837±0.189 |
| Nitric oxide (µmol/L) | 75.67 ± 8.626 | *44.31±7.811 |
| Homocystein (µmol/L) | 6.256 ± 1.629 | *18.37 ± 3.192 |

*P < 0.001; Data are reported as means ± SD.
BP: Blood Pressure; HDL-C: High Density Lipoprotein Cholesterol; LDL-C: Low Density Lipoprotein Cholesterol; hsCRP: High sensitive C Reactive Protein; ADMA: Asymmetric dimethylarginine

Table 1. Clinical and laboratory data of patients with CKD and healthy subjects.

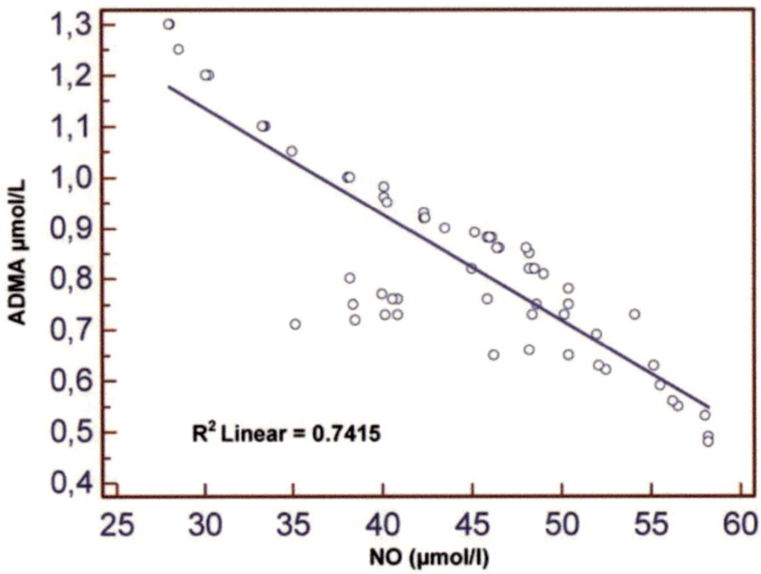
1,3
1,2
1,1
1,0
0,9
0,8
0,7
0,6
0,5
0,4
ADMA µmol/L
$R^2$ Linear = 0.7415
25
30
35
40
45
50
55
60
NO (µmol/l)

(a)

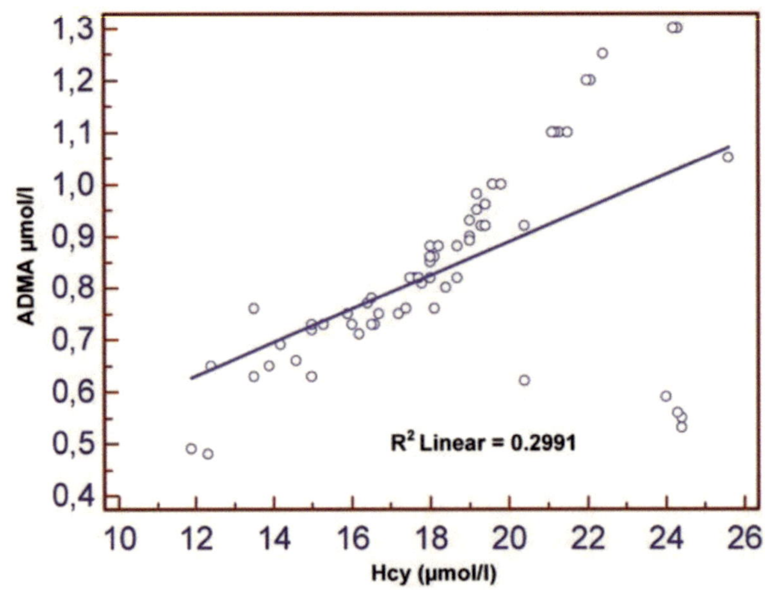
1,3
1,2
1,1
1,0
0,9
0,8
0,7
0,6
0,5
0,4
ADMA µmol/l
$R^2$ Linear = 0.2991
10
12
14
16
18
20
22
24
26
Hcy (µmol/l)

(b)

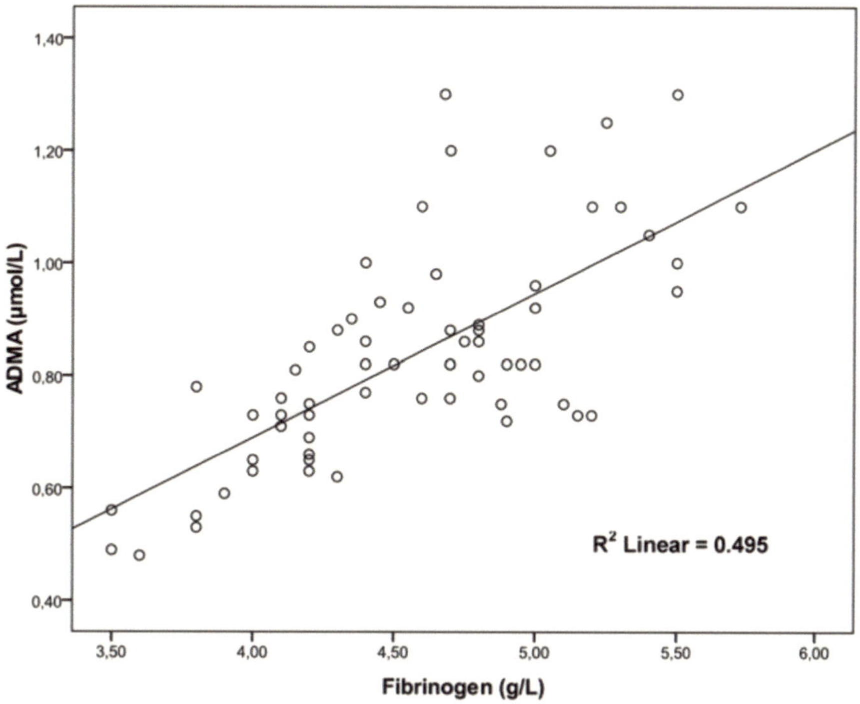


(c)

Fig. 2. Correlation between asymmetric dimethylarginine (ADMA) and **(A)** nitric oxide (NO), **(B)** homocysteine (Hcy), and **(C)** fibrinogen.

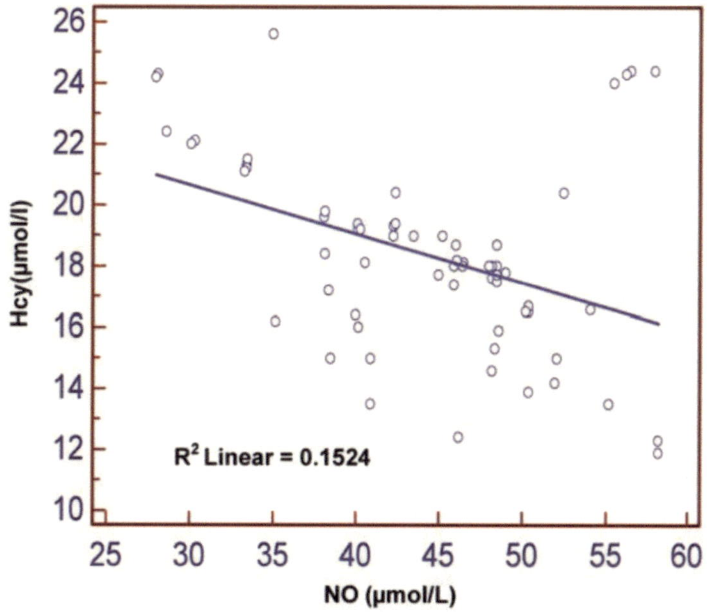


Fig. 3. Correlation between nitric oxide (NO) and homocysteine (Hcy).

vasodilation and plaque rupture with thrombus formation (8). In addition, increased ADMA level in circulation is a combined result of decreased elimination and reduced activity of ADMA catabolism by dimethylarginine dimethylaminohydrolase (DDAH) (8,9). Elevated plasma levels of ADMA in patients with end stage renal disease (ESRD) were first reported by Vallance et al. (15). Several recent studies have already indicated that elevated plasma ADMA levels could cause cardiovascular morbidity and mortality in progressive chronic kidney disease (4-13). Mihout et al. (9) demonstrated that high plasma ADMA levels contribute to the development of hypertension, oxidative stress, and interstitial and glomerular fibrosis, and peritubular capillary rarefaction. This may be involved in the decline of renal function. Serum levels of ADMA in CKD are predictive of renal survival and of cardiovascular damage. High ADMA levels are associated with endothelial dysfunction and oxidative stres (12). In the study by Young et al. (8) , there was a strong association of ADMA with prevalent cardiovascular disease and a modest association with all-cause and cardiovascular disease mortality. ADMA is strongly associated with intima-media thickness of the carotid artery and left ventricular mass, particularly concentric left ventricular hypertrophy (11).

Coen et al. (12) suggested that ADMA levels could be influenced by the severity of hyperparathyroidsm and contribute to cardivascular death linked to parathyroid hormone (PTH) of hemodialysis patients. Another study conducted by Shi et al (5) has shown that the circulating level of ADMA is an important risk factor of LVH and predicts CVD in pre-dialysis CKD patients.

Selcoki et al. (10) reported that ADMA level was to be one of the strongest risk markers for atherosclerosis in patients with mild and moderate CKD. Ninety percent of ADMA has been metabolized by DDAH, while the other small portion, 10 %, is excreted by urinary system. Potential mechanisms of elevated plasma ADMA levels in renal failure are increased protein methylation, increased proteolysis, impaired renal excretion and impaired metabolism by DDAH (18). These results are consistent with data from our study. Our results suggest that high ADMA level can be a significant risk factor for progression of renal dysfunction in the earlier stages of CKD.

Several recent studies found markedly elevated plasma ADMA levels not only in patients with ESRD, but also in patients with progressive CKD (2). It is of note that our results are in line with a recent study by Nakamura et al. (28), who found that elevation of serum ADMA levels play a role in the progression of atherosclerosis and CKD in high-risk patients.

Studies in both the general population and the dialysis population showed a strong and independent link between ADMA, all-cause mortality, and cardiovascular events (11,12,21,24). As a consequence, elevated serum levels of ADMA may be of relevance not only in vascular pathology but also in the pathophysiology of hypertension, and in paralel, in the development of renal damage (13).

When ADMA accumulates in CKD due to defective inactivation and excretion, it is a factor of impaired NO synthesis. The decrease in the generation of NO lead to endothelial malfunction and damage (12). Nitric oxide is an important molecule which has many physiological functions, such as mediating vasodilation, inhibiting atherosclerosis, and modulating the growth of the myocardium (5). Nitric oxide is produced from its precursor L-arginine via a reaction catalyzed by endothelial NO synthase (NOS) (8,9). Endothelium-derived nitric oxide is a potent endothelial vasodilator which balances constrictors to regulate blood pressure and vascular tone (9). Leone et al. (35) suggested that NO may play a role in blood pressure regulation. NO is a cardiovascular protective substance because it causes vasodilation and leucocyte aggregation (10). Nitric oxide also plays a role in regulating renal sodium excretion and renin release (30). Nitric oxide, synthesised from L-arginine, contributes to the regulation of blood pressure and to host defence (29). As an endogenous vasodilator it contributes to renal arteriolar tone and modulates relaxation of the mesangium, thus contributing to regulation of glomerular microcirculation. It has antiplatelet and antithrombogenic effects and thus helps prevent thrombosis within the glomerular capillaries (30).

Clinical and experimental evidence suggest that the elevation of ADMA may cause a low production of NO (11,14-17,29,30). Synthesis of NO can be blocked by inhibition of nitric oxide synthase (NOS) activities with guanidino-substituted analogues of L-arginine such as ADMA (28). Accumulation of endogenous ADMA, leading to impaired NO synthesis, might contribute to the hypertension and immune dysfunction associated with chronic renal failure (29). Reduced bioavailability of NO, increased systemic blood pressure, endothelial cell injury and dysfunction are thought to play an important role in progressive kidney damage (7). Endothelial dysfunction due to reduced availability of NO is an early step in the course of atherosclerotic vascular disease (7). Increased ADMA blood levels may contribute to this process. In addition, NO inhibits key processes of atherosclerosis, such as monocyte endothelial adhesion, platelet aggregation, and vascular smooth muscle cell poliferation (31).

In our study, while serum ADMA and Hcy levels were significantly higher in the patients with CKD than in healthy subject, the NO level was significantly lower. Our findings were in agreement with previous studies (7,9,10,18). Low NO is a major feature of chronic kidney diseases. We examined the relationship of ADMA with NO and with Hcy in CKD patients. In this prospective study, high ADMA level was associated with both decreased NO and increased Hcy. Similarly, Strong relationships between increased serum Hcy, fibrinogen, ADMA and decreased NO, GFR and mortality from cardiovascular events have recently been demonstrated. Several prospective clinical studies have shown that ADMA, fibrinogen, Hcy, LDL-C and other cardiovascular risk parameters are effected in patients with CKD, atherosclerosis, hypertension, diabetes and other clinical entities (14-18,22).

The major factor for high plasma ADMA levels in renal failure seems to be a decrease DDAH activity, which in turn may be due to increased oxidative stress and/or hyperhomocysteinemia (18). Recent studies show contradictory data regarding the role of hyperhomocysteinemia on cardiovascular morbidity and mortality in CKD patients (32). Rasmussen et al. (22) suggested that elevated homocysteine level is an independent predictor of cardiovascular events in patients with ESRD. Ninomiya et al. (33) suggested that baseline Hcy level showed a significantly inverse association with rate of change in kidney function during the 5 years after being adjusted for confounding factors, including baseline kidney function.

One study indicates a linkage between hyperhomocysteinemia, oxidative stress and ADMA metabolism (32). Recently, it was hypothesized that some of the deleterious effects of hyperhomocysteinemia may involve ADMA-related cardiovascular effect in CKD (18-20). Hyperhomocysteinemia, elevated plasma ADMA concentrations have first been described in patients with renal failure (18). Plasma levels of homocysteine and ADMA are elevated in patients with renal failure and both have been associated with cardiovascular events, possibly due to their negative effects on endothelial function. ADMA in methylation of homocystein plays an important role. Elevated homocysteine level is strongly related to renal function and probably due to decreased metabolic clearance (18-20). Homocysteine and ADMA are aminoacids which are biochemically linked by a common synthetic pathway. Homocysteine inhibits DDAH, the enzyme responsible for the breakdown of ADMA. Homocysteine may enhance protein degradation by destabilizing protein structure or by increasing oxidative stress, resulting in ADMA release (18).

Contraversely, Simic-Ogrizovic et al. (24) suggested that although total serum Hcy level was not found to be a predictor of overall and cardiovascular mortality, the role of hyperhomocysteinemia as risk factor for cardiovascular disease cannot be excluded in hemodialysis patients.

We found a strong association between ADMA levels and hyperfibrinogenemia, and hyperhomocysteinemia in our study. In addition, as inflammation index, CRP and fibrinogen were increased. Our results show that increased ADMA, Hcy, hsCRP and fibrinogen levels contribute to the progression of renal disease. Serum levels of ADMA and Hcy may interact and modulate the effect of each other, thus contributing to a common mechanism leading to cardiovascular diseases in CKD. These findings are similar to observations from previous studies (18-21).

The level of serum fibrinogen (an inflammation marker) is increased in CKD. Increased serum fibrinogen level independently predicts cardiac events (20). Shishehbor et al. (19) suggested that Hcy and fibrinogen levels can explain nearly 40% of the attributable mortality risk from CKD. Bostom et al. (21) suggested that Hcy, lipoprotein(a) (Lp(a)), and fibrinogen interact to promote atherothrombosis, combined hyperhomocysteinemia, hyperfibrinogenemia, and, Lp(a) excess may contribute to the high incidence of vascular disease sequelae experienced by dialysis patients, which is inadequately explained by traditional cardiovascular disease risk factors. In our present study, the serum level of LDL-C was significantly higher in the patients with CKD than in the healthy subjects. In addition, the ADMA level was positively correlated with LDL-C. The association of increased LDL-C with increased risk of coronary heart disease may be thought as a covariable in the oxidative activation of ADMA synthesis.

Descamps-Latscha et al. (23) thought that CRP, fibrinogen and advanced oxidation protein products (AOPP) levels independently predict atherosclerotic cardiovascular events in patients with CKD in the predialysis phase and might directly contribute to the uremia-associated accelerated atherogenesis. These findings lend support to the hypothesis that accumulation of ADMA is an important risk factor for cardiovascular events in CKD (2).

Our findings suggest that high ADMA, fibrinogen and Hcy levels and NO deficiency may contribute to the process of atherosclerotic cardiovascular disease and other consequeces of uremia in predialysis patients with CKD. In addition, the ADMA level was associated with hyperhomocysteineamia and hyperfibrinogenemia.

## 5. References


[1] Zawada ET. Indications for dialysis. Handbook of Dialysis. Daugirdas JT, Ing TS (eds).Little, Brown and Company, Boston 1994: 604-622.

[2] Zoccali C, Mallamaci F, Tripepi G. Traditional and emerging risk factors in end-stage renal disease. Kidney Int 2003;63(suppl85):S105-S110.

[3] Busch M, Franke S, Miller A, et al. Potential risk factors in chronic kidney disease: EGEs, total homocysteine and metabolites, and the C-reactive protein. Kidney Int 2004;66:338-347.

[4] Fujimi-Hayashida A, Ueda S, Yamagishi S, et al. Association of asymmetric dimethylarginine with severity of kidney injury and decline in kidney function in IgA Nephropathy. Am J Nephrol 2011; 33: 1-6.

[5] Shi B, Ni Z, Zhou W, et al. Circulating levels of asymmetric dimethylarginine are an independent risk factor for left ventricular hypertrophy and predict cardiovascular events in pre-dialysis patients with chronic kidney disease. Eur J Intern Med 2010;21(5):444-8.

[6] Abedini S, Meinitzer A, Holme I, et al. Asymmetrical dimethylarginine is associated with renal and cardiovascular outcomes and all-cause mortality in renal transplant recipients. Kidney Int 2010;77(1): 44-50.

[7] Fliser D, Kielstein JT, Haller H, and Bode-Böger SM. Asymmetric dimethylarginine: A cardiovascular risk factor in renal disease? Kidney Int (Supp) 2003;(84):37–40.

[8] Young JM, Terin N, Wang X, et al. Asymmetric dimethylarginine and mortality in stages 3 to 4 chronic kidney disease. Clin J Am Soc Nephrol 2009;4(6):1115–1120.

[9] Mihout F, Shweke N, Big´e N, et al. Asymmetric dimethylarginine (ADMA) induces chronic kidney disease through a mechanism involving collagen and TGF-β1 synthesis. J Pathol 2011; 223(1) : 37–45.

[10] Selcoki Y, Aydın M, İkizek M, Armutcu F, Eryonucu B, Kanbay M. Association between asymmetric dimethylarginine and the severity of coronary artery disease in patients with chronic kidney disease. Turk Neph Dial Transpl 2011;20(1):58-64.

[11] Kielstein JT, Simmel S, Bode-Böger SM, et al. Subpressor dose asymmetric dimethylarginine modulates renal function in humans through nitric oxide synthase inhibition. Kidney Blood Pres Res 2004;27(3):143-147.

[12] Coen G, Mantella D, Sardella D, et al. Asymmetric dimethylarginine, vascular calcifications and parathyroid hormone serum levels in hemodialysis patients. J Nephrol 2009;22(5):616-622.

[13] Kielstein JT, Böger RH, Bode-Böger SM, et al. Low dialysance of asymmetric dimethylarginine (ADMA)- in vivo and in vitro evidence of significant protein binding. Clin Nephrol 2004;62(4):295-300.

[14] Vallance P, Leiper J. Blocking NO synthesis: How, where and why? Nature Reviews Drug Discovery 2002;1(12):939-950

[15] Vallance P, Leone A, Calver A, Collier J, Moncada S. Accumulation of an endogenous inhibitor of nitric oxide synthesis in chronic renal failure. Lancet 1992;339(8793):572-575.

[16] Schmidt RJ, Baylis C. Total nitric oxide production is low in patients with chronic renal disease. Kidney Int 2000;58:1261-1266.

[17] Baylis C. Nitric oxide deficiency in chronic kidney disease. Am J Physiol Renal physiol 2008;294(1):F1-F9.

[18] van Guldener C, Nanayakkara PW, Stehouwer CD. Homocysteine and asymmetric dimethylarginine (ADMA): biochemically linked but differently related to vascular disease in chronic kidney disease.Clin Chem Lab Med. 2007;45(12):1683-7.

[19] Shishehbor MH, Oliveira LP, Lauer MS, et al. Emerging cardiovascular risk factors that account for a significant portion of attributable mortality risk in chronic kidney disease. Am J Cardiol. 2008 Jun 15;101(12):1741-6. Epub 2008 Apr 9.

[20] Weiner DE, Tighiouart H, Elsayed EF, et al. The relationship between nontraditional risk factors and outcomes in individuals with stage 3 to 4 CKD.Am J Kidney Dis. 2008 Feb;51(2):212-23.

[21] Bostom AG, Shemin D, Lapane KL, et al. Hyperhomocysteinemia, hyperfibrinogenemia, and lipoprotein (a) excess in maintenance dialysis patients: a matched case-control study. Atherosclerosis. 1996 Aug 23;125(1):91-101

[22] Rasmussen LE, Svensson M, Jørgensen KA, et al. The content of docosahexaenoic acid in serum phospholipid is inversely correlated with plasma homocysteine levels in patients with end-stage renal disease. Nutr Res. 2010 Aug;30(8):535-40.

[23] Descamps-Latscha B, Witko-Sarsat V, Nguyen-Khoa T,et al. Advanced oxidation protein products as risk factors for atherosclerotic cardiovascular events in nondiabetic predialysis patients. Am J Kidney Dis. 2005 Jan;45(1):39-47

[24] Simic-Ogrizovic S, Stosovic M, Novakovic I, et al. Fuzzy role of hyperhomocysteinemia in hemodialysis patients' mortality. Biomed Pharmacother. 2006 May;60(4):200-7.

[25] Cockcroft DW and Gault MH: Prediction of creatinine clearance from serum creatinine. Nephron 1976, 16: 31-41.

[26] Chen BM, Xia LW, Zhao RQ. Determination of NG, NG-dimethylarginine in human plasma by high performance liquid chromatography. J Chromatogr B Biomed Sci Appl 1997;692:467-471.

[27] Bories PN, Bories C. Nitrate determination in biological fluids by an enzymatic one-step assay with nitrate reductase. Clin Chem 1995;41:904-907.

[28] Nakamura T, Sato E, Fujiwara N. Ezetimibe decreases serum levels of asymmetric dimethylarginine (ADMA) and ameliorates renal injury in non-diabetic cronic kidney disease patients in a cholesterol-independent manner. Pharm Res 2009;60(6):525-528.

[29] Leone A, Moncada S, Vallance P, Calver A and Collier J. Accumulation of an endogenous inhibitor of nitric oxide synthesis in chronic renal failure. 1992; 339(8793): 572-575.

[30] Raij L, Jaimes E, del Castillo D, Guerra J and Westberg G. Pathophysiology of the vascular wall: the role of nitric oxide in renal disease. Prostaglandins, Leukotrienes and Essential Fatty Acids 1996;54(1):53-58.

[31] Fliser D, Kronenberg F, Kielstein JT. Asymmetric dimethylarginine and progression of chronic kidney disease: The Mild to Moderate Kidney Disease Study. J Am Soc Nephrol 2005;16:1-6.

[32] Schmitt B, Wolters M, Kressel G, et al. Effects of combined supplementation with B vitamins and antioxidants on plasma levels of asymmetric dimethylarginine (ADMA) in subjects with elevated risk for cardiovascular disease.Atherosclerosis. 2007 Jul;193(1):168-76.

[33] Ninomiya T, Kiyohara Y, Kubo M. Hyperhomocysteinemia and the development of chronic kidney disease in a general population: The Hisayama study. Am J Kid Dis 2004;44(3):437-445.

# 13

# Neutrophil Activation and Erythrocyte Membrane Protein Composition in Stage 5 Chronic Kidney Disease Patients

Elísio Costa[1,2], Luís Belo[2,3] and Alice Santos-Silva[2,3]
[1]*Instituto de Ciências da Saúde da Universidade Católica Portuguesa*
[2]*Instituto de Biologia Molecular e Celular da Universidade do Porto*
[3]*Faculdade de Farmácia da Universidade do Porto*
*Portugal*

## 1. Introduction

Anaemia is a frequent complication associated with stage 5 chronic kidney disease (CKD), and is mainly due to insufficient production of erythropoietin by the kidneys. Accumulation of uremic toxins, excessive toxic storage of aluminium in the bone marrow (Miyoshi, 2006), blood loss (either iatrogenic, from the puncture sites of the vascular access and blood sampling, or from other sources, such as the gastrointestinal tract), and premature erythrocyte destruction have also been frequently associated with anaemia in stage 5 CKD patients (Medina, 1994; Pisoni, 2004).

The erythrocyte, presenting a limited biosynthesis capacity, suffers and accumulates physical and/or chemical changes, which become more pronounced with cell aging, and whenever an unusual physical or chemical stress develops (Locatelli, 2004a). Erythrocytes are physically stressed during the haemodialysis process, and metabolically stressed by the unfavourable plasmatic environment, due to metabolite accumulation, and by the high rate of haemoglobin autoxidation, due to the increase in haemoglobin turnover, a physiologic compensation mechanism triggered in case of anaemia (Lucchi, 2000; Stoya, 2002). The erythrocytes are, therefore, continuously challenged to sustain haemoglobin in its reduced functional form, as well as to maintain the integrity and deformability of the membrane.

Leukocytosis is essential as the primary host defence, and neutrophils, the major leukocyte population of blood in adults, play a primordial role. It is well known that neutrophils have mechanisms that are used to destroy invading microorganisms. These cells use oxygen-dependent and oxygen-independent microbicidal artillery to destroy and remove infectious agents (Witko-Sarsat, 2000). Activated neutrophils also undergo degranulation, with the release of several components, namely, proteases and cationic proteins (Witko-Sarsat, 2000).

In this book chapter we review the cross-talk between changes in erythrocyte membrane protein composition and the release of neutrophil activation products.

## 2. Erythrocyte membrane protein composition

Erythrocyte membrane proteins can be classified into three categories, according to their functional properties in the membrane struture (An & Mohandas, 2008; Mohandas & Gallagher, 2008). The first includes cytoskeletal proteins, as spectrin (α and β chains), protein 4.1, and actin; the second includes integral/transmembrane proteins of which the representative proteins are band 3 and glycophorins; the third includes anchoring/linker proteins, namely, ankyrin (also known as band 2.1) and protein 4.2. The anchoring/linker membrane proteins mediate the attachment of cytoskeletal proteins to integral proteins (Fig. 1) (Lucchi, 2000; Gallagher, 2005; Mohandas & Gallagher, 2008).

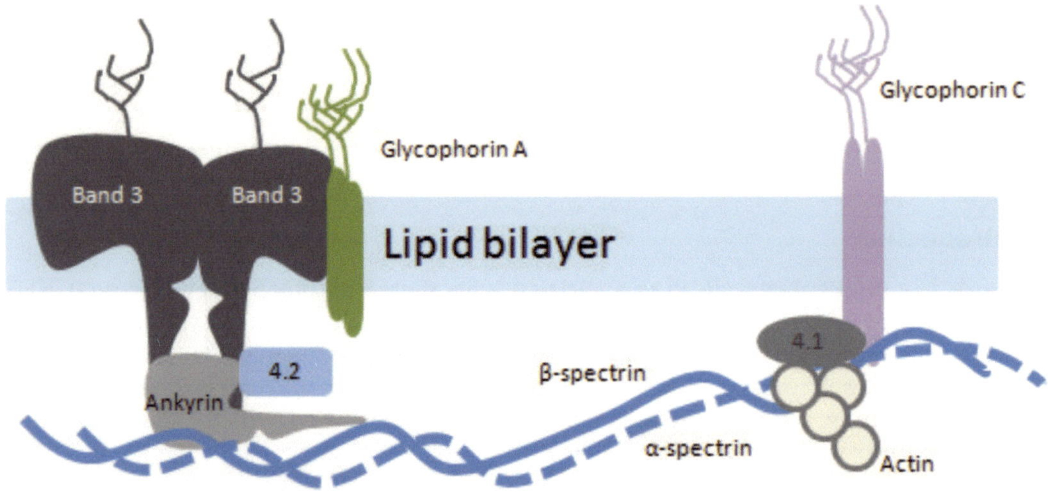


Fig. 1. Schematic representation of red blood cell membrane, showing the topographical localization of proteins and their interactions. The membrane is a complex structure in which a plasma membrane envelope composed of amphiphilic lipid molecules is anchored to a two dimensional elastic network of skeletal proteins through tethering sites (transmembrane proteins) embedded in the lipid bilayer. Adapted from An & Mohandas, 2008.

The cytoskeleton is a 3-dimensional network of proteins that covers the cytoplasmatic surface of the erythrocyte membrane and is responsible for its biconcave shape and the properties of elasticity and flexibility. It comprises approximately half the membrane protein mass and is primarily composed of spectrin, protein 4.2 and actin. Spectrin is the major protein of the cytoskeleton, and, therefore, the primary cause of erythrocyte shape, integrity and deformability. It is linked to the lipid bilayer, by vertical protein interactions with the transmembrane proteins, band 3 and glicophorin A (Lucchi, 2000). In the vertical protein interaction of spectrin with band 3 there are also ankyrin (also known as band 2.1) and protein 4.2 involved. A normal linkage of spectrin with the other proteins of the cytoskeleton assures normal horizontal protein interactions. The vertical and horizontal interactions between membrane constituents account for the integrity, strength, and deformability of the cell (An & Mohandas, 2008; Mohandas & Gallagher, 2008). Disruption of vertical interactions because of membrane protein deficiencies favours membrane vesiculation with loss of surface area and development of spherocytic cells, with increasing rigidity of the cell membrane that may lead to premature spleen sequestration and destruction (An & Mohandas, 2008).

## 3. Neutrophil activation

Leukocytosis and recruitment of circulating leukocytes into the affected areas are hallmarks of inflammation. Leukocytes are chimio-attracted to inflammatory regions and their transmigration from blood to the injured tissue is primarily mediated by the expression of cell-adhesion molecules in the endothelium, which interact with surface receptors on leukocytes (Muller, 1999; Sullivan, 2000). This leukocyte-endothelial interaction is regulated by a cascade of molecular steps that lead to the morphological changes that accompany adhesion. At the inflammatory site, leukocytes release their granular content and may exert their phagocytic capacities.

In acute inflammation, the leukocyte infiltration is predominantly of neutrophils, whereas in chronic inflammation an infiltration predominantly of macrophages and lymphocytes is observed. Leukocyte-endothelial cell interactions are important for leukocyte transmigration and trafficking in physiological conditions. There is increasing evidences that changes in those leukocyte-endothelial interactions, due to endothelium damage or dysfunction, might be implicated in the pathogenesis of diseases, such as inflammatory diseases (Harlan, 1985; Ley, 2007).

Leukocytosis is essential as the primary host defence, and neutrophils, the major leukocyte population of blood in adults, play a primordial role. It is well known that neutrophils have mechanisms that are used to destroy invading microorganisms. These cells use an extraordinary array of oxygen-dependent and oxygen-independent microbicidal weapons to destroy and remove infectious agents (Witko-Sarsat, 2000). Oxygen-dependent mechanisms involve the production of reactive oxygen species (ROS), which can be microbicidal (Roos, 2003), and lead to the development of oxidative stress. Oxygen-independent mechanisms include chemotaxis, phagocytosis and degranulation. The generation of microbicidal oxidants by neutrophils results from the activation of a multiprotein enzyme complex, known as the reduced nicotinamide adenine dinucleotide phosphate (NADPH) oxidase, which catalyzes the formation of superoxide anion ($O_2^{\cdot-}$). Activated neutrophils also undergo degranulation, with the release of several components, namely, proteases (such as elastase) and cationic proteins (such as lactoferrin) (Saito, 1993; Brinkmann, 2004).

Elastase is a member of the chymotrypsin superfamily of serine proteinases, expressed in monocytes and mast cells, but mainly expressed by neutrophils, where it is compartmentalized in the primary azurophil granules. The intracellular function of this enzyme is the degradation of foreign microorganisms that are phagocytosed by the neutrophil (Brinkmann, 2004). Elastase can also degrade local extracellular matrix proteins (such as elastin), remodel damaged tissue, and facilitate neutrophil migration into or through tissues. Moreover, elastase also modulates cytokine expression at epithelial and endothelial surfaces, up-regulating the production of cytokines, such as IL-6, IL-8, transforming growth factor β (TGF-β) and granulocyte-macrophage colony-stimulating factor (GM-CSF); it also promotes the degradation of cytokines, such as IL-1, TNF-α and IL-2. There is evidence in literature that high levels of elastase are one of the major pathological factors in the development of several chronic inflammatory lung conditions (Fitch, 2006).

Plasma lactoferrin is predominantly neutrophil derived and its presence in the specific granules is often used to identify these types of granules. Lactoferrin is also found in other granules, in the tertiary granules, though in lower concentrations (Olofsson, 1977; Baynes 1986; Halliwell & Gutteridge, 1990; Saito, 1993). Lactoferrin is a multifunctional iron glycoprotein, which is known to exert a broad-spectrum primary defence activity against bacteria, fungi, protozoa and viruses. It can bind to large amounts of free iron. The iron-bound lactoferrin is taken up by activated macrophages, which express specific lactoferrin receptors. During inflammation, this contributes to iron deprivation of the erythroid precursors, which do not express lactoferrin receptors (Bárány, 2001). Other mechanisms in which lactoferrin is implicated include a growth regulatory function in normal cells, coagulation, and perhaps cellular adhesion modulation (Levay and Viljoen, 1995).

In a recent study of our group (Pereira, 2010), we found that stage 5 CKD patients present a decreased expression of the CXCR1 neutrophil surface marker, which plays an important role in neutrophil migration (Fig. 2); a higher elastase plasma levels was also found, as compared to a control group (table 1).

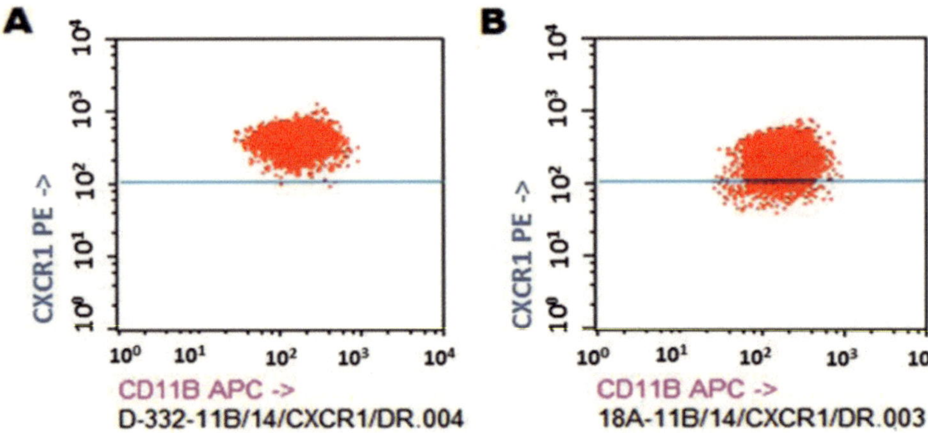


Fig. 2. Decreased expression of the CXCR1 neutrophil surface markers in stage 5 CKD patients. A - Control; B - Stage 5 CKD patient. Cells were stained with allophycocyanin (APC) conjugated anti-CD11B and phycoerythrin (PE) conjugated anti-CXCR1.

CXCR1 is a receptor that recognizes CXC chemokines, particularly, the pro-inflammatory IL-8 (Pay, 2006; Sherry, 2008). The decreased expression of this receptor in neutrophil surface is associated to the release of components of neutrophil granules and is correlated with the need for inotropic support. Recently, it was reported that the levels of the neutrophil chemoattractant receptor, CXCR1, is mildly diminished in CKD pediatric patients, as a consequence of the end stage renal disease itself, and that the recurrent serial bacterial infections they suffered was markedly exacerbated by CXCR1 neutrophil loss (Sherry, 2008). This loss of CXCR1 on neutrophils might be due to the uremic state, to changes in leukocyte adhesion molecule expression or membrane microvilli and/or to cross-desensitization of this receptor, due to prior exposure to several unrelated chemoattractants, including N-formylated peptides and the complement cleavage product C5a (Sherry, 2008). Chronic exposure of circulating inflammatory cells to these mediators may lead to loss of chemokine receptor expression and/or function via cross-desensitization.

| | Controls (n=26) | All patients (n=63) |
|---|---|---|
| Hb (g/dL) | 13.90 (13.2-15.00) | 10.90 (10.30-12.30)* |
| White cell counts (x $10^9$/L) | 5.78 ± 1.59 | 6.23 ± 2.10 |
| Lymphocytes (x $10^9$/L) | 2.35 ± 0.75 | 1.47 ± 0.60* |
| Monocytes (x $10^9$/L) | 0.25 ± 0.08 | 0.38 ± 0.16* |
| Neutrophils (x $10^9$/L) | 3.03 ± 1.02 | 4.14 ± 1.79* |
| Albumin (g/dL) | NM | 3.8 ± 0.4 |
| CRP (mg/dL) | 1.75 (0.76-4.70) | 5.75 (1.90-14.01)* |
| Elastase (µg/L) | 28.29 (26.03-34.74) | 36.11 (29.69-50.65)* |
| Elastase/Neutrophil ratio | 10.86 (7.44-12.12) | 8.91 (7.43-13.78) |
| Lactoferrin (µg/L) | 236.56 (193.56-295.03) | 239.35 (165.64-332.60) |
| Lactoferrin/Neutrophil ratio | 72.11 (55.52-111.83) | 60.32 (42.82-99.45) |

Table 1. Haematological data and neutrophil activation markers, for controls and for stage 5 CKD patients.* $p<0.05$, *vs* controls. NM: not measured. Results are presented as mean ± standard deviation or as median (interquartile ranges). Hb: Haemoglobin; CRP: C-reactive protein. Adapted from Costa, 2008a.

The haemodialysis procedure, itself, seems to lead to neutrophil activation (Costa, 2008a). By evaluating CKD patients before and after haemodialysis procedure (Costa, 2008b), we found a higher haemoglobin concentration and erythrocyte count after haemodialysis (Table 2). This increase in circulating erythrocytes, has been associated (Dasselaar, 2007) to a

| | Stage 5 CKD Patients (n=20) | |
|---|---|---|
| | Before | After |
| Hb (g/dL) | 12.10 (10.95-12.80) | 13.20 (11.15-14.60)* |
| White cell counts (x $10^9$/L) | 5.86 ± 1.5 1 | 5.93 ± 2.19 |
| Neutrophils (x $10^9$/L) | 3.82 ± 1.24 | 3.97 ± 1.77 |
| Monocytes (x $10^9$/L) | 0.24 ± 0.38 | 0.17 ± 0.12 |
| Lymphocytes (x $10^9$/L) | 1.64 ± 0.69 | 1.66 ± 0.64 |
| Elastase (µg/L) | 36.16 (29.71-47.13) | 51.69 (40.08-71.68)* |
| Elastase/Neutrophil ratio | 10.66 (7.32-13.54) | 14.66 (13.34-18.95)* |
| Lactoferrin (µg/L) | 198.61 (137.81-216.97) | 236.56 (171.28-363.63)* |
| Lactoferrin/Neutrophil ratio | 48.33 (33.88-64.31) | 60.72 (51.81-94.81)* |
| CRP (mg/dL) | 3.06 (1.39-5.22) | 3.53 (1.54-5.56) |

Table 2. Hematological data and neutrophil activation markers for stage 5 CKD patients, before and after haemodialysis procedure. *$p<0.05$, *vs* before haemodialysis. Results are presented as mean ± standard deviation or as median (interquartile ranges). Hb: haemoglobin; CRP: C-reactive protein. Adapted from Costa, 2008b.

translocation of erythrocytes from the splanchnic circulation (and possibly from the splenic circulation) in order to compensate the hypovolemic stress during dialysis ultrafiltration. We also found, after haemodialysis, an increase in mean cell hemoglobin concentration and a decrease in mean cell volume that could be related to erythrocyte membrane protein loss during the hemodialysis procedure (Costa, 2008b). Markers of neutrophil activation were also found to be increased after haemodialysis. In fact, a decrease in CXCR1 neutrophil expression was observed after the haemodialysis procedure [before haemodialysis: 252.25 ± 45.14 MFI (mean fluorescence intensity) vs after haemodialysis: 239.71 ± 47.62 MFI; $p$=0.04], as well as an increase in elastase and lactoferrin plasma levels (Table 2). The enhanced neutrophil activation state after haemodialysis could result from different mechanisms; namely, complement activation, direct interaction with haemodialysis membrane, and from the passage into the blood of bacterial fragments, such as LPS, from contaminated dialysate through the dialyzer membrane.

## 4. Erythrocyte senescence and/or damage

In stage 5 CKD patients, the erythrocytes are metabolically stressed by the unfavourable plasmatic environment, due to metabolite accumulation; by the high rate of haemoglobin autoxidation, due to the increase in haemoglobin turnover, a physiologic compensation mechanism triggered to compensate anaemia (Lucchi, 2000; Stoya, 2002). The erythrocytes will be further stressed during the haemodialysis procedure. Therefore, the erythrocytes are continuously challenged to sustain haemoglobin in its reduced functional form and to maintain the integrity and deformability of the membrane.

When haemoglobin is denatured, it links to the cytoplasmic pole of band 3, triggering its aggregation and leading to the formation of strictly lipidic portions of the membrane, poorly linked to the cytoskeleton. These cells are, probably, more prone to undergo vesiculation (loss of poorly linked membrane portions) whenever they have to circulate through the haemodialysis membranes or the microvasculature. Vesiculation may, therefore, lead to modifications in the erythrocyte membrane of stage 5 CKD patients (Reliene, 2002; Rocha, 2005).

Erythrocytes that develop intracellular defects earlier during their life span are removed prematurely from circulation (Santos-Silva, 1998; Rocha-Pereira, 2004). The removal of senescent or damaged erythrocytes seems to involve the development of a senescent neoantigen on the membrane surface, marking the cell for death. This neoantigen is immunologically related to band 3 (Kay, 1994). The deterioration of the erythrocyte metabolism and/or of its antioxidant defences may lead to the development of oxidative stress within the cell, allowing oxidation and linkage of denatured haemoglobin to the cytoplasmatic domain of band 3, promoting its aggregation, the binding of natural anti-band 3 autoantibodies and complement activation, marking the erythrocyte for death. The band 3 profile [high molecular weight aggregates (HMWAg), band 3 monomer and proteolytic fragments (Pfrag)] is used in order to differentiate younger, damaged and/or senescent erythrocytes. Older and damaged erythrocytes present with higher HMWAg and lower Pfrag. Younger erythrocytes show reduced HMWAg and higher Pfrag (Santos-Silva, 1998). Several diseases, known as inflammatory conditions, present an abnormal band 3 profile, suggestive of oxidative stress development (Santos-Silva, 1998; Belo, 2002; Rocha-Pereira, 2004).

Leukocyte activation is part of an inflammatory response, and is an important source of ROS and proteases, both of which may impose oxidative and proteolytic damages to erythrocyte and plasma constituents. Actually, oxidative stress has been reported to occur in stage 5 CKD patients and has been proposed as a significant factor in haemodialysis-related shortened erythrocyte survival.

In literature, there are few reports about the effect of CKD and haemodialysis procedure in erythrocyte membrane protein composition (Matos, 1997; Wu, 1998; Ibrahim, 2002). Studies performed in erythrocytes from stage 5 CKD patients, using cuprophane and polyacrylonitrile dialysis membranes, showed some changes in the membrane proteins, namely, a reduction in spectrin and band 3, and an isolated reduction in band 3, respectively (Sevilhano, 1990; Delmas-Beauvieux, 1995). Wu et al (Wu, 1998) and Ibrahim et al (2002) showed that stage 5 CKD patients presented a median osmotic fragility higher than the controls, and, after the haemodialysis procedure, that osmotic fragility decreased.

Recently, we reported for the first time, changes in the erythrocyte membrane band 3 profile in stage 5 CKD patients. These patients presented a decrease in HMWAg and in HMWAg/band 3 monomer ratio (Fig. 3 and table 3). These changes seem to reflect a younger erythrocyte population; however, CKD presented also a decrease in Pfrag and in Pfrag/band 3 monomer ratio, both suggesting a rise in erythrocyte damage. Thus, it seems that the band 3 profile observed in CKD patients is associated both to an increase in younger erythrocytes and to an increase in damaged erythrocytes (Costa, 2008c). This study also showed that the haemodialysis procedure *per se* does not lead to an increase in the studied markers of erythrocyte damage. Actually, no differences were found after haemodialysis, in band 3 profile.

| | **Controls (n=26)** | **Stage 5 CKD patients (n=63)** |
|---|---|---|
| HMWAg (%) | 19.90 (15.42-21.12) | 15.23 (13.38-19.40)* |
| Band 3 monomer (%) | 55.28 (53.39-57.41) | 61.84 (56.87-64.41)* |
| Pfrag (%) | 26.29 ± 4.78 | 22.70 ± 6.01* |
| HMWAg/ Band 3 monomer | 0.33 ± 0.07 | 0.27 ± 0.07* |
| Pfrag/ Band 3 monomer | 0.48 ± 0.11 | 0.38 ± 0.13* |

* $p<0.05$ *vs* controls. HMWAg; high molecular weight aggregates; Pfrag: proteolytic fragments. Results are presented as mean ± standard deviation or as median (interquartile ranges).

Table 3. Band 3 profile for controls and stage 5 CKD patients.

Some changes in erythrocyte membrane protein composition of stage 5 CKD patients using high-flux polysulfone FX-class dialysers of Fresenius, were also observed (Costa, 2008b; Costa, 2008d). A decrease in spectrin was the most significant change (table 4). This reduction in spectrin may account for a poor linkage of the cytoskeleton to the membrane, favoring membrane vesiculation, and, probably, a reduction in the erythrocyte lifespan of

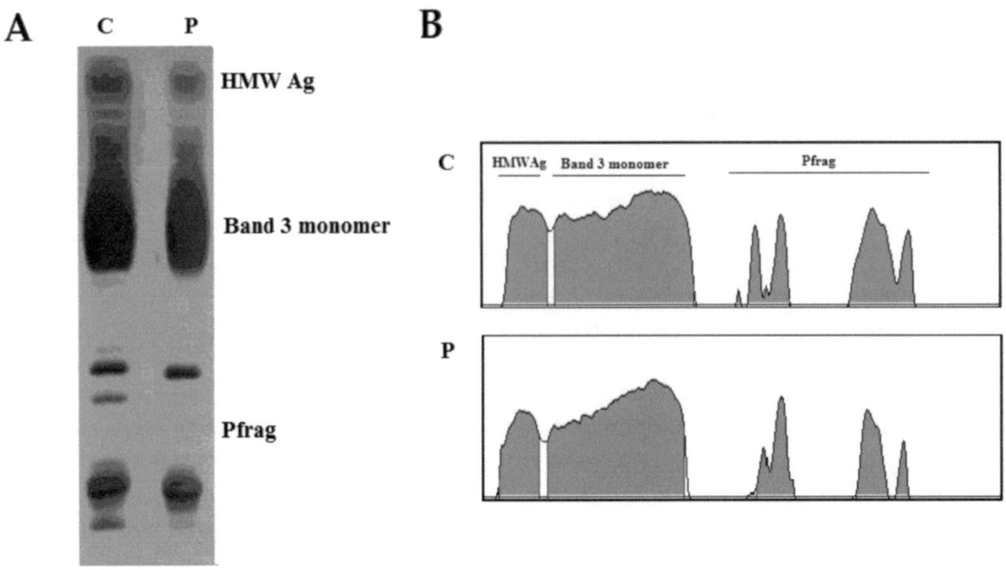


Fig. 3. A- Illustration of two band 3 profiles, one presented by a control (C), and the other presented by a stage 5 CKD patient (P). B- Examples of densitometer tracing of immunoblots for band 3 profile, C- Control; P – stage 5 CKD patient. HMWAg; high molecular weight aggregates; Pfrag: proteolytic fragments.

| | **Controls (n=26)** | **CKD stage 5 Patients (n=63)** |
|---|---|---|
| Spectrin (%) | 27.63 (26.41-28.79) | 24.27 (19.39-26.13)* |
| Ankyrin (%) | 6.97±1.62 | 6.53 ±1.90 |
| Band 3 (%) | 38.57 ± 3.99 | 39.29±4.03 |
| Protein 4.1 (%) | 7.56±1.45 | 7.24 ±1.49 |
| Protein 4.2 (%) | 5.51±0.72 | 5.44 ±1.44 |
| Band 5 (%) | 6.82±0.86 | 6.87 ±1.03 |
| Band 6 (%) | 5.19±1.04 | 6.98±1.37* |
| Band 7 (%) | 2.20±0.65 | 3.32 ±1.24* |
| Protein 4.1/Spectrin | 0.276 ± 0.624 | 0.330 ± 0.120a) |
| Protein 4.1/Band 3 | 0.192 (0.154-0.227) | 0.183 (0.155-0.208) |
| Protein 4.2/Band 3 | 0.149 (0.125-0.162) | 0.138 (0.110-0.163) |
| Spectrin/Band 3 | 0.707 (0.649-0.822) | 0.569 (0.512 -0.686)* |
| Ankyrin/Band 3 | 0.185 ± 0.585 | 0.169 ± 0.057 |
| Spectrin/Ankirin | 4.18 ± 1.07 | 3.77 ± 1.84 |

Table 4. Erythrocyte membrane protein profile for controls and stage 5 CKD patients.* $p<0.05$, *vs* controls. Results are presented as mean ± standard deviation or as median (interquartile ranges). HMWAg; high molecular weight aggregates; Pfrag: proteolytic fragments. Adapted from Costa, 2008d.

these patients (Reliene, 2002). Significant increases in protein bands 6 and 7 were also observed, which may further reflect an altered membrane protein interaction and destabilization of membrane structure. This membrane destabilization was further strengthened by the significant changes observed for spectrin/band 3 ratio (Costa, 2008b; Costa, 2008d). These membrane protein changes may be due to a higher erythrocyte metabolic stress and/or to changes resulting from the haemodialysis procedure *per se*.

Studying the effect of the haemodialysis procedure on erythrocyte membrane protein composition in stage 5 CKD patients, by evaluating membrane protein composition before and immediately after haemodialysis procedure (table 5), some trends towards the control profile were observed for some of the membrane proteins - band 3, band 6 and band 7; spectrin showed an even lower value after haemodialysis, and ankyrin, protein 4.1, protein 4.2 and band 5 also presented a trend to decrease. Comparing the ratios before and after haemodialysis, only the ratio spectrin/band 3 showed a statistically significant value, reflecting a vertical membrane protein disturbance.

| | **Stage 5 CKD patients (n=20)** | |
|---|---|---|
| | **Before haemodialysis** | **After haemodialysis** |
| Spectrin (%) | 25.58 (24.10-27.07) | 24.47 (22.31-26.95)* |
| Ankyrin (%) | 6.39 ± 1.55 | 6.23 ± 1.28 |
| Band 3 (%) | 38.10 ± 3.78 | 41.13 ± 2.44* |
| Protein 4.1 (%) | 6.48 ± 1.60 | 6.39 ± 1.69 |
| Protein 4.2 (%) | 4.34 ± 0.99 | 4.84 ± 1.04 |
| Band 5 (%) | 6.56 ± 0.91 | 6.71 ± 0.59 |
| Band 6 (%) | 6.46 ± 0.87 | 6.17 ± 1.15 |
| Band 7 (%) | 2.09 ± 0.43 | 2.37 ± 0.34 |
| Protein 4.1/Spectrin | 0.243 ± 0.070 | 0.251 ± 0.081 |
| Protein 4.1/Band 3 | 0.170 (0.138-0.206) | 0.163 (0.121-0.202) |
| Protein 4.2/Band 3 | 0.114 (0.101-0.133) | 0.118 (0.101-0.147) |
| Spectrin/Band 3 | 0.685 (0.626-0.796) | 0.647 (0.566-0.689)* |
| Ankyrin/Band 3 | 0.171 ± 0.049 | 0.152 ± 0.330 |
| Spectrin/Ankirin | 4.48 ± 1.361 | 4.45 ± 1.49 |

* $p$<0.05, *vs* before haemodialysis. Results are presented as mean ± standard deviation or as median (interquartile ranges). HMWAg; high molecular weight aggregates; Pfrag: proteolytic fragments. Adapted from Costa, 2008b.

Table 5. Erythrocyte membrane protein profile for stage 5 CKD patients, before and immediately after haemodialysis procedure.

Haemodialysis procedure seems to have an important role in the changes observed for erythrocyte membrane protein composition; however, their exact origin(s) are not yet fully understood. An hypothesis is that the increased plasma levels of elastase found in stage 5

CKD patients could induce changes in erythrocyte membrane proteins, leading to a decrease in erythrocyte lifespan, and, consequently, to an increase in the degree of the anaemia. This hypothesis was tested (Pereira, 2011), by performing some *in vitro* assays using erythrocytes from 18 stage 5 CKD patients (10 responders and 8 non-responders to recombinant human erythropoietin therapy) and from 8 healthy controls; erythrocyte suspensions in phosphate buffered saline, pH 7.4, were incubated at 37º C, under gentle rotation, in the presence of 0.03, 0.1 and 0.5 µg/mL of neutrophil elastase. These assays used erythrocytes collected before and immediately after the haemodialysis procedure.

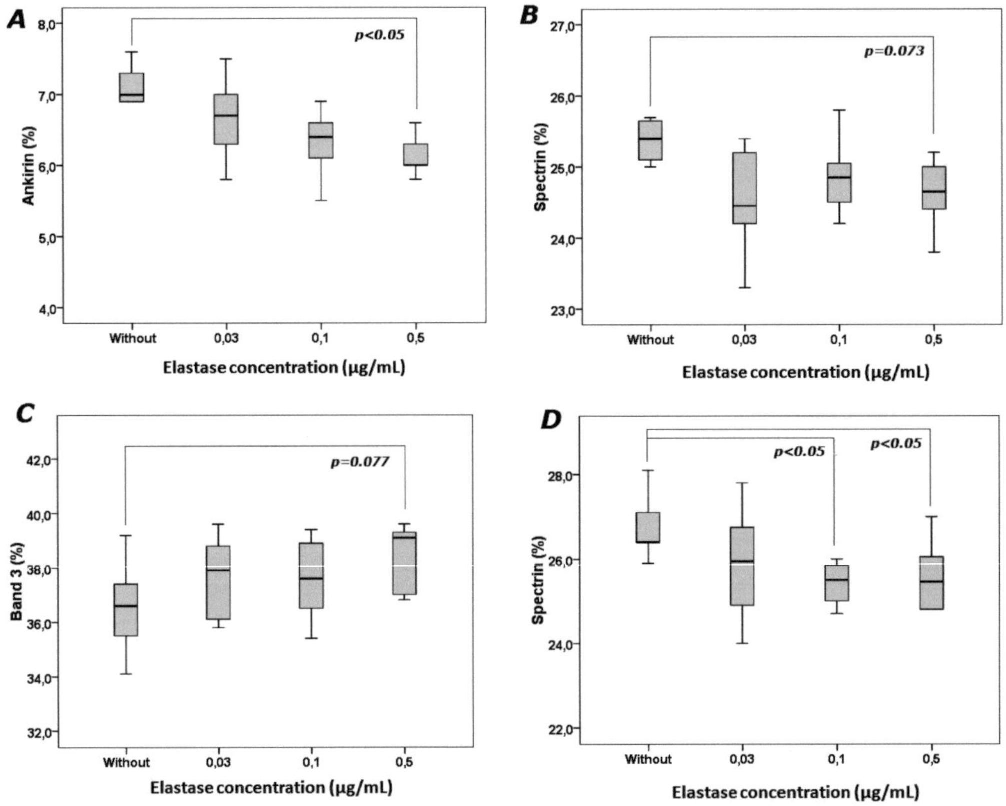


Fig. 4. Changes in ankyrin (A), spectrin (B) and band 3 (C) observed for erythrocytes from responder stage 5 CKD patients before haemodialysis, when incubated without and with elastase; changes in spectrin presented by erythrocytes from non-responder stage 5 CKD patients before haemodialysis, when incubated without and with elastase (D). Adapted from Pereira, 2011.

No significant differences were found between the protein composition of the erythrocyte membranes from healthy controls and from stage 5 CKD patients, when their erythrocytes, collected after the haemodialysis procedure, were incubated without and with different elastase concentrations. However, the erythrocytes from stage 5 CKD patients, collected before the haemodialysis procedure, showed some susceptibility to elastase; the erythrocytes from responders stage 5 CKD patients, incubated with 0.5 µg/mL of elastase showed a significant decrease in ankyrin [7.0 (6.5-7.5%) *vs* 6.0 (5.9-6.5%), $p$=0.024], and trends towards a decrease in spectrin [25.6 (25.1-26.9%) *vs* 24.7 (24.4-25.6%), $p$=0.073) and an increase in band 3 [36.6 (34.8-37.6%) *vs* 39.1 (36.9-39.4%), $p$=0.077), as compared with erythrocytes incubated without elastase. Similar changes were found for the erythrocytes incubated with 0.1 µg/mL of elastase. In non-responders stage 5 CKD patients, the erythrocytes incubated with 0.1 and 0.5 µg/mL of elastase, showed a significant decrease in spectrin [25.5 (24.9-25.9%) and 25.3 (24.8-26.2%), respectively *vs* 26.4 (26.0-27.3%), $p$=0.011 for both], as compared to erythrocytes incubated without elastase (Fig. 4).

These findings suggest that the erythrocytes from stage 5 CKD patients, before the haemodialysis procedure, are more susceptible to the proteolytic action of elastase upon the membrane. Considering that after the haemodialysis procedure the composition of the erythrocyte membrane from stage 5 CKD patients did not change, it seems that the more susceptible erythrocytes were removed during the haemodialysis procedure. Moreover, the release of neutrophil activation products, such as elastase, during haemodialysis may contribute to the removal of the more damaged cells, by enhancing membrane protein changes.

## 5. Other pathologies associated with neutrophil activation and erythrocyte damage

Several physiological (physical exercise, pregnancy) and pathological (hereditary spherocytosis, cardiovascular disease, preeclampsia, psoriasis) conditions presenting with neutrophilic leukocytosis have been associated to an altered erythrocyte membrane protein composition and to other changes reflecting erythrocyte damage. Moreover, they have been associated to increased neutrophil activation products, suggesting that leukocyte activation may trigger injuries in the neighboring erythrocytes.

In Hereditary Spherocytosis (HS), mutations in genes encoding for some membrane proteins - band 3, spectrin, protein band 4.2 and ankyrin - may result in their partial or inaccurate assembly to the membrane. Deficiencies in one or more of those proteins cause a decrease in membrane stability that, in turn, leads to loss of membrane surface area through membrane vesiculation. By losing membrane vesicles, the cell will become spherocytic and the membrane more rigid, triggering the sequestration of cell in the spleen and, therefore, the reduction of the erythrocyte lifespan and the development of anemia (Mohandas & Gallagher, 2008).

Two distinct pathways lead to the reduction in membrane surface area: i) deficiencies in spectrin, ankyrin, or protein 4.2 reduce the density of the membrane cytoskeleton, causing a weaker linkage to the lipid bilayer, favoring the loss of membrane vesicles containing lipids and band 3; ii) deficiency in band 3 favors the development of band 3 deficient areas in the membrane, with loss of the lipid-stabilizing effect of band 3, and therefore, the release of band 3-free microvesicles, from the membrane (Iolascon, 2003; Perrotta, 2008). In a recent work by our group (Rocha, 2010), studying 160 HS patients, the analysis of erythrocyte membrane protein profile showed that 109 patients presented a primary deficiency in band 3, 35 patients a primary ankyrin deficiency, 14 patients an isolated deficiency in spectrin and 2 patients an isolated deficiency in protein 4.2. Furthermore, severe HS patients presented with higher neutrophil count and higher levels of TNF-α, IFN-γ, elastase, lactoferrin and ferritin. Our data show HS as a disease linked to enhanced erythropoiesis that is disturbed in the more severe forms, to which inflammation, at least in part, seems to contribute.

Patients with cardiovascular disease, namely, with recent myocardial infarction (within the last 48 h), survivors for at least 3 months of myocardial infarction and hypertensive individuals, presented besides a neutrophilic leukocytosis a different band 3 profile, with higher values of HMWAg and lower values of band 3 monomer and of Pfrag (Santos-Silva, 1995). Ischemic stroke patients presented the same altered band 3 profile, associated with increased plasma levels of leukocyte activation products - elastase and lactoferrin - when compared with controls (Santos-Silva, 1998).

Band 3 profile in normal pregnancy in the first trimester of pregnancy, when compared with healthy controls, presented significantly reduced HMWAg and increased Pfrag. Comparing the third with the first trimester, a significant reduction in band 3 and a significant rise in Pfrag was also described. These results suggest band 3 profile as a marker of erythrocyte changes in normal pregnancy, which are independent of the 'physiological anemia' of pregnancy. These changes suggest an increase in damaged erythrocytes, but also an increase in younger erythrocytes in the maternal circulation. We also found alterations in the markers of erythrocyte damage in preeclampsia, in both umbilical cord blood and maternal circulation. In preeclamptic pregnancies in the third trimester of gestation, a significantly higher level of elastase and a significantly higher elastase to neutrophil ratio was also described, suggesting an increased neutrophil activation in these patients (Belo, 2002; Belo, 2003).

Psoriasis was also associated with plasma neutrophil activation, showing increased plasma levels of elastase and lactoferrin, associated with alterations in band 3 profile (Rocha-Pereira, 2004).

## 6. Conclusions

Stage 5 CKD is associated with an altered structure of erythrocyte membrane proteins, which may be due to the disease itself and/or to the interaction of blood cells with haemodialysis membranes. Haemodialysis procedure seems to contribute to a disturbance in the erythrocyte membrane protein structure, as showed by the significant reduction in spectrin, the most striking change observed.

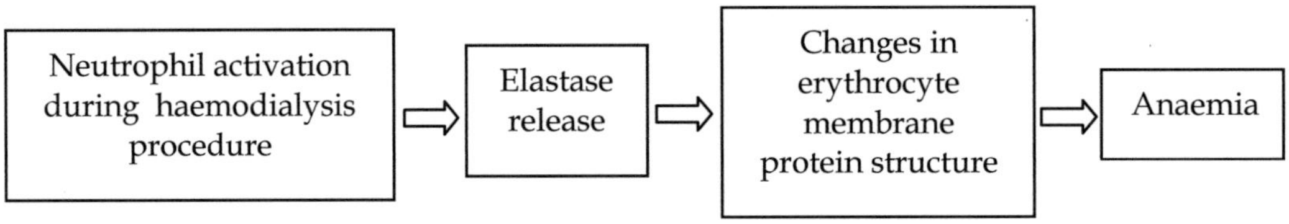


Fig. 5. In stage 5 CKD patients, the increased plasma levels of elastase can induce changes in erythrocyte membrane proteins, leading to a decrease in the erythrocyte lifespan and, consequently, to increase the degree of anaemia in these patients.

Moreover, stage 5 CKD patients under haemodialysis also present higher elastase plasma levels, which might reflect the rise in neutrophils and the enhanced inflammatory process found in these patients. Haemodialysis procedure seems to be associated with neutrophil activation, with subsequent elastase release that seems to induce changes in the erythrocyte membrane protein composition, probably contributing to a decrease in the erythrocyte half-life, and, therefore to the anemia found in stage 5 CKD patients (Fig. 5).

## 7. Acknowledgments

This work was supported by national funds - "Fundação Portuguesa para a Ciência e Tecnologia" (FCT: PIC/IC/83221/2007) and co-financed by FEDER (FCOMP-01-0124-FEDER-008468).

## 8. References

An, X.; Mohandas, N. (2008). Disorders of red cell membrane. *Br J Haematol*, vol. 141, pp. 367-375, ISSN 0007-1048

Bárány, P. (2001). Inflammation, serum C-reactive protein, and erythropoietin resistance. *Nephrol Dial transplant*, vol. 16, pp. 224-227, ISSN 0931- 0509

Baynes, R.; Bezwoda, W.; Bothwell, T.; Khan, Q.; Mansoor, N. (1986). The non immune inflammatory response: serial changes in plasma iron, iron binding capacity, lactoferrin, ferritin and C reactive protein. *Scan J Clin Lab Invest,* vol. 46, pp. 695-704, ISSN 0036-5513

Belo, L.; Rebelo, I.; Castro, E.M.; Catarino, C.; Pereira-Leite, L.; Quintanilha, A.; Santos-Silva, A. (2002). Band 3 as a marker of erythrocyte changes in pregnancy. *Eur J Haematol*, vol. 69, pp.145-151, ISSN 0902- 4441

Belo, L.; Santos-Silva, A.; Caslake, M.; Cooney, J.; Pereira-Leite, L.; Quintanilha, A.; Rebelo, I. (2003). Neutrophil activation and C-reactive protein concentration in preeclampsia. *Hypertens Pregnancy*, vol. 22, pp.129-141, ISSN 1064-1955

Brinkmann, V.; Reichard, U.; Goosmann, C.; Fauler, B.; Uhlemann, Y.; Weiss, D.S.; Weinrauch, Y. & Zychlinsky, A. (2004). Neutrophil extracellular traps kill bacteria. *Science*, vol. 303, pp.1532-1535, ISSN 0036-8075

Costa, E.; Rocha, S.; Rocha-Pereira, P.; Nascimento, H.; Castro, E.; Miranda, V.; Faria, M.S.; Loureiro, A.; Quintanilha, A.; Belo, L. & Santos-Silva, A. (2008a). Neutrophil activation and resistance to recombinant human erythropoietin therapy in hemodialysis patients. *Am J Nephrol*, vol. 28, pp. 935-940, ISSN 1046-6673

Costa, E.; Rocha, S.; Rocha-Pereira, P.; Castro, E.; Miranda, V.; Sameiro-Faria, M.; Loureiro, A.; Quintanilha, A.; Belo, L. & Santos-Silva, A. (2008b). Changes in red blood cells membrane protein composition during hemodialysis procedure. Ren Fail, vol. 30, pp. 971-975, ISSN 0886- 022

Costa, E.; Rocha, S.; Rocha-Pereira, P.; Castro, E.; Miranda, V.; Sameiro-Faria, M.; Loureiro, A.; Quintanilha, A.; Belo, L. & Santos-Silva, A. (2008c). Band profile as a marker of erythrocyte changes in chronic kidney disease patients. *The Open Clinical Chemistry Journal*, vol. 1, pp. 57-63, ISSN 1874-2416

Costa, E.; Rocha, S.; Rocha-Pereira, P.; Castro, E.; Miranda, V.; Sameiro-Faria, M.; Loureiro, A.; Quintanilha, A.; Belo, L. & Santos-Silva, A. (2008d). Alterated erythrocyte membrane protein composition in chronic kidney disease stage 5 patients under haemodialysis and recombinant human erythropoietin therapy. *Blood Purif*, vol. 26, pp. 267-273, ISSN 0253-5068

Dasselaar, J.J.; Hooge, M.N..; Pruim, J.; Nijnuis, H.; Wiersum, A.; Jong, P.E.; Huisman, R.M.; Franssen, C.F.M. (2007). Relative blood volume changes underestimated total blood volume changes during hemodialysis. *Clin J Am Soc Nephrol* 2:669-674, ISSN 1555-9041

Delmas-Beauvieux, M.C.; Combe, C.; Peuchant, E.; Carbonneau, M.A.; Dubourg, L.; de Précigout, V.; Aparicio, M.; Clerc, M. (1995). Evaluation of red blood cell lipoperoxidation in hemodialysed patients during erythropoietin therapy supplemented or not with iron. *Nephron*, vol. 69, pp. 404-410, ISSN 0028-2766

Fitch, P.M.; Roghanian, A.; Howie, S.E.M. & Sallenave, J.M. (2006). Human neutrophil elastase inhibitors in innate and adaptive immunity. *Biochemical Society Transactions*, vol. 34, pp. 279-282, ISSN 0300-5127

Gallagher, P.G. (2005). Red cell membrane disorders. Hematology. *Am Soc Hematol Educ Program*, pp. 13-18, ISSN 1520-4383

Halliwell, B.; Gutteridge, J.M.C. (1990). The antioxidants of human extracelular fluids. *Arch Biochem Biophys*, vol. 280, pp. 1-8, ISSN 0003- 9861

Harlan, J.M. (1985). Leukocyte-endothelial interactions. *Blood*, vol. 65, pp. 513- 525, ISSN 0006-4971

Ibrahim, F.F.; Ghannam, M.M.; Ali, F.M. (2002). Effect of dialysis on erythrocyte membrane of chronically hemodialyzed patients. *Renal failure*, vol. 24, pp. 779-790, ISSN 0886-022X

Iolascon, A.; Perrota, S.; Steward, G.W. (2003). Red blood cell membrane defects. *Rev Clin Exp Hematol*, vol. 7, pp. 22-56, ISSN 1127-0020

Kay, M.M.; Wyant, T. & Goodman, J. (1994). Autoantibodies to band 3 during aging and disease and aging interventions. *Ann N Y Acad Sci*, vol. 719, pp. 419- 447, ISSN 0077-8923

Levay, P.F.; Viljoen, M. (1995). Lactoferrin: a general review. *Haematologica*, vol. 80, pp. 252-267, ISSN 0390-6078

Ley, K.; Laudanna, C.; Cybulsky, M.I. & Nourshargh, S. (2007). Getting to the site of inflammation: the leukocyte adhesion cascade updated. *Nature Reviews Immunology*, vol. 7, pp. 678-689, ISSN 1474-1733

Locatelli, F.; Aljama, P.; Barany, P.; Canaud, B.; Carrera, F.; Eckardt, K.U.; Horl, W.H.; Macdougal, I.C.; Macleod, A.; Wiecek, A. & Cameron, S. (2004a). European Best Practice Guidelines Working Group. Revised European best practice guidelines for the management of anemia in patients with chronic renal failure. *Nephrol Dial Transplant*, vol. 19, Suppl 2, pp. ii1-ii47, ISSN 0931- 0509

Lucchi, L.; Bergamini, S.; Botti, B.; Rapanà, R.; Ciuffreda, A.; Ruggiero, P.; Ballestri, M.; Tomasi, A. & Albertazzi, A. (2000). Influence of different hemodialysis membrane on red blood cell susceptibility of oxidative stress. *Artif Organs*, vol. 24, pp. 1-6, ISSN 1525-1594

Martos, M.R.; Hendry, B.M.; Rodrígues-Puyol, M.; Dwight, J.; Díez-Marqués, M.L.; Rodríguez-Puyol, D. (1997). Haemodialyser biocompatibility and erythrocyte struture and function. *Clin Chim Acta*, vol. 265, pp. 235-246, ISSN 0009-8981

Medina, A.; Ellis, C.; Levitt, M.D. (1994). Use of alveolar carbon monoxide measurements to assess red blood cell survival in hemodialysis patients. *Am J Hematol*, vol. 46, pp.91-94, ISSN 0361-8609

Miyoshi, I.; Saito, T.; Bandobashi, K.; Ohtsuki, .;, Taguchi, H. (2006). Concomitant deposition of aluminum and iron in bone marrow trabeculae. *Intern Med*, vol. 45, pp. 117-118, ISSN 0365-4362

Mohandas, N.; Gallagher, P.G. (2008). Red Cell membrane: past, present, and future. *Blood*, vol. 112, pp. 3939-3948

Muller, W.A. (1999). Leukocyte-endothelial cell adhesion molecules in transendothelial migration, pp. 585-592, In: *Inflammation: basic principles and clinical correlates*, Gallin, J.I.; Snyderman, R.; Fearon, D.T.; Haynes, B.F. & Nathan C. (Ed.), 585-592, Lippincott Williams and Wilkins, ISBN 978-039-7517-59-6, Philadelphia, USA

Olofsson, T.; Olsson, I.; Venge, P.; Elgefors, B. (1977). Serum myeloperoxidase and lactoferrin in neutropenia. *Scand J Haematol,* vol. 18, pp. 73-80, ISSN 0036-553X

Pay, S.; Musabak, U.; Simşek, I.; Pekel, A.; Erdem, H.; Dinç, A. & Sengül, A. (2006). Expression of CXCR-1 and CXCR-2 chemokine receptors on synovial neutrophils in inflammatory arthritides: does persistent or increasing expression of CXCR-2 contribute to the chronic inflammation or erosive changes? *Joint Bone Spine*, vol. 73, pp. 691-6, ISSN 1778-7254

Pereira, R.; Costa, E.; Gonçalves, M.; Miranda, V.; Sameiro-Faria, M.; Quintanilha, A.; Belo, L.; Lima, M. & Santos-Silva, A. (2010). Neutrophil and monocyte activation in chronic kidney disease patients under hemodialysis and its relationship with resistance to recombinant human erythropoietin and to the hemodialysis procedure. *Hemodial Int*, vol. 14, pp. 295-301, ISSN 1492-7535

Pereira, R.; Rocha, S.; Borges, A.; Nascimento, H.; Reis, F.; Miranda, V.; Sameiro-Faria, M.; Quintanilha, A.; Belo, L.; Costa, E.; Santos-Silva, A. (2011). Elastase release during the hemodialysis procedure seems to induce changes in red blood cell membrane proteins. *Hemodial Int, in press*, ISSN 1492-7535

Perrota, S.; Gallagher, P.G.; Mohandas, N. (2008). Hereditary spherocytosis. Lancet, vol. 372, pp. 1411-1426, ISSN 0140-6736

Pisoni, R.L.; Bragg-Gresham, J.L.; Young, E.W.; Akizawa, T.; Asano, Y.; Locatelli, F.; Bommer, J.; Cruz, J.M.; Kerr, P.J.; Mendelssohn, D.C.; Held, P.J.; Port, F.K. (2004). Anemia management and outcomes from 12 countries in the dialysis outcomes and practice patterns study (DOPPS). *Am J Kidney Dis,* vol. 44, pp. 94-111, ISSN 0272-6386

Reliene, R.; Marini, M.; Zanella, A.; Reinhart, W.H.; Ribeiro, M.L.; del Giudice, E.M.; Perrotta, S.; Ionoscon, A.; Eber, S. & Lutz, H.U. (2002). Splenectomy prolongs in vivo survival of erythrocytes differently in spectrin/ankyrin- and band 3-deficient hereditary spherocytosis. *Blood*, vol. 100, pp. 2208-2215, ISSN 0006-4971

Rocha, S.; Costa, E.; Rocha-Pereira, P.; Ferreira, F.; Cleto, E.; Barbot, J.; Quintanilha, A.; Belo, L.; Santos-Silva, A. (2010). Erythrocyte membrane protein destabilization versus clinical outcome in 160 Portuguese Hereditary Spherocytosis patients.*Br J Haematol*, vol. 149, pp.785-794, ISSN 00071048

Rocha, S.; Rebelo, I.; Costa, E.; Catarino, C.; Belo, L.; Castro, E.M.B.; Cabeda, J.M.; Barbot, J.; Quintanilha, A. & Santos-Silva, A. (2005). Protein deficiency balance as a predictor of clinical outcome in hereditary spherocytosis. *Eur J Haematol*, vol. 74, pp. 374-80, ISSN 0902- 4441

Rocha-Pereira, P.; Santos-Silva, A.; Rebelo, I.; Figueiredo, A.; Quintanilha, A. & Teixeira, F. (2004). Erythrocyte damage in mild and severe psoriasis. *Br J Dermatology*, vol. 150, pp. 232–44, ISSN 0007-0963

Roos, D.; Van Bruggen, R. & Meischl, C. (2003). Oxidative killing of microbes by neutrophils. *Microbes Infect*, vol. 5, pp. 1307–1315, ISSN 1286-4579

Saito, N.; Takemori, N.; Hirai, K.; Onodera, R.; Watanabe, S.; Naiki, M. (1993). Ultrastructural localization of lactoferrin in the granules other than typical secondary granules of human neutrophils. *Human Cell,* vol. 6, pp. 42-48, ISSN 0914-7470

Santos-Silva, A.; Castro, E.; Teixeira, N.; Guerra, F.; Quintanilha, A. (1995). Altered erythrocyte membrane band 3 profile as a marker in patients at risk for cardiovascular disease. *Atherosclerosis*, vol. 116, pp.199-209, ISSN 0021-9150

Santos-Silva, A.; Castro, E.M.B.; Teixeira, N.A.; Guerra, F.C. & Quintanilha, A. (1998). Erythrocyte membrane band 3 profile imposed by cellular aging, by activated neutrophils and by neutrophilic elastase. *Clin Chim Acta*, vol. 275, pp.185–196, ISSN 0009-8981

Sevillano G, Rodrígues-Puyol M, Martos R, Duque I, Lamas S, Diez-Marques ML, Lúcio J, Rodriguez-Puvol D. (1990). Cellulose acetato membrane improves some aspects of red blood cell function in hemodialysis patients. *Nephrol Dial Transplant,* vol. 5, pp. 497-499, ISSN 0931- 0509

Sherry, B.; Dai, W.W.; Lesser, M.L. & Trachtman, H. (2008). Dysregulated chemokine receptor expression and chemokine-mediated cell trafficking in pediatric patients with ESRD. *Clin J Am Soc Nephrol*, vol. 3, pp. 397-406, ISSN 1555-9041

Stoya, G.; Klemm, A.; Baumann, E.; Vogelsang, H.; Ott, U.; Linss, W. & Stein, G. (2002). Determination of autofluorescence of red blood cells (RBCs) in uremic patients as a marker of oxidative damage. *Clin Nephrol*, vol. 58, pp.198-204, ISSN 0301- 0430

Sullivan, G.W.; Sarembock, I.J. & Linden, J. (2000). The role of inflammation in vascular diseases. *J Leukoc Biol*, vol. 67, pp. 591-602, ISSN 0741-5400

Witko-Sarsat, V.; Rieu, P.; Descamps-Latscha, B.; Lesavre, P.; Halbwachs-Mecarelli, L. (2000). Neutrophils: molecules, functions and pathophysiological aspects. *Lab Invest,* vol. 80, pp. 617–653, ISSN 0023-6837

Wu, S.G.; Jeng, F.R.; Wei, S.Y.; Su, C.Z.; Chung, T.; Chang, W.J.; Chang, H.W. (1998). Red blood cell osmotic fragility in chronically hemodialyed. *Nephron,* vol.78, pp. 28-32, ISSN 0028-2766

# 14

# Assessing Iron Status in CKD Patients: New Laboratory Parameters

Eloísa Urrechaga[1], Luís Borque[2] and Jesús F. Escanero[2]
[1]*Laboratory, Hospital Galdakao, Usansolo Galdakao, Vizcaya*
[2]*Department of Pharmacology and Physiology, Faculty of Medicine University of Zaragoza, Zaragoza*
*Spain*

## 1. Introduction

Chronic kidney disease (CKD) affects millions of people worldwide, with high incidence and prevalence and increasing costs. Anemia, a common observation in CKD, can develop in the early phases of the disease and contributes to a poor quality of life (Eknoyan *et al.*, 2004).

Anemia in patients with CKD is due to many factors. Erythropoiesis and iron homeostasis are impaired as a result of a complex chain of events, including the relative deficiency of erythropoietin, chronic inflammation, blood loss, decreased iron absorption and utilization, exogenous iron and erythropoietin acquisition via biologically unregulated mechanisms (blood transfusions and medicinal erythropoietin and iron administration) (Weiss, 2009; Guidi & Santonastaso, 2010; Lankhorst & Wish, 2010).

The advent of erythropoiesis stimulating agents (ESA) and various intravenous iron preparations has resulted in a much more effective management of anemia of CKD, allowing us to maintain hemoglobin levels in certain desired ranges and to effectively treat iron deficiency. Among the emerging challenges are the risks associated with administering high ESA and iron doses, leading to elevated hemoglobin levels and iron overload (Zager *et al.*, 2002).

Recombinant human erythropoietin (rHuEpo) has been available for treatment of renal disease anemia since 1989. However, rHuEpo therapy results in iron deficiency due to insufficient iron stores for the accelerated erythropoiesis. Iron deficiency is the main cause of suboptimal response to erythropoietin in dialysis patients (Cavill & Macdougall, 1993). Maintenance iron supplementation is required to successfully treat anemia; intravenous iron compounds are used to treat dialysis patients who become iron deficient.

Monitoring erythropoietin treated patients' iron status is important to detect iron deficiency and avoid the adverse effects of iron medication. The assessment of iron requirements and monitoring of therapy require accurate markers. New alternative markers for iron status that may be useful when serum ferritin and transferrin saturation are insufficient. These newer tests include reticulocyte hemoglobin content, percentage of hypochromic red cells and soluble transferrin receptor, all of which have shown some promise in recent studies (Goodnough *et al.*, 2010).

The percentages of hypochromic red cells (%Hypo) and reticulocyte hemoglobin content (CHr) are reported by the Siemens analyzers (Siemens Medical Solutions Diagnostics, Tarrytown NY, USA).

Two other parameters correlate to %Hypo and CHr, erythrocyte hemoglobin equivalent (RBC-He) and reticulocyte hemoglobin equivalent (Ret-He), reported by the Sysmex XE-2100 analyzer (Sysmex Corporation, Kobe, Japan); percentages of hypochromic red cells (% Hypo He) are now available on the Sysmex analyzer XE 5000 (Sysmex Corporation, Kobe, Japan.

Beckman Coulter (Beckman Coulter Inc., Miami, Fl, USA) has introduced on the LH series analysers a new parameter, low hemoglobin density (LHD%), related to the iron availability for erythropoiesis in the previous weeks; derived from mean cell hemoglobin concentration (MCHC). In this chapter the potential clinical utility of this parameter in the assessment of iron status in CKD patients is discussed.

### 1.1 Iron homeostasis

The normal Western diet contains 15–20 mg iron in Hem (10%) and non-Hem (ionic, 90%) forms. Only 1–2 mg of iron is absorbed and lost every day. Importantly, the total amount of iron in the body can be regulated only by absorption, whereas iron loss occurs only passively from sloughing of skin and mucosal cells as well as from blood loss. Iron absorption is balanced against iron loss so daily iron absorption may increase in response to increased iron demand (eg, growth, pregnancy or blood loss) (Conrad *et al.*, 2002; (Miret *et al.*, 2003).

Nearly all absorption of dietary iron occurs in the duodenum. Several steps are involved, including the reduction of iron to a ferrous state, apical uptake, intracellular storage or transcellular trafficking, and basolateral release. Molecular participants in each of these processes have been identified.

The non-Hem iron mainly exists in the $Fe^{3+}$ state. The ferric iron is reduced to ferrous iron before it is transported across the intestinal epithelium. The reduction of iron from the ferric to the ferrous state occurs at the enterocyte brush border by means of a duodenal ferric reductase (Dcytb). Once the insoluble $Fe^{3+}$ is converted to $Fe^{2+}$. Ferrous iron is then transported across the apical plasma membrane of the enterocyte by divalent metal transporter 1 (DMT1) DMT1 is expressed at the duodenal brush border where it controls uptake of dietary iron, and also traffics other metal ions such as zinc, copper and cobalt by a proton-coupled mechanism (Conrad *et al.*, 2002).

Iron taken up by the enterocyte may be stored intracellularly as ferritin (and excreted in the feces when the senescent enterocyte is sloughed) or transferred across the basolateral membrane to the plasma. This iron is transferred out of the enterocyte by the basolateral transporter ferroportin; this process is facilitated by the ferroxidase activity of the ceruloplasmin homologue hephaestin (Fleming *et al.*, 2005).

There are no substantial physiologic mechanisms that regulate iron loss. Accordingly, iron homeostasis is dependent on regulatory feedback between body iron needs and intestinal iron absorption.

Iron stores, erythropoietic activity, hemoglobin, oxygen content, and inflammation modulates the dietary iron absorption (Nemeth *et al.*, 2004).

Essentially all circulating plasma iron normally is bound to transferrin. The liver synthesizes transferrin and secretes it into the plasma. The chelation of ferric iron serves three purposes: it renders iron soluble under physiologic conditions, it prevents iron-mediated free radical toxicity, and it facilitates transport into cells. Transferrin is the most important physiological source of iron for red cells (Ponka, 1998).

Although transferrin was characterized fifty years ago, its receptor eluded investigators until the early 1980s.

The molecule is a transmembrane homodimer linked by disulfide bonds. This disulfide-linked homodimer has subunits containing 760 amino acids each. Oligosaccharides account for about 5% of the 90 kDa subunit molecular mass. A broad body of literature now supports the concept that the iron-transferrin complex is internalized by receptor-mediated endocytosis. (Beaumont *et al.*, 2009).

Most of the body iron is associated to hemoglobin in circulating erythrocytes. Erythropoiesis is a very active process that takes place in the bone marrow and leads to the daily production of 200 billion new erythrocytes to compensate for the destruction of senescent red cells by tissue macrophages. The control of erythropoiesis depends mostly on erythropoietin production by the kidney and on the availability of iron.

Macrophages play a central role in the organism as they recycle iron after phagocytosis of senescent erythrocytes. This mechanism mainly occurs in the spleen and bone marrow and to a lesser extent in the Küpffer cells of the liver.

During aging, erythrocytes accumulate multiple modifications (cell shrinkage, externalization of phosphatidyl-serine, peroxydation of the membrane). The fixation and ingestion of red cells by macrophages are triggered by cellular receptor-mediated phagocytosis (through recognition of externalized phosphatidyl-serine or neoantigens of senescence) (Lang *et al.*, 2005).

Iron can be stored in the macrophages associated to ferritin or hemosiderin or exported to the plasma. Iron export from macrophages to transferrin is accomplished by ferroportin, the same iron-export protein as expressed in the duodenal enterocyte, and reoxydized by ceruloplasmin (Knutson *et al.*, 2005).

Metabolically inactive iron, is stored in ferritin and hemosiderin. Normally, 95% of the stored iron in liver tissue is found in hepatocytes as ferritin. The level of serum ferritin parallels the concentration of storage iron within the body, regardless of the cell type in which it is stored.

The control of iron homeostasis acts at both the cellular and the systemic level and involves a complex system of different cell types, transporters, and signals. To maintain systemic iron homeostasis, communication between cells that absorb iron from the diet (duodenal enterocytes), consume iron (mainly erythroid precursors), and store iron (hepatocytes and tissue macrophages) must be tightly regulated (Swinkels *et al.*, 2006).

In the last 10 years, understanding of the regulation of iron homeostasis has changed substantially. A small peptide hormone, hepcidin, emerged as the central regulator of iron absorption, plasma iron levels, and iron distribution. Hepcidin is secreted by mainly by hepatocytes, and to a lesser extent by macrophages and adipocytes. The hormone inhibits iron flows into plasma from macrophages involved in recycling of senescent erythrocytes, duodenal enterocytes engaged in the absorption of dietary iron, and hepatocytes that store iron.( Ganz & Nemeth, 2009).

The human hepcidin gene is located on chromosome 19q13.1, encodes a precursor protein of 84 amino acids. During its export from the cytoplasm, this full-length pre-prohepcidin undergoes enzymatic cleavage, resulting in a 64 amino acids prohepcidin. Next, the 39 amino acids pro-region peptide is probably post-translationally removed, renders bioactive hepcidin-25. In human urine also are identified hepcidin-22 and hepcidin-20, which are N-terminally truncated iso-forms of hepcidin-25 (Kemna *et al.,* 2008).

Hepcidin expression is controlled by various stimuli: iron, inflammation, erythropoiesis, and hypoxia. iron and inflammation induce hepcidin production, while iron deficiency, hypoxia, and stimulation of erythropoiesis completely inhibit its production. Hepcidin is secreted into the circulation, where it down-regulates the ferroportin-mediated release of iron from enterocytes, macrophages and hepatocytes and is the key for the regulation of systemic iron homeostasis (Fleming *et al.,* 2005), reduces the quantity of circulating iron by limiting the egress of the metal from both intestinal and macrophage cells; the cellular process by which hepcidin acts, through its binding to ferroportin, thereby inducing internalization and subsequent degradation of the exporter (Bergamaschi & Villani., 2009).

In the intestine, delivery of dietary iron to plasma transferrin is inhibited by increasing concentrations of hepcidin, and iron is subsequently removed from the body, through the elimination of enterocytes (desquamation process). In macrophages, degradation of ferroportin by hepcidin results in the trapping of iron inside the cells, thereby limiting the acquisition of iron by erythroid cells (Nemeth *et al.,* 2004).

Figure 1 shows and summarizes the information contained on the previous section.

### 1.2 Anemia in CKD

Anemia of chronic disease (ACD), the most frequent anemia among hospitalized patients, occurs in chronic inflammatory disorders, such as chronic infections, cancer and autoimmune diseases; is a hypoproliferative anemia, defined by low plasma iron concentrations in the presence of high reticuloendotelial iron stores. Cytokines are implicated in the ACD increasing iron sequestration in the reticuloendothelial system (Weiss & Goodnough, 2005), results in hyposideremia. This results in limited availability of iron for erythroid progenitor cells and iron restricted erythropoiesis.

A particular case of ACD is represented by anemia of chronic kidney disease (CKD).

CKD is becoming a major public health problem worldwide; the incidence and prevalence of this disease is increasing and the costs of treatment lead to a large burden for the health care systems, particularly in developing countries (Guidi & Santonastaso, 2010).

The severity of kidney disease is classified into five stages according to the glomerular filtration rate (GFR). It is estimated that approximately half of the patients in stage 3 CKD (GFR: 30–59 mL/min/1.73 $m^2$) are anemic (Eknoyan *et al.,* 2004).

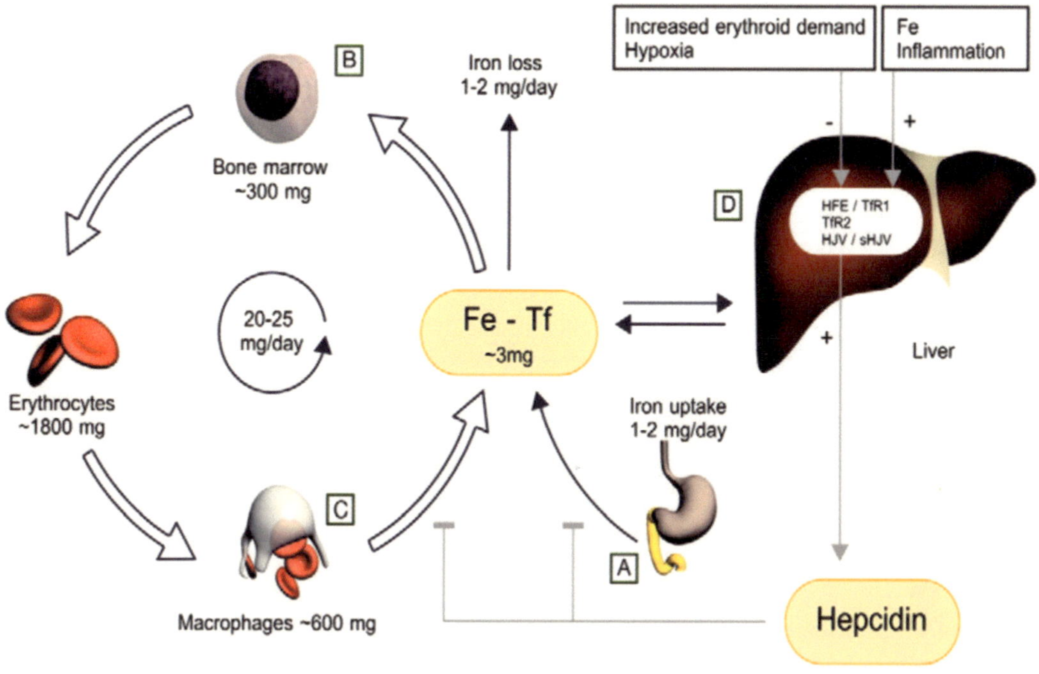


Fig. 1. Iron is absorbed from the diet by duodenal enterocytes and then bound to plasma transferrin (Tf). Fe-Tf is distributed to the bone marrow for erythropoiesis. At the end of their lifespan, senescent erythrocytes are phagocytosed by tissue macrophages and heme iron is recycled back to plasma transferrin.
Hepcidin regulates the systemic iron homeostasis; synthesized by the liver is secreted into the circulation, where it down-regulates the ferroportin-mediated release of iron from enterocytes, macrophages, and hepatocytes.
Swinkels, D. W. et al. Clin Chem 2006;52:950-968.

Anemia, a common observation in CKD, can develop in the early phases of the disease is associated to poor outcomes and contributes to a reduced quality of life, with symptoms including dyspnea, headache, light-headedness, and fatigue. Anemia in patients with CKD is due to many factors. The most well-known cause is inadequate production of erythropoietin. As renal failure progresses, the contribution of erythropoietin deficiency to anemia increases (Lankhorst & Wish, 2010).

Other causes which lead to impaired erythropoiesis contribute to anemia include diversion of iron traffic, diminished erythropoiesis, blunted response to erythropoietin, erythrophagocytosis, reduced proliferative activity of erythroid precursors in bone marrow, reduced survival of red cells, the decreased iron availability lead to impaired erythropoiesis (Weiss, 2009).

Absolute iron deficiency is defined as a decreased total iron body content. Iron deficiency anemia (IDA) occurs when iron deficiency is sufficiently severe to diminish erythropoiesis and cause the development of anemia. Functional iron deficiency describes a state where the total iron content of the body is normal or even elevated, but the iron is "locked away" and unavailable for the production of red blood cells. This condition is observed mainly in patients with chronic renal failure who are on hemodialysis.

Functional iron deficiency is defined as an imbalance between the iron needs for erythropoiesis and the iron supply, with the latter not maintained at sufficient rate for adequate hemoglobinization of reticulocytes and mature erythrocytes (Cavil & Macdougal, 1993).

In iron deficiency anemia (IDA) iron supply depends on the quantity of iron storage in the body, while in functional iron deficiency (iron restricted erythropoiesis) supply depends on the rate of mobilization of iron from the stores. The diagnosis of iron deficiency or functional iron deficiency is particularly challenging in patients with acute or chronic inflammatory conditions because most of the biochemical markers for iron metabolism are affected by acute phase reaction. This is the case of the anemia of chronic disease (ACD) and the anemia associated to chronic renal failure (CKD).

Recombinant human erythropoietin (rHuEpo) has been available for treatment of renal disease anemia since 1989 (Esbach *et al.*, 1989). However, rHuEpo therapy results in functional iron deficiency due to insufficient iron stores for the accelerated erythropoiesis. Iron deficiency is the main cause of suboptimal response to erythropoietin in dialysis patients. Maintenance iron supplementation is required to successfully treat anemia. Long term orally administered iron therapy is limited by noncompliance, gastrointestinal side effects, insufficient absorption and drug interaction; intravenous iron compounds are used to treat dialysis patients who become iron deficient (Macdougal, 1995).

Monitoring erythropoietin treated patients' iron status is important to detect iron deficiency and avoid the adverse effects of iron medication (Sunder-Plassmann & Hörl, 1997; Kletzmayr *et al.*, 2002; Zager *et al.*, 2002).

Biochemical indicators of iron metabolism (iron levels, transferrin, transferrin saturation, ferritin) although widely used, may be influenced by the acute phase response, which complicates clinical interpretation of the test results. Serum ferritin, an indicator of iron storage but not of iron supply, is an acute phase reactant and its levels are affected by inflammation. Because cytokines are commonly increased in CKD, serum ferritin levels might not reflect true iron stores (Mast, 2001; Coyne, 2006).

Transferrin is a negative acute phase reactant, rendering the calculation of transferrin saturation unreliable in this case. Transferrin fluctuates due to the diurnal variation of serum iron and is affected by nutritional status, leading to a lack of sensitivity and specificity in assessing iron's availability (Fishbane *et al.*, 1996). For these reasons, an iron deficient erythropoietic response to rHuEpo may occur despite normal serum ferritin and transferrin values.

### 1.2.1 Guidelines for diagnosis of anemia

After considerable review of the literature, Kidney Disease Outcomes Quality Initiative (K/DOQI) anemia work groups in 1997, 2001, and 2006 decided that the serum ferritin and the transferrin saturation (TSAT) should be the primary tools for assessing iron management in patients with anemia and chronic kidney disease, including end- stage renal disease. For patients with chronic kidney disease, absolute iron deficiency may be diagnosed when TSAT is

< 20% and serum ferritin is < 100 ng/mL. Functional iron deficiency may be more difficult to diagnose since iron status parameters may indicate adequate iron stores. There are different criteria in defining functional iron deficiency, one of them is published by the Kidney Disease Outcomes Quality Initiative- K/DOQI (Eknoyan *et al.* 2001).

The serum ferritin reflects storage iron, and absolute iron deficiency, according to the K/DOQI guidelines, correlates with serum ferritin <100 ng/mL. Absolute iron deficiency, the iron deficiency that is characterized by low or absent bone marrow staining for iron, is to be distinguished from functional or relative iron deficiency, which is defined as a response to intravenous iron with an increase in hemoglobin (Hb) or a decrease in erythropoiesis-stimulating agent requirement.

In 2004, European Best Practice Guidelines suggested an Hb target of 110 g/L (Locatelli *et al.*, 2004); values of >140 g/L were considered undesirable in general, and the limit for patients with cardiovascular disease was set at 120 g/dL. Caution of not exceeding the value of Hb concentrations 120 g/L was recommended to be given also for patients with diabetes, especially if they had concurrent peripheral vascular disease.

Assessment of anemia should include the laboratory measurement of the following parameters:

- Hb concentration, to assess the degree of anemia
- Red blood cell indices (mean cell volume MCV, mean cell hemoglobin MCH), to assess the type of anemia
- absolute reticulocyte count , to assess erythropoietic activity
- plasma ferritin concentration, to assess iron stores
- To assess iron available for erythropoiesis
    - percentage of hypochromic red cells
    - plasma transferrin Saturation
    - reticulocyte hemoglobin content
- Plasma C reactive protein, to assess inflammation

### 1.2.2 New parameters for the diagnosis of anemia

The question regarding anemia therapy in those patients is which are the best parameters to assess the iron available for erythropoiesis. New laboratory parameters are reported by different manufacturers as potential tools for anemia and iron restricted erythropoiesis diagnosis. These tests include reticulocyte hemoglobin content, percentage of hypochromic red cells and soluble transferrin receptor (Wish, 2006; Goodnough *et al.*, 2010).

Serum transferrin receptor (sTfR) is a useful test for this purpose because it is not affected by inflammation so is a reliable marker of iron deficiency in mixed situations (Punnonen *et al.*, 1997; Beguin, 2003; Skikne, 2008).

The sTfR test is based on the fact that erythroblasts in the bone marrow will increase the presentation of membrane transferrin receptor in the setting of iron deficiency. If a patient is not receiving sufficient iron and erythropoiesis is being stimulated by an ESA, then increased transferrin receptors will become expressed on the erythroblasts, some of which come off and will be detectable in the circulation. The sTfR correlates with this membrane expression of the transferrin receptor and also tends to be elevated in the presence of increased erythroid activity. It does seem to be a reasonable index of erythropoietic activity (Chiang *et al.*, 2002; Tarng & Huang, 2002) and reflects the effect of stimulating bone marrow red cells production, before an increase in reticulocytes is noted and well before the Hb rises; therefore an increase in the sTfR may be the first detectable measure. It is not affected by inflammation (Beerenhout *et al.*, 2002) and this reason would make sTfR a more reliable test than serum ferritin.

Direct consequence of an imbalance between the erythroid marrow iron requirements and the actual supply is a reduction of red cell hemoglobin content, which causes hypochromic mature red cells and reticulocytes. Interest has been generated in the use of erythrocyte and reticulocyte parameters, available on the modern analysers based on flow cytometry technology.

The modern hematological parameters contribute to the advanced study of the anemia and depend on the technology employed; the debate about other parameters with the same clinical meaning and potential utility as reticulocyte hemoglobin content and percentage of hypochromic red cells is open.

### 1.3 Technology at a glance

The Hemogram is one of the more required tests by the clinicians; the analysis nowadays is totally automated and the correct interpretation of the results requires to unite the knowledge about the characteristics of the equipment and the clinical meaning of the results. The suppliers contribute innovations, providing new parameters that can help the clinicians to make a diagnosis in a fast, cheap and useful manner (Buttarello & Plebani, 2008).

The professionals of the Clinical Laboratory must obtain the maximum yield of the new technologies obtaining as much information as possible.

Automated blood cell counters have changed substantially during the last 20 years. Technological progress has meant that in recent years modern analyzers, fully automated, have been available. These analyzers report new parameters that provide further information from the traditional count; this information must be evaluated to prove the potential clinical utility in different clinical situations.

When a state of iron deficiency proceeds red blood cells are continuously produced in the bone marrow and as the iron stores progressively decrease, mean cell volume (MCV), mean cell hemoglobin (MCH) and red blood cell count (RBC) count tend to decline. In iron deficient erythropoiesis, synthesis of hemoglobin (Hb) molecules is severely impaired leading to the production of erythrocytes with low Hb concentration (hypochromic cells). Because of their long life span of approximately 3 months, several cohorts of normochromic and increasingly hypochromic red cells coexist in the peripheral blood leading to anisocytosis; red cell distribution width (RDW) reflects the variation of size of the red cells.

Flow cytometry provides information about individual cell characteristics. This is in contrast to previous measurements of MCV, MCH, and MCHC which only calculate mean indices for the total red cell population.

MCV is the mean of the volumes of all erythrocytes; RDW refers to the variety of volumes present in the red cell population, so the whole picture is clear and the contribution of marginal sized subpopulations to the calculated mean value can be assessed.

This is not the case for MHC. MCH is calculated from red blood cell count and hemoglobin and represents the average; the percentage subsets of erythrocytes can give complementary information of the contribution of cell with extreme values (hypochromic and hyperchromic cells) to the mean values, reflecting the fluctuations of iron availability to the erythron in the previous weeks.

Modern counters provide information about the reticulocyte counts but also about the characteristics of these cells (size or hemoglobin content) related to the quality of the erythropoiesis.

Nevertheless, each Company applies the technology in a different way in the analyzers, with different algorithms to translate the electronic signals to graphs and numerical values. For this reason these new parameters are exclusive of each manufacturer and they are patented.

### 1.3.1 Siemens

On last decades, several new red blood cell and reticulocyte parameters have been reported having utilities in detection of iron deficiency and functional iron deficiency. Two of these parameters are hypochromic red cells (referred to as %Hypo) and CHr (reticulocyte hemoglobin content) reported by the Siemens ADVIA 120 hematology analyzer (Thomas & Thomas, 2002).

Reticulocyte hemoglobin content (CHr) and the percentage of hypochromic red blood cells (%Hypo) reflect iron availability and are reliable markers of functional iron deficiency (Cullen *et al.*, 1999).

CHr is defined by the formula (CHr = MCVr X CHCMr), wherein MCVr is the mean reticulocyte cell volume and CHCMr is the mean hemoglobin concentration of reticulocytes, which is obtained by an optical cell-by-cell hemoglobin measurement.

Reticulocytes are immature red blood cells with a life span of only 1 to 2 days. When these are first released from the bone marrow, measurement of their hemoglobin content can provide the amount of iron immediately available for erythropoiesis. A less than normal hemoglobin content in these reticulocytes is an indication of inadequate iron supply relative to demand. The amount of hemoglobin in these reticulocytes also corresponds to the amount of hemoglobin in mature red blood cells. CHr has been evaluated recently in numerous studies as a test for iron deficiency and functional iron deficiency and has been found to be highly sensitive and specific. However, exact threshold values have not been established, as the threshold values vary (28-30 pg), depending on the laboratory and instrument used.

The measurement of CHr is a direct assessment of the incorporation of iron into erythrocyte hemoglobin and thus an estimate of the recent functional availability of iron into the erythron; due to the life span of the reticulocytes CHr is a sensitive indicator of iron deficient erythropoiesis (Fishbane *et al.*, 1997; Mast *et al.*, 2002; Brugnara 2003).

Epoetin is effective in stimulating production, of red blood cells, but without an adequate iron supply to bind to heme, the red blood cells will be hypochromic, i.e., low in hemoglobin content. Thus, in states of iron deficiency, a significant percentage of red blood cells leaving the bone marrow will have a low hemoglobin content. By measuring the percentage of red blood cells with hemoglobin concentration <280 g/L, iron deficiency can be detected.

Hypochromic red cells percentages have been correlated with iron deficiency. %Hypo is reported by Siemens Advia 120 hematology analyzer based on the optical cell-by-cell hemoglobin measurement (Figures 2 and 3).

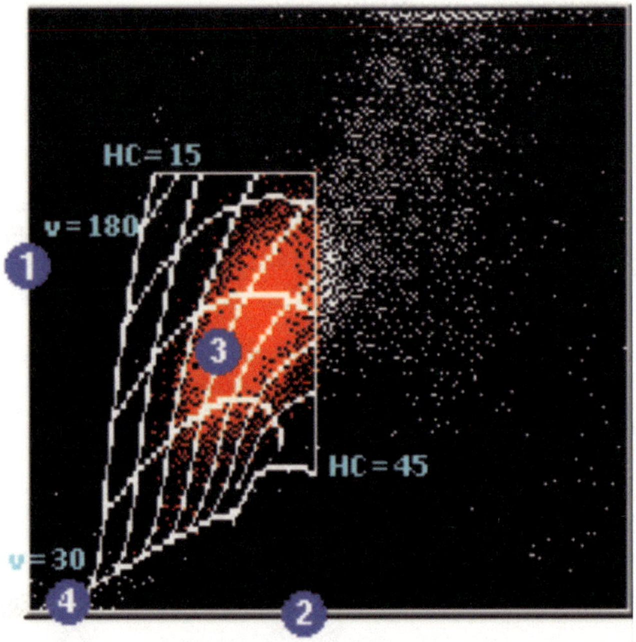


Fig. 2. RBC Scatter Cytogram.

1. Low-angle light scatter (2° to 3°)
2. High-angle light scatter (5° to 15°)
3. Mie map containing RBCs
4. Platelets detected in RBC method

The RBC Scatter cytogram is the graphical representation of two light-scatter measurements: the high-angle light scatter (5° to 15°) is plotted along the x axis, and the low-angle light scatter (2° to 3°) is plotted along the y axis. (Figure 2).

The RBC map shows the relationship between the light-scatter measurements and the cell-by-cell characteristics of volume and hemoglobin concentration. The map grid encompasses RBC volumes between 30 fL and 180 fL and hemoglobin concentrations between 190 g/L and 490 g/L. (Figure 3).

The measurement of %Hypo (defined as the percentage of red blood cells with Hb concentration less than 280 g/L) is a sensitive method for quantifying the hemoglobinization of mature red cells. Because of the long circulating life span of mature erythrocytes %Hypo values are related to iron status in the last 2-3 months, and have been recognised as an indicator of iron deficiency (Macdougal 1998; Bovy *et al.*, 2005; Bovy *et al.*, 2007). %Hypo < 5% is considered normal. Two different criteria, more specifically, %Hypo >5% and >10% have been used. %Hypo >10% has been more commonly used for defining absolute iron deficiency and functional iron deficiency (Locatelli *et al.*, 2004).

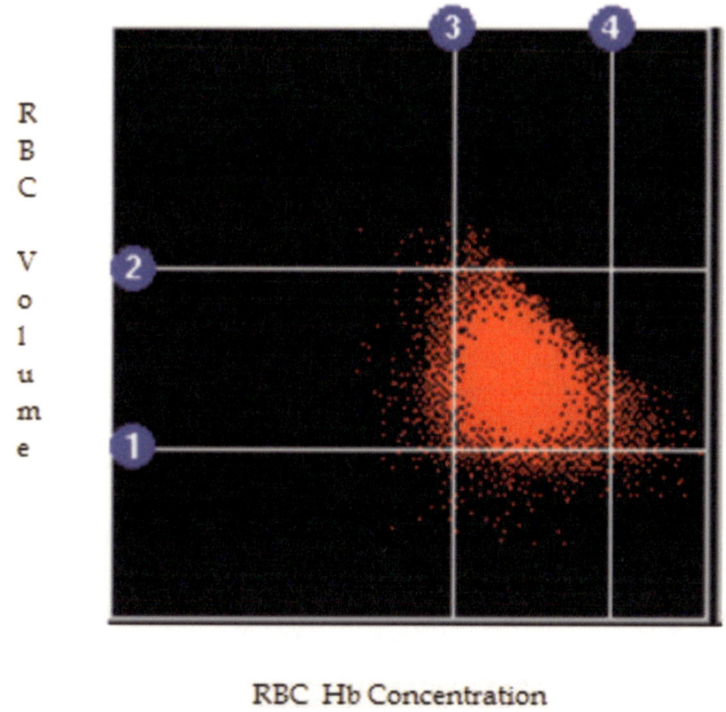


Fig. 3. Volume/Hemoglobin Concentration (V/HC) cytogram (Mie Map) is a linear version of the RBC scatter cytogram. Hemoglobin concentration is plotted along the x axis and cell volume is plotted along the y axis. Only red blood cells appear on this cytogram.
Markers organize the cytogram into 9 distinct areas of red blood cell morphology.
On the x axis, hemoglobin concentration markers are set at 280 g/L (3) and 410 g/L (4).
Red blood cells with a hemoglobin concentration less than 280 g/L are hypochromic, while cells with a hemoglobin concentration greater than 410 g/L are hyperchromic.
On the y axis, RBC volume markers are set at 60 fL (1) and 120 fL (2).
Red blood cells with a volume less than 60 fL are microcytic, while cells with a volume greater than 120 fL are macrocytic.

CHr and %Hypo have been used as a diagnostic tool, together with biochemical markers, to distinguish IDA from ACD, and are incorporated to the guidelines for the monitoring of recombinant human erythropoietin rHuEpo therapy (Macdougall *et al.*, 2000; Kotisaari 2002; Locateli *et al.*, 2004).

### 1.3.2 Sysmex

Sysmex XE analyzers (Sysmex Corporation, Kobe, Japan) employ flow cytometry technology. In the reticulocyte channel blood cells are stained by a polymethine dye, specific for RNA/DNA, and analysed by flow cytometry using a semiconductor laser. A bi-dimensional distribution of forward scattered light and fluorescence is presented as a scattergram, indicating mature red cells and reticulocytes (Figure 4).

Forward scatter correlates with erythrocyte and reticulocyte hemoglobin content (Ret He, RBC He).

Ret He is the mean value of the forward light scatter histogram within the reticulocyte population obtained in a reticulocyte channel on the Sysmex XE-2100 hematology analyzer. Measurements of Ret He provides useful information in diagnosing anemia, iron restricted erythropoiesis and functional iron deficiency and response to iron therapy during r-HuEpo (Buttarello *et al*, 2004; Canals *et al*, 2005; Brugnara *et al*, 2006; Thomas *et al*, 2006; Garzia *et al.*, 2007).

Ret He, generated by all Sysmex XE analysers (Sysmex Corporation, Kobe, Japan), has been recognised as a direct assessment of the incorporation of iron into erythrocyte hemoglobin and a direct estimate of the recent functional availability of iron into the erythron, thus provides the same information as CHr (Thomas *et al.*, 2005; David *et al.*, 2006). Twenty nine pg is the cut off value that defines deficient erythropoiesis Several studies have demonstrated that Ret He and CHr have the same clinical meaning (Mast *et al*, 2008; Maconi *et al.*, 2009; Miwa *et al.*, 2010).

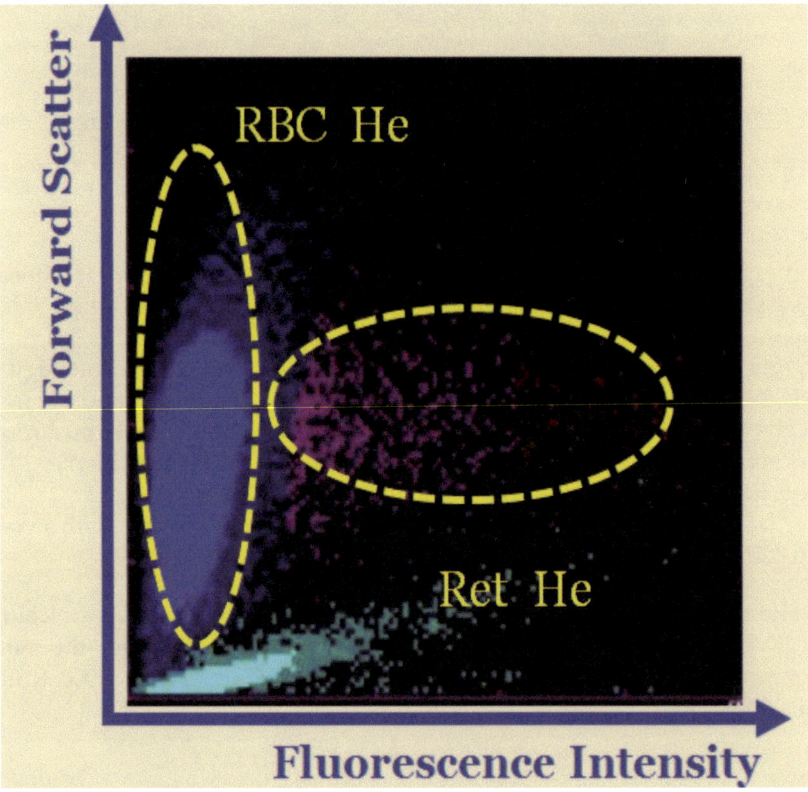


Fig. 4. In the reticulocyte channel blood cells are stained by a polymethine dye, specific for RNA/DNA, and analysed by flow cytometry using a semiconductor laser. A bi-dimensional distribution of forward scattered light and fluorescence is presented as a scattergram, indicating mature red cells and reticulocytes. Forward scatter correlates with erythrocyte and reticulocyte hemoglobin content (RBC He, Ret He).

The Sysmex XE 5000 analyzer incorporates flow fluorescence cytometry technology, which enables independent measurement of the volume and hemoglobin content of individual red cells. Derived from this technology four new RBC extended parameters or erythrocyte subsets are now available in this analyzer.

%Hypo-He indicates the percentage of hypochromic red cells with a Hb content < 17 pg.
%Hyper-He indicates the percentage of hyperchromic red cells with a Hb content > 49 pg.
%Micro R indicates the percentage of microcytic red cells with a volume less than 60 fL.
%Macro R indicates the percentage of macrocytic red cells with a volume greater than 120 fL.

The new Symex XE 5000 analyzer reports the percentages of hypochromic red cells; the reference range and the values in different types of anemia have been published (Urrechaga *et al.*, 2009).

%Hypo-He indicates the percentage of hypochromic red cells with an Hb content equivalent to less than 17pg. Recent studies confirm the clinical reliability of the hypochromic red cells, reported by the Sysmex XE 5000 counter, as markers of iron deficiency in hemodialysis patients; 2.7 % is the cut off value which defines iron deficiency (Buttarello *et al.*, 2010).

Figure 5 shows s a scattergram of the reticulocyte channel.

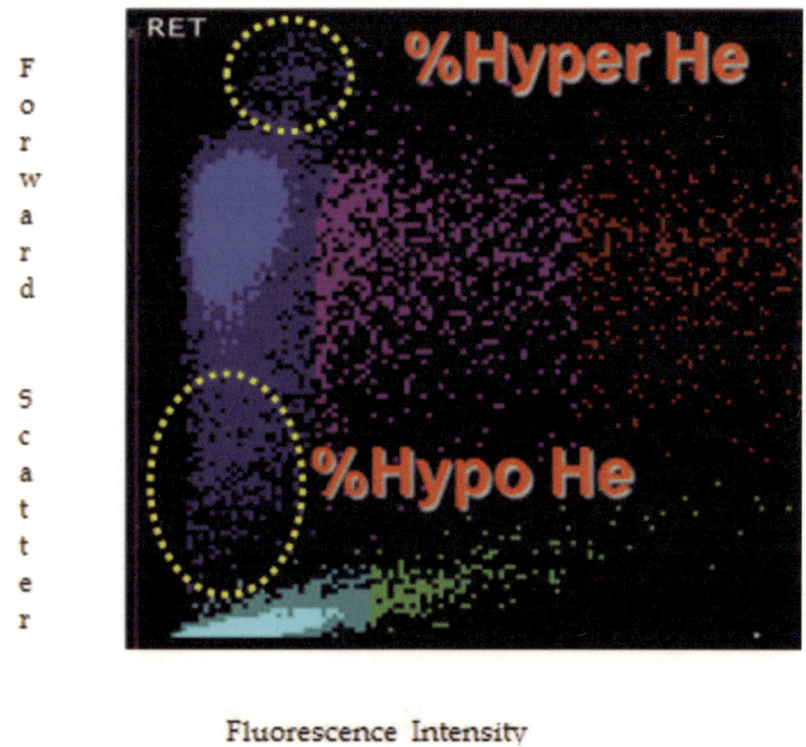


Fig. 5. A bi-dimensional distribution of forward scattered light and fluorescence is presented as a scattergram, indicating mature red cells and reticulocytes. Forward scatter correlates with the hemoglobin content. A new algorithm divides the RBC He signal in three areas.

The percentages of red cells subsets can be calculated and the new parameters %Hypo-He and %Hyper-He obtained.

%Hypo-He indicates the percentage of hypochromic red cells with a Hb content < 17 pg.
%Hyper-He indicates the percentage of hyperchromic red cells with a Hb content > 49 pg.

### 1.3.3 Beckman-Coulter

The percentage of hypochromic red cells are only available on Siemens analyzers (Siemens Medical Solutions Diagnostics, Tarrytown N.Y., USA) and on the new Sysmex analyzer XE 5000 (Sysmex Corporation, Kobe, Japan); this fact limits its generalized use. Beckman Coulter (Beckman Coulter Inc. Miami, Fl, USA) applies the Volume Conductivity Scatter technology to this field and new parameters are now available on the LH series analyzers.

Low hemoglobin density (LHD %) derives from the traditional mean cell hemoglobin concentration (MCHC), using the mathematical sigmoid transformation

$$\text{LHD}\,\% = 100 \times \sqrt{1 - \left[1/\left(1 + \text{e}\,1.8\,(30 - \text{MCHC})\right)\right]}$$

MCHC is an all inclusive measure of both the availability of iron over the preceding 90–120 days, and of the proper introduction of iron into intracellular hemoglobin. In the same way LHD% is related to iron availability and the hemoglobin concentration of the mature red cells. In this equation defining LHD %, in addition to the standard sigmoid function, a square root is applied to further enhance numerical resolution in the region corresponding to the lower end, to improve the differentiation between the normal and the abnormal among the blood samples having relatively low values of LHD %.

The reference range for LHD % and the values in normal population and different types of anemia have been established (Urrechaga, 2010). Then a study was conducted to investigate its clinical usefulness in the assessment of iron status in terms of correlation with %Hypo (Urrechaga *et al.*, 2010) and sTfR (Urrechaga *et al.*, 2011).

Cells are identified and classified by simultaneous three-dimensional analysis using Volume, Conductivity, and Light Scatter (Figure 6). Volume, as measured by direct current, is used to identify the size of the cell. Conductivity, or radio frequency measurements, provides information about the internal characteristics of the cell. Light scatter measurements, obtained as cells pass through the helium-neon laser beam, provide information about cell surface characteristics and cell granularity.

## 2. Materials and methods

### 2.1 Criteria for selecting the groups of patients

Samples from 120 healthy individuals, 72 iron deficiency anemia (IDA), 60 IDA with acute phase response (IDA APR), 71 chronic kidney disease (CKD) and 58 anemia of chronic disease (ACD) were randomly extracted from the routine workload and run sequentially on both LH 750 (Beckman Coulter Inc. Miami, Fl, USA) and Advia 2120 (Siemens Medical Solutions Diagnostics, Tarrytown N.Y., USA) analyzers within 6 hours of collection.

Healthy group: 54 male and 66 female adult subjects, with no clinical symptoms of disease and with results of the complete blood count and biochemical iron metabolism markers within reference ranges.

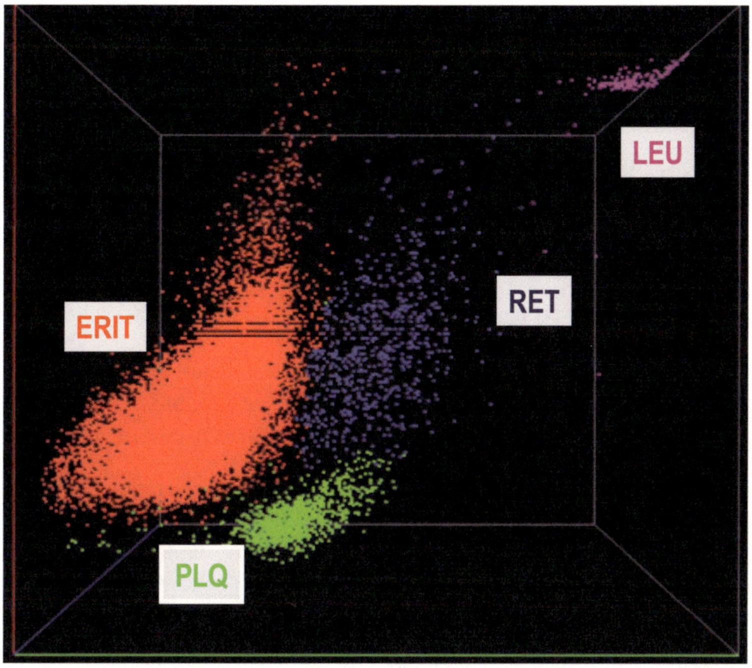


Fig. 6. the Beckman -Coulter cube in which the cells are classified according to the volume, conductivity and laser scatter signals. ERIT , erythrocytes; PLQ, platelets; RET, reticulocytes; LEU, leucocytes.

A group of 132 IDA patients fulfilled traditional diagnostic criteria for iron deficiency anemia diagnosis, serum iron < 7.5 µmol/L, transferrin saturation < 20 %, ferritin < 50 µg/L, and Hb < 110 g/L (Cook, 2005), were included before iron treatment. This group was divided into a non acute phase response group (n=72, CRP < 5 mg/L) and acute phase response group (n=60, CRP > 5 mg/L). Acute phase response included inflammation or infectious conditions, in addition to ferropenic status.

CKD patients were managed according to the recommendations of the NKF-K/DOQI guidelines (Locatelli *et al.*, 2004). All patients were treated with a variety of erythropoietin doses, the majority of them were treated with a maintenance dose of intravenous iron weekly, in order to maintain Hb at the recommended level 110 - 120 g/L.

ACD group included patients with a variety of diseases: chronic infections (tuberculosis); neoplasic disorders (Hodgkin's disease, breast carcinoma); non infectious inflammatory diseases (rheumatoid arthritis, systemic lupus erythematosus). ACD patients received treatment to maintain normal erythropoiesis and presented the traditional diagnostic criteria for 'Functional iron-deficiency' diagnosis Transferrin saturation < 20%, Hb < 110 g/L and serum ferritin values normal or over the reference range (Weiss & Goodnough, 2005).

In a second phase of the study ACD group was extended to 85 patients. This group was further subdivided based on sTfR levels. ACD patients with sTfR higher than 21 nmol/L were considered to have storage iron depletion (iron deficiency associated, n=24) and patients with normal sTfR were considered to have functional iron deficiency (n=61).

sTfR was measured with Access sTfR assay in the Access immunochemical analyzer (Beckman Coulter Inc., Miami Fl, USA).

### 2.2 Statistical evaluation of analytical results

Statistical software package SPSS (SPSS; Chicago, IL, USA) version 17.0 for Windows was applied for statistical analysis of the results.

Reference ranges were calculated from the results obtained in the group of healthy subjects (95 central percentiles of the distribution). Kolmogorov - Smirnoff test was applied to verify the Gaussian distribution of LHD% values.

When the parameters under study presented a non Gaussian distribution non parametric tests were applied. Correlation coefficients were calculated by Spearman method; independent samples Mann-Whitney U test was performed; p values less than 0.05 were considered to be statistically significant.

Receiver operating characteristic (ROC) curve analysis was utilized to illustrate the diagnostic performance of LHD% and other Laboratory tests in the detection of iron deficiency status; two analysis were performed; first iron deficiency was defined by %Hypo > 5 %, and second , including 85 ACD patients, the gold standard was sTfR > 21 nmol/L.

Cut off values were established based on the optimal combination of sensitivity and specificity.

Cohen's Kappa Index of Inter-rater Reliability (κ index) was calculated to determine the concordance between LHD% and sTrR.

κ has a range from 0-1.0, the larger values indicate better reliability; κ > 0.7 is considered satisfactory.

| | RBC $10^{12}$/L | Hb g/L | MCV fL | MCH pg | MCHC g/L | Iron µmol/L | Transf g/L | Ferritin µg/L | Sat % |
|---|---|---|---|---|---|---|---|---|---|
| Healtł | 4.9 (0.27) | 154 (6.4) | 91.1 (2.55) | 31.3 (1.53) | 343 (5.2) | 16.5 (0.62) | 2.53 (0.2) | 75 (2.8) | 31 (1.9) |
| IDA | 4.6 (0.61) | 95 (14.2) | 70 (10.3) | 22.5 (4.23) | 320 (17.3) | 4.8 (2.15) | 3.31 (0.53) | 14 (9) | 6 (3.6) |
| IDA APR | 4.4 (0.43) | 96 (12.1) | 75.8 (3.7) | 21.5 (1.3) | 327 (9.2) | 5.1 (3.5) | 2.78 (0.28) | 37 (25) | 9 (5.6) |
| ACD | 3.5 (0.48) | 101 (11) | 93.2 (6.0) | 31.9 (2.23) | 343 (10) | 10.0 (6.8) | 2.68 (0.66) | 522 (704) | 15 (5) |
| CKD | 3.5 (0.45) | 112 (8.5) | 95.6 (6.67) | 31.1 (2.23) | 325 (8) | 9.8 (4.47) | 1.87 (0.43) | 335 (204) | 21 (10) |

Table 1. shows the hematological and biochemical data, mean and (standard deviation), of the different groups. 120 healthy individuals, 72 iron deficiency anemia (IDA), 60 IDA with acute phase response (IDA APR), 71 chronic kidney disease (CKD) and 58 anemia of chronic disease (ACD).

RBC, red blood cells; Hb, hemoglobin; MCV, mean cell volume; MCH, mean cell hemoglobin; MCHC, mean cell hemoglobin concentration; Transf, transferrin; Sat, % transferrin saturation.

## 3. Results

Table 1 shows the hematological and biochemical data, mean and (standard deviation). The parameters presented are of general use for every Laboratory in the evaluation of anemia.

The patients included in the study sufferered common clinical situations in our daily practice: anemia of chronic disease (ACD), chronic kidney disease (CKD), iron deficiency anemia (IDA) iron deficiency anemia and acute phase response (IDA APR)

The healthy group was recruited to assess the reference range for the new parameter LHD %.

LHD % values in a population of 120 healthy adult subjects were not normally distributed and showed a non Gaussian distribution (Kolmogorov-Smirnoff test, p=0.034; figure 7). Reference range 0 - 4.4 %.

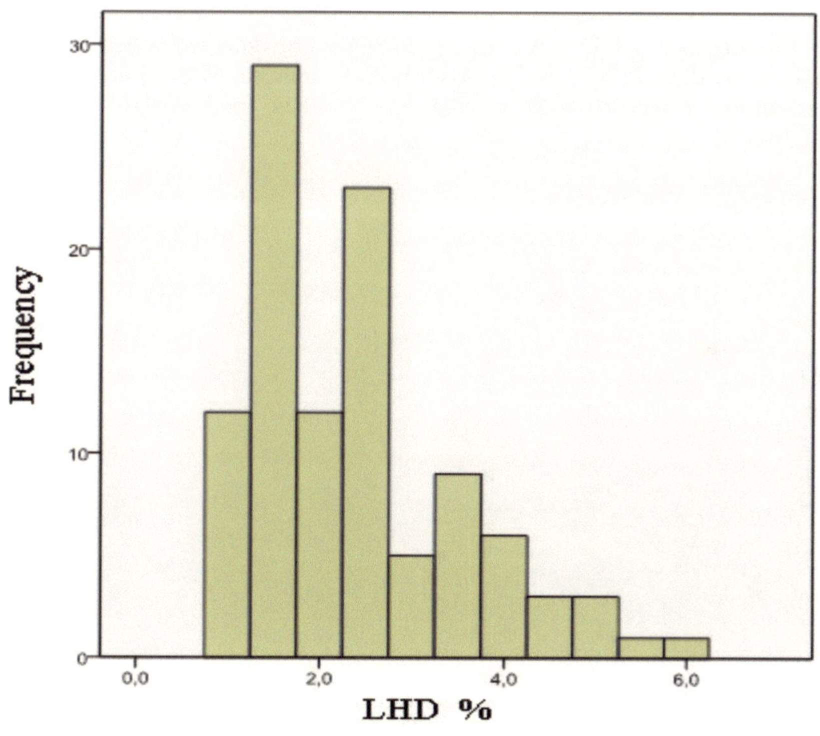


Fig. 7. Low hemoglobin density (LHD %) values in a population of 120 healthy adult subjects. The values showed a non Gaussian distribution (Kolmogorov-Smirnoff test, p=0.034).

Table 2 exhibits %Hypo values, mean and standard deviation (SD) and LHD % values, median and 5th - 95th interquartiles (IQ), in the variety of anemias and healthy subjects included in the study.

| | % Hypo<br>Mean (SD) | LHD %<br>Median (IQ) |
|---|---|---|
| Healthy | 0.13 (0.15) | 2.1 (0.9-4.1) |
| IDA | 17.2 (17.4) | 29.6 (7.5-76) |
| IDA APR | 16.8 (15.5) | 27.3 (8.3-71.2) |
| ACD | 4.1 (4.4) | 7.3 (5.1-30) |
| CKD | 5.1 (6.7) | 9.6 (5.6-27) |

Table 2. %Hypo values, mean and standard deviation (SD) and LHD % values, median and 5th - 95th interquartiles (IQ), in the variety of anemias and healthy subjects included in the study.

IDA, iron deficiency anemia; IDA APR, iron deficiency anemia and acute phase response; ACD, anemia of chronic disease; CKD, chronic kidney disease.

Correlation between %Hypo and LHD% values, $r = 0.869$ (Spearman method) ($p<0.001$). $y = 1.338\,x + 4.40$ (Figure 8).

Independent samples U test was performed in order to detect statistical deviations between the groups of patients.

Significant differences in LHD % values ($p<0.001$) were detected when groups with iron deficiency (IDA, median 29.6 % and IDA with APR, median 27.3 %) were compared with patients undergoing therapy (ACD, median 7.3 %; CKD, median 9.6 %) and the healthy subjects (median 2.1 %).

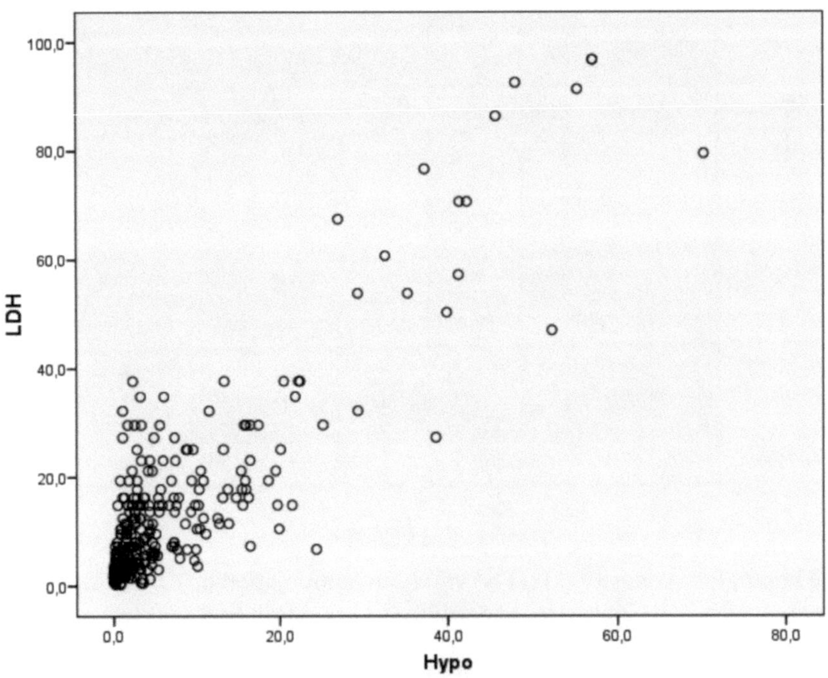


Fig. 8. Relationship between %Hypo and LHD% values (Spearman correlation) $r = 0.869$ $y = 1.338\,x + 4.4$.

No statistic difference was found between IDA group and IDA patients with acute phase response (p=0.578).

Receiver operating characteristic (ROC) curve analysis for LHD% in the diagnosis of iron deficiency, defined by %Hypo > 5% AUC 0.954, cut off 6.0 %, sensitivity 96.6%, specificity 83.3% (Figure 9).

Discriminant efficiency of biochemical parameters and classical erythrocyte indices: mean cell hemoglobin (MCH), AUC 0.89; mean cell volume, (MCV), AUC 0.822; serum ferritin, AUC 0.722; serum iron, AUC 0.683 (Figure 9).

In the group including 85 ACD patients, significant differences were detected when iron replete ACD patients (LHD% 10.5 %) were compared to the group with both ACD and IDA (LHD% 24.1 %, p<0.0001).

Table 3 exhibits sTfR values, mean and standard deviation (SD) and LHD % values, median and 5th - 95th interquartiles in these patients.

ROC analysis for LHD% in the detection of iron deficiency rendered area under curve (AUC) 0.903; at a threshold value 5.5 % sensitivity was 88.6 % and specificity 76.9 %. The ferropenic state was defined by a sTfR > 21 nmol/L.

Using the cut off 5.5 % for LHD% the k index obtained in comparison to sTfR was 0.65.

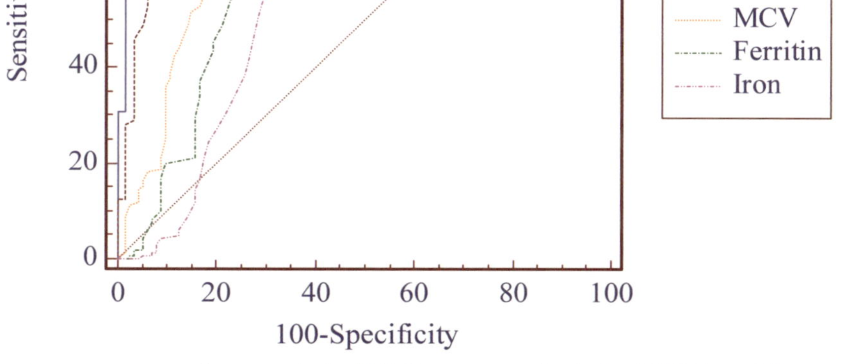


Fig. 9. Receiver operating characteristic (ROC) curve analysis for LHD% and Biochemical parameters and classical erythrocyte indices in the diagnosis of iron deficiency, defined by %Hypo >5%. LHD% Ares under curve (AUC) 0.954; mean cell hemoglobin (MCH), AUC 0.89; mean cell volume, (MCV), AUC 0.822; serum ferritin, AUC 0.722; serum iron, AUC 0.683.

| | Healthy | ACD | ACD/ IDA | ACD/ Iron replete |
|---|---|---|---|---|
| LHD% | 2.1<br>(0.9-4.1) | 14.2<br>(4.5-68.9) | 24.1<br>(5.1-68.9) | 10.5<br>(4.5-14.0) |
| sTfR (nmol/L) | 15.1<br>(2) | 20.3<br>(6.6) | 30.8<br>(8.3) | 17.9<br>(6.1) |

Table 3. sTfR values, mean and standard deviation (SD) and LHD % values, median and $5^{th}$ - $95^{th}$ interquartiles in a group of 120 healthy subjects, 85 anemia of chronic disease patients (ACD), 61 of them iron replete and 24 iron deficient (ACD/IDA).

## 4. Discussion

CKD is a widespread health problem in the world and anemia is a common complication. Anemia conveys significant risk for cardiovascular disease, faster progression of renal failure and decreased quality of life.

Ferrokinetic studies provided on last decades important insights into human iron homeostasis in vivo. More recently, modern molecular biology and genetic studies of model organisms have extended our knowledge of normal iron biology and led to the identification of new key players in iron homeostasis and the detailed understanding of human iron disorders.

New insights in iron metabolism and the understanding of iron homeostasis, erythropoietin production and regulation and the relationships between mediators of inflammation and bone marrow erythropoiesis are modifying the traditional view on anemia, in special anemia of chronic disease. The anemia of CKD is among them, with the added burden of erythropoietin deficiency. Recent elucidations of specifically disrupted points of erythroid marrow function by inflammatory mediators, especially proinflammatory cytokines and inflammation-mediated induction of hepcidin, have improved our understanding of erythropoiesis-stimulating agents (ESAs) hyporesponsiveness.

These patients require a thorough evaluation to identify and correct causes of anemia other than erythropoietin deficiency. The mainstay of treatment of anemia secondary to CKD has become ESAs. The use of ESAs does carry risks and these agents need to be used judiciously. Iron deficiency often co-exists in this population and must be evaluated and treated. Correction of iron deficiency can improve anemia and reduce ESA requirements. Partial, but not complete, correction of anemia is associated with improved outcomes in patients with CKD.

Undoubtedly, the advent of ESA and various intravenous iron preparations has resulted in a much more effective management of anemia of CKD, allowing clinicians to maintain hemoglobin levels in certain desired ranges and to effectively treat iron deficiency. Among the emerging challenges are the risks associated with administering high ESA and iron doses, leading to elevated hemoglobin levels and iron overload. Goal-oriented treatment strategies targeting "desirable" hemoglobin and iron levels are now the norm in clinical nephrology.

The treatment of renal anemia with rHuEpo has improved the quality of life and outcome of hemodialysis patients. The efficacy of this therapy depends on the identification and correction of resistance factors, such as vitamin deficiency, inflammation, hyperparathyroidism. The major cause of resistance to rHuEpo is iron deficiency. The assessment of functional iron deficiency remains a daily challenge for nephrologists and their need to be careful of an appropriate use of the resources and the need to optimize patient treatment.

A better understanding of iron homeostasis enhance treatments for anemia. Subsequently, evidence-based diagnostic strategies must be developed, using both conventional and innovative laboratory tests, to differentiate between the various causes of distortions of iron metabolism.

Efforts have been made to evaluate some readily available and relatively inexpensive laboratory parameters as indirect markers of iron restricted erythropoiesis and iron availability in a clinical context influenced by inflammation and acute phase reaction.

The assessment of iron requirements and monitoring of therapy require accurate markers. It is desirable to seek alternative markers for iron status widely available. LHD% is related to iron availability for erythropoiesis in the previous weeks, derived from MCHC, it could be calculated in different hematological counters.

The data exposed show the reliability of LHD% in distinguishing iron deficient patients with and without inflammation. This parameter could help to the correct classification of patients with iron deficiency when the traditional markers become unreliable: it is particularly challenging the accurate assessment of iron status in chronically ill patients such as CKD.

LHD % correlates with the percentage of hypochromic erythrocytes as reported by Siemens analyzers (%Hypo) and comparing the results obtained for LHD% with those of sTfR the reliability of LHD% in distinguishing iron deficient patients with and without inflammation has been stated.

In conclusion, these results show that the new LHD% parameter is useful for diagnosing iron deficiency and a reliable parameter recognizing subsets of patients and therefore improving the diagnosis and management of anemia.The analysis of LHD% can be performed simultaneously in the course of routine blood counts, with no incremental costs and no additional needs of more blood sampling. In conjunction with standard blood cell counts and iron parameters could enable the diagnosis to be made rapid and accurately.

More prospective and longitudinal studies are needed in order to verify the results obtained, to determine their reliability for clinical purposes or whether the additional information provided could be used in managing the iron requirements of patients in different clinical situations.

## 5. Conclusion

Iron metabolism is a dynamic process which cannot be defined by one laboratory test only. The analysis of these new parameters can be performed simultaneously in the course of routine blood counts, with no incremental costs and no additional needs of more blood sampling. In conjunction with standard blood cell counts and iron parameters could enable the diagnosis to be made rapid and accurately.

Prospective and longitudinal studies are needed in order to verify the published results, to determine their reliability for clinical purposes or whether the additional information provided could be used in managing the iron requirements of patients, allowing better evaluation of the causes underlying apparently similar conditions of anemia and improving the collaboration between laboratory professionals and clinicians.

## 6. References


Beaumont, C. & Delaby, C. (2009). Recycling iron in normal and pathological states. *Seminars in Hematology* 46, 328-338.

Beerenhout, C., Bekers, O., Kooman, J.P., van der Sande, F.M. & Leunissen, K.M. (2002). A comparison between the soluble transferrin receptor, transferrin saturation and serum ferritin as markers of iron state in hemodialysis patients. *Nephron* 92, 32-35.

Beguin, Y. (2003). Soluble transferrin receptor for the evaluation of erythropoiesis and iron status. *Clinica Chimica Acta* 329, 9-22.

Bergamaschi, G. & Villani, L. (2009). Serum hepcidin: a novel diagnostic tool in disorders of iron metabolism *Haematologica* 94, 1631-1633.

Bovy, C., Gothot, A., Krzesinski, J.M., & Beguin, Y. (2005). Mature erythrocyte indices: new markers of iron availability. *Haematologica* 90, 549-551.

Bovy, C., Gothot, A., Delanaye, P., Warling, X., Krzesinski, J.M., & Beguin, Y. (2007). Mature erythrocyte parameters as new markers of functional iron deficiency in hemodialysis: sensitivity and specificity. *Nephrology Dialysis Transplantation* 22(1), 1156-1162.

Brugnara, C. (2003). Iron deficiency and erythropoiesis: New diagnostic approaches. *Clinical Chemistry* 49, 1573-1578.

Brugnara, C., Schiller, B., & Moran, J. (2006). Ret He and assessment of iron deficient states. *Clinical and Laboratory Haematology* 28(5), 303-308.

Buttarello, M., Temporin, V., Ceravolo, R., Farina, G. & Burian, P. (2004). The new reticulocyte parameter RET Y of the Sysmex XE 2100. Its use in the diagnosis and monitoring of post treatment sideropenic anemia. *American Journal of Clinical Pathology* 121, 489-495.

Buttarello, M., Plebani, M. (2008). Automated blood cell counts. State of the art. *American Journal of Clinical Pathology* 130, 104-116.

Buttarello, M., Pajola, R., Novello, E., Robeschini, M., Cantaro, S., Oliosi, F., Naso, A., & Plebani, M. (2010). Diagnosis of iron deficiency diagnosis of iron deficiency in patients undergoing hemodialysis. *American Journal of Clinical Pathology* 133, 949-954.

Canals, C., Remacha, A.F., Sarda, M.P., Piazuelo, J.M., Royo, M.T., & Romero, M.A. (2005). Clinical utility of the new Sysmex XE 2100 parameter - reticulocyte hemoglobin equivalent in the diagnosis of anemia. *Haematologica* 90, 1133-1134.

Cavill, I., & Macdougall, I.C. (1993). Functional iron deficiency. *Blood* 82, 1377.

Chiang, W.C., Tsai, T.J., Chen, Y.M., Lin, S.L. & Hsieh, B.S. (2002). Serum soluble transferrin receptor reflects erythropoiesis but not iron availability in erythropoietin-treated chronic hemodialysis patients. *Clinical Nephrology 58, 363-* 369.

Conrad, M.E. & Umbreit , J.N. (2002). Pathways of iron absorption. *Blood Cells Molecular Disorders* 29, 336-355.

Coyne, D. (2006). Iron indices: what do they really mean? *Kidney International* Supp 101, S4-8.

Cullen, P., Söffker, J., Höpfl, M., Bremer, c., Schlaghecken, R., Mehrens, T., Assmann, G., & Schaefer, R.M. (1999). Hypochromic red cells and reticulocyte haemglobin content as markers of iron-deficient erythropoiesis in patients undergoing chronic haemodialysis. *Nephrology Dialysis Transplantation* 14, 659-665.

David, O., Grillo, A., Ceoloni, B., Cavallo, F., Podda, G., Biancotti, P.P., Bergamo, D., & Canavese, C. (2006). Analysis of red cell parameters on the Sysmex XE 2100 and Advia 120 in iron deficiency and in uraemic chronic disease. *Scandinavian Journal of Clinical and Laboratory Investigation* 66, 113-120.

Eknoyan G, *et al.* (2001). Continuous quality improvement: DOQI becomes K/DOQI and is updated. National Kidney Foundation's Dialysis Outcomes Quality Initiative. *American Journal of Kidney Disease* 37(1), 179-194.

Eknoyan, G., Lameire, N., Barsoum, R., Eckardt, K., Levin, A., Levin, N., *et al.* (2004). The burden of kidney disease: improving global outcomes. *Kidney International* 66, 1310–1314.

Eschbach, J.W., Downing, M.R., Egrie, J.C., Browne, J.K., & Adamson, J.W. (1989). USA multicenter clinical trial with recombinant human erythropoietin. *Contributions to Nephrology* 76, 160-165.

Fishbane, S., Imbriano, L.J., Kowalski, E.A., & Maesaka, J.K. (1996). The evaluation of iron status in patients receiving recombinant human erythropoietin. *Journal of the American Society of Nephrology* 7, 654-657.

Fishbane, S., Galgano, C., Langley, R.C. Jr, Canfield, W., & Maesaka, J.K. (1997). Reticulocyte hemoglobin content in the evaluation of iron status of hemodialysis patients. *Kidney International* 52, 217-222.

Fleming, R.E. & Bacon, B.R. (2005). Orchestration of iron homeostasis. *New England Journal of Medicine* 352, 1741-1744.

Ganz, T. & Nemeth, E. (2009). Iron sequestration and Anemia of Inflammation. *Seminars in Hematology* 46, 387-393.

Garzia, M., Di Mario, A., Ferraro, E., Tazza, L., Rossi, E., Luciani, G., & Zini, G. (2007). Reticulocyte Hemoglobin Equivalent: an indicator of reduced iron availability in chronic kidney diseases during erythropoietin therapy. *Laboratory Haematology* 13, 6-11.

Goodnough, L.T., Nemeth, E., & Ganz, T. (2010). Detection, evaluation and management of iron-restricted erythropoiesis. *Blood* 116, 4754-4761.

Guidi, G.C., & Santonastaso, C.L. (2010). Advancements in anemias related to chronic conditions. *Clinical Chemistry and Laboratory Medicine* 48, 1217-1226.

Kemna, E.H.J.M., Tjalsma, H., Willems, H.L. & Swinkels, D.W. (2008). Hepcidin: from discovery to differential diagnosis. *Haematologica* 93(1), 90-97.

Kletzmayr, J., Sunder-Plassmann, G., & Hörl, W.H. (2002). High dose intravenous iron: a note of caution. *Nephrology Dialysis Transplantation* 17, 962-965.

Knutson, M.D., Oukka, M., Koss, L.M. *et al.* (2005). Iron release from macrophages after erythrophagocytosis is up-regulated by ferroportin 1 overexpression and down-regulated by hepcidin. *Proceedings of the Academy of Natural Sciences USA* 102, 1324-1328.

Kotisaari, S., Romppanen, J., Penttila, I., & Punnonen, K. (2002). The Advia 120 red blood cell and reticulocyte indices are useful in diagnosis of iron-deficiency anemia. *European Journal of Hematology* 68, 150-156.

Lang, K.S., Lang, P.A. & Bauer, C. (2005). Mechanisms of suicidal erythrocyte death. Cell Physiology and Biochemistry 15,195-202.

Lankhorst, C.E., & Wish, J.B. (2010). Anemia in renal disease: diagnosis and management. *Blood Reviews* 24, 39–47.

Locateli, F., Aljama, P., Barany, P., Canaud, B., Carrera, F., Eckardt, K., Horl, W.H., MacDougall, I.C., MacLeod, A., Wiecek, A., & Cameron, S. (2004). European Best Practice Guidelines Working Group. Revised European best practice guidelines for the management of anaemia in patients with chronic renal failure. *Nephrology Dialysis Transplantation* 19 (suppl 2), 1-47.

Macdougall, I.C. (1995). Poor response to EPO: practical guidelines on investigation and management. *Nephrology Dialysis Transplantation* 10, 607-614.

Macdougall, I.C. (1998). Merits of hypochromic red cells as a marker of functional iron deficiency. *Nephrology Dialysis Transplantation* 13, 847-849.

Macdougall, I.C., Horl, W.H., Jacobs, C., Valderrabano, F., Parrondo, I., Thompson, K., & Cremers, S. (2000). European best practice guidelines 6–8: assessing and optimizing iron stores. *Nephrology Dialysis Transplantion* 15, 20-32.

Maconi, M., Cavalca, I., Danise, P., Cardarelli, F., & Brini, M. (2009). Erythrocyte and reticulocyte indices in chronic kidney diseases: comparison of two methods. *Scandinavian Journal of Clinical and Laboratory Investigation* 69, 365-370.

Mast, A. (2001). The clinical utility of peripheral blood tests in the diagnosis of iron deficiency anemia. *Bloodline* 1, 7-9.

Mast ,A.E., Blinder, M.A., Lu, Q., Flax, S., & Dietzen, D.J. (2002). Clinical utility of the reticulocyte hemoglobin content in the diagnosis of iron deficiency. *Blood* 99, 1489-1491.

Mast, A.E., Blinder, M.A., & Dietzen, D.J. (2008). Reticulocyte haemoglobin content. *American Journal of Hematology* 83(4), 307-310.

Miret, S., Simpson, R.J. & McKie, A.T. (2003). Physiology and molecular biology of dietary iron absorption. *Annu Rev Nutr.* 23, 283-301.

Miwa, N., Akiba, T., Kimata, N., Hamaguchi, Y., Arakawa, Y., Tamura, T., Nitta, K., & Tsuchiya, K. (2010). Usefulness of measuring reticulocyte hemoglobin equivalent in the management of haemodialysis patients with iron deficiency. *International Journal of Laboratory Hematology* 32, 248-255.

Nemeth, E., Tuttle, M.S., Powelson, J., Vaughn, M.B., Donovan, A., Ward, D.M., Ganz, T. & Kaplan, J. (2004). Hepcidin regulates cellular iron efflux by binding to ferroportin and inducing its internalization. *Science* 306, 2090-2093.

Ponka, P., Beaumont, C. & Richardson, D.R. (1998). Function and regulation of transferrin and ferritin. *Seminars in Hematology* 35, 35-54.

Punnonen, K., Irjala, K., & Rajamaki, A. (1997). Serum transferrin receptor and its ratio to serum ferritin in the diagnosis of iron deficiency. *Blood* 89, 1052-1057.

Skikne, B.S. (2008). Serum transferrin receptor. *American Journal of Hematology* 83, 872-875.

Sunder-Plassmann, G., Spitzauer, S., & Hörl, W.H. (1997). The dilemma of evaluating iron status in dialysis patients - limitations of available diagnostic procedure. *Nephrology Dialysis Transplantation* 12, 1575-1580.

Swinkels, D.W., Janssen, M.C.H., Bergmans, J. & Marx, J.J.M. (2006). Herediatary hemochromatosis: genetic complexity and new diagnostics approaches. *Clinical Chemistry* 52(6), 950-968.

Tarng, D.C. & Huang, T.P. (2002). Determinants of circulating soluble transferrin receptor level in chronic haemodialysis patients. *Nephrology Dialysis Transplantation* 17,*1063*–1069.

Thomas, C., & Thomas,L. (2002). Biochemical markers and hematologic indices in the diagnosis of functional iron deficiency. *Clinical Chemistry* 48, 1066-1076.

Thomas, L., Franck, S., Messinger, M., Linssen, J., Thome, M., & Thomas, C. (2005). Reticulocyte hemoglobin measurement - comparison of two methods in the diagnosis of iron-restricted erythropoiesis. *Clinical Chemistry and Laboratory Medicine* 43, 1193-1202.

Thomas, C., Kirschbaum, A., Boehm, D., & Thomas, L. (2006). The diagnostic plot. *Medical Oncology* 23(1), 23-36.

Urrechaga, E., Borque, L., & Escanero, J.F. (2009). Potential utility of the new Sysmex XE 5000 red blood cell extended parameters in the study of disorders of iron metabolism. *Clinical Chemistry and Laboratory Medicine* 47(11), 1411-1416.

Urrechaga, E. (2010). The new mature red cell parameter, low haemoglobin density of the Beckman-Coulter LH750: clinical utility in the diagnosis of iron deficiency. *International Journal of Laboratory Hematology* 32, e144-150.

Urrechaga, E., Borque, L., & Escanero J.F. (2010). Erythrocyte and reticulocyte indices on the LH 750 as potential markers of functional iron deficiency. *Anemia* DOI 10:1155/2010/625919.

Urrechaga, E., Borque, L., & Escanero J.F. (2011).Low Hemoglobin density potential marker of iron availability. *International Journal of Laboratory Hematology* DOI 10.1111/j.1751-553x.2011.01355.x.

Weiss, G., Goodnough, L.T. (2005). Anemia of chronic disease. *New England Journal of Medicine* 352, 1011-1023.

Weiss, G. (2009). Iron metabolism in the anemia of chronic disease. *Biochimica and Biophysica Acta* 1790, 682-693.

Wish, J.B. (2006). Assessing Iron status: beyond serum ferritin and transferrin saturation. *Clinical Journal of the American Society of Nephrology* 1, S4-S8.

Zager, R.A., Johnson, A.C.M., Hanson, S.Y., & Wasse, H. (2002). Parenteral iron formulations: a comparative toxicologic analysis and mechanisms of cell injury. *American Journal of Kidney Disease* 40, 90-103.

# 15

# Exogenous Fluorescent Agents for the Determination of Glomerular Filtration Rate

Raghavan Rajagopalan and Richard B. Dorshow
*Covidien Pharmaceuticals, Hazelwood, Missouri, USA*

## 1. Introduction

Glomerular filtration rate (GFR) is now widely accepted as the best indicator of renal function in the state of health and illness.[1,2] Current clinical guidelines advocate its use in the staging of chronic kidney disease as well as in assessing the risk of kidney failure under acute clinical, physiological, and pathological conditions.[3-6] Acute renal failure (ARF) is a major cause of complications in the post-surgical and post-intervention vascular and cardiac procedure patient populations. ARF is also a major public health issue because it may lead to chronic renal failure. Real-time, continuous monitoring of GFR in patients at the bedside is particularly important in the case of critically ill or injured patients, and those undergoing organ transplantation because most of these patients face the risk of multiple organ failure (MOF) resulting in death.[7-10] MOF is a sequential failing of lung, liver, and kidneys and is incited by one or more severe causes such as acute lung injury (ALI), adult respiratory distress syndrome (ARDS), hypermetabolism, hypotension, persistent inflammation, or sepsis. The transition from early stages of trauma to clinical MOF is marked by the extent of liver and renal failure and a change in mortality risk from about 30% to about 50%.[10] Accurate determination of GFR is also necessary for monitoring patients undergoing cancer chemotherapy with nephrotoxic anticancer drugs,[11] or those at risk for contrast media induced nephropathy (CIN).[12] Finally, GFR measurement is also useful for patients with chronic illness such as diabetes, hypertension, obesity, hyperthyroidism, cystic fibrosis, etc. who are at risk for renal impairment.[13-15]

## 2. Current GFR markers

In order to assess the status and to follow the progress of renal disease, there is a need to develop a simple, accurate, and continuous method for the determination of renal function by non-invasive procedures. At present, endogenous serum creatinine (**1**) (Fig. 1) concentration measured at frequent intervals over a 24-hour period has been the most common method of assessing renal function despite the well known serious limitations.[16-18] The results from this analysis are frequently misleading since the value is affected by age, state of hydration, renal perfusion, muscle mass, dietary intake, and many other anthropometric and clinical variables. Theoretical methods for estimating GFR (eGFR)[19-21] from body cell mass and plasma creatinine concentration have also been developed, but these methods also rely on the above anthropomorphic variables. Moreover, creatinine is

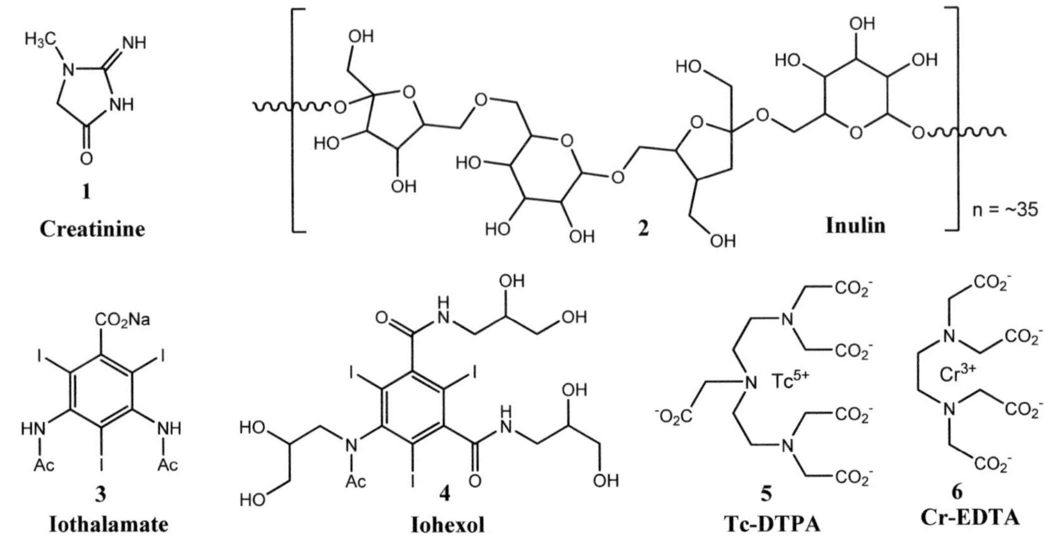


Fig. 1. Structures of Currently Known Exogenous GFR Markers.

partially cleared by tubular secretion along with glomerular filtration, and, as Diskin[17] recently remarked, "Creatinine clearance is not and has never been synonymous with GFR, and all of the regression analysis will not make it so because the serum creatinine depends upon many factors other than filtration." More recently, endogenous cystatin-C has been suggested as an improvement over creatinine,[15,20] but this marker also suffers from the same limitations as creatinine, and thus it remains questionable whether it is really an improvement.

In the past several decades, exogenous tracers such as inulin (**2**), iothalamate (**3**), iohexol (**4**), $^{99m}$Tc-DTPA (diethylenetriaminepentaacetate) (**5**), and $^{51}$Cr-EDTA (ethylenediamine-tetraacetate) (**6**) (Fig.1), have been developed to determine GFR, but all of them require either radiometric, HPLC (high performance liquid chromatography), or X-ray fluorescence methods for detection and quantification.[22-29] Unfortunately, all of these markers suffer from various undesirable properties including the use of radioactivity, ionizing radiation, and the laborious ex-vivo handling of blood and urine samples, and the use of HPLC method that render them unsuitable for continuous monitoring of renal function in the clinical setting. Furthermore, inulin as well as other polysaccharides are polydisperse polymers, and availability of these substances in a reliable, uniform batches is a serious limiting factor for their use as GFR markers. Currently, iothalamate and iohexol are the accepted standard for the assessment of GFR. However, iothalmate requires the collection of blood samples and requires HPLC method, which is not well suited for continuous monitoring. Continuous monitoring of GFR has been accomplished via radiometric[12] and magnetic resonance imaging[30] techniques, but these are not suitable at the bedside. Hence, the availability of an exogenous marker for the measurement of GFR under specific yet changing circumstances would represent a substantial improvement over any currently available or widely practiced method. Moreover, a method that depends solely on the renal elimination of an exogenous chemical entity would provide an absolute and continuous pharmacokinetic measurement requiring less subjective interpretation based upon age, muscle mass, blood pressure, etc.

## 3. Development of fluorescent tracer agents

Accordingly, there has been some effort on developing exogenous GFR tracer agents that absorb and emit in the visible or near infrared (NIR) region, which includes small molecules as well as macromolecular bioconjugates such FITC (fluorescien isothicyanate)-inulin and FITC- and Texas Red-dextrans.[31-37] The key requirements for an ideal fluorescent tracer agent are: (a) must be excited at and emit in the visible region ($\lambda \geq \sim425$ nm); (b) must be highly hydrophilic; (c) must be either neutral or anionic; (c) must have very low or no plasma protein binding; (d) must not be metabolized in vivo, and (e) must clear exclusively via glomerular filtration as demonstrated by equality of plasma clearance with and without a tubular secretion inhibitor such as probenecid.[38] The selection of the lead clinical candidate(s) may be based on secondary considerations such as the ease of synthesis, lack of toxicity, and stability. The secondary screening criteria should further take into account the tissue optics properties and the degree of extracellular distribution of the fluorescent tracers. Volume of distribution is an important parameter in the assessment of hydration state of the patient, whereas the absorption/emission properties provide essential information for the design of the probe.

This chapter focuses on the most recent development on luminescent tracers for GFR measurement. There are basically two principal pathways for the design of fluorescent tracers for GFR determination. The first method involves enhancing the fluorescence of known renal agents that are intrinsically poor emitters such as lanthanide metal complexes; and the second involves transforming highly fluorescent dyes (which are intrinsically lipophilic) into hydrophilic, anionic species to force them to clear via the kidneys.[32] In the first approach, several europium-DTPA complexes endowed with various molecular 'antenna' to induce ligand-to-metal fluorescence resonance energy transfer (FRET) were prepared and tested.[32] Some of metal complexes (e.g. compound **7** exhibited high (c.a. 2000-fold) enhancement of europium fluorescence and underwent clearance exclusively through the kidneys, but whether they cleared exclusively via glomerular filtration remains uncertain. Moreover, the excitation maxima of these complexes remained in the violet or UV-A region.

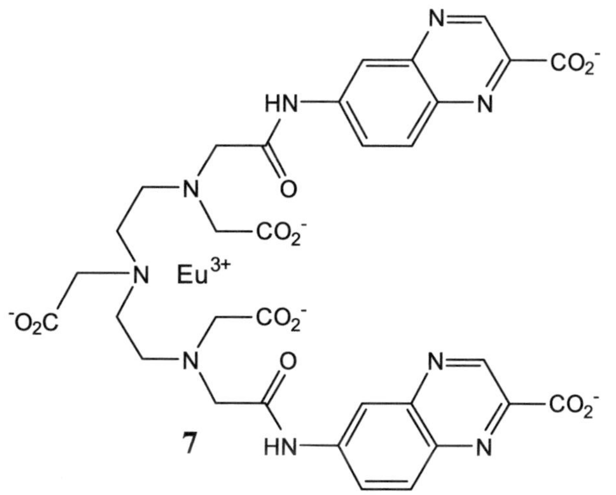


**7**

Fig. 2. Eu-DTPA-Quinoline Complex.

Pyrazines (Fig. 3) are one the very few classes of photostable small molecules having highly desirable properties for various biomedical and non-medical optical applications.[39-41] Pyrazine derivatives **8** containing electron donating groups (EDG) in the 2,5 positions and electron withdrawing groups (EWG) in the 3,6 positions such as compounds **9-11** are shown to absorb and emit in the visible region with a large Stokes shift on the order of ~ 100 nm and with fluorescence quantum yields of about 0.4.[39,40] For example, conversion of the carboxyl group in **8** to the secondary amide derivatives **9** produces a bathochromic (red) shift of about 40 nm, and alkylation of the amino group in **9** produces further red shift of about 40 nm. Thus, the pyrazine nucleus offers considerable opportunity to 'tune' the electronic properties by even simple modifications. Furthermore, the relative small size of pyrazine renders it an ideal scaffold to introduce hydrophilic substituents to bring about renal clearance.

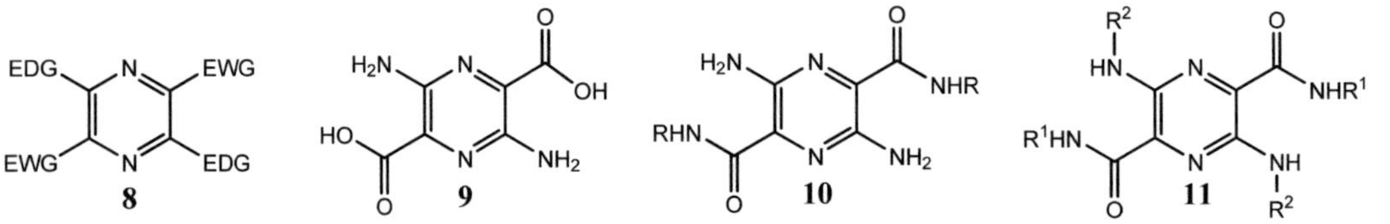


EDG = $NR_2$, OR, etc.
EWG = $CO_2H$, CN, etc.

$\lambda_{abs}$: 410 nm
$\lambda_{em}$: 480 nm

$\lambda_{abs}$: 430-450 nm
$\lambda_{em}$: 550-560 nm

$\lambda_{abs}$: 480-500 nm
$\lambda_{em}$: 585-605 nm

Fig. 3. Pyrazine Derivatives.

Based on the structure and properties of known GFR tracer agents, and on the primary and secondary considerations stated earlier, the set of GFR tracer agents can be divided finto our categories as outlined in Table 1. The upper and lower quadrants address the tissue optics differences, and the left and right quadrants address volume of distribution ($V_d$) differences. ($V_d$) is important not only in affecting clearance rates, but also in the assessment of hydration state of a patient. Tissue optics parameters are important in instrument design in that the longer the wavelength of light, the deeper the penetration into the tissue. Recently, low and high molecular weight hydrophilic pyrazine derivatives **12-15** (Fig. 4) bearing neutral and anionic side chains such as alcohols, carboxylic acids, and polyethylene glycol (PEG) units were reported.[41] The structures of the candidates from each of the four quadrants above are shown in Fig. 2. Unlike inulin, dextran, and other polymers, compounds **13** and **15** are monodisperse. The photophysical and biological properties of these compounds are given in Table 2. Both plasma protein binding and urinary clearance properties are superior to iothalamate, which is a currently used 'gold standard' for clinical GFR measurement. Furthermore, all four compounds displayed insignificant biodegradation.

| | Volume of Distribution | |
|---|---|---|
| **Tissue Optics** | *Short Wavelength*<br>*Low Molecular Weight* | *Short Wavelength*<br>*High Molecular Weight* |
| | *Long Wavelength*<br>*Low Molecular Weight* | *Long Wavelength*<br>*High Molecular Weight* |

Table 1. Design of Exogenous Fluorescent GFR Tracers.

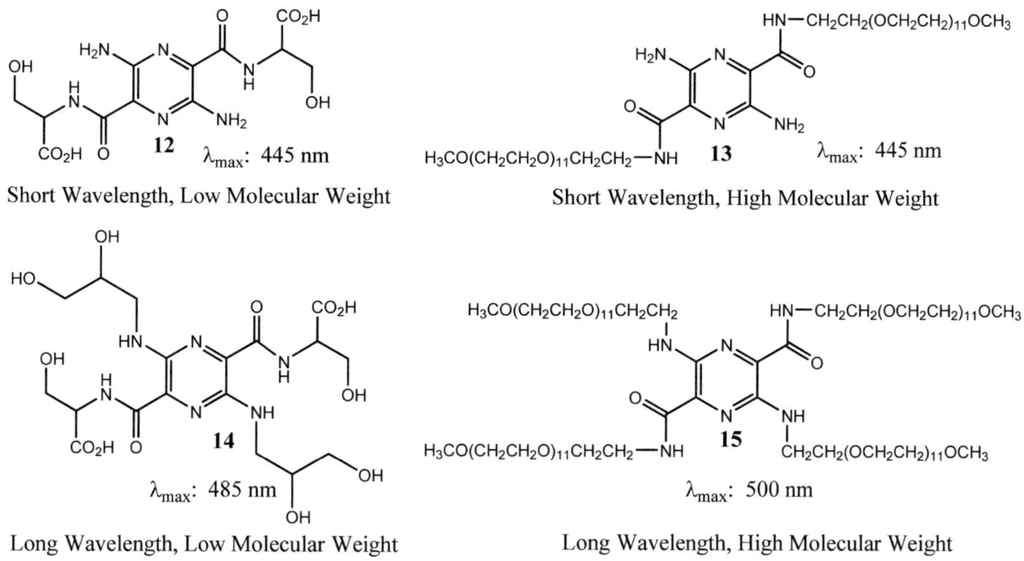


Fig. 4. Hydrophilic Pyrazine Derivatives.

| | 12 | 13 | 14 | 15 | Iothalamate |
|---|---|---|---|---|---|
| Absorption Maxima, ($\lambda_{max}$, nm) | 435 | 437 | 488 | 499 | NA |
| Emission Maxima, ($\lambda_{max}$, nm) | 557 | 558 | 597 | 604 | NA |
| Plasma Protein Binding (%) | 0 | 0 | 0 | 3 | 10 |
| Plasma Clearance Half-Life (min) | 29 | 25 | 20 | 19 | 32 |
| Injected Dose Recovered in Urine at 6 Hrs (%) | 90 | 71 | 88 | 97 | 80 |
| Clearance - No probenecid (mL/min) | 2.5 | NA | 3.0 | 3.1 | 2.5 |
| Clearance - Probenecid, 70 mg/kg (mL/min) | 2.6 | NA | 2.4 | 3.3 | 2.2 |

Table 2. Physicochemical and Pharmacokinetic Properties of Pyrazine Tracers.

An in vivo fluorescence image of the renal clearance of compound **13** is shown in Fig. 5. The panel contains images of three mice. The mouse in the middle was administered 300 μL of a 2 mM solution in phosphate-buffered saline (PBS) of compound **13**. The other mice served as controls where the mice received only PBS. Compound **13** distributed throughout the body and then concentrated in one spot in the abdomen. Surgery after the 60 minute time point verified that this highly fluorescent spot in the abdomen was the bladder. Thus, this observation of fluorescence only appearing at the bladder is a visual demonstration of the high percent of injected dose recovered in urine given in Table 2.

## 4. Real-time monitoring of renal clearance

In vivo noninvasive real-time monitoring of renal clearance, with eventual translation to commercial development, has been demonstrated in the rodent model. A schematic of an apparatus is shown in Fig. 6. A 445 nm solid state laser was directed into one leg of a silica

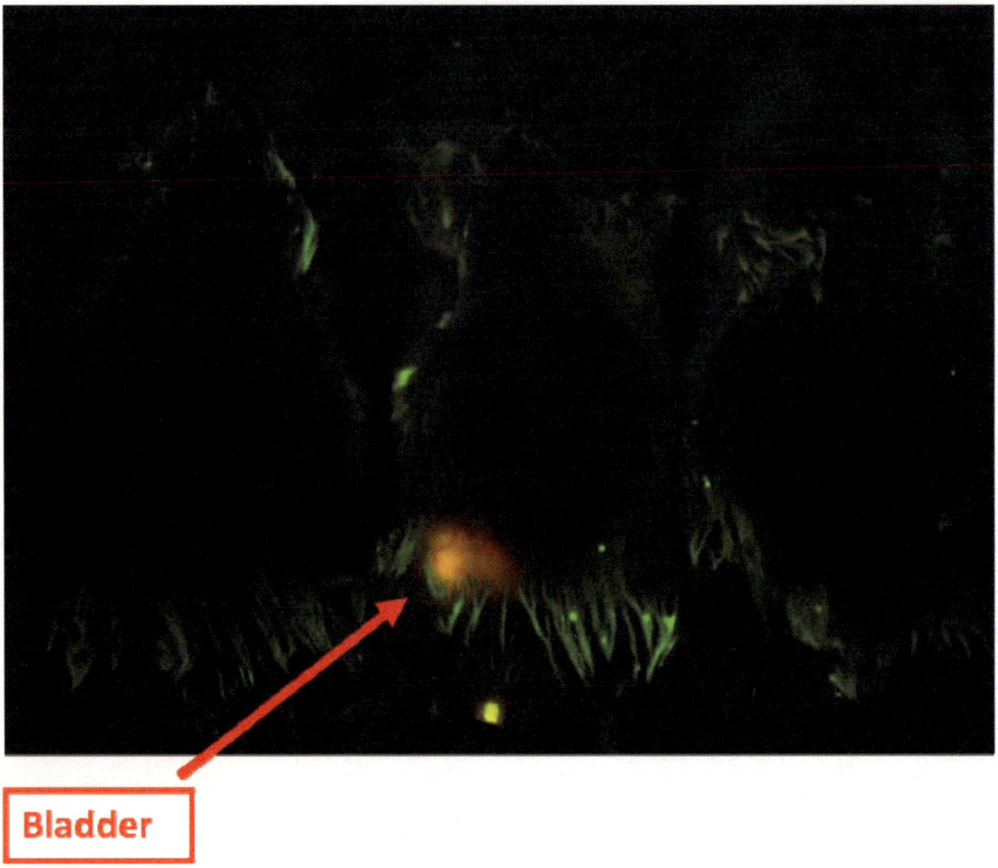


Fig. 5. Optical Image of Pyrazine **13** at 1 Hour Post Administration.

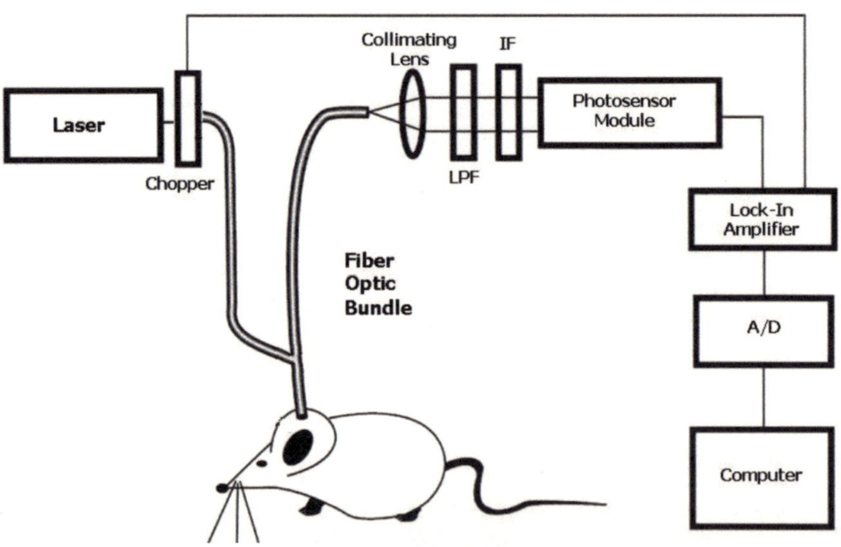


Fig. 6. Apparatus for non-invasive in vivo detection of fluorescence.

bifurcated fiber optic bundle, with the common end of this bifurcated bundle placed approximately 2 mm from the rat ear. The second leg of the bifurcated fiber optic bundle was fitted with a collimating beam probe. A long pass filter and narrow band interference filter were placed in front of a photosensor module. A chopper was placed after the laser and before the launch into the bifurcated cable. The output of the photosensor was connected to a lock-in amplifier. The lock-in output was digitized and the digitized data was acquired by computer using data acquisition software.

Anesthesized Sprague-Dawley rats of weight ~ 400 g were used. A volume of 1 mL of a 0.4 mg/mL concentration in PBS of compound 12 was administered to a rat with normal functioning kidneys and to a rat with a recent bi-lateral nephrectomy. The continuously monitored fluorescent signal is shown in Figure 5. An increase in fluorescence at the ear is immediately seen in both rats. In the normal rat, the fluorescence decreases back to baseline as the kidney removes compound 12 from the body. In the ligated rat, the fluorescence remains elevated with time as the body is unable to remove compound with the kidneys not functioning.

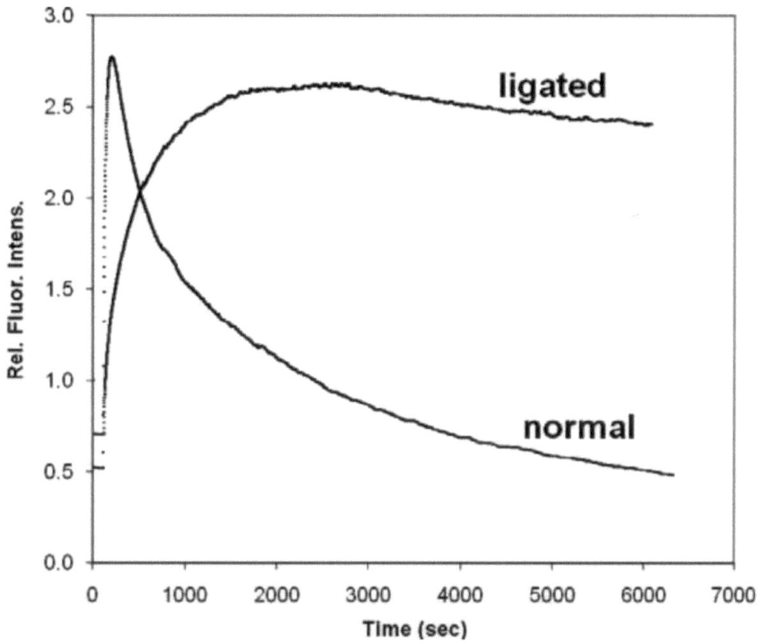


Fig. 7. Continuous Monitoring of Pyrazine **12** in Normal and Partially Nephrectomized Rats.

## 5. Conclusions

On the basis of the fluorescence properties, plasma protein binding data, the injected dose recovered in urine, the plasma clearance data, and the renal tubular secretion studies, the pyrazine deriviatives **12-15** are promising candidates as exogenous fluorescent tracer agents for the determination of GFR under both chronic and acute settings. In the rat model, these compounds display superior properties compared to iothalamate, which is currently an accepted standard for the measurement of GFR.

A prototype instrument for clinical trials has been developed based on the apparatus in Figure 4. A clinical trial with one of the pyrazine compounds is currently being planned.

The clinical trial will test the safety and efficacy of the tracer agent, as well as refine the instrumentation. Optimization parameters for the instrument include incident light power and power density, light delivery and collection fiber optics, light source and detector, placement of detector on body, and the data acquisition and analysis algorithm.

The addition of a fluorescent GFR tracer agent would be a major addition to the armament of fluorescent compounds in clinical use today. Indocyanine green (ICG) is FDA-approved for use in angiography, cardiac output, and liver function.[42] Currently, there are on-going clinical trials for lymph node mapping and melanoma imaging using ICG.[43] Fluorescein is the only other FDA appoved fluorescent agent, used for angiography.[42] A near-infrared dye for attachment to targeting vectors for optical imaging has been studied for safety and pharmacology, and may soon be ready for human clinical trials too.[44]

## 6. References

[1] Ekanoyan, G.; Levin, N. W. In Clinical Practice Guidelines for Chronic Kidney Disease: Evaluation, Classification, and Stratification (K/DOQI), National Kidney Foundation: Washington, D.C., 2002; pp 1–22.

[2] Stevens, L.A.; Coresh, J.; Greene, T.; Levey, A.S. Assessing kidney function - Measured and estimated glomerular filtration rate. *The New England Journal of Medicine* 2006, *354*, 2473-2483.

[3] C.A. Rabito, L.S.T. Fang, and A.C. Waltman, "Renal function in patients at risk with contrast material-induced acute renal failure: Noninvasive real-time monitoring," *Radiology* 1993, *186*, 851-854.

[4] N.L. Tilney, and J.M. Lazarus, "Acute renal failure in surgical patients: Causes, clinical patterns, and care," *Surgical Clinics of North America* 1983, *63*, 357-377.

[5] B.E. VanZee, W.E. Hoy, and J.R. Jaenike, "Renal injury associated with intravenous pyelography in non-diabetic and diabetic patients," *Annals of Internal Medicine* 1978, *89*, 51-54.

[6] S. Lundqvist, G. Edbom, S. Groth, U. Stendahl and S.-O. Hietala, "Iohexol clearance for renal function measurement in gynecologic cancer patients," *Acta Radiologica* 1996, *37*, 582-586.

[7] Baker, L. Oppenheimer, and B. Stephens, "Epidemiology of trauma deaths," *American Journal of Surgery* 1980, *140*, 144-150.

[8] R.G. Lobenhoffer, and M. Grotz, "Treatment results of patients with multiple trauma: An analysis of 3406 cases treated between 1972 and 1991 at a German level I trauma center," *Journal of Trauma* 1995, *38*, 70-77.

[9] J. Coalson, "Pathology of sepsis, septic shock, and multiple organ failure," in *New Horizons: Multiple Organ Failure*, D.J Bihari and F.B. Cerra, Eds., pp 27-59, Society of Critical Care Medicine, Fullerton, CA, 1986.

[10] F.B. Cerra, "Multiple organ failure syndrome," in *New Horizons: Multiple Organ Failure*, D.J Bihari and F.B. Cerra, Eds., pp 1-24, Society of Critical Care Medicine, Fullerton, CA, 1989.

[11] Jennings, S.; de Lemos, M.L.; Levin, A.; Murray, N. Evaluation of creatinine-based formulas in dosing adjustment of cancer drugs other than carboplatin. *Journal of Oncology Pharmacy Practice* 2010, *16*, 113-119.

[12] C.A. Rabito, L.S.T. Fang, and A.C. Waltman, "Renal function in patients at risk with contrast material-induced acute renal failure: Noninvasive real-time monitoring," *Radiology* 1993, *186*, 851-854.

[13] Chagnac, A.; Herman, M.; Zingerman, B.; Erman, A.; Rozen-Zvi, B.; Hirsh, J.; Gafter, U. Obesity-induced glomerular hyperfiltration: its involvement in the pathogenesis of tubular sodium reabsorption. *Nephrology, Dialysis, and Transplantation* 2008, *23*, 3946-3952.

[14] van Hoek, I.; Lefebvre, H.P.; Peremans, K.; Meyer, E.; Croubles, S.; Vandermeulen, E.; Koositra, H.; Saunders, J.H.; Binst, D.; Daminet, S. Short- and long-term follow-up of glomerlular and tubular renal markers of kidney function in hyperthyroid cats after treatment with radioiodine. *Domestic Animal Endocrinology* 2009, *36*, 45-56.

[15] Beringer, P.M.; Hidayat, L.; Heed, A.; Zheng, L.; Owens, H.; Benitez, D.; Rao, A.P. GFR estimates using cystatin C are superior to serum creatinine in adult patients with cystic fibrosis. *Journal of Cystic Fibrosis* 2009, *8*, 19-25.

[16] Bellomo, R.; Ronco, C.; Kellum, J. A.; Mehta, R. L.; Palevsky, P. Acute Dialysis Quality Initiative workgroup. Acute renal failure - definition, outcome measures, animal models, fluid therapy, and information technology needs: the Second International Consensus Conference of the Acute Dialysis Quality Initiative (ADQI) Group. *Crit. Care* 2004, *8*, R204–R212.

[17] Diskin, C. J. Creatinine and GFR: an imperfect marriage of convenience. *Nephrol. Dial. Transplant.* 2006, *21*, 3338–3339.

[18] Carrie, B. J.; Goldbetz, H. V.; Michaels, A. S., Myers, B. D. Creatinine: an inadequate filtration marker in glomerular disease. *Am. J. Med.* 1980, 69, 177–182.

[19] Donadio, C.; Consani, C.; Ardini, M.; Caprio, F.; Grassi, G.; Lucchesi, A. Prediction of glomerular filtration rate from body cell mass and plasma creatinine. Current Drug *Discovery Technologies* 2004, *1*, 221-228.

[20] C. White, A. Akbari, N. Hussain, L. Dinh, G. Filler, N. Lepage, and G. Knoll, "Estimating glomerular filtration rate in kidney transplantation: A comparison between serum creatinine and cystatin C-based methods," *J. Am. Soc. Nephrol*, 2005, *16*, 3763-3770 and references cited therein.

[21] Stevens, L. A.; Levey, A. S. Measured GFR as a confirmatory test for estimated GFR. *J. Am. Soc. Nephrol.* 2009, *20*, 2305–2313.

[22] Sturgeon, C.; Sam, A. D.; Law, W. R. Rapid determination of glomerular filtration rate by single-bolus inulin: a comparison of estimation analyses. *J. Appl. Physiol.* 1998, 84, 2154–2162.

[23] Wilson, D. M.; Bergert, J. M.; Larson, T. H.; Leidtke, R. R. GFR determined by nonradiolabeled iothalamate using capillary electrophoresis. *Am. J. Kidney Dis.* 1997, 39

[24] P. Guesry, L. Kaufman, S. Orloff, J.A. Nelson, S. Swann, and M. Holliday, "Measurement of glomerular filtration rate by fluorescent excitation of non-radioactive meglumine iothalamate," *Clinical Nephrology* 1975, *3*, 134-138.

[25] Finco, D.R.; Measurement of glomerular filtration rate via urinary clearance of inulin and plasma clearance of technetium Tc-99m pentetate and exogenous creatinine in dogs. *American Journal of Veterinary Research* 2005, *66*, 1046-1055.

[26] Miyagawa, Y.; Takemura, N.; Hirose, H. Evaluation of a single sampling method for estimation of plasma iohexol clearance in dogs and cats with various kidney functions. *Journal of Veterinary Medical Science* 2010, *72*, 271-278.

[27] Berg, U.; Baeck, R.; Celsi, G.; Halling, S.E.; Homberg, I.; Krmar, R.T.; Monemi, K.A.; Oeborn, H; Herthelius, M. Comparison of plasma clearance of iohexol and urinary clearance of inulin for measurement of GFR in children. *American Journal of Kidney Diseases* 2010, *57*, 55-61.

[28] Schwartz, G.J.; Cole, S.R.; Warady,B.; Munoz, A. Glomerular filtration rate via plasma iohexol disappearance: pilot study for chronic kidney disease in children. *Kidney International* 2006, *69*, 2070-2077

[29] Arsos, G.; Moralidis, E.; Tsechelidis, I.; Sakagiannis, G.; Sidiropolou, V.; Psarouli, E. Measurement of glomerular filtration rate with chromium-51 ethylene diamino tetraacetic acid in the presence of gallium-67 citrate: a novel method for the solution of the problem. *Nuclear Medicine Communications* 2011, *32*, 227-232.

[30] Choyke, P.L.; Austin, H.A.; Frank, J.A.; Girton, M.E.; Diggs, R.L.; Dwyer, A.J.; Miller, L.; Nussenblatt, R.; McFarland, H.; Simon, T. Hydrated clearance of gadolinium-DTPA as a measurement of glomerular filtration rate. *Kidney International* 1992, *41*, 1595-1598.

[31] Rajagopalan, R.; Neumann, W.L.; Poreddy, A.R.; Fitch, R.M.; Freskos, J.N.; Asmelash, B.; Gaston, K.R.; Galen, K.P.; Shieh, J-J.; Dorshow, R.B. Hydrophilic pyrazine dyes as exogenous fluorescent tracer agents for real-time poin-of-care measurement of glomerular filtration rate. *Journal of Medicinal Chemistry* 2011, *54*, 5048-5058.

[32] Chinen, L.; Galen, K. P.; Kuan, K. T.; Dyszlewski, M. E.; Ozaki, H.; Sawai, H.; Pandurangi, R. S.; Jacobs, F. G.; Dorshow, R. B.; Rajagopalan, R. Fluorescence-enhanced europium complexes for the assessment of renal function. *J. Med. Chem.* 2008, 51, 957–962.

[33] Rabito, C .A.; Chen, Y.; Schomacker, K. T.; Modell, M. D. Optical, real-time monitoring of the glomerular filtration rate. *Appl. Opt.* 2005, *44*, 5956–5965.

[34] Yu, W.; Sandoval, R. M.; Molitoris, B. A. Rapid determination of renal filtration using an optical ratiometric imaging approach. *Am. J. Physiol. Renal Physiol.* 2007, 292, F1873–F1880.

[35] Schock-Kusch, D.; Sadick, M.; Henninger, N.; Kraenzlin, B.; Claus, G.; Kloetzer, H. -M.; Weiss, C.; Pill, J.; Gretz, N. Transcutaneous measurement of glomerular filtration rate using FITC-sinistrin in rats. *Nephrol. Dial. Transplant.* 2009, 24, 2997–3001.

[36] Wang, E.; Sandoval, R.M.; Campos, S.B.; Molitoris, B.A. Rapid diagnosis and quantification of acute kidney injury using fluorescent ratio-metric determination of glomerular filtration rate in rat. *American Journal of Physiology* 2010, 299(5, Pt. 2), F1048-F1055.

[37] Qi, Z.; Breyer, M.D. Measurement of glomerular filtration rate in conscious mice. *Methods in Molecular Biology* 2009, *466(Kidney Research)*, 61-72.

[38]Fritzberg, A. R.; Kasina, S.; Eshima, D.; Johnson, D. L. Synthesis and biological evaluation of technetium-99m-$MAG_3$ as a hippuran replacement. *J. Nucl. Med.* 1986, 27, 111–116.

[39] Shirai, K.; Yanagisawa, A.; Takahashi, H.; Fukunishi, K.; Matsuoka, M. Synthesis and fluorescent properties of 2,5-diamino-3,6-dicyanopyrazine dyes. *Dyes and Pigments* 1998, 39, 49–68.

[40] Kim, J. H.; Shin, S. R.; Matsuoka, M.; Fukunishi, K. Self-assembling of aminopyrazine fluorescent dyes and their solid state spectra. *Dyes and Pigments* 1998, 39, 341–357.

[41] Poreddy, A. R.; Asmelash, B.; Neumann, W. L.; Dorshow, R. B. A highly efficient method for the N-alkylation of aminopyrazines: Synthesis of hydrophilic red fluorescent dyes. *Synthesis* 2010, 2383–2392.

[42] Alford, R.; Simpson, H. M.; Duberman, J.; Hill, C.G.; Ogawa, M.; Regino, C.; Kobayashi, H.; Choyke, P.L. Toxicity of organic flurophores used in molecular imaging: Literature review. *Molecular Imaging* 2009, *8*, 341-354.

[43] http://clinical trials.gov

[44] Marshall, M.V.; Draney, D.; Sevick-Muraca, E.M.; Olive, D.M. Singe-dose intravenous toxicity study of IRDye 800CW in Sprague-Dawley rats. Molecular Imaging and Biology 2010, 12, 583-594.

# 16

# Modern Surgical Treatments of Urinary Tract Obstruction

Bannakij Lojanapiwat
*Faculty of Medicine, Chiang Mai University*
*Thailand*

## 1. Introduction

Obstructive nephropathy is a term describing the damage to the renal parenchyma that results from the obstruction to the flow of urine anywhere along the urinary system. Long term obstruction causes chronic renal disease. Obstruction coexisting with infection and impaired renal function, when complicated by elevated temperature and leukocytosis that can lead to septic shock, are an absolute indication for urinary diversion such as percutaneous nephrostomy. This particular patient needs emergency diversion. One of the most common indications of nephrostomy placement is ureteric obstruction causing uremia. It is therefore necessary to make the patients fit enough for the designated surgery.

Percutaneous nephrostomy involving supravesicle drainage is one of the most common procedures in urologic practice. Goodwin described a trocar nephrostomy technique in a markedly dilated kidney in 1955. (Goodwin et al., 1955). Percutaneous nephrostomy is performed for temporary or permanent supravesicle urinary diversion. The treatment goals in patients with malignant ureteric obstruction are symptom relief and avoidance of any complications from renal insufficiency. Permanent nephrostomy has been used in patients with obstruction from uncorrectable causes such as inoperable tumors. (Table 1)

The indication of nephrostomy tube placement depends on whether the procedure is elective or urgent. The purpose of nephrostomy tube placement in obstructive renal disease is to preserve kidney function and drain infected urine. Establishing a safe and reliable nephrostomy tract is key that range from simple urinary drainage to intrarenal surgical operation. (Fig. 1-4)

| |
|---|
| Complications of obstruction as sepsis and pain. |
| Improve renal function. |
| Localized disease that additional therapy may prolong survival. |
| Improve quality of life. |
| Independent existence at home possible. |

Table 1. Indication for palliative diversion.

Careful discussion between patients, relatives and health care professionals about nephrostomy tube placement must be undertaken before the intervention because patients will require a drainage bag which reduces the quality of life.

Renal function in several patients recover following temporary percutaneous nephrostomy tube placement. The definite treatment is need prior nephrostomy tube removal. Advance in endourologic instrumentation and techniques, endourologic operations as the minimally invasive surgery (percutaneous nephrolithotomy, endopyelotomy, infundibulotomy and endoureterotomy) are the procedure of choice for these patients. The nonfunctioning kidneys following the diversion usually require nephrectomy.

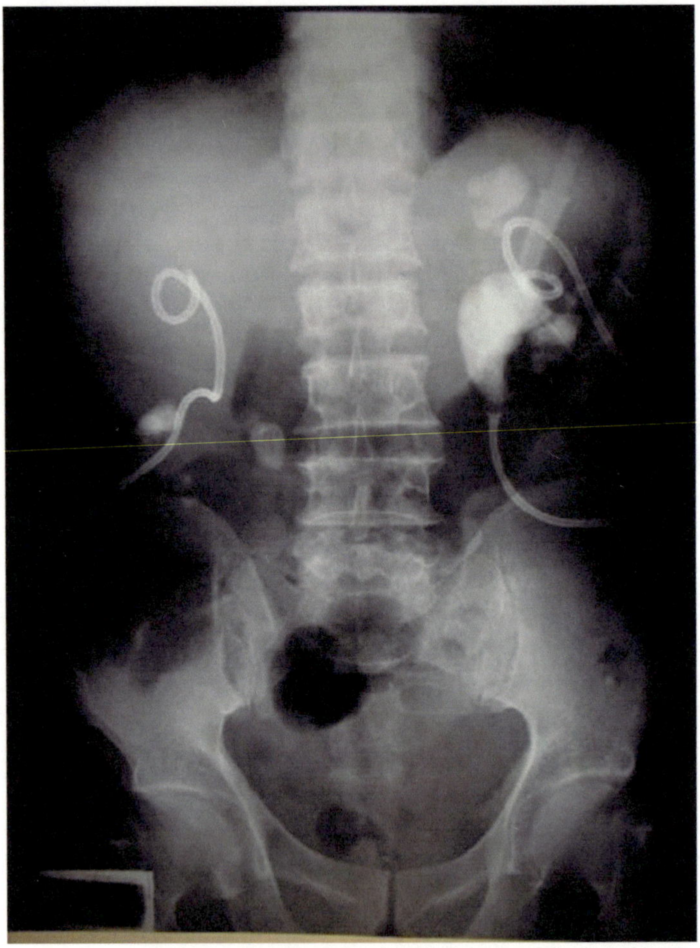

Fig. 1. Bilateral percutaneous nephrostomy in a patient with right upper ureteral calculi and bilateral renal calculi presenting of anuria.

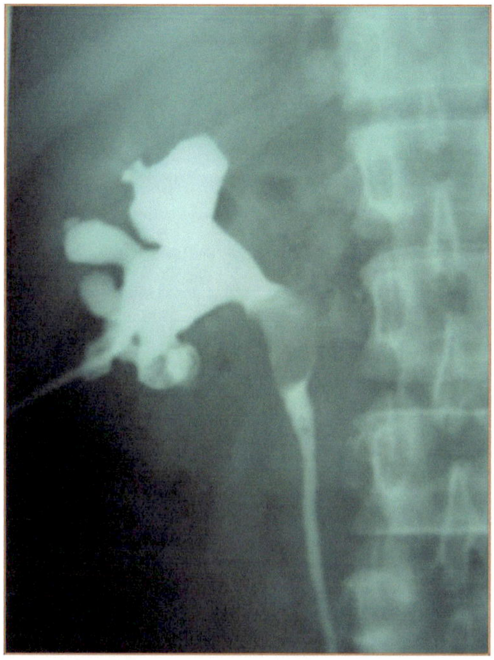

Fig. 2. Nephrostogram following nephrostomy tube placement due to azotemia and pyonephrosis demonstrated impacted upper ureteric calculi.

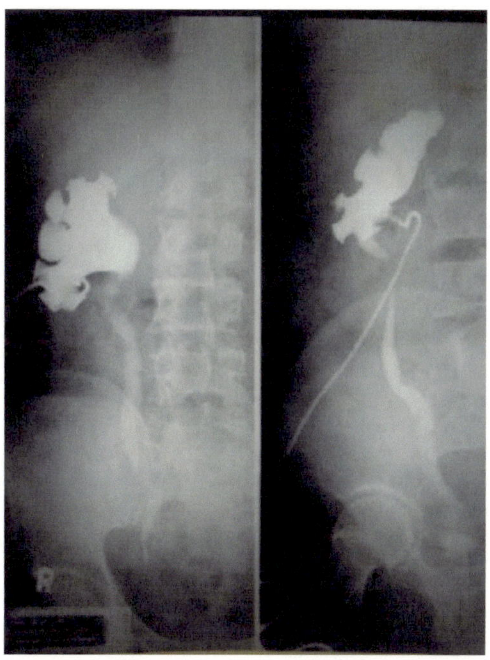

Fig. 3. Percutaneous nephrostomy in patient with complete distal ureteral obstruction from advanced cervical cancer.

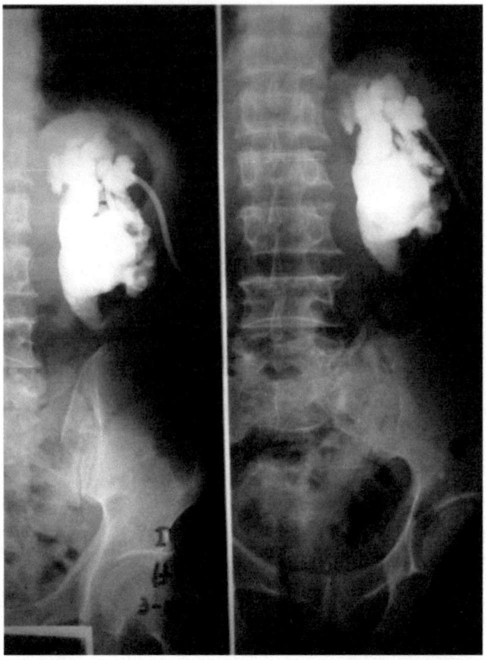

Fig. 4. Percutaneous nephrostomy at upper calyx due to complete upper ureteral obstruction from previous surgery. (single kidney)

## 2. Urinary tract obstruction

The peak incidence of urinary tract obstruction in males is in the eighth and ninth decades secondary to benign prostatic hyperplasia and prostatic carcinoma, whereas the peak incidence in females is in the fourth to six decades secondary to pregnancy and carcinoma of the cervix or uterus. (Gulmi et al., 1998)

### 2.1 Etiology of urinary tract obstruction

The etiology of urinary tract obstruction can be divided into intrinsic and extrinsic causes. (Table 2)

#### 2.1.1 Extrinsic causes

Extrinsic causes of urinary tract obstruction are the diseases of genitourinary system, gastrointestinal system, vascular system, retroperitoneal pathology and biologic agents such as actinomycosis. (Curhan & Zeidel, 1996)

The common causes of extrinsic processes are tumor of the kidney, ureter and bladder and other gastrointestinal pathologies such as Crohn's disease, appendicitis and diverticulitis.

#### 2.1.2 Intrinsic causes

The common intrinsic causes are from intraluminal obstructions such as nephrolithiasis / ureterolithiasis, papillary necrosis, blood clot, fungal ball and urethral strictures.

| | | |
|---|---|---|
| **Extrinsic causes** | : Genitourinary system | |
| | | - Tumor of kidney, bladder, ureter |
| | | - Prostatic hyperplasia, prostatic carcinoma |
| | | - Carcinoma of cervix and uterus |
| | : Gastrointesinal system | |
| | | - Crohn's disease |
| | | - Appendicitis |
| | | - Diverticulitis |
| | : Vascular system | |
| | | - Aneurysm of aorta and iliac artery |
| | : Retroperitoneal pathology | |
| | | - Retroperitoneal fibrosis |
| **Intrinsic causes** | : | - Nephrolithiasis |
| | | - Ureterolithiasis |
| | | - Uretero-pelvic junction obstruction |
| | | - Ureteral stricture |
| | | - Urethral stricture |

Table 2. Common etiologies of urinary tract obstruction.

### 2.2 Clinical presentation

Signs, symptoms and degree of obstructive nephropathy depended on the following factors:

- The time interval in which the obstruction occurs
- Unilateral or bilateral obstruction
- Etiology of the obstruction (intrinsic or extrinsic)
- Degree of the obstruction (complete or partial)

The presenting symptoms of bilateral and chronic obstruction can be nonspecific such as increases in abdominal girth, ankle edema, malaise, anorexia, headache, weight gain, fatigue and shortness of breath.

### 2.3 Radiographic assessment

#### 2.3.1 Ultrasound

Ultrasound is the most valuable tool of radiologic assessment of obstructive uropathy in patients with azotemia, even in pregnant and pediatric patients. This investigation provides information about both renal parenchyma and the collecting system. Hydronephrosis is demonstrated as a dilated collecting system separating the normally echogenic renal sinus. Echoes within the collecting system may indicate pyonephrosis, hemorrhage or a lesion of the transitional mucosa. The thickness of the renal parenchyma can be represented the duration of obstruction.

Ultrasonography for diagnosing obstruction can provide false positive (overdiagnosis) and false negative (missing an obstruction) results. The conditions that can cause false negatives with ultrasonography are acute onset of obstruction, an intrarenal collecting system, dehydration, and the misinterpretation of caliectasis for renal cortical cyst. (LeRoy., 1996) . False positive imaging for the obstruction can be caused by parapelvic cyst, intrarenal pelvis, high urine flow state and vesicoureteral reflux. (Stables et al., 1978)

### 2.3.2 Retrograde pyelography

Retrograde pyelography may be needed to demonstrate the cause of obstruction that is either intrinsic and extrinsic. This assessment can evaluate the site, severity of obstruction and degree of hydronephrosis especially in patients with poor kidney function.

### 2.3.3 Computer tomography (CT scan)

Computer tomography (CT scan) can demonstrate the information of obstruction and hydronephrosis without contrast media. All kinds of urinary calculi and other intraperitoneal / extraperitoneal pathology can be detected by this assessment.

## 3. Surgical approach

Nephrostomy can be performed either by open operation or by closed percutaneous methods. With the development of endourologic and imaging techniques, percutaneous nephrostomy is widely used. Recently, the percutaneous nephrostomy placement became the standard of care, replacing surgical nephrostomy. (Banner et al., 1991 & Sherman et al., 1985)

Establishing safe and reliable nephrostomy tract is very important. The aim of the nephrostomy tract ranges from simple urinary drainage to intrarenal surgical operation. For percutaneous renal surgeries, some surgeons prefer a two stage surgery which can limit bleeding, provide a clear field and let the nephrostomy tract mature.

A successful outcome without complications is the goal of this procedure, which requires careful preoperative planning and proper techniques. The preoperative anatomy of the patient, the nature of the urologic procedure planned and available equipment are very important.

### 3.1 Open nephrostomy technique

Explore the kidney and open the renal pelvis and choose the calix which is suitable for nephrostomy. The catheter is introduced through thinned cortex into the renal pelvis.

### 3.2 Percutaneous nephrostomy techniques

### 3.2.1 Preoperative patient preparation

All patients need appropriate hemostasis evaluation and urine bacteriologic assessment. Careful review and assessment of the degree of hydronephrosis, anatomic variance of the pelvicaliceal system, and relative position of the kidney are key factors for success and will reduce any potential complication of nephrostomy tube placement. This can be evaluated by previous or currents plain Kidney-Urinary–Bladder (KUB) radiography, intravenous pyelography, retrograde pyelography, computed tomogram and ultrasonographic studies. These radiographic investigations demonstrate size, number and location of renal and ureteral calculi as well as establishing baseline renal function and other pathology.

The evaluation of choice to detect urolithiasis and intraabdominal anatomy in patients with emergent or complex medical conditions is a computer tomography (CT scan) of the whole abdomen. Pre-nephrostomy placement with CT scan is recommended in selected patients with splenomegaly, colonic malposition and marked colonic distention. (LeRoy., 1996)

Patients who have urinary tract infection are treated with bacteriologically specific antibiotics and these patients need parenteral antibiotics for 36 to 48 hours before surgery to ensure adequate serum levels of effective antibiotics. The recommended regimen is ciprofloxacin 400 mg IV every 12 hr, ampicillin 1 gm IV every 6 hr with gentamicin 1 mg/kg every 8 hr or third generation cephalosporin.

Laboratory testing of any bleeding problem such as PT, PTT (Prothrombin time, Partial thromboplastin time) and platelet count should be done with appropriate adjustments especially in patients with a history of prolonged bleeding, liver disease, clinically easy brusisability or other conditions predisposing to a coagulopathy. A platelet count should be above 80,000 cells per ml prior to the procedure. Aspirin therapy should be discontinued 1 week prior to the procedure. Caumadin as an anticoagulants must be discontinued. Subcutaneous heparin can be administered for high risk patients with venous thrombosis.

### 3.2.2 Patient's position

Nephrostomy tube placement can be preferred in both prone and supine positions with highly successful outcome. Most patients usually undergo the procedure in the prone position with abdominal support. Supine position is selected for patients with high surgical risks such as seriously ill patients, patients with endotracheal tubes with or without ventilation, patients with congestive heart failure, patients with complicated fractures and patients who have undergone a major surgical procedure.

The advantages of prone or prone oblique with body side of targeted kidney slightly elevated are operator's hands are outside the vertical x-ray beam. (Fig. 5) With supine position with the body side of targeted kidney elevated slightly off the tabletop, the renal access can be performed with ultrasound or CT guidance.

### 3.2.3 Anesthetic

Most patients need only local anesthesia, but some may need intravenous sedation or general anesthesia, the latter specifically for pediatric patients. The type of anesthesia administered depends on the individual patient and indication of nephrostomy tube placement. Simple percutaneous external drainage can be tolerated with local anesthesia or intravenous analgesia with sedation. General anesthesia is preferable in children with all indications of nephrostomy tube placement.

### 3.2.4 Imaging guidance

The imaging guidance equipment is very important in renal access. The guidance system for urinary tract interventions are fluoroscopic guidance, real-time ultrasonography and CT scan.

#### 3.2.4.1 Ultrasound guidance

The puncture of the desired calix can be done in dilated systems. If only the renal pelvic can be identified, initial puncture can be done at renal pelvic following with antegrade

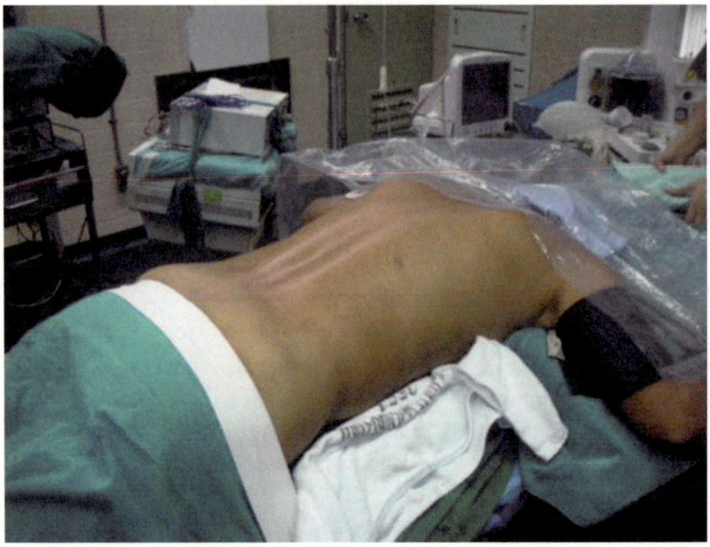

Fig. 5. Patient in prone position for renal access.

pyelography for secondary definitive caliceal puncture. Ultrasound guidance is helpful in determining the depth and the angle of approach. (Juul et al., 1985 & LeRoy et al., 1984). Real time ultrasound is widely used for percutaneous access of a dilated collecting system and is beneficial in infants, pregnant women and patients following renal transplantation. (Falahatkar et al., 2010). The disadvantage of percutaneous nephrostomy access by ultrasound guidance, this guidance system may be compromised by rib artifacts. (Fig. 6, 7)

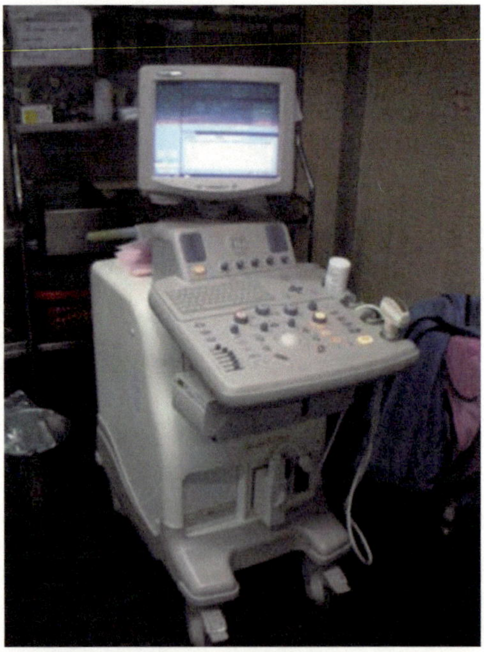

Fig. 6. Ultrasound machine as imaging guidance.

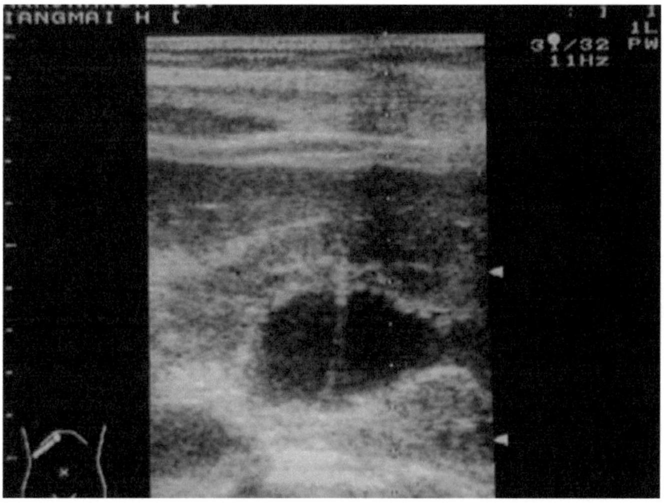


Fig. 7. Ultrasound imaging demonstrated a guidewire in dilated pelvis.

### 3.2.4.2 Fluoroscopic guidance

Fluoroscopic guidance is essential for guidewire manipulation especially in patients with non or mild dilatation of renal pelvis. Collecting system can be opacified with contrast following cystoscopic retrograde ureteral catheter placement, injection of intravenous contrast material and direct percutaneous puncture with 22 gauge needle. Pyelotubular and pyelosinus backflow can be avoided by not overinjecting the collecting system.

In difficult cases, with non-dilated collecting system, the collecting system can be distended with retrograde ureteral balloon catheter. Fluoroscopy can demonstrate the position of the nephrostomy tube in the most desirable position (renal pelvis), minimizing the number of complications. To avoid radiation exposure to operator's hand, Amplatz needle holder can be used. (LeRoy., 1996). This equipment keeps the operator's hand out of the x-ray beam. The patient's table should be not so high that the operator's neck and face are too far from the patient. (Fig. 8-11)

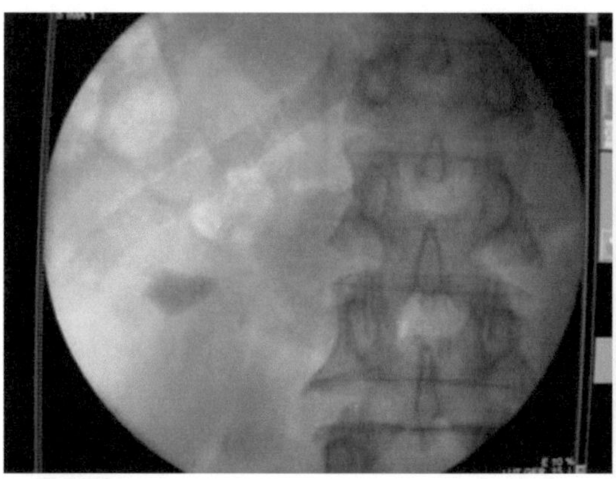

Fig. 8. Right renal pelvic stone in patient of right flank pain.

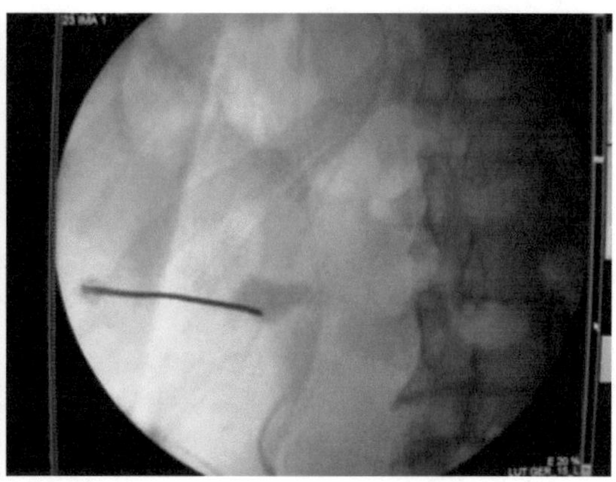

Fig. 9. 21-gauge needle was introduced toward the stone.

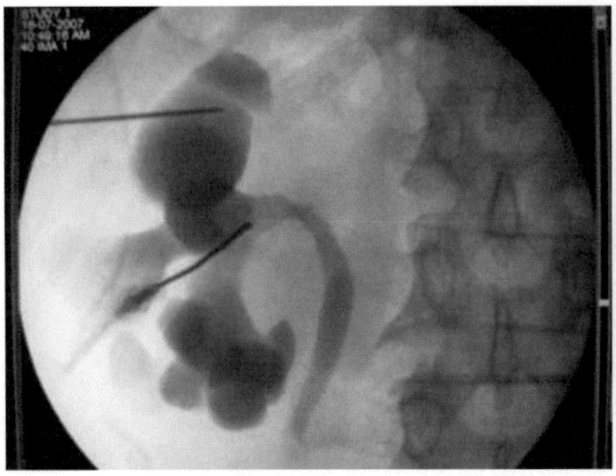

Fig. 10. Nephostogram via access needle demonstrated hydronephrosis of right kidney. The second needle was introduced toward the upper calyx for upper pole percutaneous nephrolithotomy.

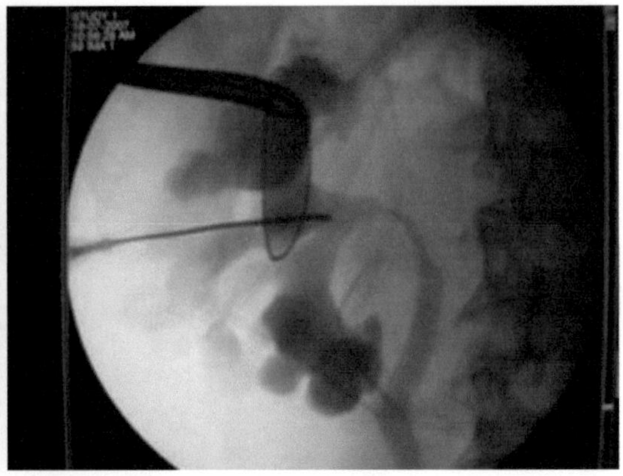

Fig. 11. The serial dilatation was done for larger access tract.

#### 3.2.4.3 Combined ultrasonography and fluoroscopy

The ideal imaging guidance technique for uncomplicated renal drainage is a combination of initial ultrasonography and followed by fluoroscopy for control of catheter and guidewire manipulation.

#### 3.2.4.4 CT guidance

The puncture can be performed into the collecting system without preoperative opacification of the collecting system. CT scan is essential in patients with organomegaly such as hepatomegaly and splenomegaly, severe skeletal abnormalities such as scoliosis and kyphosis, morbid obesity, and previous major intraabdominal surgical interventions. (Haaga et al., 1977)

### 3.2.5 Access equipment

Two commercial access systems are available, namely, trocar with a cannula and needle-guidewire-catheter techniques. The trocar technique is dangerous if the collecting system is not entered at the first pass. Currently, the Seldinger-based needle-guidewire equipment is much more popular due to its safety. This equipment has two common needle sizes 18-gauge and 21-gauge.With needle size 18-gauge, 0.035 or 0.038 inch guidewire is accepted to pass into the collecting system. The 0.018-inch guidewire is for needle size 21-gauge. (Fig. 12-15)

The advantage of 18 gauge trocar needle is minimal deviation along the course of the needle. The advantages of 21-gauge needle are decreased risk of parenchymal damage, optimal size for nondilated collecting system.The soft tip of 0.018 inch guidewire is rarely perforated the collecting system. A special nephrostomy tube kit is available, containing an 18-gauge needle, guidewire, dilators, a percutaneous nephrostomy catheter size 8 Fr or 10 Fr. Angiographic method is preferable to the trocar technique because of its safety.

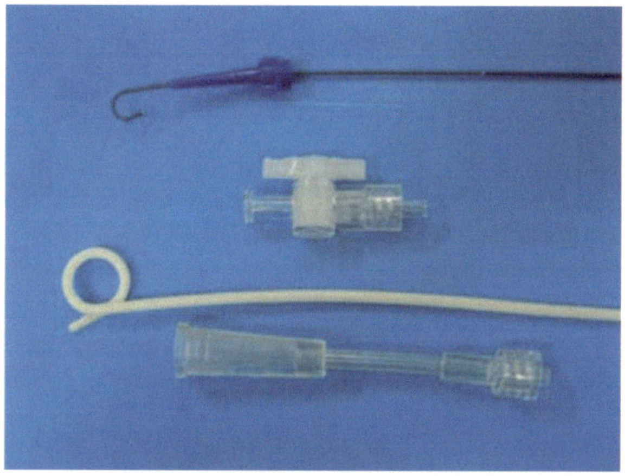

Fig. 12. Commercial access systems of needle-guidewire-catheter techniques.

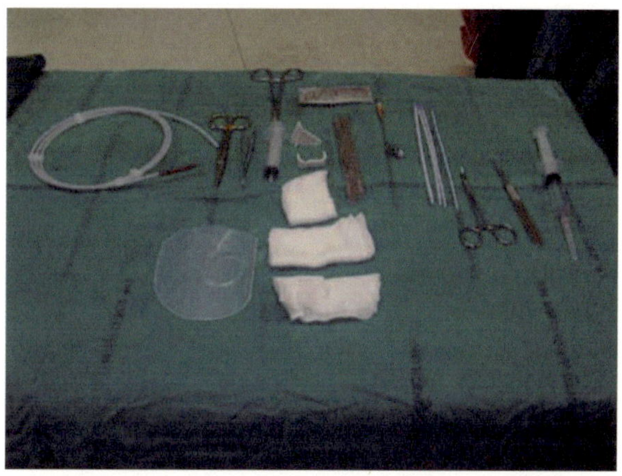

Fig. 13. Basic instruments for percutaneous nephrostomy tube placement.

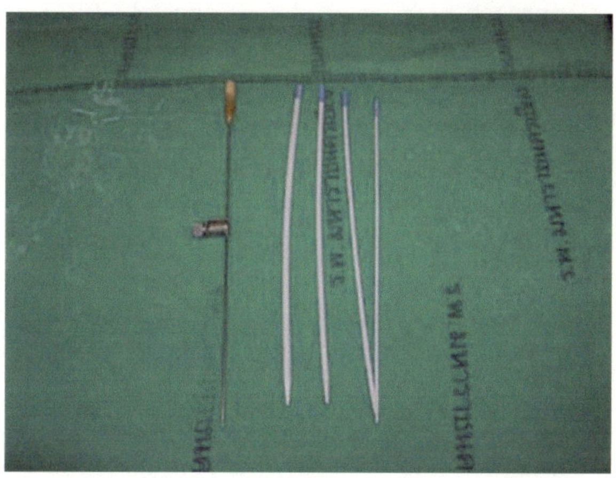

Fig. 14. Needle and dilators.

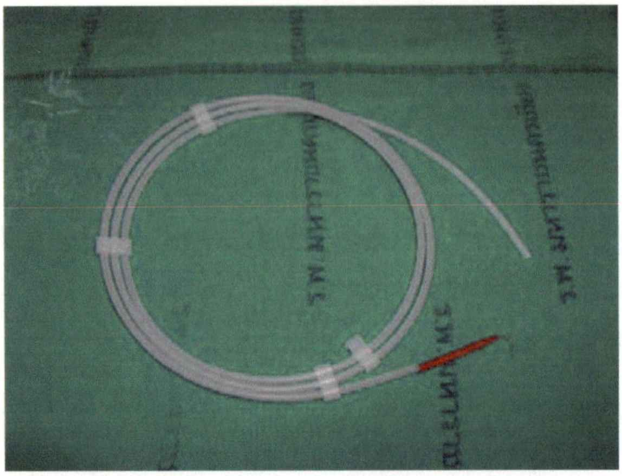

Fig. 15. Benson guidewire.

### 3.2.6 Access route

Choosing the point of entry is a very important step which can influence the final position of the nephrostomy tube. The ideal percutaneous access tract into the collecting system should begin at the posterior axillary line. The tract courses through renal parenchyma into the tip of the posterolateral calyx, and then into the middle portion of renal pelvis. This puncture line provides the stabilization of the nephrostomy tract and seals the tube that prevents urine extravasation into the perinephric space.

This technique can avoid the major bleeding due to fewer number of blood vessels at caliceal tip and this position aids subsequent endourologic manipulation such as percutanous nephrolithotomy (PCNL) or endopyelotomy. The more medially sited tract nephrostomy tube causes more discomfort for the patient in the supine position due to the compression the external portion of PNT tube with the back.

If possible, the puncture should be performed subcostally for prevention of pleural complication. In special situations, the intercostal approach may be used due to the anatomy of kidney. Upper pole approach may be needed in special situations. In ephostomy tract placement for endourologic procedures via the upper pole, the incidence of hydrothorax or hydropneumothorax is 5 to 12 percent. (Lojanapiwat & Prasopsuk, 2006). Chest tube drainage is required for patient with significant amounts of hydrothorax.

The advantages of lateral puncture are avoiding access through the bulky paraspinal muscle, ensuring the placement through the parenchyma and less chance of damaging a major vessel. Pleural complication following lateral intercostal tract is less than vertical tracts.

#### 3.2.6.1 The site of puncture depends on the indication of nephrostomy tube placement

- Simple renal drainage

  Percutaneous nephrostomy placement can be performed through nearly any tract. But if the patient needs permanent nephrostomy, the nephrostomy tube should be an ideal percutenous access tract for the patient's comfort.

- Further endourologic procedures.
  - Percutaneous nephrolithotomy (PCNL)
    : Pelvic stone
      - ideal tract is through any middle or lower calyx.

    : Calyceal stone
      - ideal tract is directly through the stone-bearing calix peripheral to the stone.

    : Staghorn stone
      - ideal tract is through upper pole calyx.

    : Upper ureteral stone
      - ideal tract is through middle pole or lower upper pole.

    : Diverticular stone
      - ideal tract is directly through diverticulum.
  - Endopyelotomy (EP) / endoureterotomy
    : Ureteropelvic junction obstruction (UPJO) and upper ureteral stricture
      - ideal tract is through middle pole or upper pole calix (Lojanapiwat, 2006).

**3.2.6.2 Upper pole access for renal access**

The upper pole of the kidney aligned medially and posterior to the lower pole, making the upper pole a shorter and easier access route. The upper-pole approach provides a straight tract along the long axis of the kidney and ensures the ability to reach most of the collecting system while providing easier manipulation of rigid instrument. The operative techniques of upper pole access need coordination with the anesthetists for controlling breathing for prevention of intercostals vessel and pulmonary complication. (Lojanapiwat & Prasopsuk, 2006) (Table 3, 4)

| |
|---|
| - Ureteropelvic junction and proximal ureteral pathology |
| - Buck of the upper pole calculi |
| - Multiple lower pole caliceal calculi |
| - Obesity or unusual body habitus |
| - Staghorn calculi |
| - Large upper ureteral calculi |

Table 3. Indication for the upper pole access.

| |
|---|
| - Need coordination with the anesthetists for controlling breathing. |
| - An intercostal puncture should be made in the lower half of the intercostal space to avoid injuring the blood vessels. |
| - During full expiration, the needle is passed through the retroperitoneum and diaphragm to prevent the injury to the lung, while needle passage through the renal parenchyma to the collecting system is done during deep inspiration for downward displacement of the kidney. |
| - An Amplatz shealth is used during the percutaneous supracostal approach to maintain low-pressure irrigation. |

Table 4. Technique of upper pole access.

#### 3.2.6.3 The causes of access failure

- Nondistended renal collecting systems
- Impacted large stone that prevent guide wire manipulation
- Obscuring the location of collecting system
- Small obstructed infundibular stone with minimal caliceal dilatation

### 3.2.7 Techniques

Follow the preparation of skin: under the ultrasonic or fluoroscopic imaging, once the pelvocalical system is clearly visible, the skin is anesthetized with one percent xylocaine or 0.25 percent bupivicaine. Xylocaine is injected into the skin, subcutaneous tissue, muscle, perinephric space and renal capsule with a small cutaneous incision. Using a needle 2 system, a 18-gauge needle is introduced toward the desired site in the renal pelvis at the more lateral point which is usually along the posterior axillary line. This can be followed and monitored by real-time ultrasound or fluoroscopy. Under fluoroscopic guidance, visualization of desired calyx is demonstrated by injection of air and contrast media. In prone position, air usually floats up to posterior calices that it is the marker for the puncture. (Fig. 16)

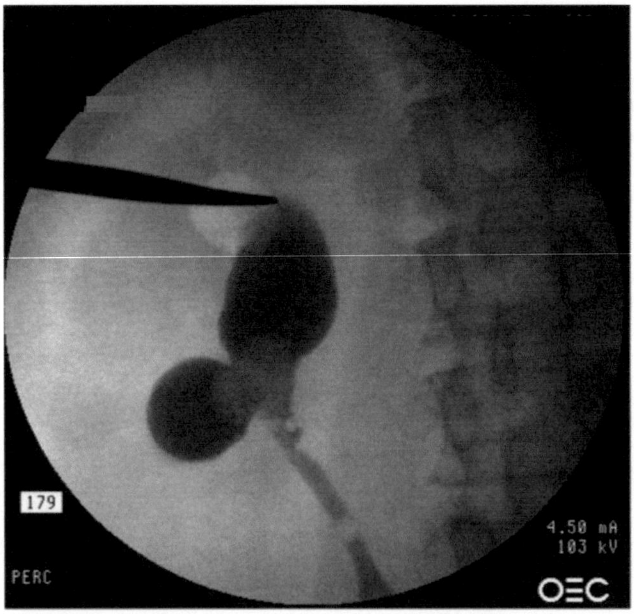


Fig. 16. Fluoroscopic imaging: air usually floats up to posterior calices in prone position that it is the marker for the puncture.

When the needle tip enters the collecting system, urine can be aspirated from the needle after the needle stylet is removed. A soft J-tipped guidewire is inserted into the needle and advanced across the caliceal infundibulum to renal pelvis. The choice of guidewires depends on the indication of nephrostomy placement. A Bentson guidewires is commonly used due to a floppy tip and coil atraumatically in collecting system.

In special situations, such as an impacted stone in the collecting system, the manipulation often requires small angled-tip catheters and hydrophilic coated wires. Then the needle is removed, and progressively larger dilators are introduced over the guidewire to dilate the access tract to facilitate the placement of soft nephrostomy tube. The size of tract dilatation depends on the goal of percutaneous access. If the goal is to provide external urinary drainage, serial dilators are inserted over the guidewire to dilate the tract to a sufficient size for the nephrostomy tube. The 8 or 10 Fr nephrostomy tube is introduced over the guidewire and optimal position is monitored by ultrasound or fluoroscopy.

The most reliable evidence for the proper placement of the nephrostomy tube can be demonstrated by nephrostogram under fluoroscopic imaging. The guidewire is withdrawn and the nephrostomy tube is secured with skin to prevent dislodging the catheter. The catheter is connected to a urine bag for drainage. (Fig. 17-20) For permanant nephrostomy tube placement, the tract can be further dilated and a regular Foley's catheter can be used.

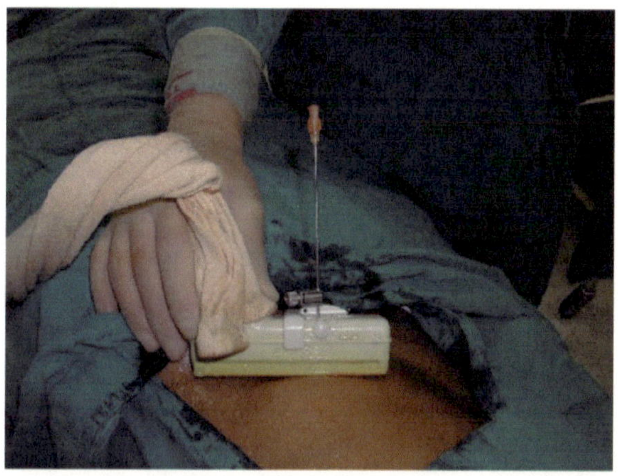

Fig. 17. Ultrasonic probe for guidance the nephrostomy tube placement.

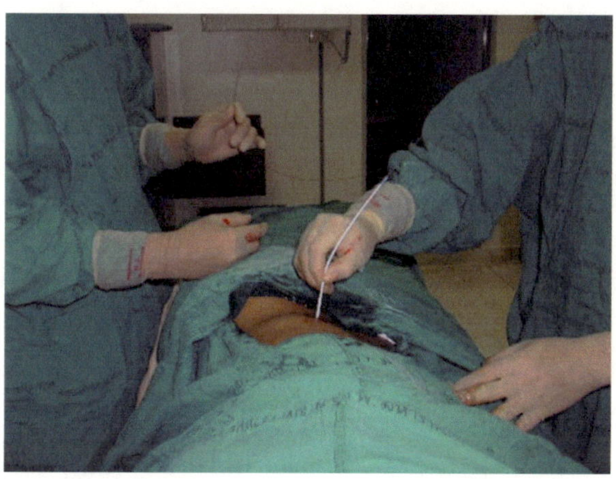

Fig. 18. Dilators over the guidewire.

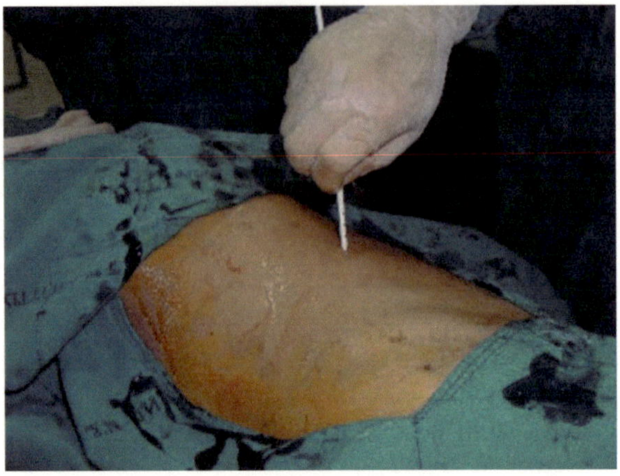

Fig. 19. 8 Fr nephostomy catheter inserted through the guidewire.

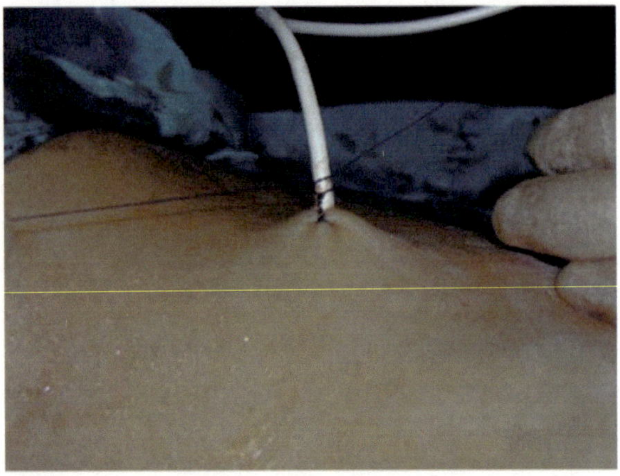

Fig. 20. The nephrostomy tube is secured with skin.

Further endourologic procedures that will follow temporary nephrostomy tube placement are percutaneous nephrolithotomy for removal of renal and upper ureteral calculi, endopyelotomy for ureteropelvic junction obstruction and infundibulotomy for infundibular stenosis. Percutaneous nephrolithotomy is effective and safe in patients with complex conditions such as underlying medical conditions and previous open nephrolithotomy. (Lojanapiwat, 2006).

Following these procedures, most patients need a larger nephrostomy tube for adequate drainage and tamponing the bleeding point from the nephrostomy tract. Recently tubeless percutaneous nephrolithotomy has been performed in uncomplicated cases with no significant bleeding, no significant extravasation, no distal obstruction and no secondary nephroscopy required. (Lojanapiwat et al., 2001) (Table 5)

- single access
- no obstructed renal unit
- no significant bleeding
- no significant extravasation
- Secondary nephroscopy is not required. (stone free)

Table 5. Criteria for tubeless percutaneous nephrolithotomy.

## 4. Results

Overall success rate of uncomplicated nephrostomy tube placement is over 97% with less success in patients who required percutaneous tract for subsequent endourologic interventions. Factors which affect the success rate of nephrostomy tube placement during endourologic operation are stone burden, degree of hydronephrosis, history of previous open nephrolithotomy, and experience of surgeon. As same as other urologic procedure, a training simulator for ultrasound-guided percutaneous nephrostomy insertion is needed for a safe, non-threatening environment, without risk to patients. Commercial and a gelatin phantoms are available. Skill is required prior to undertaking procedures in patients. (Rock et al., 2010)

## 5. Complications

Complications following simple nephrostomy tube drainage are minor with a rate approaching 4%. (LeRoy, 1996). The common complications are hemorrhage, infection, improper catheter placement, nephrostomy tube dislodging after initial proper placement, nephrocutaneous fistula, stone formation and post-obstructive diuresis. Initial hematuria is common, but should be cleared in 24 - 48 hours post operatively.

Small subcapsular hematoma is found about 3% of cases, a complication that is usually resolved without sequelae. Bleeding from iatrogenic arteriovenous-caliceal fistulas occurs in less than 2% and can be managed with angioembolization. (Fig. 21, 22) Pulmary

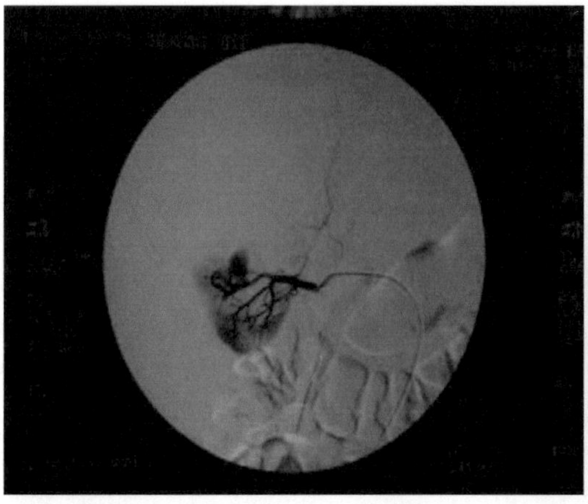

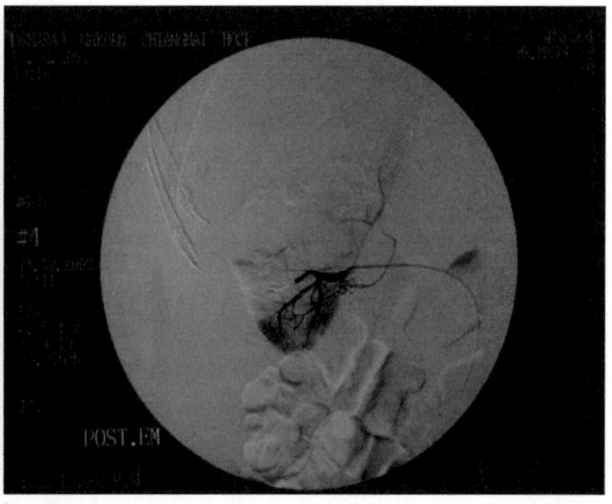


Preoperative and postoperative angioembolization of arteriovenous fistula follow percutaneous nephrolithotomy.

Fig. 21. Arteriovenous fistula at middle part of kidney.

Fig. 22. Disappear of fistula after angioembolization.

complication is found in endourologic procedure via upper pole access. Patients with significant hydrothorax usually need intercostal drainage. (Lojanapiwat & Prasopsuk, 2006). (Fig. 23, 24) Other minor complications are small perforations with collection, malfunction of nephrostomy tube, persistence nephrocutaneous fistula and sepsis in patients with infected urine. (de la Rosette et al., 2011) (Fig. 25)

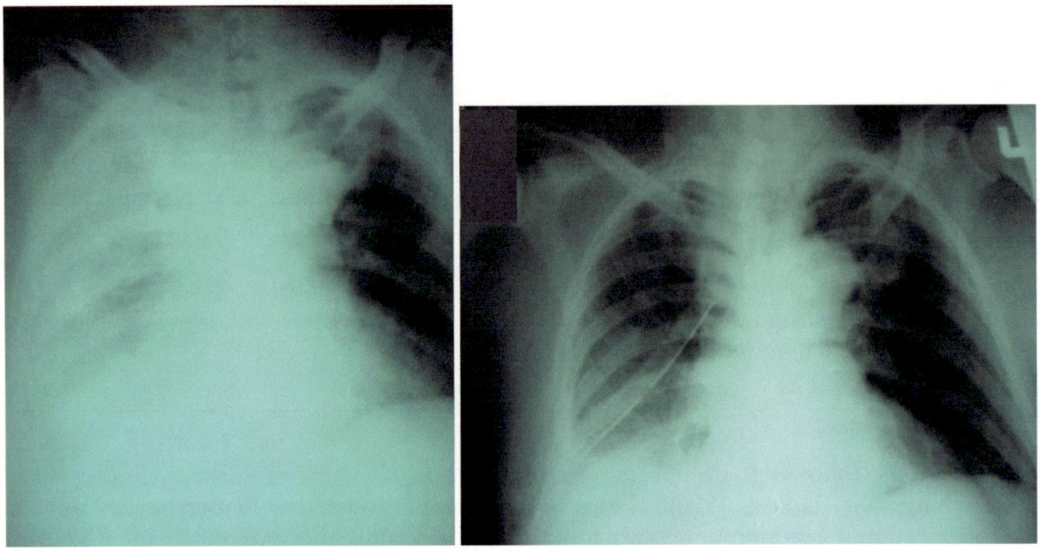

Fig. 23, 24. Hydrothorax: Immediate post-operative and post intercostal tube drainage chest x-ray of patient following upper pole percutaneous nephrolithotomy.

Patients who develop postobstructive diuresis (POD > 3 liters per day or > 200 ml/hr for 12 to 24 hours) following urinary diversion should be treated with intravenous fluid of 0.45 percent NaCI at a two hourly rate equal to one half the previous two hours urine output. (Gulmi et al., 1998)

Nephrostomy tube dislodgement from the skin can be undertaken even when carefully fixed to the skin with silk suture. Zhou and colleges reported a new technique to reinforce the nephrostomy tube in 48 patients by using 2 cm long rubber drainage tube as the outer tube to encase the nephrostomy tube and suturing the longitudinal cutting edges together with the skin suture. This technique can significantly decrease the dislodgement incidence of nephrostomy tube. (Zhou et al., 2011)

Prevention of nephrocutaneous fistula, a nephrostogram should show radio-opaque contrast medium passing freely down the ureter into the bladder. Clamping the catheter should be done before removing the catheter and should cause no pain and no leakage around the catheter.

Foreign-body calculi at nephrostomy tube can occur after long term placement. Dalton et al reviewed the inducement of foreign-body calculi in laboratory animals as 1) Stone may develop on foreign bodies in absence or presence of infection, 2) Urea-splitting organisms enhance the formation of foreign-body stones, 3) Diuresis and urinary acidification inhibits foreign-body stone formation. Iatrogenic foreign body stones lead to a significant proportion of this urologic problem such as ureteral catheters or nephrostomy tubes. (Dalton et al., 1975).

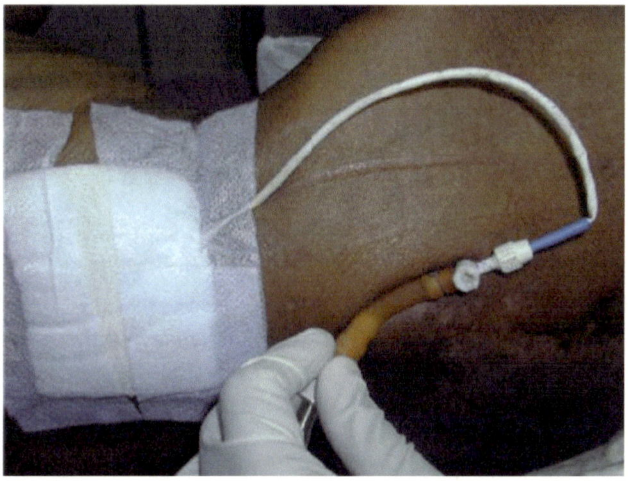

Fig. 25. Kinking of tube follow long term nephrostomy tube placement.

## 6. Percutaneas nephrostomy placement in special situations

### 6.1 Renal anomalies

Due to abnormal anatomy of patients with renal anomalies such as horseshoe kidney; in prone position, the site of access is relatively median often at paraspinous area.

### 6.2 Transplanted kidney

In supine position, the percutanous access can be achieved through extraperitoneal approach under ultrasound guidance. The puncture site start at medial to the anterior superior iliac crest. Occasionally, CT guidance is needed especially when there is bowel loops between anterior abdominal wall and kidney.

### 6.3 Pelvic kidney

Access nephrostomy tube to pelvic kidney is challenging due to significant complications such as bleeding and urine extravasation. This technique requires combined transabdominal laparoscopic and transurethral retrograde access creation.

### 6.4 Pediatric kidney

Access to the pediatric kidney is more complex than the adult kidney in terms of fluid management and the appropriate size of the nephrostomy tube. Long term stabilization the nephrostomy tube in children is often difficult.

## 7. Summary

Percutaneous nephrostomy is performed for temporary or permanent supravesicle urinary diversion. The successful outcome without complication is the goal of this procedure and this requires careful preoperative planning and proper techniques. The guidance system for urinary tract intervention are fluoroscopic guidance, real-time ultrasonography and CT scan. The ideal nephrostomy tract should course through renal parenchyma into the tip of posterolateral calix then into the middle portion of renal pelvis. The complication following simple nephrostomy tube drainage is minor.

## 8. References


Banner, MP.; Ramchandani, P. & Pollack, HM. (1991). Interventional procedures in the upper urinary tract. Cardiovasc Intervent Radiol, 14(5):267-84.

Curhan, CG. & Zeidel, ML. (1996). Urinary tract obstruction, In BM Brenner(ed): The kidney. 5th ed. Philadelphia, WB Saunders CO, Vol 2 Chap41, 1391.

Dalton, DL.; Hughes, J. & Glenn, JF. (1975). Foreign bodies and urinary stones Urology, 6: 1

de la Rosette, J.; Assimos, D.; Desai, M.; Gutierrez, J.; Lingeman, J.; Scarpa, R. & Tefekli, A. (2011). CROES PCNL Study Group. The Clinical Research Office of the Endourological Society Percutaneous Nephrolithotomy Global Study: indications, complications, and outcomes in 5803 patients. J Endourol. 25(1):11-7.

Falahatkar, S.; Asgari, SA.; Nasseh, H.; Allahkhah, A.; Farshami, FJ.; Shakiba, M. & Esmaeili, S. (2010). Totally ultrasound versus fluoroscopically guided complete supine percutaneous nephrolithotripsy: a first report. J Endourol, 24(9):1421-6.

Goodwin, WE.; Casey, WC. & Woolf, W. (1955). Percutaneous trocar (needle) nephrostomy in hydronephrosis. J Am Med Assoc, 12; 157(11):891-4.

Gulmi, FA.; Felsen, D. & Vaughan, ED. (1998). Management of post-obstructive diuresis, AUA update series , Vol 17:178-83.

Haaga, JR.; Zelch, Mg.; Alfids, RJ.; Steward, BH. & Daugherty, JD. (1977). Interventional CT scanning. Radiol Clin North Am. 15(3):449-56.

Juul, N.; Nielsen, V. & Torp-Pederson, S. (1985). Percutaneous balloon catheter nephrostomy guided by ultrasound. Results of a new technique. Scand J Urol Nephrol, 19(4):291-4.

LeRoy, AT. (1996). Percutaneous access, In: Smith, AD. & Badlani, GH. & Bagley, DH. (eds): Smith's textbook of Endourology. 1st ed. St Louis, Missouri, Quality Medical Publishing, Inc, Chap 14, P 199-223.

LeRoy, AJ.; May, GR.; Bender, CE.; Williams, HJ Jr.; Mc Gough, PF.; Segura, JW. & Patterson, DF. (1984). Percutaneous nephrostomy for stone removal. Radiology, 151(3):607-12.

Lojanapiwat, B. & Prasopsuk, S. (2006). Upper-pole access for percutaneous nephrolithotomy: comparison of supracostal and infracostal approaches. J Endourol, 20(7):491-4.

Lojanapiwat, B. (2006). Previous open nephrolithotomy: does it affect percutaneous nephrolithotomy techniques and outcome? J Endourol, 20(1):17-20.

Lojanapiwat, B.; Soonthornpan, S. & Wudhikarn, S. (2001). Tubeless percutaneous nephrolithotomy in selected patients. J Endourol, 15(7):711-3.

Rock, BG.; Leonard, AP. & Freeman, SL. (2010). A training simul ator for ultrasound-guided percutaneous nephrostomy insertion. Br J Radiol, 83:612-4.

Stables, DP.; Ginsberg, NJ. & Johnson, ML. (1978). Percutaneous nephrostomy: a series and review of the literature. AJR Am J Roentgenol, 130(1):75-82.

Sherman, JL.; Hopper, KD.; Greene, AJ. & Johns, TT. (1985). The retrorenal colon on computed tomography: a normal variant. J Comput Assist Tomogr, 9(2):339-41.

Zhou, T.; Gao, X.; Yang, C.; Peng, Y.; Xiao, L.; Xu, C, et al. (2011). Reforcement for percutaneous nephrostomy tubes with a new technique. J Endourol, 25:41-4.

17

# Extra-Anatomic Urinary Drainage for Urinary Obstruction

Michael Kimuli, John Sciberras and Stuart Lloyd
*St. James's University Hospital, Leeds*
*UK*

## 1. Introduction

Long-term drainage of the urinary tracts of patients with impassable ureteric strictures remains a major challenge to the urologist. Until the mid 1970's the only viable, minimally invasive treatment was a permanent nephrostomy with all its sequelae, loss of quality of life, risk of tube dislocation, infection, and recurrent obstruction (Marberger, 2006). For decades, researchers experimented with different prosthetic ureteric replacements with minimal success. with minimal success. The breakthrough came in 1976 with a case report of the first successful prosthetic replacement of both ureters in a patient with malignant obstruction. The authors proved that not only were prosthetic materials possible replacements for ureters, peristaltic activity was not needed for permanent normal function of the upper urinary tract (Schulman, et al., 1976). This landmark study resulted in rapid progress in the investigation for potential materials for ureteric replacement that could be used without need for major reconstructive surgery. However, it was not until 1994 that the first viable 7F double-pigtail prosthetic extra-anatomic bypass system was developed (Lingam et al., 1994). Despite several series reporting excellent outcomes during the last two decades, extra-anatomic stenting is not yet universally offered to candidate patients.

Conventionally, such patients are offered a minimally invasive procedure in the form of a percutaneous nephrostomy or alternatively reconstructive surgery. Percutaneous nephrostomy, though minimally invasive, is far from ideal for long-term use. Reconstructive surgery overcomes some of the problems related to long-term nephrostomy use; however, it requires patients to undergo major surgery. Unfortunately, the majority of impassable ureteric strictures are due to malignant disease, which has been reported to carry a poor prognosis with a resulting median survival of 3 to 7 months (Kouba et al., 2008). This prognosis highlights the importance of maintaining quality of life in this group of patients and major reconstructive surgery with all its potential sequelae, should ideally be avoided.

An ideal urinary diversion should provide symptomatic relief for the required duration without requiring multiple changes and should be associated with minimal or no morbidity. Several authors have reported their experience of using extra-anatomical stents (EAS) for temporary or permanent drainage of obstructed urinary tracts (Ahmadzadeh, 1991; Lingam et al., 1994; Nakada et al., 1995; Desgrandchamps et al., 1998a 1998b; Minhas et al., 1999; Lloyd et al., 2007). In this chapter, we describe the indications for and the technique of inserting the EAS, and a review of the results from the major series.

## 2. Patient indications

The main indication for insertion of an EAS is malignant ureteric obstruction that has failed management with internal ureteric stenting or nephrostomy (Fig 1a-b). Patients with benign ureteric obstruction that have either failed open reconstructive surgery or are unfit or unwilling to undergo open surgery can also be considered for EAS. Increasing experience with EAS has been paralleled by an expansion in it is indications. At our institution for example, we have successfully used EAS to treat intractable urinary incontinence due to ureteric fistulae in patients otherwise unfit for open surgical repair. In some patients, it has been used as a temporary measure for ureteric fistula before definitive repair is carried out. Lastly, EAS is increasingly being used in transplanted kidneys (Olsburgh , 2007) as well as in patients with ileal conduit (own series).

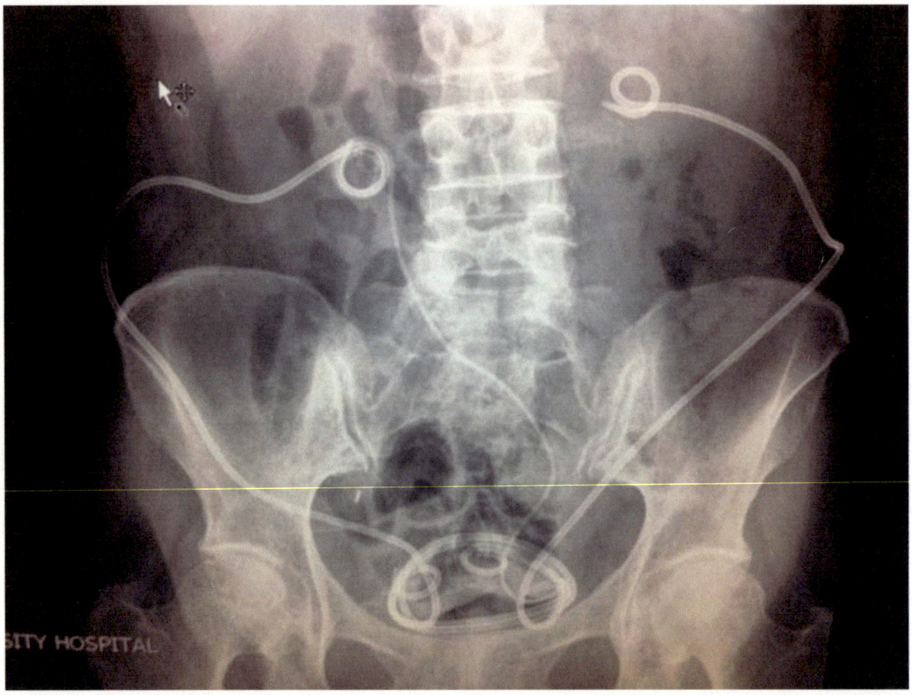


Fig. 1a. Bilateral Extra-anatomic stents of the Paterson Forrester type (short-term). There is also trans-ureteric ureterostomy stent seen in-situ to be removed. Patient had bilateral strictures and fistula after reconstruction in a post-irradiated abdomen and several attempts at corrective surgery without success.

The only absolute contraindications are uncorrected coagulopathies and active malignancy, either arising or invading the bladder. Tumour seeding along the track may occur if the stent is placed near a tumour (Fig. 2). Bowel stomas and multiple abdominal scars make stent placement more challenging but are not a contraindication. Likewise, patients with a small capacity bladder require appropriate counseling regarding potential increased urinary frequency especially if they have been managed with nephrostomy for a long time. Patients should be warned of the risk of subcutaneous infection that will usually respond to a course of appropriate antibiotic. Rarely, the infection may necessitate removal of the stent with a

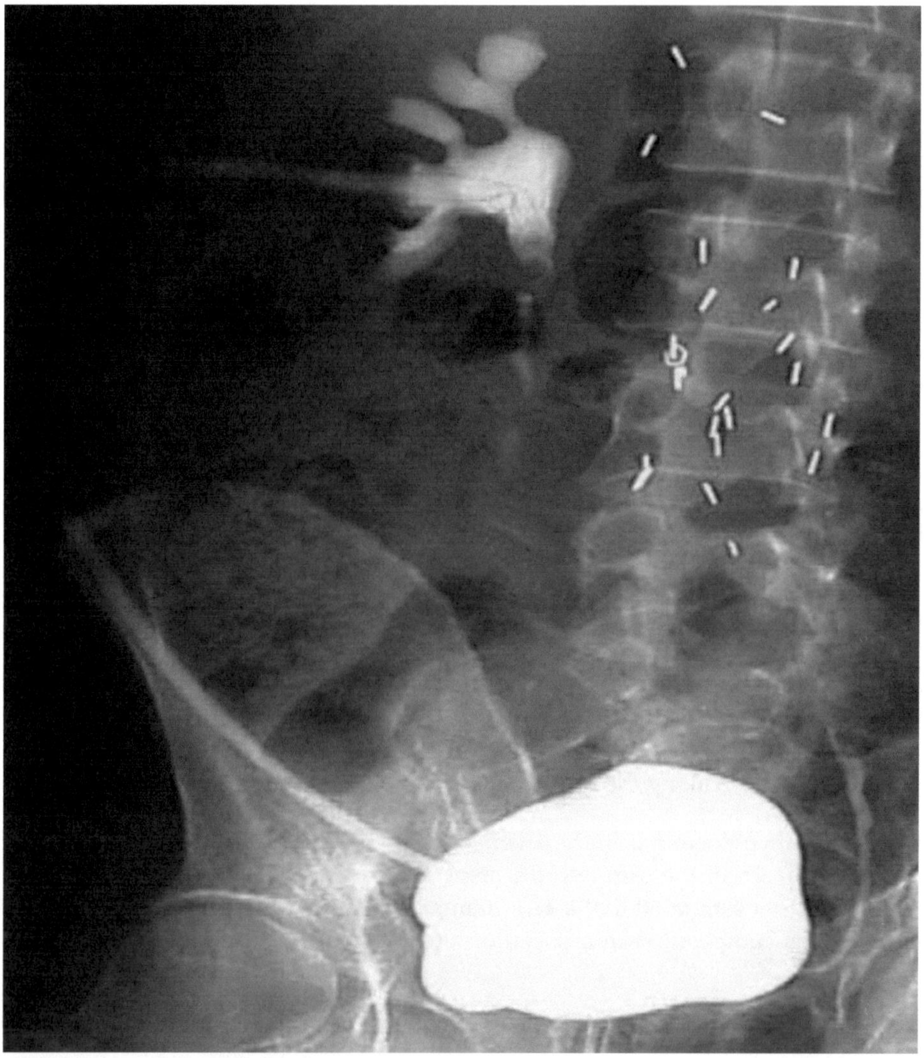

Fig. 1b. Cystogram in a patient with a Detour extra-anatomic stent (permanent type) for ureteric obstruction after sarcoma excision.

temporary conversion of the proximal end to a nephrostomy. Rarely still, stent blockage may occur requiring change before 12 months. In our experience, storage bladder symptoms from the stent are exceptionally rare and no stent was ever removed at our institution due to this problem.

## 3. Stents

Different types of EAS have been developed and used successfully by different authors (Lingam, 1994; Minhas, 1999; Desgrandchamps, 1998a;, Lloyd, 2007). The designs have varied with the materials used, length of stent, diameter of stent and on whether one or composite stent/s are utilized. They however, all have a common objective of establishing a

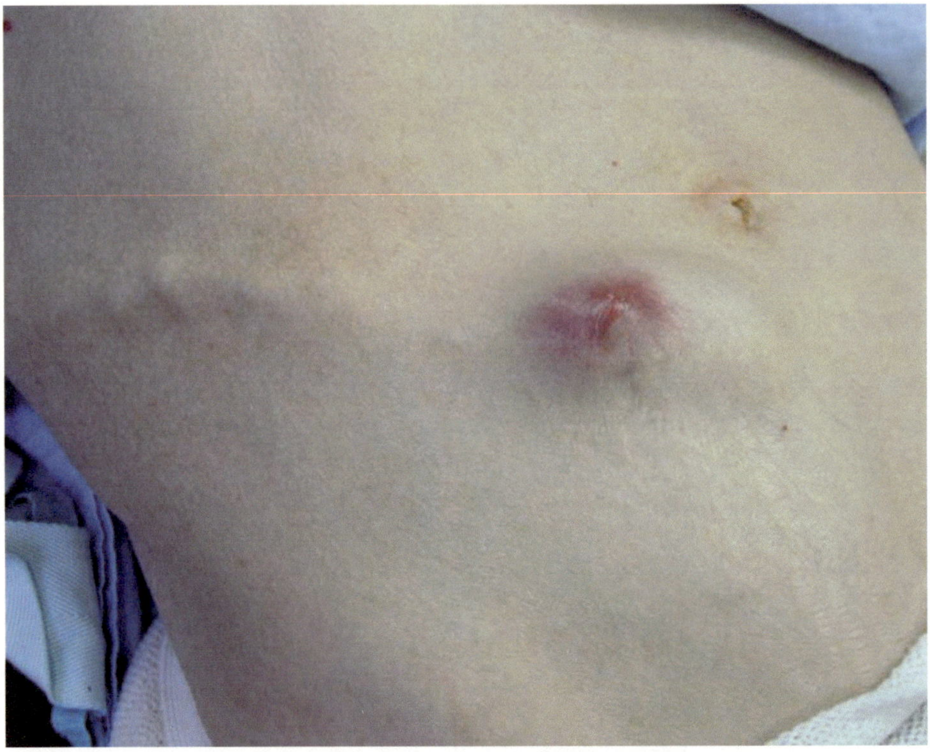

Fig. 2. Tumour invasion along the route of an extra-anatomic stent.

nephro-vesical subcutaneous urinary diversion. The diameter of the stent is thought to be the main determinant of the duration the stent may remain in situ without encrustation or blocking. It has been estimated that a 17 F diameter is required to prevent stent encrustation irrespective of its composition in association with increased fluid intake (Andonian, et al. 2005).

To this end, we utilize two types of stents in our practice. One is a short-term 8.5F 65cm EAS without side holes except at either end. We offer to all patients with malignant disease and in patients with poor general health and benign disease where there is concern regarding the functionality of the bladder. If they survive the first change and have a good prognosis, we will usually discuss conversion to a more long-term 29F Detour EAS. The latter stent requires a more invasive technique including an open cystostomy but has the advantage of potentially being a permanent diversion with a single procedure. We use it as a primary option in patients with a long life expectancy. Below, we describe our technique of inserting both types of stents.

## 4. The Paterson-Forrester stent

### 4.1 Equipment

The Paterson-Forrester 65cm, 8.5F polyurethane stent (Cook Ireland Ltd)

Cystoscopy tray for either (flexible or rigid cystoscopy)

Percutaneous nephrostomy track placement tray with telescopic metal dilators to size 3 (18F).

Contrast solution in a luer lock syringe

Minor operation tray with scalpel, tissue forceps and clips

Dissecting scissors

Needle holder and absorbable sutures

Nephrostomy needle and 0.38F j tip wire

12 F peel away sheath

0.38F floppy tip stiff core Sensor wire (Microvasive)

*Extra equipment for exchange of stent*

6F end flushing ureteric catheter

Flexible rat-toothed stent removing forceps if flexible cystoscope is used

### 4.2 First time insertion PF stent

The procedure for insertion involves three steps:

1. Insertion of stent in the kidney via a new or existing nephrostomy tract. Our preferred option is to use the track of an existing nephrostomy tube after a minimum of 5 days insertion.
2. Creation of a subcutaneous tunnel and tunneling of the stent to reach the supra-pubic region.
3. Creation of a supra-pubic tube cystostomy and insertion into the bladder in the bladder.

*Step 1*

For unilateral placement, the patient is positioned in the Lloyd-Davis position, with the ipsi-lateral leg in extension and the affected side elevated to approximately $20^0$ with 3 litre saline bags. Gram-negative antibiotic prophylaxis is given - usually Gentamicin 2mg/Kg. The skin is prepared with aqueous iodine and draping applied to leave the abdomen and nephrostomy tube exposed (Fig. 3). The C-arm is positioned at the opposite side of the stent insertion while the camera with stack is placed near the foot of the table opposite the operator. An assistant needs to be able to perform a cystoscopy at the same time the operator places the upper end of the stent as detailed below.

Ideally the patient already has a nephrostomy tube in place and thus the following steps are undertaken. However, it is possible to create a new track and deliver the proximal end of the stent into the kidney de-novo. Local anaesthetic is injected into the skin around the nephrostomy tube and contrast is injected to opacify the collecting system. A 0.38F Sensor guide wire (Microvasive) is passed through the existing nephrostomy tube and the tube removed under screening leaving the wire in the system. The tapered end of the EAS is placed into the collecting system over the wire producing a good coil in the kidney. The skin incision is extended in a transverse direction for 2cm and the existing cutaneous aspect of the existing fistulous track is excised and dissected free from the rest of the tract in order to allow the stent to sit below the skin cutaneous margin (Fig. 4).

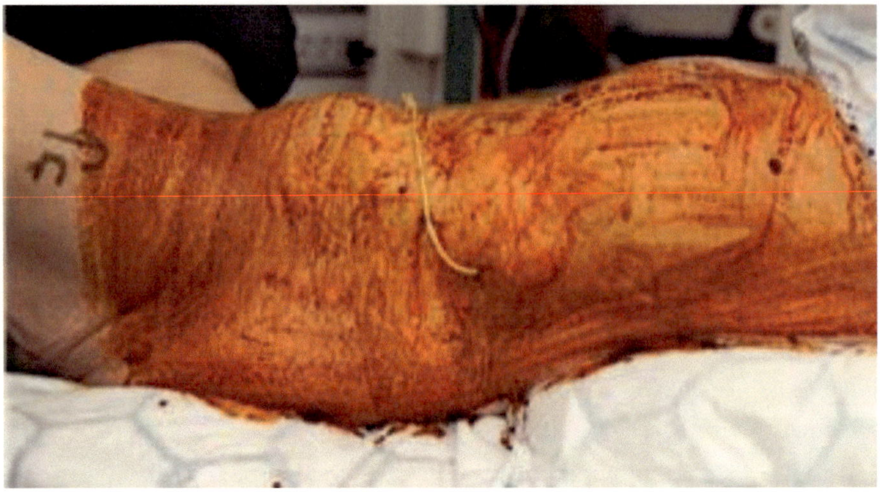

Fig. 3. Patient positioning over the edge of the operating table with fluid bags elevating the side and the nephrostomy tube included in skin preparation.

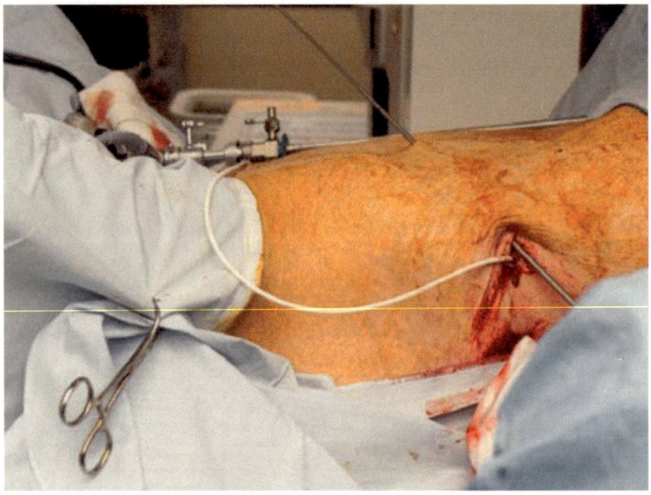

Fig. 4. The Paterson-Forrester extra-anatomic stent is passed over a guide wire and replaces the nephrostomy tube. The skin bridge is dissected free.

*Step 2*

The Alken PCNL coaxial metal dilators are used to create a multi-stage subcutaneous tunnel (Fig. 5). The 9F long metal guide rod is passed in the subcutaneous fat layer obliquely towards the iliac fossa. The tract is sequentially dilated to 18F. After injection with local anaesthetic the skin is incised over the tip of the dilators at a point that allows control of both ends of the dilators. The smaller dilators are retrieved from the new incision leaving only the 18F dilator in place through which the EAS is passed towards the bladder. The metal dilator is then retrieved distally leaving the stent in a new subcutaneous tunnel. The procedure is repeated two or three times depending upon the route taken to the supra-pubic area avoiding scars and or stomas.

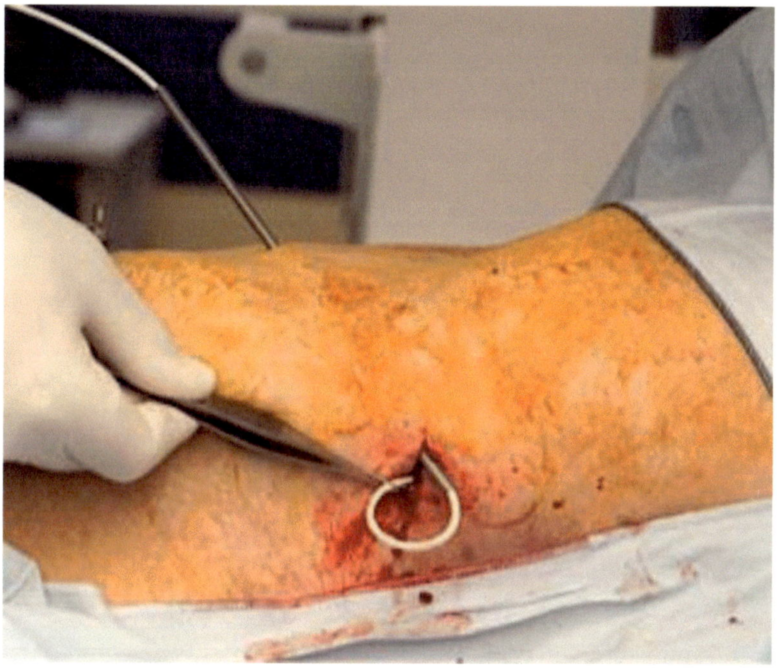

Fig. 5. The Alken dilators used to create a subcutaneous tunnel down to the supra-pubic region.

*Step 3*

The site of the last skin incision should be in the supra-pubic region but lateral to the midline. An assistant performs a cystoscopy to allow visualization of the stent as it is inserted into the bladder using a modified Seldinger technique with the aid of a 12 F peel-away sheath. Before the stent is finally delivered into its final subcutaneous tunnel the position of proximal end of the stent is checked with x ray screening (Fig. 6). The presence of a cystoscope should prevent distal stent migration out through the urethra. The skin is closed with absorbable sutures and skin glue.

### 4.3 Exchange of PF stent

Stents are changed routinely at 12 months (although licensed for 3 months), using the following technique:

A clip is used to identify a suitable position to incise the skin anteriorly, ideally half way along the stent but any position proximal to the bladder is acceptable. It is better to be able to see this site and the proximal coil in the kidney in the same fluoroscopic image. Making a small transverse incision at the appropriate site exposes the stent. The stent is then cut and a Sensor guide-wire passed through the proximal portion of the stent, which is then removed. The new stent is passed over the guide-wire before withdrawing the wire. The guide-wire is then passed into the bladder via the distal end of the old stent, which is then removed. The distal end of the new stent is passed over the wire into the bladder and the guide-wire removed endoscopically from the distal end of the stent (Minhas et al., 1999).

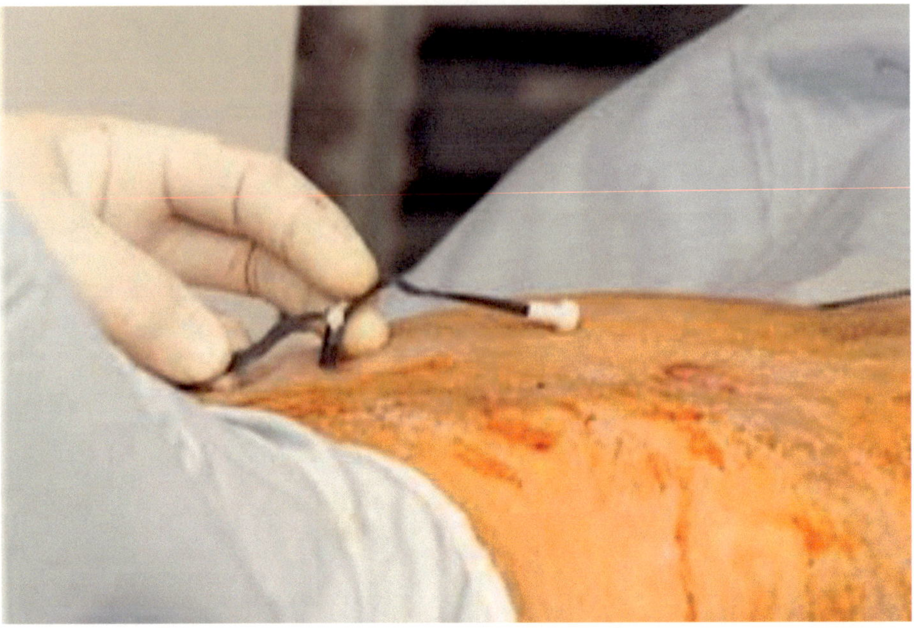

Fig. 6. Supra-pubic puncture and peel-away sheath used to deliver stent into the bladder under cystoscopic control.

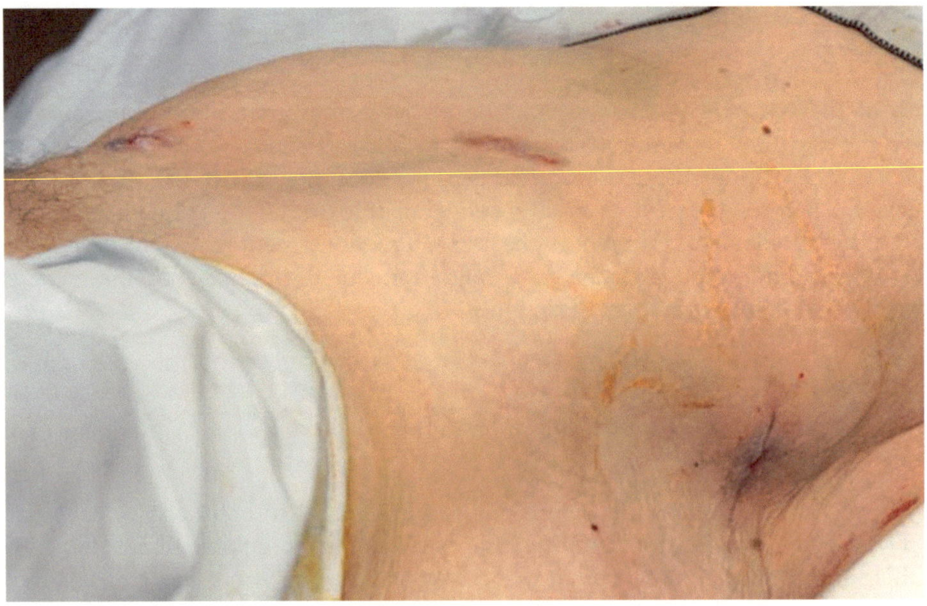

Fig. 7. Wounds closed with subcutaneous absorbable sutures and skin glue.

## 5. Insertion of the detour stent

The equipment required are provided as a kit and include the 29F PTFE-silicone stent and the dilator (Coloplast, UK). In addition, a surgical set suitable for a lower abdominal transverse incision is required. Insertion of the permanent Detour stent follows the same principals described above but because it is a bigger stent (29F), it requires the tract to be dilated to 30F (Lloyd et al., 2007). This is achieved with a 30F renal Amplatz sheath and a large-bore plastic subcutaneous tunneling device, which are included in the kit (Fig. 8a-f). A lower abdominal transverse incision is undertaken before a 1cm open cystostomy is performed via which the stent is placed into the bladder and secured with 4-0 Vicryl sutures to the bladder serosa. The large bore subcutaneous stent can be easily palpated and seen in the thin patient (Fig. 9).

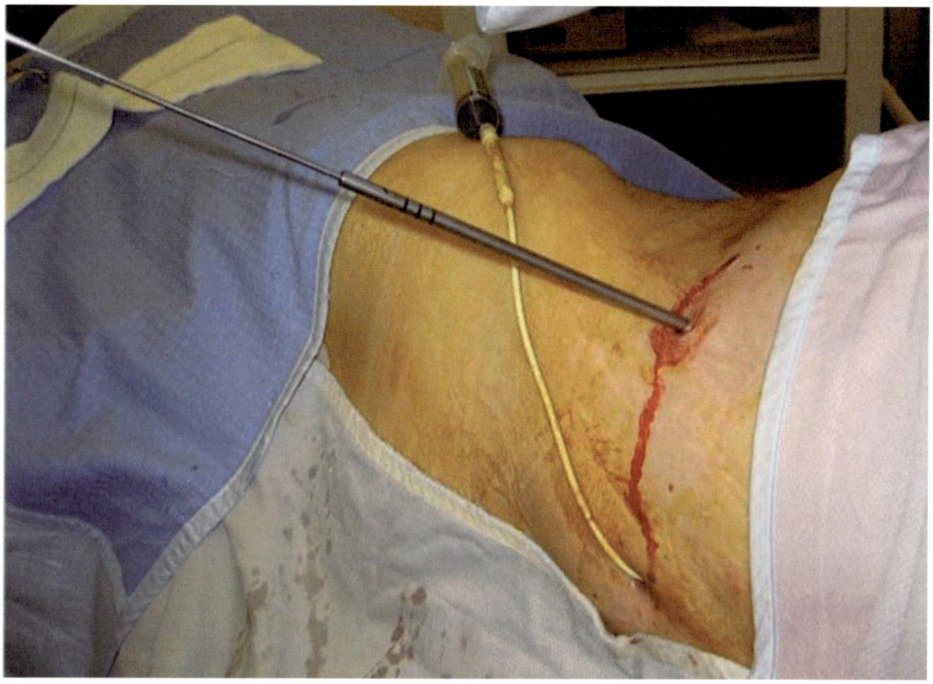

Fig. 8a. Lateral percutaneous track using the existing nephrostomy to inject contrast to outline and dilate the pelvi-calyceal system

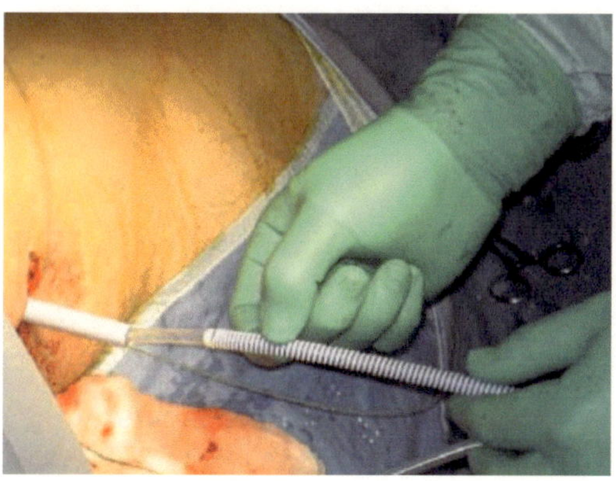

Fig. 8b. Insertion of the proximal end of the Detour stent through the Amplatz sheath into the kidney (note yellow radiolucent ring to aid positioning).

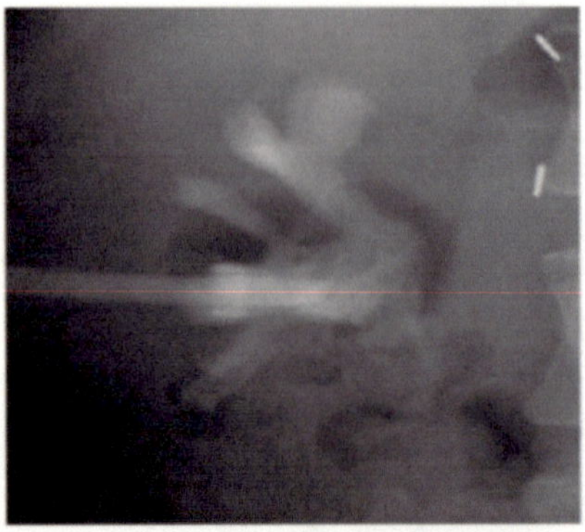

Fig. 8c. Opaque contrast medium injected through the stent to ensure correct positioning.

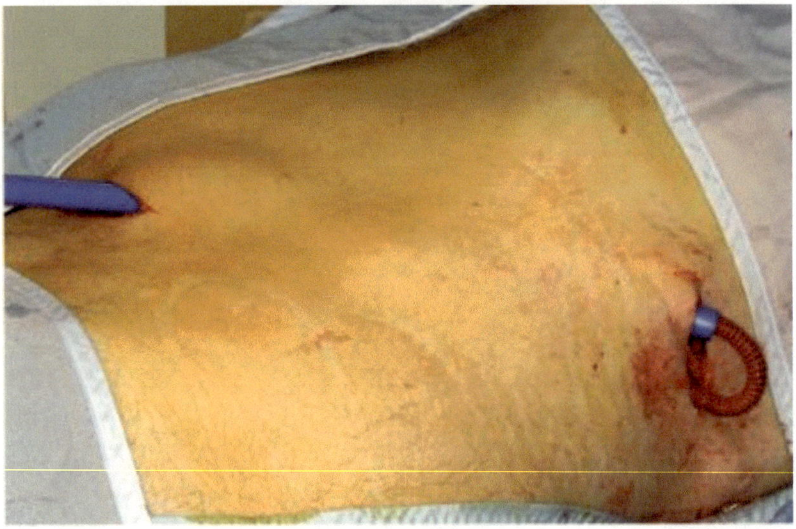

Fig. 8d. Subcutaneous tunneling device (blue) and Detour stent being positioned from renal puncture site to supra-pubic region prior to bladder suture

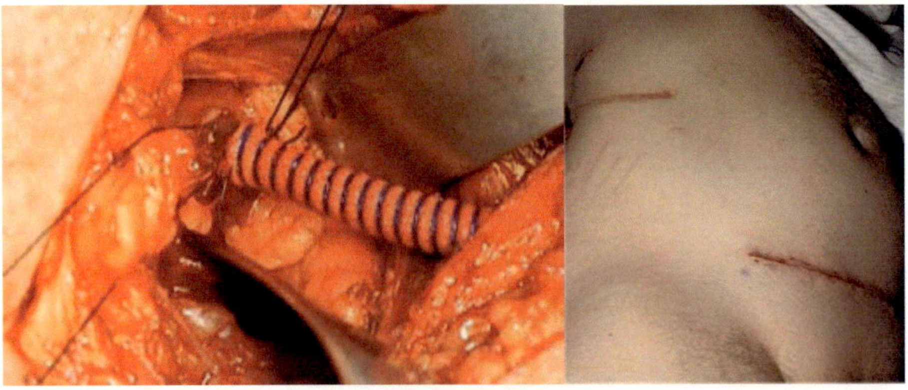

Fig. 8e,f. Sutured cystostomy after shortening the stent, skin glue is applied to wounds after subcutaneouse sutures and glue.

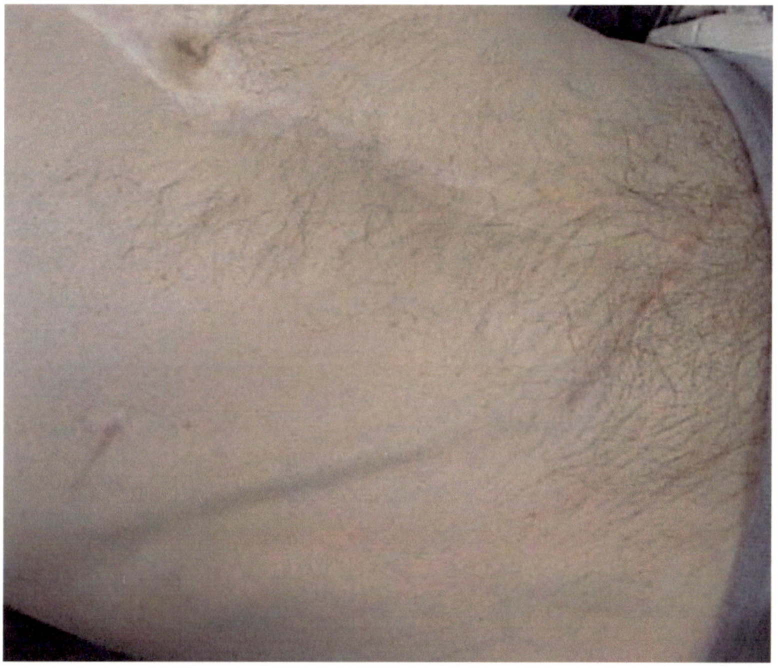

Fig. 9. Wide bore Detour stent may be palpable in thin patients. Healed incisions are visible.

## 6. Post-operative management and follow-up

A Foley catheter may be left in the bladder for a few hours to observe fluid balance but it is not essential following insertion of the short term EAS. Patients are usually discharged home on the day of surgery or the following day. The referring physician monitors the renal function. The patients are instructed to seek medical help immediately if they develop any signs of local or systemic sepsis. Following placement of the Detour stent, an indwelling catheter is left in situ for 1 week, and a cystogram is performed to check the integrity of the suture line before catheter removal (Fig. 10). Flexible cystoscopic view may show some mucosal oedema at the site of implantation (Fig. 11).

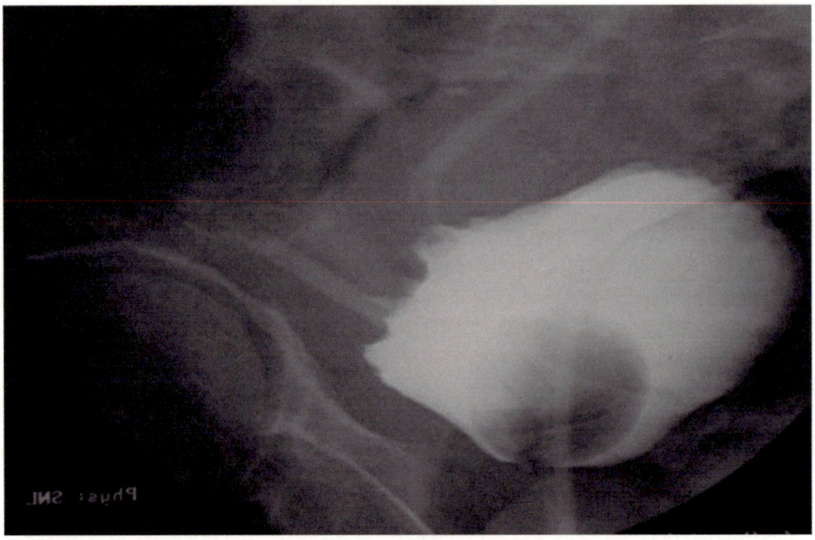

Fig. 10. Cystogram used to check for suture line integrity.

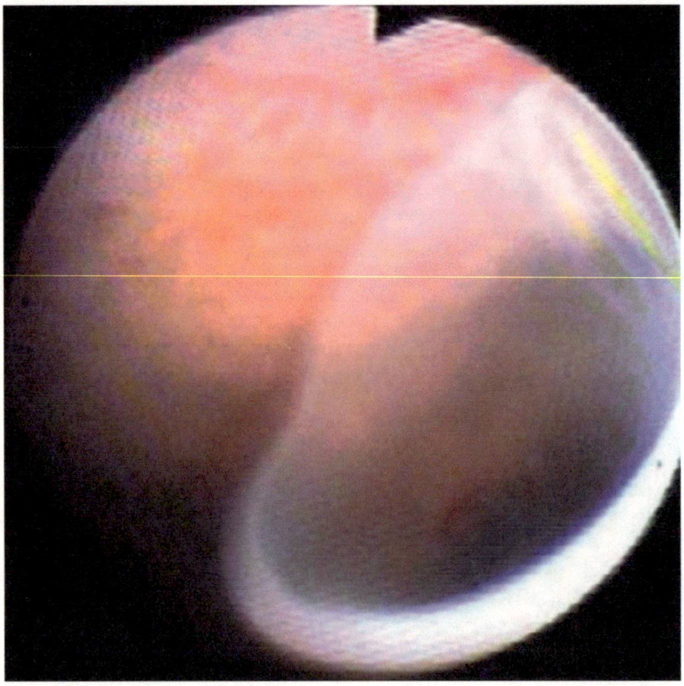

Fig. 11. Cystoscopic appearance of the silicone part of the Detour stent.

## 7. Discussion of results

End-stage ureteric obstruction, which has failed ureteric stenting, presents a significant challenge the urologist. Most of our patients have terminal cancer and are therefore not ideal candidates for major reconstructive surgery. The remainder of the patients have either failed or declined reconstructive surgery, or are too frail for major surgery. The conventional practice of managing this group of patients is with external percutaneous nephrostomy drainage. Unfortunately long-term nephrostomy drainage presents significant compromises to the patient's quality of life in addition to requiring regular changes.

In 1991, Ahmadzadeh reported short-term results in 8 patients with ureteric obstruction who underwent subcutaneous urinary diversion using a specially designed stent. The procedure had the advantage of being simple whilst at the same time avoided the complications and social effects of other methods of palliative treatment by urinary diversion (Ahmadzadeh 1991). Since this pioneering article, several authors have reported their experience with different types of EAS for urinary diversion. In 1994 Lingam and colleagues reported their series of 5 patients who had EASs inserted during a 15-month period. The diversion was created using a specially designed 7F double pigtail stent, which they routinely changed at 4-month intervals. They found it to be a safe, effective and an acceptable alternative to nephrostomy drainage that improved quality of life (Lingam et al., 1994). A year later, another small study reported a marked improvement in patients' overall comfort and quality of life following conversion of nephrostomies to EASs using a similar but slightly larger 8.5F stent (Nakada et al., 1995). In the same year, Desgrandchamps introduced another stent prototype, which was a one-piece, self-retaining expanded polytetrafluoroethylene-silicone tube that was successfully assembled as an EAS in 19 patients with a mean follow-up of 7.2 months. All patients expressed an improvement in the quality of life although in one case, a conversion to a conventional percutaneous nephrostomy was necessary (Desgrandchamps et al., 1995).

In 1999, our group published results of 13 patients treated with EAS. Urinary diversion was successful in all patients; two survived for more than 1 year, with changes at six monthly intervals. In three patients the stents were replaced by percutaneous nephrostomies because of problems with leakage or infection. The remaining patients died with functioning EAS in situ. For the first time long-term follow up was reported. This study showed that the mean (range) time from stent placement to death was 7.5 (3–18) months. It was also the first time in the literature that an EAS had been used in a patient with a benign stricture of a native ureter. The patient remained well and was alive to the end of the study at 24 months (Minhas et al., 1999). Since this original publication, we have implanted over one hundred EAS in candidate patients at our institution with equally excellent results (unpublished series).

One drawback of this one-piece stent was its long length of 70-cm, which some found to be complex to implant, time-consuming, and cumbersome for the patient (Schmidbauer et al., 2006). Nissenkorn and Gdor developed a two 14F 50-cm polyurethane J stents joined by a connector. After stent placement was confirmed by injecting a contrast agent through the tube, the stents were intra-operatively shortened as needed before linking them together. They used the stents successfully in eight patients with a mean follow up of mean 5.5 months (Nissenkorn & Gdor, 2000). In 2006, Schmidbauer et al. reported their successful results using a composite prosthesis set composed of two 12F polyurethane J-tubes, a 58-cm percutaneous nephrostomy part and a 56-cm percutaneous cystostomy part, malleable tunnelers, and a metal connector for joining the two tubes. In 27 patients followed up for 12 months (2 - 54 months) an improvement in mean quality of life score from 3.4+/-1.4 pre-operatively to 7.6+/-

1.0 post-operatively was reported. In five patients (17.9%) the system had to be replaced due to occlusion at a mean follow-up of 10.2 months. In three out of these five patients only the distal part of the two-piece bypass was exchanged (Schmidbauer et al., 2006).

Desgrandchamps et al. were the first authors to report use of a permanent PTFE-silicone EAS (Detour). They reported 3 patients who underwent successful EAS for ureteric necrosis, a rare complication of renal transplantation (Desgrandchamps et al., 1998). In 2001, the same group, reported use of the PTFE-silicone EAS in 27 patients with neoplastic (22) or benign (5) ureteric strictures. The mean follow-up was 6.3 months for the deceased patients and 47 months for the surviving ones, the longest follow-up being 84 months. In 3 cases, the EAS had to be removed due skin erosion in one and local tumour progression with bladder fistulae in two patients. Otherwise, five patients survived with the prosthesis in situ and a follow-up as long as 84 months without encrustation, infection, obstruction, or skin problems and with normally functioning kidneys (Jabbour et al., 2001). A prospective evaluation of their patients' quality using the EORTC QLC-30 questionnaire following insertion of the Detour EAS demonstrated an improvement of the function scale as a result of the elimination of the external percutaneous tube and a parallel worsening of the symptom scale secondary to the progression of disease (http://groups.eortc.be/qol/questionnaires_qlqc30.htm). Patient ratings of the global quality of life and satisfaction with the urinary diversion were high because of the absence of the percutaneous tube (Desgrandchamps et al., 2007). Other authors have since reported equally excellent results with the Detour EAS (Lloyd et al., 2007; Olsburgh et al., 2007; Burgos et al., 2009).

Aminsharifi A et al. recently described a promising simple modification of using percutaneous access to the bladder utilizing a split Amplatz sheath, and thus obviating the need for open cystostomy incision (Aminsharifi et al., 2010).

The main long-term complication reported is tumour invasion along the stent and active bladder cancer is the main contraindication to EAS insertion. One case report reported a patient presenting with acute obstruction of the Detour system secondary to a Candida infection that was managed successfully with short term nephrostomy and systemic anti-mycotic therapy without removing the stent (Bynens et al., 2006).

## 8. Conclusion

The long term data show that EAS offers an excellent temporary or permanent internalization of urinary drainage with a minimally invasive method where open surgery has been tried and failed or was not considered feasible, and avoids the need for long-term nephrostomy drainage.

An ideal EAS should be associated with minimal or no peri-operative morbidity; whilst at the same time does not require regular changes. Such a stent does not currently exist but it is likely that the rapid advancement in tissue engineering and biomaterials will make it possible to design one soon.

## 9. References

Ahmadzadeh, M. (1991). Clinical experience with subcutaneous urinary diversion: new approach using a double pigtail stent. *Br J Urol*, 67, 596-599.

Aminsharifi, A., Taddayun, A., Jafari, M. & Ghanbarifard, E. (2010). Pyelovesical bypass graft for palliative management of malignant ureteric obstruction: optimizing the technique by percutaneous access to the bladder using a split Amplatz sheath. *Urology*, 76, 993-995.

Andonian, S., Zorn, K.C., Paraskevas, S. & Anidjar, M. (2005). Artificial ureters in renal transplantation. *Urology*, 66, 1109.

Burgos, F.J., Bueno, G., Gonzalez, R., Vazquez, J.J., Diez-Nicolas, V., Marcen, R., Fernandez, A. & Pascual, J. (2009). Endourologic implants to treat complex ureteral stenosis after kidney transplantation. *Transplant Proc*, 41, 2427-2429.

Bynens, B.G., Ampe, J.F., Denys, H. & Oyen, P.M. (2006). Case report: relief of acute obstruction of the Detour subcutaneous pyelovesical bypass. *J Endourol*, 20, 669-671.

Desgrandchamps, F., Cussenot, O., Meria, P., Cortesse, A., Teillac, P. & Le Duc, A. (1995). Subcutaneous urinary diversions for palliative treatment of pelvic malignancies. *J Urol*, 154, 367-370.

Desgrandchamps, F., Duboust, A., Teillac, P., Idatte, J.M. & Le Duc, A. (1998a). Total ureteral replacement by subcutaneous pyelovesical bypass in ureteral necrosis after renal transplantation. *Transpl Int*, 11 Suppl 1, S150-151.

Desgrandchamps, F., Leroux, S., Ravery, V., Bochereau, G., Menut, P., Meria, P., Ballanger, P. & Teillac, P. (2007). Subcutaneous pyelovesical bypass as replacement for standard percutaneous nephrostomy for palliative urinary diversion: prospective evaluation of patient's quality of life. *J Endourol*, 21, 173-176.

Desgrandchamps, F., Paulhac, P., Fornairon, S., De Kerviller, E., Duboust, A., Teillac, P. & Le Duc, A. (1998b). Artificial ureteral replacement for ureteral necrosis after renal transplantation: report of 3 cases. *J Urol*, 159, 1830-1832.

Jabbour, M.E., Desgrandchamps, F., Angelescu, E., Teillac, P. & Le Duc, A. (2001). Percutaneous implantation of subcutaneous prosthetic ureters: long-term outcome. *J Endourol*, 15, 611-614.

Kouba, E., Wallen, E.M. & Pruthi, R.S. (2008). Management of ureteral obstruction due to advanced malignancy: optimizing therapeutic and palliative outcomes. *J Urol*, 180, 444-450.

Lingam, K., Paterson, P.J., Lingam, M.K., Buckley, J.F. & Forrester, A. (1994). Subcutaneous urinary diversion: an alternative to percutaneous nephrostomy. *J Urol*, 152, 70-72.

Lloyd, S.N., Tirukonda, P., Biyani, C.S., Wah, T.M. & Irving, H.C. (2007). The detour extra-anatomic stent--a permanent solution for benign and malignant ureteric obstruction? *Eur Urol*, 52, 193-198.

Marberger, M. 2006. Prosthetic nephrovesical bypass. *Eur Urol*, 50, 879-883.

Minhas, S., Irving, H.C., Lloyd, S.N., Eardley, I., Browning, A.J. & Joyce, A.D. (1999). Extra-anatomic stents in ureteric obstruction: experience and complications. *BJU Int*, 84, 762-764.

Nakada, S.Y., Gerber, A.J., Wolf, J.S., Jr., Hicks, M.E., Picus, D. & Clayman, R.V.(1995). Subcutaneous urinary diversion utilizing a nephrovesical stent: a superior alternative to long-term external drainage? *Urology*, 45, 538-541.

Nissenkorn, I. & Gdor, Y. (2000). Nephrovesical subcutaneous stent: an alternative to permanent nephrostomy. *J Urol*, 163, 528-530.

Olsburgh, J., Dorling, A., Tait, P. & Williams, G. (2007). Extra-anatomic stents for transplant ureteric stenosis. *Br J Radiol*, 80, 216-218.

Schmidbauer, J., Kratzik, C., Klingler, H.C., Remzi, M., Lackner, J. & Marberger, M. (2006). Nephrovesical subcutaneous ureteric bypass: long-term results in patients with advanced metastatic disease-improvement of renal function and quality of life. *Eur Urol*, 50, 1073-1078.

Schulman, C.C., Vandendris, M., Vanlanduyt, P. & Abramow, M. (1976). Total replacement of both ureters by prostheses. *Eur Urol*, 2, 89-91.

# 18

# Percutaneous Nephrostomy

Rameysh D. Mahmood, Lee Yizhi and Mark Tan M.L.
*Dept of Diagnostic Radiology, Changi General Hospital*
*Singapore*

## 1. Introduction

Percutaneous nephrostomy (PCN) is a passageway that is introduced percutaneously into the renal pelvicalyces that can later be maintained by a tube, stent or catheter. Following its introduction by Wickbom in 1954 who described percutaneous puncture of the renal pelvis as a diagnostic procedure, Goodwin and Casey first described its therapeutic use for relief of urinary tract obstruction the following year in 1955 (Goodwin, Casey et al. 1955; Stables, Ginsberg et al. 1978). Since then, this now commonplace procedure has undergone significant progress in both its technical and imaging aspects, with improvisation of puncture devices and techniques, coupled with the advancing imaging modalities used to guide the procedure. Thanks to its good safety profile, percutaneous nephrostomy is the preferred technique for treatment of various urological conditions, and its pioneering role for relief of urinary tract obstruction remains in good use until today.

This chapter aims to review the clinical use of percutaneous nephrostomy as well as the background technical aspects involved in carrying out the procedure. Some emphasis will be placed in the anatomical considerations that are crucial in determining approach as well as risk profile for an individual case. The associated known complications of the procedure will also be discussed, along with the therapeutic options available for the relevant complications.

## 2. Indications and contraindications of percutaneous nephrostomy

In essence, percutaneous nephrostomy may be performed for diagnostic or therapeutic purposes. For example, an antegrade pyelography can be performed following percutaneous nephrostomy to diagnose urinary tract obstruction. Its therapeutic uses on the other hand, can be seen to fall under two broad groups. Typically, the procedure is carried out to provide urinary diversion, and for a large number of cases this is related to urinary tract obstruction due to various causes. Secondly, the nephrostomy can be used to provide access to the urinary tracts for further intervention such as endopyeloscopy and nephrolithotomy. This is usually performed in collaboration with a urologist.

### 2.1 Indications

The following is a list of indications recognised by the Society of Interventional Radiology (SIR) (Ramchandani, Cardella et al. 2003):

1. Provision of urinary diversion in cases of urinary tract obstruction, which may be secondary to intrinsic or extrinsic ureteral obstruction. This may be related to urinary calculi, malignancy or iatrogenic causes. The obstruction may be diagnosed incidentally on imaging studies, or patients may present with features of obstructive uropathy.
2. In cases of pyonephrosis, where there is urgency in providing immediate drainage as these patients are at risk of developing fulminant sepsis and shock. This may be suspected in patients with clinical features of sepsis, accompanied by flank pain and evidence of urinary tract obstruction on imaging.
3. Urinary diversion in cases of urinary leakage or fistula, which may in turn be related to trauma for example.
4. Urinary diversion for hemorrhagic cystitis.
5. Providing access for urological interventions and endoscopy (nephrolithotomy and removal of urinary calculus, ureteral stent placement, delivery of chemotherapeutic agents e.g. for upper tract transitional cell carcinoma, foreign body retrieval e.g. migrated ureteral stents). Percutaneous nephrostomy has been shown to provide adequate treatment of various types of urinary calculi including staghorn calculi.

The above indications can be applied to both native as well as transplanted kidneys.

### 2.2 Contraindications

Percutaneous nephrostomy has a good safety profile, and there is no single recognizable absolute contraindication (Ramchandani, Cardella et al. 2003). Relative contraindications however do exist, for which the benefits and potential risk must be weighed for each individual case.

Patients with known renal vascular malformations or arterial aneurysm are at risk of severe hemorrhage should there be accidental injury to these affected vessels. Nevertheless these patients may still require emergent decompression particularly in cases of urinary tract obstruction complicated by pyonephrosis. Careful preprocedural planning is vital, taking into account the nature of vascular malformations or aneurysm in detail by using the appropriate imaging method such as CT when determining approach and puncture tract. The performing physician should be aware of the potential need for angiographic embolization in these cases, particularly if bleeding becomes difficult to control and there is risk of hemodynamic instability. Similarly, patients with severe coagulopathy or bleeding diathesis are exposed to risks of severe hemorrhage. For these patients, thorough assessment of their coagulation profile as well as appropriate correction of coagulopathy may be necessary prior to the procedure.

Electrolyte imbalances such as severe hyperkalaemia may frequently be encountered particularly in cases of background chronic renal disease, and in whom the concomitant urinary tract obstruction may need to be urgently treated. In these cases, appropriate medical therapy is required to correct the electrolyte imbalance in order to reduce the risk of developing complications such as cardiac arrhythmia or cardioplegia (Ramchandani, Cardella et al. 2003).

Special attention should also be made to those patients with significant underlying morbidity or terminal illness who are deemed unsuitable for conventional surgery but yet there may be a role for percutaneous nephrostomy to provide a temporary measure. Risks of complications are higher in these patients, and they are ideally treated as an inpatient to ensure adequate planning prior to the procedure as well as providing periprocedural monitoring.

Fluoroscopic or CT-guided percutaneous nephrostomy may be contraindicated in pregnant patients in the first trimester in order to minimize radiation exposure to the fetus. Percutaneous nephrostomy performed using only ultrasound guidance has been described with good success rates (Gupta, Gulati et al. 1997; Ozden, Yaman et al. 2002), with Gupta reporting an overall success rate of 98.5%. However minimum radiation exposure should always be borne in mind even in non-pregnant patients in accordance with ALARA (As Low As Reasonably Achievable) principle.

## 3. Anatomical considerations

Following assessment of the primary diagnosis and indication for percutaneous nephrostomy for each particular case, the procedure should not be performed without adequate review of all relevant imaging performed prior to the procedure. Percutaneous nephrostomy is usually performed using ultrasound or fluoroscopic guidance, although in many cases, CT may have been performed to arrive at the diagnosis prior to the procedure and correlation with these images may prove to be beneficial.

The primary diagnosis should be reviewed thoroughly, and this should include the cause and level of obstruction, degree of pelvicalyceal dilatation, as well as the most accessible renal calyx for catheter placement. If urinary calculi are present within the renal pelvis, their exact nature and location must be elucidated. The success rate for percutaneous nephrostomy has been reported to be lower in patients with a non-dilated collecting system, complex calculus disease and staghorn calculus (Ramchandani, Cardella et al. 2003). The kidney itself must also be assessed for the presence of anatomical variants or congenital anomalies such as horseshoe kidney.

Equally important to note is the vascular anatomy of the target kidney. Its precise delineation, as well as the presence of abnormal vascular malformations or aneurysmal dilatation should be noted. Injury to the first order segmental renal arteries may occur in the region of the renal pelvis, particularly if the puncture is made too medially. To prevent vascular injury and bleeding complications, the safest approach has been described by approaching the cusp of the papilla as far peripherally as possible, and by entering the kidney via the Brodel's line (Dyer, Regan et al. 2002). Brodel's line is a zone of relative avascularity and watershed territory, which is located just posterior to the lateral convex margin of the kidney, between the major anterior and posterior divisions of the renal artery. Care should be taken to avoid a through-and-through two-wall puncture of the renal pelvis as this runs the risk of injury to the anterior segmental renal artery.

The position of the affected kidney relative to the surrounding abdominal viscera should be thoroughly assessed as this has a bearing in determining the safest and most effective approach for renal puncture. Under normal circumstances, the posterolateral margins of the kidneys are immediately adjacent to the posterolateral aspects of the abdominal wall with no organs to interpose in between. Hence, a posterior approach is advantageous in avoiding the surrounding organs (Hruby 1990). Although the spleen, liver, pancreas and the adrenal glands are in close proximity to the kidneys, they are usually not shown to interpose between the posterior aspect of the kidney and the adjacent abdominal wall. Hruby described no injury to these organs in their retrospective review of 3100 patients who underwent percutaneous nephrostomy. However trans-splenic puncture has been reported in a series of patients who underwent percutaneous nephrostomy for nephrolithotomy (Carey, Siddiq et al. 2006).

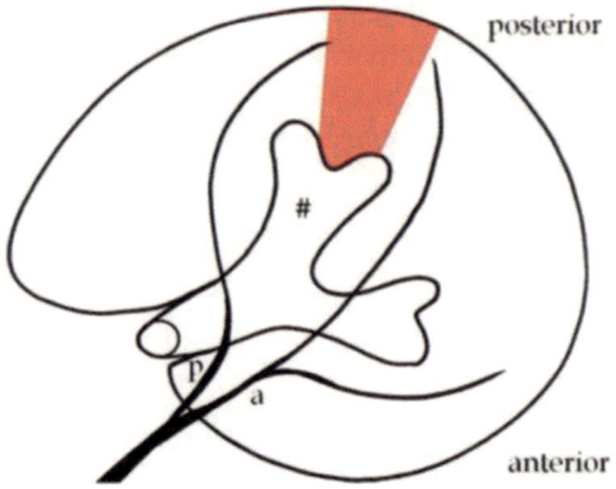


Fig. 1. Axial diagram of a kidney as seen in a prone patient illustrating the relations of the relatively avascular zone of Brodel (shaded) with the posterior (p) and anterior (a) branches of the main renal artery as well as the posterior calyx (#).

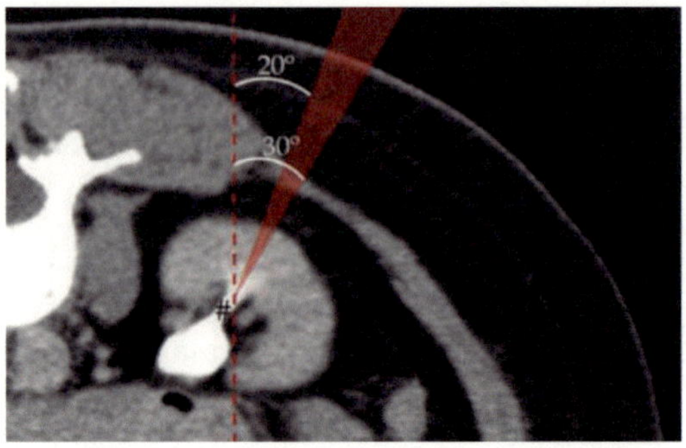


Fig. 2. The shaded wedge represents an ideal approach through Brodel's avascular zone. This approach of approximately 20°–30° from the sagittal plane (dotted line) into the posterior calyx (#) minimizes the risk of bleeding. A CT pyelogram is used to better illustrate the pelvicalyceal system.

There are exceptions to the above, as parts of the pleura lie in the posterior costodiaphragmatic recess that may overlap with the anterior pole of the kidney. Under normal circumstances, the lower line of the pleura usually crosses the 12$^{th}$ rib at the lateral border of the erector spinae muscle, and part of the 12$^{th}$ rib posterior to this point lies above the pleural line. This is important to note as a transpleural puncture may result in pneumothorax or hydrothorax, and for this reason, a subcostal approach should be used. Hruby described the best subcostal approach to be below the 12$^{th}$ rib, approximately 2 fingerbreadth lateral to the lateral border of the paraspinal musclature, which is approximately along the posterior axillary line.

It is important to note however that the position of the kidneys in relation to the pleura varies according to respiration and individual anatomical variations, and this may be best assessed by using fluoroscopy just prior to puncture. The lower pole calyx is therefore the most likely to lie below the pleural line, and may in this way provide the safest approach. This is even more so in the right kidney, which is normally lower in position as compared to the left. However the upper pole calyx may have to be punctured in such cases where there is limited access to the lower pole calyx, for example due to presence of a large calculus. In such cases, a supracostal approach may have to be used with care.

In addition to the pleura, the colon is frequently found in close contact with the anteromedial aspect of the kidney, and too medial an approach may run the risk of colonic perforation. Occasionally, a retrorenal colon may also be encountered, and approach should therefore be negotiated accordingly. Although uncommon, cases of colonic perforation has been reported and this will be discussed further later in this chapter.

## 4. Patient preparations, procedure and technique

### 4.1 Patient preparations

As described, a patient who is about to undergo percutaneous nephrostomy should be thoroughly assessed for current physical status and presence of comorbidities that may affect the risk of developing complications following the procedure. Hyperkalaemia, should be corrected appropriately. Patients who are coagulopathic will have to be managed with plasma or platelet transfusion. Acceptable platelet and INR (International Normalised Ratio) levels vary between institutions, but INR values of less than 1.3 or platelet levels of more than 80,000/dL have been considered acceptable (Ramchandani, Cardella et al. 2003).

Prophylactic antibiotics have been widely used in preparing patients for percutaneous nephrostomy, although no clinical trial has published reports of its benefits to date. A prospective controlled study of patients undergoing percutaneous nephrolithotomy (Mariappan, Smith et al. 2006) reported significant reduction in the risk of upper tract infection and urosepsis following 1 week of prophylactic ciprofloxacin. However this may not be extrapolated in cases of percutaneous nephrostomy not related to underlying calculus or nephrolithotomy, as the presence of calculus is known to be associated with increased risk of infection. On a similar note, McDermott et al regarded the genitourinary tract as being contaminated in the presence of advanced age, diabetes, bladder dysfunction, indwelling urinary catheter, prior manipulation, ureterointestinal anastomosis, bacteriuria and calculi particularly of the struvite variety (McDermott, Schuster et al. 1997). This is particularly so in the presence of clinical signs of infection. It has been recommended that patients with low risk of infection receive a single dose of 1g of intravenous cefazolin or ceftriaxone prior to the procedure (Ramchandani, Cardella et al. 2003). If these patients do not develop continuing signs of infection following the procedure, no further antibiotic treatment is necessary. Patients who are septic or with the above risk factors and at risk of developing infections, are recommended to prophylactically receive 1g of intravenous ceftriaxone 8-hourly or 1g of IV sulbactame 6-hourly, along with 80mg of IV gentamycin 8-hourly (Ramchandani, Cardella et al. 2003). Antibiotics are given for 5-7 days in the peri-procedure period, and should be adjusted according to the results of urine culture obtained from the procedure.

Other aspects of patient preparation are common to most other interventional procedures performed in a hospital setting, and this entail obtaining informed consent regarding the procedure as well as adequate fasting if conscious sedation is considered. Certain groups of patients such as young children may have to undergo general anaesthesia, in which case collaboration with an anaesthetist may be necessary.

### 4.2 Technique

The patient is traditionally positioned in the prone or prone-oblique position, with the target puncture side elevated by approximately 20-30 degrees. The prone technique was originally adopted by Goodwin probably to avoid the colon and has since gained acceptance. The supine anterolateral position has also been recently suggested (Cormio, Annese et al. 2007) as being a safe and effective technique, with the benefits of greater patient comfort as well as causing less respiratory and circulatory difficulties in obese patients. Regardless, the target kidney should be reimaged and reassessed, and this is most commonly performed with ultrasonography. The target renal calyx should be identified and a planned approach should be clearly delineated. The puncture site should then be identified and marked at this stage of the procedure. As described above, the target renal calyx's position relative to the diaphragm during respiration should be observed, and ideally, a subcostal approach targeting Brodel's line should be utilized.

The site of renal puncture is determined by the indication for the procedure. A lower pole posterior calyx for instance, would be best used for simple urinary drainage (Dyer, Regan et al. 2002), while those of the upper and middle poles provide better access to the renal pelvis and ureter, especially if ureteral interventions are being considered. A puncture posterior to a calculus may assist in the treatment of calculus disease. These calyces are best identified by administration of intravenous iodinated contrast with visualization of contrast within the renal collecting system under fluoroscopic guidance. The anterior calyces are usually seen tangentially, while the posterior calyces are seen en face due to the orientation of the kidney about its horizontal axis. This would be contraindicated if the patient has prior history of contrast allergy or an underlying poor renal function, and it is probably not ideal in a severely obstructed system where poor contrast excretion can be expected.

After the patient has been adequately cleaned and draped using sterile methods, the puncture site should be infiltrated with an acceptable local anaesthesia such as 1% xylocaine. Instruction should be given to the patient to breathhold while a 21G diagnostic needle (e.g Accustick System - Boston Scientific, Neff Set - Cook Medical) is used to puncture the skin, which is then advanced posteroanterioly at an angle towards the intended calyx. Alternatively, a three-part co-axial needle may also be used, where there is an outer blunt cannula, an inner 22G needle as well as a stylet. As the renal fibrous capsule of the kidney is punctured, a finer needle may then be introduced via the coaxial needle to puncture the collecting system.

Movement of the needle that follows the kidney as the patient resumes respiration, as well as spontaneous drainage of urine from the needle as the needle stylet is removed, can be used to confirm successful renal entry. Spontaneous urine drainage is particularly seen in an obstructed system. If urine is not spontaneously draining, it may be aspirated from the needle instead. Sampled urine can be sent for culture and further analysis. Renal entry can be further confirmed by administration of contrast medium into the collecting system via the diagnostic needle.

A skin incision at the puncture site may now be performed, appropriately sized according to the catheter width that is to be used. A 0.018-inch guidewire is then passed through the needle to enter the renal pelvis (Figure 3). Over the guidewire, the tract is dilated to an appropriate size with a sheath/dilator assembly to later receive nephrostomy catheters, which can be up to 14Fr (French catheter scale) in size. The dilator and the 0.018 inch guide-wire can now be removed, leaving the sheath in place (Figure 4). Subsequently, a 0.038inch guide-wire is advanced through the sheath and placed as distally into the ureter as possible to stabilize the tract (Figure 5). The nephrostomy catheter is then inserted over the guidewire (e.g. an 8Fr Navarre pig-tail catheter - Bard Nordic. Figures 6 and 7). The use of a metal cannula may be considered to stabilize the tube during its passage towards the kidney across the perirenal soft tissue.

Smaller-bore catheters (7-8Fr) are sufficient for drainage of non-infected and less viscid urine, while a larger-bore 14Fr catheter may be considered for drainage of infected urine or pus. Once the catheter is placed, its position can be further confirmed by administration of contrast to opacify the collecting system via the tube. The collecting system may be seen to decompress if the catheter is appropriately placed. Care should be taken to avoid over-distension of the collecting system so as to prevent bacteremia and risk of sepsis. To avoid catheter dislocation or dislodgement, self-retaining catheters should be used, and this should be placed as far into the collecting system as possible. Care must however be taken not to obstruct the ureter if a larger-bore catheter is used. Once firmly placed, the catheter is secured externally with retention sutures or other securing devices such as a skin disc.

Further urological intervention may follow the above puncture technique. The tract can be dilated further to allow passage of other instruments such as ureteroscope, balloon-dilatation system or nephrolithotomy instruments. A ureteral stent may also be placed through the percutaneous puncture. A larger-bore catheter may be considered by the urologist to allow for better drainage.

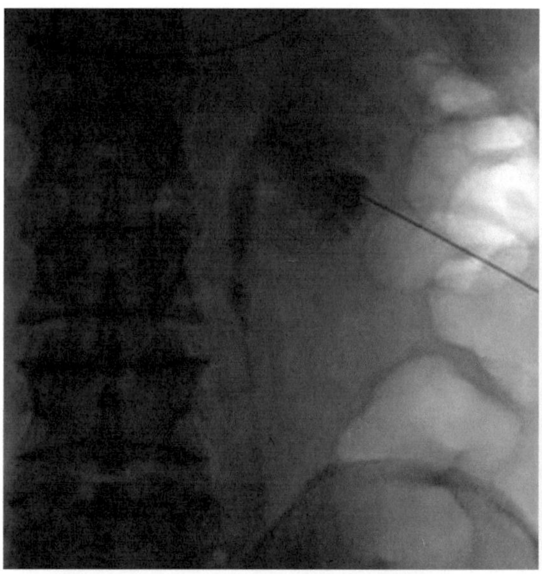

Fig. 3. A lower pole puncture was made with a 21 gauge Accustick needle into the lower pole calyx of the left kidney, with opacification of the collecting system by contrast. The obstructing calculus (c) can be seen along the proximal left ureter, causing upstream dilatation.

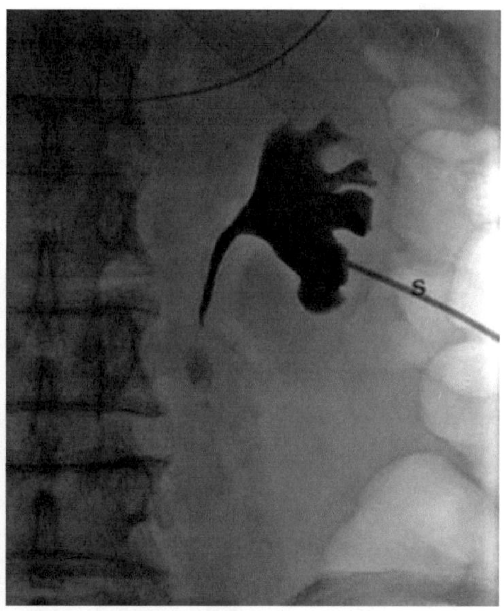


Fig. 4. A 0.018 inch guidewire was introduced through the needle into the renal pelvis as distally as possible. The sheath/dilator assembly was then advanced over the guidewire (not shown). The dilator and the 0.018-inch guidewire were then removed, leaving the sheath (s) in place. More contrast was instilled to delineate the collecting system.

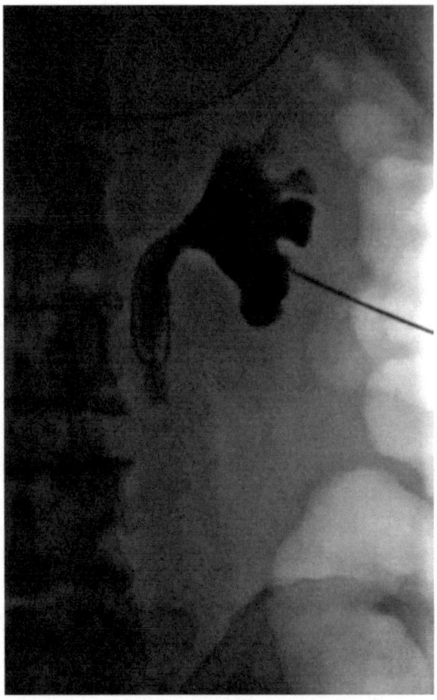

Fig. 5. Subsequently a 0.038 inch guidewire was advanced through the sheath and placed as distally into the ureter as possible for stability.

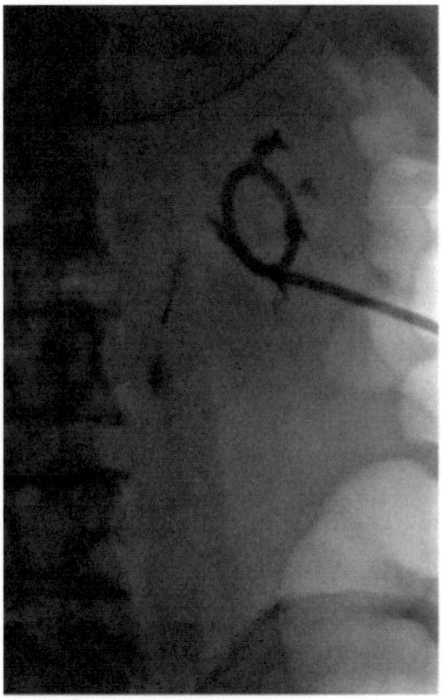

Fig. 6. An 8Fr Navarre catheter was then inserted over the 0.038 inch guidewire and secured in place.

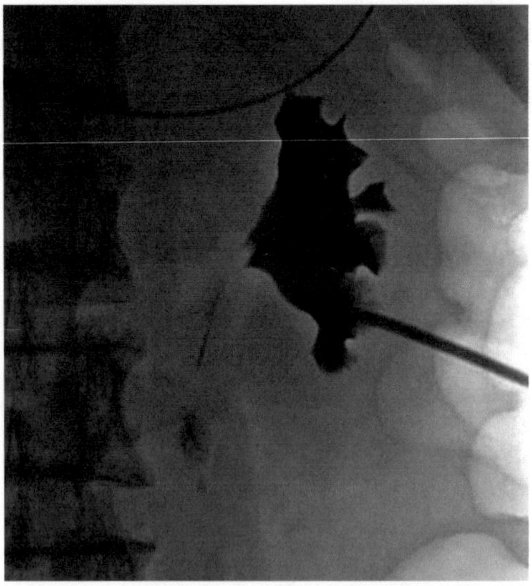

Fig. 7. The final image showing contrast opacification of the left renal collecting system. Note the reduced caliber of the upper ureter following successful drainage.

### 4.3 Post-procedure care

Post-procedure care is essential and may be crucial for early detection as well as reducing the risk of deterioration should complications occur during the procedure. High-risk patients may also require hospitalization for adequate monitoring. Frequent monitoring of vital signs should be routinely performed during initial recovery as signs of hemorrhage or sepsis may present suddenly and would require immediate attention. This should be accompanied by routine charting of the catheter output, noting the degree of hematuria as well as the output volume. Although commonly seen in virtually all patients, hematuria should resolve within 24-48 hours (Dyer, Regan et al. 2002). Prolonged hematuria should alert the physician to the possibility of persistent bleeding from vascular injury.

Catheter care is useful to reduce rate of catheter dislodgement and clogging, and it should be flushed with normal saline and aspirated routinely. Catheter clogging is a commonly occurring complication however, and this may even necessitate a change of catheter.

Antibiotics may be discontinued if there is low-risk of infection, although this should be continued in high-risk patients as described above. This should ideally be adjusted according to the urine culture results if available.

## 5. Complications

According to SIR, the reported success rate for percutaneous nephrostomy is 98-99%, and this is defined as successful placement of catheter of sufficient size to allow for adequate drainage of the urinary tract or to allow successful tract dilatation for further interventional procedure. The success rates have been reported to be lower in cases of non-dilated collecting system or complex calculus disease (e.g. staghorn calculus) where a success rate of about 85% was reported (Ramchandani, Cardella et al. 2003). Despite the high success rates however, complications are frequently encountered, be it minor or major, with a reported incidence of approximately 10% of cases (Ramchandani, Cardella et al. 2003).

Several factors are associated with increased risk of complications. Patients at the extremes of age may develop complications from the procedure itself or even that related to the use of general anaesthesia, should this become necessary particularly in young children. Patient's coexisting comorbidities such as obesity, scoliosis, hepatomegaly and extremely mobile kidneys may necessitate greater manipulation, resulting in a technically challenging and thereby risky procedure. Further, in patients with chronic lung diseases and poor respiratory reserve such as emphysema, particular attention should be paid to the use of a subcostal approach to minimize risk of respiratory complications such as pneumothorax.

### 5.1 Minor complications

Minor complications are defined as complications occurring in relation to the procedure that are of no consequence and can be managed conservatively, or those requiring nominal therapy with no consequences (Ramchandani, Cardella et al. 2003). These patients may still require overnight hospitalization for observation. According to published reports, minor complications have been reported to occur in the range of 15-28% of cases (Stables 1982; Lee, Smith et al. 1987; Dyer, Regan et al. 2002).

Post-procedure bleeding varies in severity, and may range from simple transient hematuria to severe hemorrhage requiring transfusion or intervention. Minor bleeding complications include transient hematuria, which occurs in virtually all patients, and small perirenal hematomas that can resolve on conservative management. Transient hematuria occurs very frequently that some authors do not regard it as a complication (Stables 1982). Clinically silent perinephric hematoma have been reported to occur fairly frequently, and is found in up to 13% of cases following percutaneous nephrostomy (Cowan 2008). These can resolve spontaneously without necessitating further interventions, leaving no serious consequences to the patient in the majority of cases. Stables also observed that in 79% of these cases, no significant renal alteration was seen. However, the presence of prolonged hematuria with or without hemodynamic instability should alert the physician for possible continuing bleeding as well as vascular injury.

Catheter-related complications such as kinking, obstruction or dislodgement may frequently be encountered and may require further intervention in 14% of cases (Cowan 2008). Published reports quoted varying rates of catheter dislodgement, from 4.8% - 11.6%. The use of larger bore catheters (for example 14Fr catheter) may reduce this rate to 1% (Cowan 2008). Stables recommended advancement of the catheter well into the renal pelvis or calyces to minimize risk of dislodgement (Stables, Ginsberg et al. 1978). However care should be taken to avoid obstructing the ureter particularly if a large bore catheter is used. A dislodged tube may have to be replaced and the new catheter may have to be inserted by creating a new tract unless if the previous tract has been well established.

To reduce the rate of catheter obstruction, routine irrigation with normal saline solution should be performed after the procedure, although the use of larger-bore catheters may reduce the rate further while providing good drainage. Debris may also be removed by manipulation with a guide wire. Occasionally however, if catheter obstruction persists despite conventional measures, catheter replacement may be necessary.

Urine leak is known to occur following percutaneous nephrostomy, with a rate of approximately 7-7.2% (Lee, Smith et al. 1987; Moskowitz, Lee et al. 1989). This is frequently minor, and contrast extravasation during or immediately after the procedure may or may not indicate ensuing complication. Also, most small leaks and tears resolve spontaneously with adequate urinary drainage or ureteral catheter insertion (Lee, Smith et al. 1987). Urine leak can also be controlled by using a larger bore catheter (Cowan 2008). However urine leak may occasionally be prolonged (lasting more than a week) and the ensuing urinoma may be large enough to require surgical intervention.

Other minor complications that may be seen following the procedure may include pain and fever. While fever can be worrisome for ensuing sepsis with potential of shock, febrile patients may require nothing more than conservative management with or without anti-pyretics. Lee reported 23% of raised temperature of more than 38.5 degrees Celsius in his published series of 582 patients who underwent percutaneous nephrolithotomy (Lee, Smith et al. 1987). These were attributed to retrograde urine flow as well as the use of irrigation fluid during the procedure. Minor wound infection has also been reported (von der Recke, Nielsen et al. 1994; Kaskarelis, Papadaki et al. 2001). These may be related to prolonged catheter use, and the use of sutures to secure the catheters to the skin (Kaskarelis, Papadaki et al. 2001). Pneumonia and atelectasis have been reported in a minority of cases, but is usually managed conservatively with antibiotics.

### 5.2 Major complications

Major complications are defined by SIR as complications that require therapy or minor hospitalization of up to 48 hours, as well as those that require major therapy, unplanned increase in level of care and prolonged hospitalization of more than 48 hours. Complications with permanent adverse sequelae or those that result in death are certainly considered to be major.

### 5.2.1 Hemorrhage

Hemorrhage requiring transfusion with or without radiological or surgical intervention is uncommon but is certainly a dreaded complication that carries a mortality risk. A number of published case series have reported major bleeding following percutaneous nephrostomy or percutaneous nephrolithotomy, and this occurs in the range of 1-4% (Lee, Smith et al. 1987; von der Recke, Nielsen et al. 1994; Dyer, Regan et al. 2002; Ramchandani, Cardella et al. 2003). This may manifest in prolonged hematuria, hemodynamic instability and perirenal hematomas. Hemorrhage may be related to vascular injury during the procedure, whether a normal vessel that are inadvertently injured, or it may be related to underlying vascular malformations or aneurysm. Hemorrhage could also be attributable to an underlying coagulopathy or bleeding diathesis. The guideline for quality improvement by SIR recommended a threshold rate of hemorrhage requiring blood transfusion to be kept below 4%.

Significant bleeding during the procedure may be controlled by a tamponade applied to the tract with a nephrostomy catheter or balloon dilatation catheter in larger tracts. If at any point that this fails, or if the patient develops subsequent significant blood loss after the procedure, angiographic evaluation would be indicated for identification of abnormal vascularity or major vascular injury with possible need for embolization. Surgical intervention may later become necessary if poor bleeding control is achieved. By this way, injured vessels may be ligated to arrest the bleeding, or as a last resort, partial or total nephrectomy may have to be performed. Lee reported 4 cases of persistent bleeding which were arrested by successful embolization, while a further 2 cases had to undergo nephrectomy or partial nephrectomy following failed embolization (Lee, Smith et al. 1987). Cowan reported 7 cases of persistent bleeding in a series of 3100 patients following percutaneous nephrostomy, and these were found to be secondary to underlying arteriovenous aneurysms that were treated successfully with embolization (Cowan 2008).

The performing physician should therefore be aware of the risk of severe blood loss, and the patient should be counseled appropriately regarding this risk during consent taking prior to the procedure. However, there are steps that can be taken during the procedure to minimise risk of hemorrhage. As described above, particular attention should be paid to the coagulation profile prior to the procedure, and any significant abnormality should be corrected accordingly. The renal vascular anatomy should be reviewed and taken into consideration when planning for puncture site and approach. The kidney should be punctured along the Brodel's avascular line as described above, and similarly, punctures too close to the inferior surface of a rib run the risk of injury to the intercostal vessels. The uses of fine needles and small-bore catheters have been associated with smaller risk of severe hemorrhage. A two-wall puncture of the renal pelvis should also be avoided to minimize risk of injury to the anterior segmental renal artery. As an additional support measure, high-risk patients should be prepared with support from the blood transfusion services should blood transfusion becomes necessary during or after the procedure.

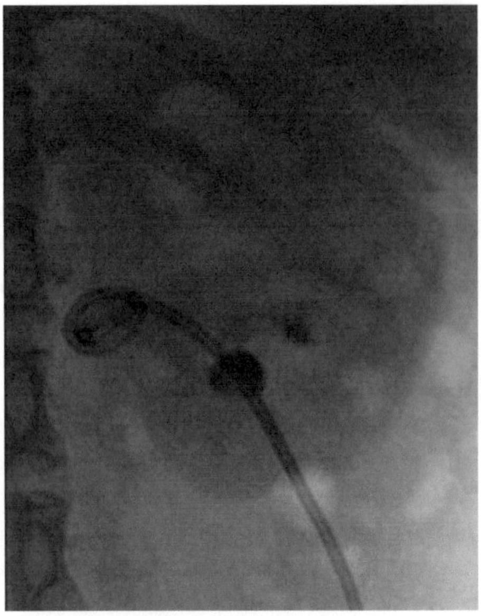

Fig. 8. An 8 Fr Navarre catheter in place with its loop apparently sited within the renal pelvis. Figures 8 to 11 are of the same patient.

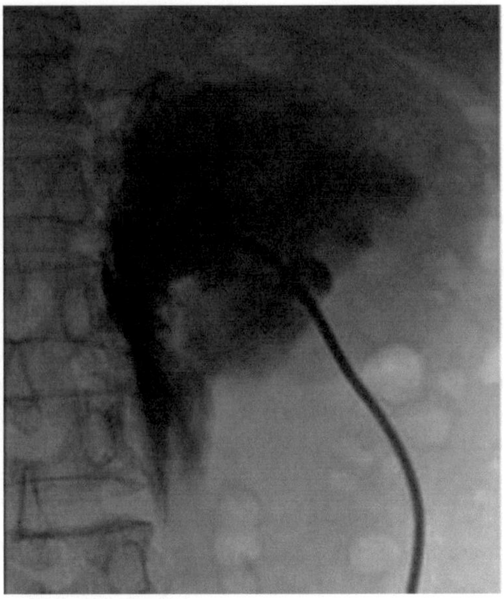

Fig. 9. Nephrogram showing contrast leakage into peripelvic fat due to transgression of the pelvicalyceal system. The patient subsequently developed flank pain and hypotension, indicating concomitant vascular injury. Sonography confirmed the presence of a peri-nephric hematoma.

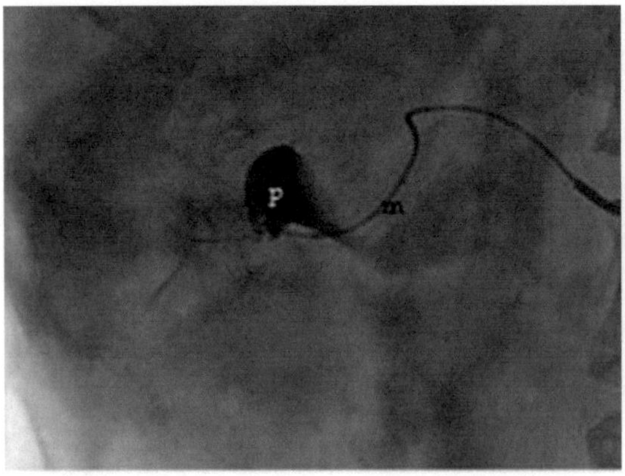


Fig. 10. Renal angiography demonstrated bleeding from a branch of the inferior segmental artery. Super-selective injection of contrast via a microcatheter (m) into the bleeding artery showed extravasation into the renal pelvis (p).

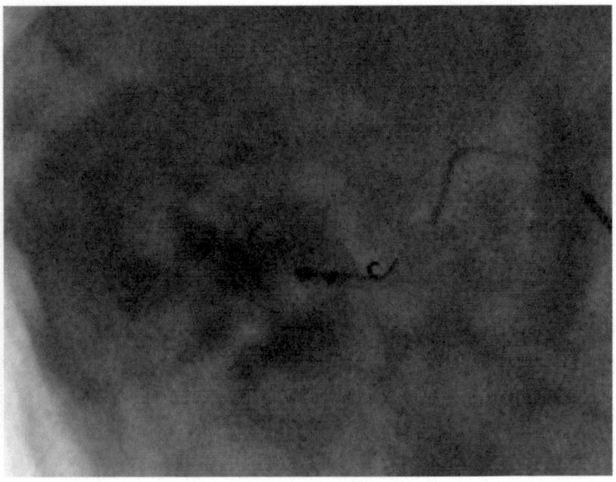


Fig. 11. Successful embolization with micro-coils (c).

### 5.2.2 Sepsis

Significant infection and sepsis following percutaneous nephrostomy is an important and well-recognised complication, with several published reports documenting its occurrence. According to SIR, sepsis related complications have been reported to occur in 1-9% of cases (Ramchandani, Cardella et al. 2003). There is a wide spectrum of severity of infection, but major sepsis may be defined as cases of septicemia requiring escalation in hospital care and longer use of antibiotics therapy, with or without shock. Transient fever is common following the procedure, occurring in almost all patients, the majority of which may settle in less than 6 hours (Lee, Patel et al. 1994). However, persistent fever with chills and signs of hemodynamic instability are worrisome signs and should be identified and treated accordingly. Septic shock is a serious complication, and has been reported to be a contributing factor towards patients mortality in some published case series. In 318 patients who underwent percutaneous nephrostomy, Lewis reported sepsis as the most common major complication, occurring in 2.2% of patients in his published case series, and it is the most severe complication necessitating intensive care (Lewis and Patel 2004). Sepsis was also considered to be a contributing factor in the death of two of these cases. Moskowitz further reported 2 cases of septicemia with shock in 11 cases of severe sepsis in his published case series of patients who underwent percutaneous nephrolithotomy (Moskowitz, Lee et al. 1989). SIR recommended a rate of septic shock of less than 4%, and a rate of less than 10% for cases of septic shock in the setting of pyonephrosis.

Several factors have been found to contribute towards increased risk of sepsis, and this includes the duration of the procedure itself, urine bacterial load, severity of urinary tract obstruction as well as presence of bacteria within the calculus (Mariappan, Smith et al. 2006). Mariappan also reported higher risk of upper urinary tract infections in patients with calculi larger than 20mm or a dilated pelvicalyceal system. Further, the puncture itself, and even the removal of calculus may reactivate underlying pre-existing infection within the urinary tract with release of bacteria into the system. Therefore, care should be taken to avoid over-distension of the renal collecting system during puncture, as this may result in bacterial reflux into the peripapillary plexus. Urine extravasation and absorption of irrigation fluid have also been found to be contributory (Lee, Patel et al. 1994).

The use of prophylactic antibiotics is therefore recommended in high-risk patients, and this has been shown to be of some benefit as reported in a prospective controlled study by Mariappan, who prescribed one week of ciprofloxacin to patients prior to percutaneous nephrolithotomy (Mariappan, Smith et al. 2006). Patients who received prophylactic ciprofloxacin were reported to have significantly reduced incidence of upper urinary tract infection as compared to the control group, with three times less risk of developing systemic inflammatory response syndrome. Antibiotics therapy may be further escalated in patients with evidence of urosepsis following the procedure, and this is best adjusted according to the results of urine culture and sensitivity.

### 5.2.3 Pleural complications

Pleural complications such as pneumo-, hydro-, or hemothorax and empyema are uncommon but have been known to occur from percutaneous nephrostomy, with a reported rate of 0.1-0.3% (Dyer, Regan et al. 2002; Ramchandani, Cardella et al. 2003). The risk of pneumo- and hydrothorax is reported to be in the range of 4-12% if a supracostal approach is used for puncture of the renal upper pole (Carey, Siddiq et al. 2006), although this may be difficult to avoid if it provides the best access to the collecting system. The use of a working sheath is an important consideration in these cases, as it may prevent leakage of fluid into the pleural cavity along the pleural tract during the procedure. Although pleural complications may be treated conservatively (Dyer, Regan et al. 2002), pleural drainage with chest tube insertion may be necessary.

#### 5.2.4 Bowel transgression and colonic perforation

Bowel transgression is another uncommon but potentially serious complication of percutaneous nephrostomy, and is reported to occur in 0.2-0.3% of cases (Ramchandani, Cardella et al. 2003; M Tan 2010). Several risk factors have been recognized that may contribute to increased risks. Patients with a markedly dilated collecting system, colonic obstruction and patients with scarce perirenal fat are more likely to have a more posteriorly located colon. This increases the risk of colonic transgression when approaching the kidney. An anatomical variant to note is the retrorenal colon which is reported to occur in 1 - 1.9% of supine patients and in up to 10 – 16% of prone patients (Hopper, Sherman et al. 1987; Tuttle, Yeh et al. 2005). This retroperitoneal bowel loop is usually gas-distended and is found mostly around the lower renal poles. Care should thus be taken to visualize this with fluoroscopy or CT before any invasive percutaneous renal procedure. Colonic perforation has also been associated with right upper calyceal punctures in patients with horseshoe kidneys (El-Nahas, Shokeir et al. 2006). Any factor contributing to poor visualization of the kidneys during image-guidance such as gross obesity, abundance of gas-filled bowel loops and mobile kidneys may also result in inadvertent colonic injury. The risk is further increased when too lateral an approach is used to puncture the kidney (Wah, Weston et al. 2004).

Most cases of reported colonic perforation due to percutaneous nephrostomy are retroperitoneal and contained, and these have been managed well conservatively with good recovery (Wah, Weston et al. 2004). However, surgical repair may be required in cases of intraperitoneal colonic perforation, or where there is ensuing hemorrhage with or without shock. M Tan described a case of inadvertent colonic injury during percutaneous nephrostomy that occurred in a thin middle-aged woman with a dilated renal pelvicalyces (M Tan 2010). The patient was asymptomatic and the perforation was only discovered 3 weeks later during a double J stent insertion when contrast was noted in the colon. The patient was managed conservatively and the percutaneous nephrostomy was later withdrawn into the colon, functioning as a percutaneous colostomy. The use of antibiotic cover would be indicated in these cases to prevent infection.

The use of image guidance is important in reducing risk of colonic perforation. The exact location of the colon relative to the kidney should be identified prior to the procedure, and as described above, too lateral an approach should be avoided in high-risk patients. In patients with risk factors leading to poor visualization of the urinary system under ultrasound guidance, CT scan should be used to look for anatomical variants, such as a retrorenal colon or horseshoe kidney, to reduce the chance of inadvertent colonic puncture (M Tan 2010).

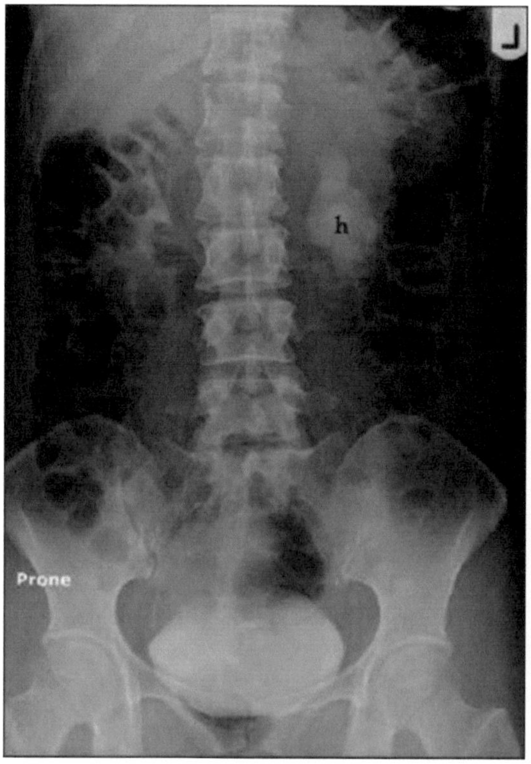


Fig. 12. Delayed phase of an intravenous urogram showing left hydronephrosis (h) due to obstruction at the pelviureteric junction. The gas-distended descending colon is in close proximity to the lateral aspect of the left kidney.

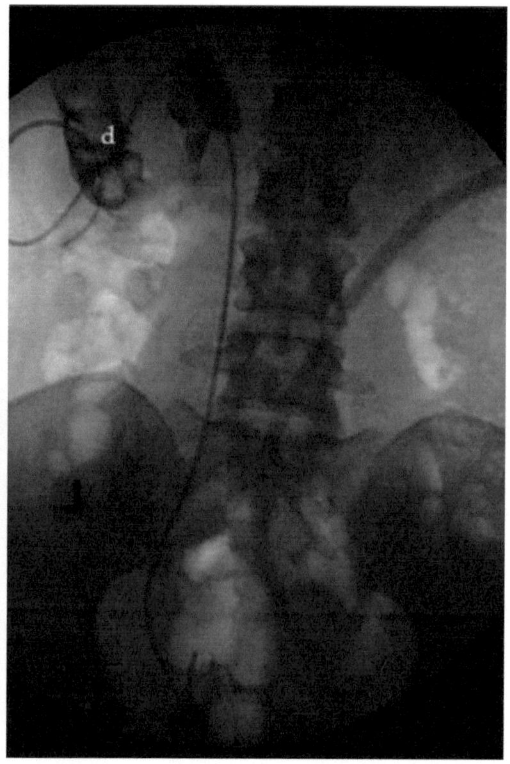


Fig. 13. Anterograde insertion of a double J stent 3 weeks later on the same patient showed extravasation of contrast through the percutaneous nephrostomy tract into the descending colon (d).

### 5.2.5 Injury to intra-abdominal viscera

Injuries to organs adjacent to the kidneys have been reported in less than 1% of cases (M Tan 2010), and of these, splenic injury is the most commonly reported. Liver laceration is less common, and seldom requires intervention (Lee, Smith et al. 1987).

The risk of splenic injury is increased if a higher supracostal approach ($10^{th}$-$11^{th}$ ribs) is used, or if the approach is made during inspiration. Should a trans-splenic tract is made, the primary concern is that of hemorrhage with risk of shock, and these may have to be managed surgically. However, conservative management may be considered in selected cases, particularly if the patient is asymptomatic and stable, and this was reported by Carey in a patient who sustained splenic injury that occurred during percutaneous nephrolithotomy (Carey, Siddiq et al. 2006). The patient was managed conservatively, with no serious consequences and the patient was discharged following removal of the nephrostomy catheter.

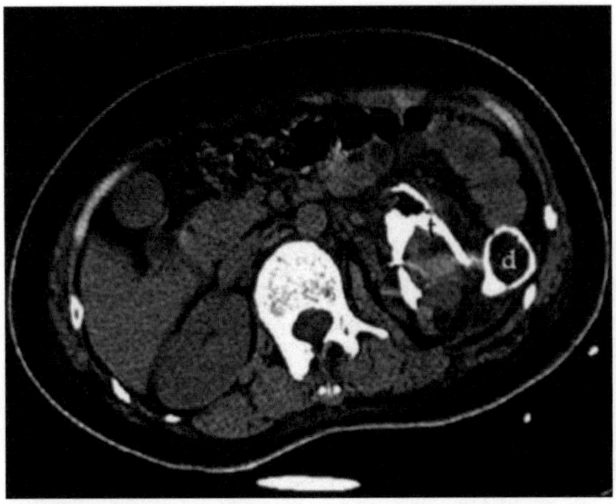

Fig. 14. Computed tomography scan showing extravasation of contrast from the dilated left collecting system through the left PCN tract (t) into the descending colon (d). In this case the tract had matured without any appreciable extravasation of contrast into the retroperitoneal space.

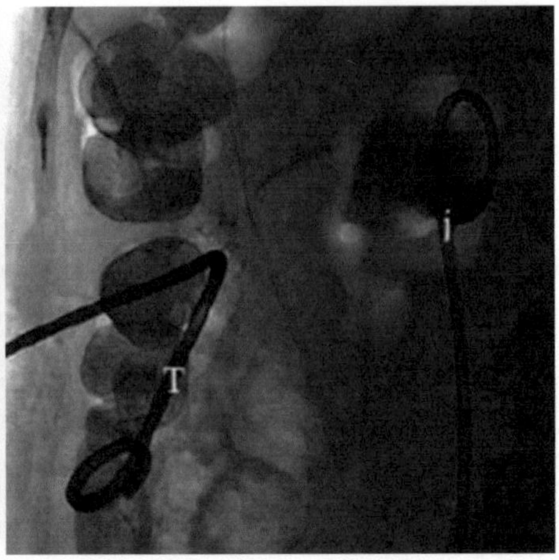

Fig. 15. Withdrawal of the PCN into the colon to be used as a percutaneous colostomy tube (T) was performed after confirmation of good anterograde urinary drainage via the double-J stent (j). Subsequent tube review confirmed closure of the colorenal fistula.

### 5.2.6 Death

Percutaneous nephrostomy has a low mortality rate, with published data reporting rates of 0.03% (Hruby 1990) and 0.3% (Lee, Smith et al. 1987). Various major complications may contribute to death following the procedure, particularly in relation to severe hemorrhage and sepsis, but it may also be contributed by other complications provoked by the procedure itself. Myocardial infarction and cardiac arrest have been reported (von der Recke, Nielsen et al. 1994). Lee reported deaths in 2 patients, one of which was attributed to respiratory failure related to underlying severe interstitial pulmonary fibrosis, while the other was due to myocardial infarction in an obese diabetic patient with hypertension. The presence of comorbidities is therefore an important predisposing factor. Patients who require general anesthesia may also be at risk of developing associated complications. However the mortality rate for percutaneous nephrostomy remains lower than conventional surgery for patients who require urological intervention but are not good candidates for conventional surgery (Lee, Patel et al. 1994).

## 6. Role of percutaneous nephrostomy in transplanted kidneys

The indications for percutaneous nephrostomy described above can be similarly adopted for transplanted kidneys, and indeed percutaneous nephrostomy has been shown to have a good safety profile in these cases (Mostafa, Abbaszadeh et al. 2008). Mostafa further demonstrated that there was no statistical difference in the 10-year survival rates of renal transplant recipients who underwent percutaneous nephrostomy when compared to other renal transplant recipients without urological complications. It also serves as a useful alternative to conventional surgery, which may pose a higher risk in these patients.

The most common urological complications in transplanted kidneys are ureteral obstruction and leakage (Mostafa, Abbaszadeh et al. 2008). These should be recognized and treated early to prevent graft failure. Ureteral obstruction is most commonly due to stricture at the ureterovesical junction anastomosis, brought about by fibrosis secondary to ischemia or rejection and therefore presents late. Mostafa reported good success rates in the treatment of these strictures, by using stents and balloon dilatations inserted via the percutaneous nephrostomy tracts. Early ureteral obstruction on the other hand may be related to other factors such as blood clots, calculus, edema or ischemic necrosis. Similarly, percutaneous interventions may be performed in the treatment of these cases.

## 7. Conclusion

Percutaneous nephrostomy is a widely used urological procedure, providing urinary diversion and access to the urinary tracts for other interventions. While demonstrating a good safety profile, many aspects of the procedure are associated with risks of complications, which may be contributed by various factors from the moment the patient is prepared until after the procedure. The performing physician must not only be well versed with the techniques involved, but he or she should also be well acquainted with the associated risks and complications so that these may be detected and treated early.

## 8. References

Carey, R. I., F. M. Siddiq, et al. (2006). Conservative management of a splenic injury related to percutaneous nephrostolithotomy. *JSLS* 10(4): 504-506.

Cormio, L., P. Annese, et al. (2007). Percutaneous nephrostomy in supine position. *Urology* 69(2): 377-380.

Cowan, N. (2008). The Genitourinary Tract; Technique and Anatomy. *Grainger & Allison's Diagnostic Radiology, A Textbook of Medical Imaging*. A. K. D. A. Adam, Churchill Livingstone. 1: 813-822.

Dyer, R. B., J. D. Regan, et al. (2002). Percutaneous nephrostomy with extensions of the technique: step by step. *Radiographics* 22(3): 503-525.

El-Nahas, A. R., A. A. Shokeir, et al. (2006). Colonic perforation during percutaneous nephrolithotomy: study of risk factors. *Urology* 67(5): 937-941.

Goodwin, W. E., W. C. Casey, et al. (1955). Percutaneous trocar (needle) nephrostomy in hydronephrosis. *J Am Med Assoc* 157(11): 891-894.

Gupta, S., M. Gulati, et al. (1997). Percutaneous nephrostomy with real-time sonographic guidance. *Acta Radiol* 38(3): 454-457.

Hopper, K. D., J. L. Sherman, et al. (1987). The variable anteroposterior position of the retroperitoneal colon to the kidneys. *Invest Radiol* 22(4): 298-302.

Hruby, W. (1990). Percutaneous Nephrostomy. *Interventional Radiology*. P. R. Robert F. Dondelinger, Jean Claude Kurdziel, Sydney Wallace, Thieme: 234 - 244.

Kaskarelis, I. S., M. G. Papadaki, et al. (2001). Complications of percutaneous nephrostomy, percutaneous insertion of ureteral endoprosthesis, and replacement procedures. *Cardiovasc Intervent Radiol* 24(4): 224-228.

Lee, W., A. Smith, et al. (1987). Complications of percutaneous nephrolithotomy. *Am. J. Roentgenol.* 148(1): 177-180.

Lee, W. J., U. Patel, et al. (1994). Emergency percutaneous nephrostomy: results and complications. *J Vasc Interv Radiol* 5(1): 135-139.

Lewis, S. and U. Patel (2004). Major complications after percutaneous nephrostomy-lessons from a department audit. *Clin Radiol* 59(2): 171-179.

M Tan, P. u., PS Jaywantraj, D Wong (2010). Colonic Perforation during Percutaneous Nephrolithotomy Treated Conservatively. *J HK Coll Radiol.* 12(3): 117-121.

Mariappan, P., G. Smith, et al. (2006). One week of ciprofloxacin before percutaneous nephrolithotomy significantly reduces upper tract infection and urosepsis: a prospective controlled study. *BJU Int* 98(5): 1075-1079.

McDermott, V. G., M. G. Schuster, et al. (1997). Antibiotic prophylaxis in vascular and interventional radiology. *AJR Am J Roentgenol* 169(1): 31-38.

Moskowitz, G. W., W. J. Lee, et al. (1989). Diagnosis and management of complications of percutaneous nephrolithotomy. *Crit Rev Diagn Imaging* 29(1): 1-12.

Mostafa, S. A., S. Abbaszadeh, et al. (2008). Percutaneous nephrostomy for treatment of posttransplant ureteral obstructions. *Urol J* 5(2): 79-83.

Ozden, E., O. Yaman, et al. (2002). Sonography Guided Percutaneous Nephrostomy: Success Rates According to the Grade of the Hydronephrosis. *Journal of Ankara Medical School* 24(2): 69-72.

Ramchandani, P., J. F. Cardella, et al. (2003). Quality improvement guidelines for percutaneous nephrostomy. *J Vasc Interv Radiol* 14(9 Pt 2): S277-281.

Stables, D. P. (1982). Percutaneous nephrostomy: techniques, indications, and results. *Urol Clin North Am* 9(1): 15-29.

Stables, D. P., N. J. Ginsberg, et al. (1978). Percutaneous nephrostomy: a series and review of the literature. *AJR Am J Roentgenol* 130(1): 75-82.

Tuttle, D. N., B. M. Yeh, et al. (2005). Risk of injury to adjacent organs with lower-pole fluoroscopically guided percutaneous nephrostomy: evaluation with prone, supine, and multiplanar reformatted CT. *J Vasc Interv Radiol* 16(11): 1489-1492.

von der Recke, P., M. B. Nielsen, et al. (1994). Complications of ultrasound-guided nephrostomy. A 5-year experience. *Acta Radiol* 35(5): 452-454.

Wah, T. M., M. J. Weston, et al. (2004). Percutaneous nephrostomy insertion: outcome data from a prospective multi-operator study at a UK training centre. *Clin Radiol* 59(3): 255-261.

# 19

# Unusual Vascular Access for Hemodialysis Therapies

Cesar A. Restrepo V

*Division of Nephrology, Department of Health Sciences, Caldas University, Manizales, Colombia*

## 1. Introduction

For many years, the arteriovenous (AV) fistula has been demonstrated to be the best vascular access for patients requiring chronical hemodialysis therapy.

The morbidity and mortality statistics for patients with AV fistula is significantly lower compared to patients with central venous catheters (1). However, many patients are found in which performing an arteriovenous fistula or implanting an AV graft is not a possibility. For these patients the usual protocol is the use of an indwelling catheter for chronic hemodialysis therapy practice.

The appearance of patients incompatible with AV fistula is due to the repetitive venous punctures in classical blood vessels, performed in the intensive care unit or for patients with chronic renal failure. These patients develop venous fibrosis making subsequent cannulations impossible.

The use of central venous catheters for initial hemodialysis therapy is also a common practice, this situation is repeated in all countries so that in the United States 60% of incident patients and 17 to 30% of prevalent patients depend on it as the only vascular access catheter despite the recommendation of the K/DOQI guides (Kidney Disease Outcomes Quality Initiative). (2)

In the year 2010, 100% of incident hemodialysis patients in our renal unit were treated with a central venous catheter. This reflects a late referral of doctors to the nephrology clinic, preventing the early practice of AV fistula.

In the same year 259 central venous catheters were implanted in our Renal Unit, 34% of them were transient in acute renal failure patients, 56% transient in patients with chronic renal failure and 10% tunneled catheters. Additionally our statistics showed that at the end of the year 2010 tunneled catheters represented 25% of vascular accesses and that in 94% of the patients using these catheters, arteriovenous fistula or AV graft implant were impossible, thus constituting the catheter tunneled the only access for the practice of chronical hemodialysis.

Traditionally, the most used vascular access is the internal jugular venous, but it can fail due to permanent thrombosis or agenesis. In these situations the usage of even more unusual routes is necessary. Routine practice of procedures through these routes can make them much more available; the purpose of this article is to familiarize physicians with these routes and the correct techniques for accomplishing safe alternative vascular accesses.

## 2. Vascular access variant

### 2.1 Upper hemithorax

Several blood vessels can be punctured in this area for the implantation of central venous catheters (Figure 1).

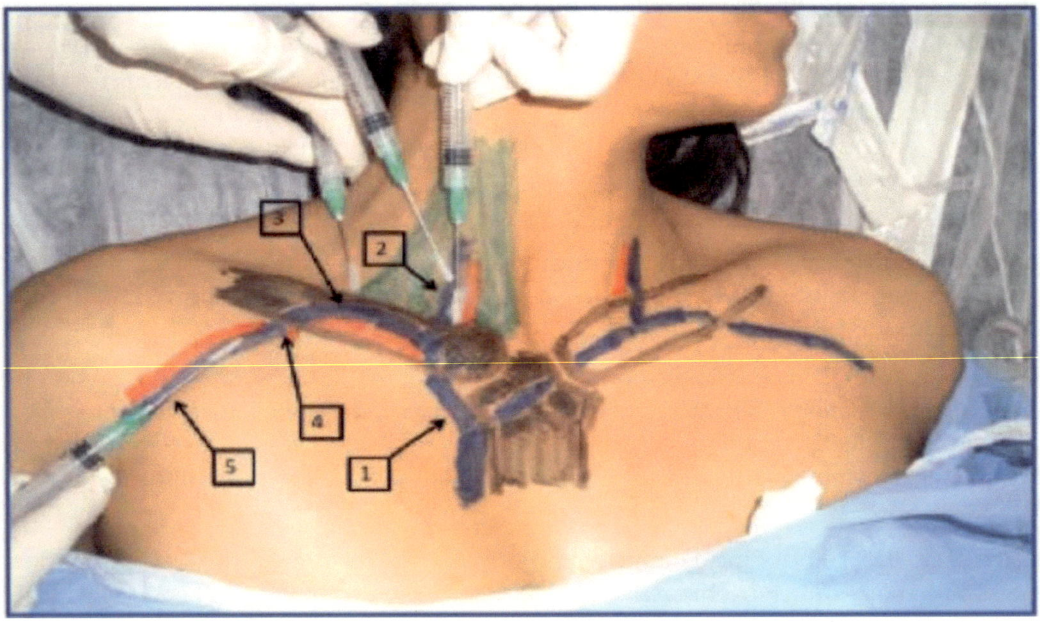


Fig. 1. 1- Innominate Vein, 2- Internal Jugular Vein, 3- Supraclavicular Vein, 4- Infraclavicular Vein, 5- Axillary Vein.

The **internal jugular** access is the most commonly used by nephrologists, but surgeons and intensive care units prefer **Infraclavicular (subclavian)** access. Subclavian access has a disadvantage; it produces subclavian vein stenosis that leads to arm edema when AV fistula is later practiced on the same side (Figure 2).

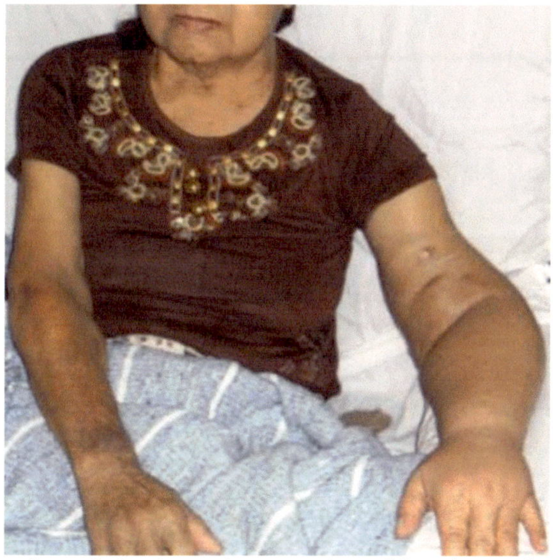

Fig. 2. Edema in left arm by subclavian vein stenosis and brachiocephalic fistula.

Catheters in the internal jugular vein kept for prolonged periods can also cause stenosis, in this case the superior vena cava (Figure 3).

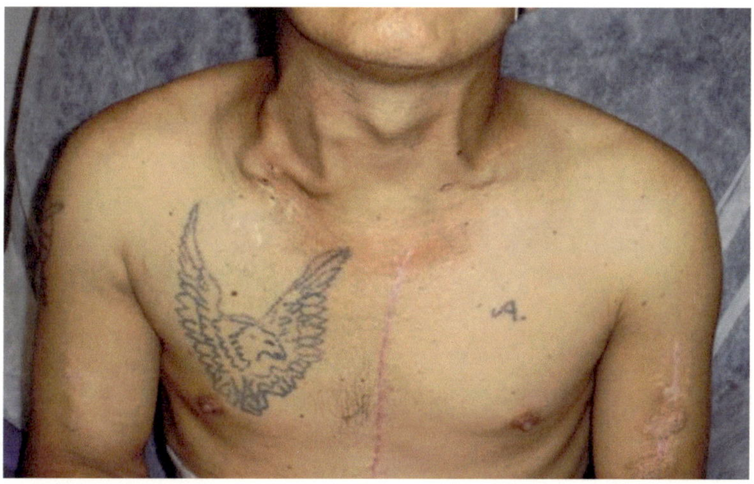

Fig. 3. Cava superior syndrome.

For patients in which the implantation of catheters in the internal jugular vein is not possible, and those in which puncturing this vein or the subclavian vein would not be convenient (for example patients with tracheostomy), an alternative not commonly used is the implantation of catheters in the **axillary vein**. (3)

This vein extends from the clavicle to the axilla (figure 4). The segment in the axillary fossa has been used for decades by pediatric surgeons especially in children with extended burns in whom this is the only preserved area. Unfortunately there are severe infectious complications due to the bacterial flora that lives in this area. (4)

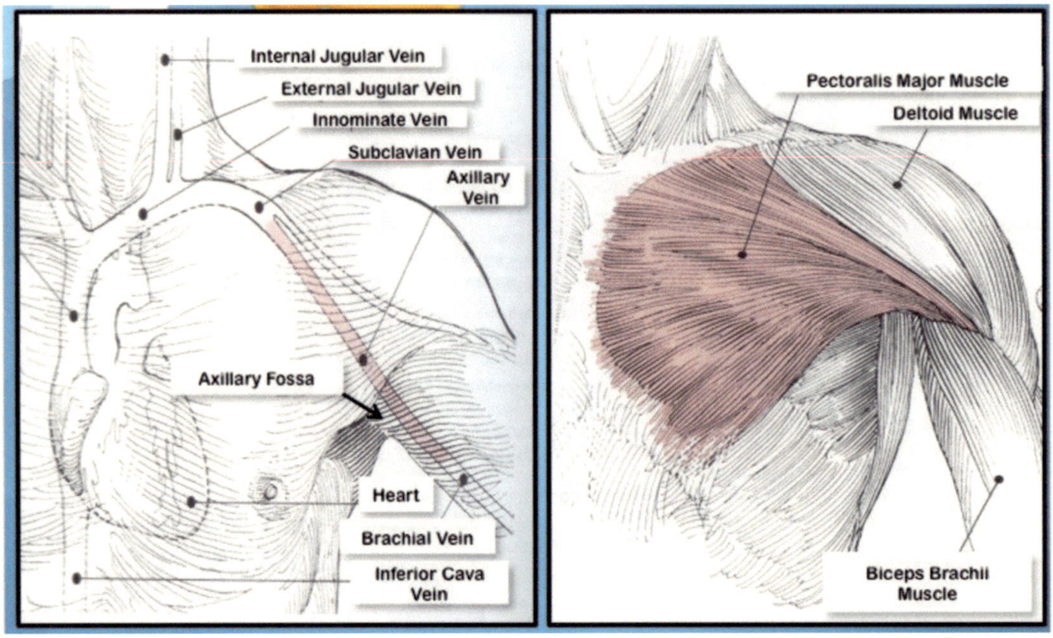


Fig. 4. Axillary Vein and muscle of anatomic area.

Other segments of the axillary vein, from the axillary fold to the clavicle have minimal risk of infection. Classically it is recommended puncturing two finger widths below the site where the coracoid process is found. (5) (Figure 5).

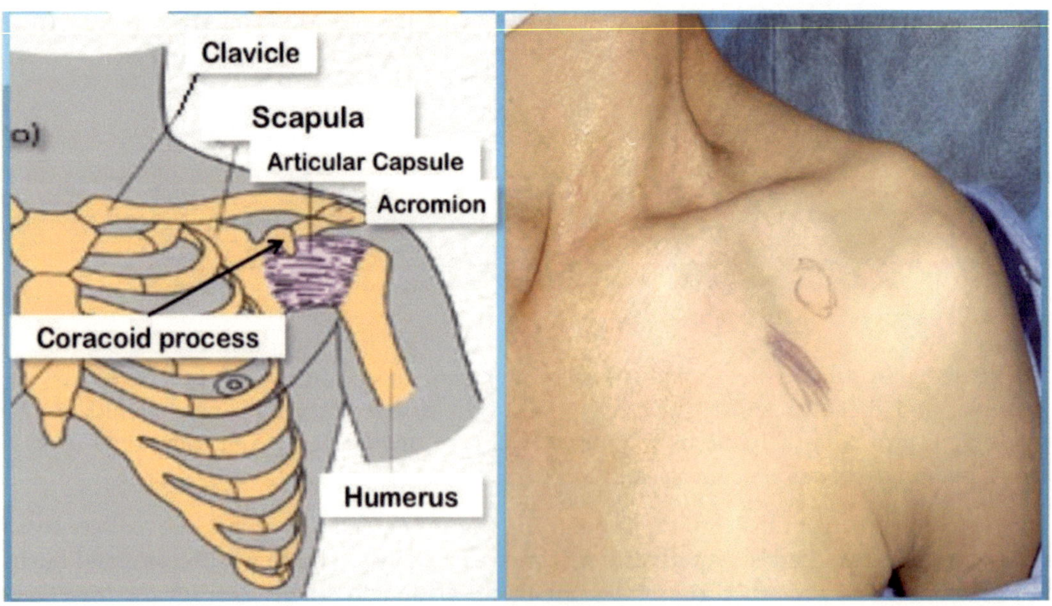


Fig. 5. Recommended place to insert axillary catheter.

In our experience and with patience it is possible to palpate the axillary artery and immediately under it puncture the axillary vein for catheter implantation. It is important to remember that in order to get to the axillary vein both pectoralis major and minor must be penetrated and hence this vessel is located in deep layers (Figure 6).

In our experience also this catheter have utility in patients in intensive care unit in which is common the presence of tracheostomy (Figure 7).

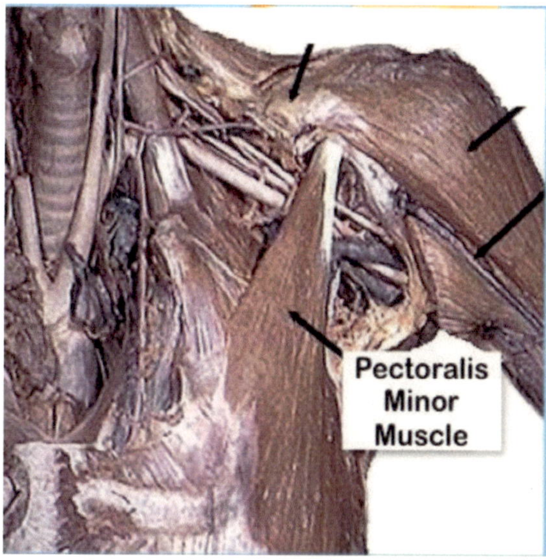


Fig. 6. Pectoralis Minor Muscle.

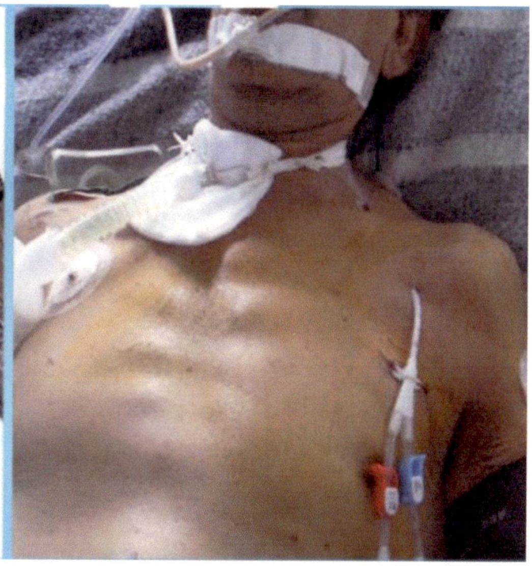

Fig. 7. Patient with tracheostomy and axillary catheter.

The use of ultrasound guidance is a very good alternative, since it allows for an easy and clear view of the vessels of the axillary region, reducing the number of punctures (Figure 8).

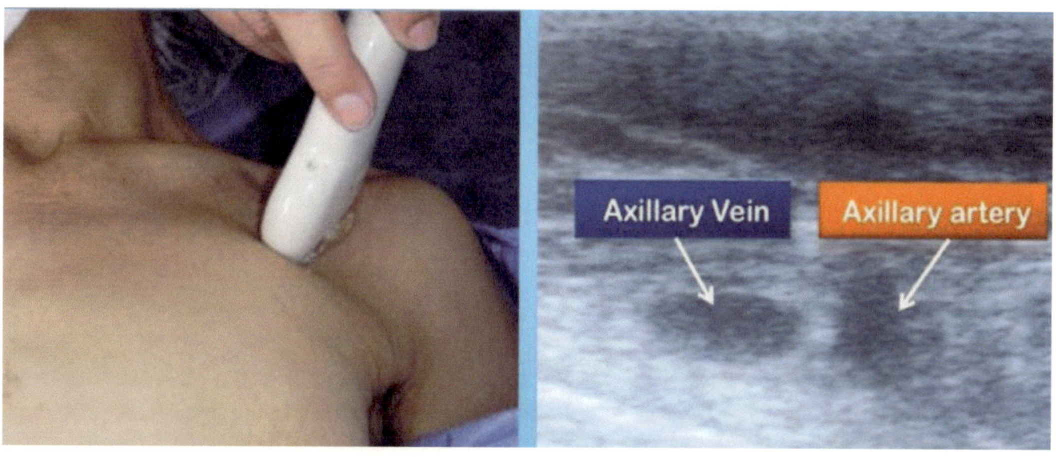


Fig. 8. Ultrasound guidance for axillary catheter implantation.

The **innominate vein** is another blood vessel rarely used for the implantation of central catheters. It is a resource most commonly used by anesthesiologists and its use has not been spread due to fear of puncturing the pleural dome. To access this vessel percutaneously an aspiration needle is introduced holding it immediately above the clavicle between the sternal and clavicular bundles of the sternocleidomastoid muscle. It is directed to the mediastinum and parallel to the anterior chest wall to obtain an abundant blood return. The vein is easily punctured and only 2 to 4 centimeters from the skin. (6) Radiologically the catheters implanted in this blood vessel can be seen riding on top of the clavicle. (Figure 9).

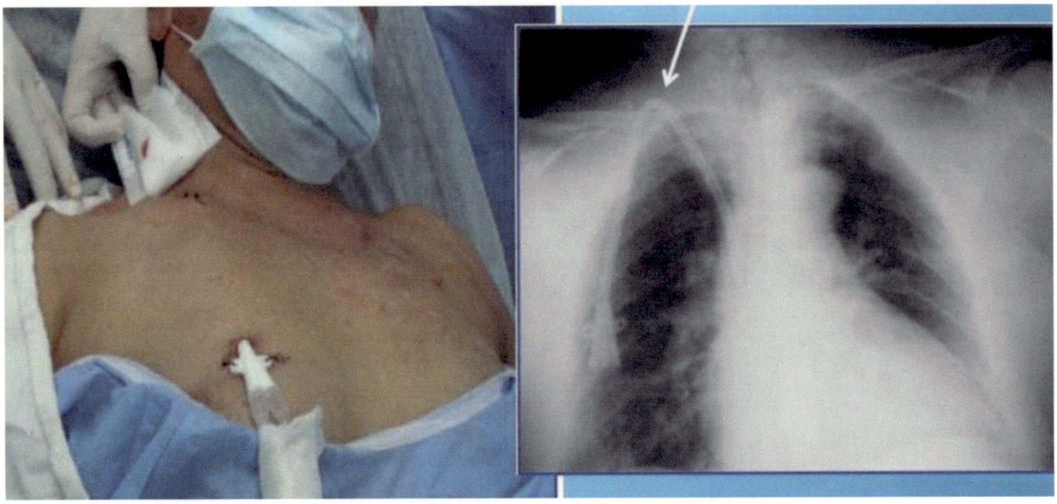

Fig. 9. Catheter inserted into the innominate vein, riding on top of the clavicle.

Innominate vein thrombosis is a rare event, but it can be seen as a complication of the extended use of catheters in this blood vessel. (Figure 10).

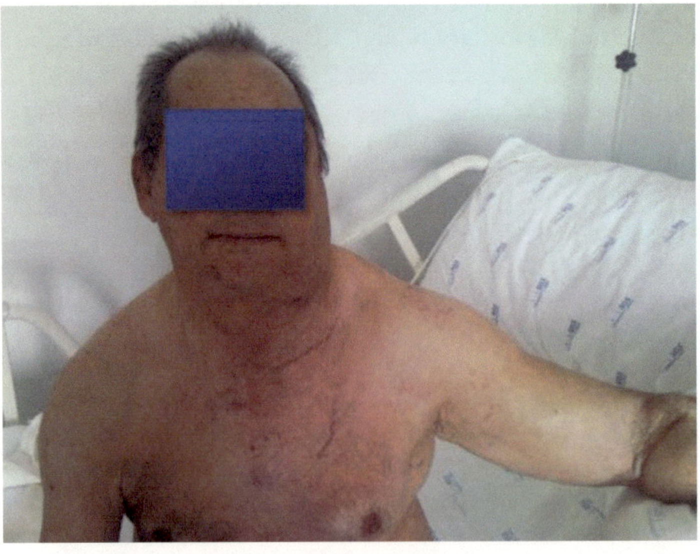

Fig. 10. Innominate vein thrombosis.

There are two final vascular accesses in the upper hemithorax for the implantation of central catheters: intracardiac and superior vena cava access. For the first, anterior thoracotomy is performed in the fifth intercostal space and the catheter is inserted into the right atrium (7). For the second, proceed with anterior right mediastonomy, incision through the third intercostal space and resecting the condrosternal union. Under direct vision puncture the superior vena cava and introduce the catheter. (8) (Figure 11) The appearance of hemothorax, pneumothorax and pneumopericardium is common in these patients, so a routine chest tube implantation is recommended during the procedure and kept for several days.

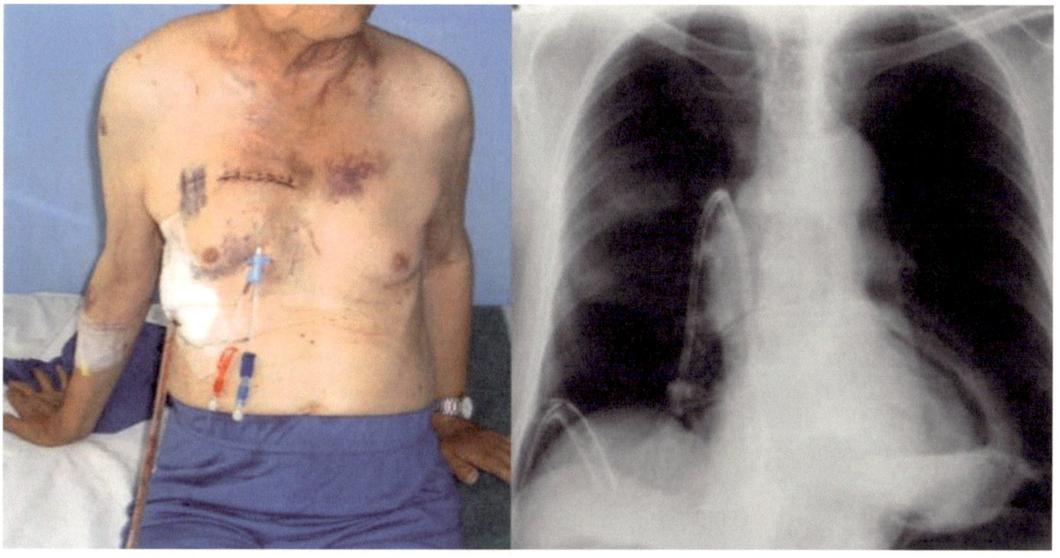

Fig. 11. Patient with catheter in superior vena cava and pneumopericardium.

### 2.2 Lower hemithorax

After exhausting the vessels of the upper hemithorax is necessary to use the lower hemithorax to continue chronic hemodialysis therapy. An alternative is to divert patients to peritoneal dialysis, but when this is not possible for various reasons it is essential to use different approaches.

In our renal unit, the first access we use is the **femoral vein** option. They are classically canalized and then tunneled either to the anterior abdominal wall or into the thigh on the same side. In our experience, this access produces complications such as frequent infections in the exiting orifice for the catheter and also thrombosis (comment pending publication). In one of our patients we managed to keep this catheter for one year only to be withdrawn when the patient received a renal transplant. (Figure 12)

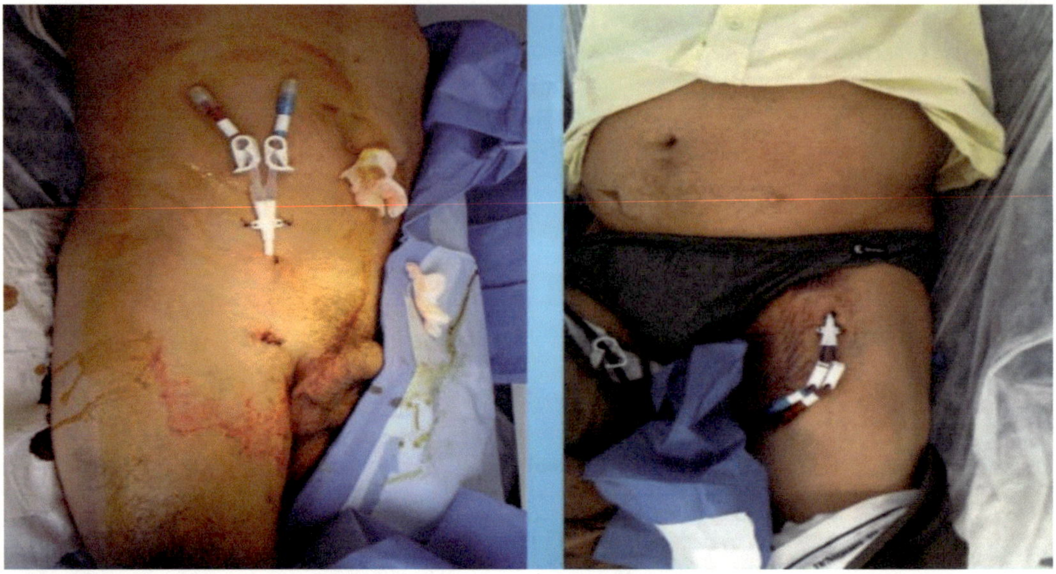

Fig. 12. Tunneled femoral catheter to anterior abdominal wall or into the thigh.

The **iliac vein** can also be used, but requires the participation of a vascular surgeon to achieve safe punctures once the ilioinguinal region has been dissected and the blood vessel exposed (Figure 13).

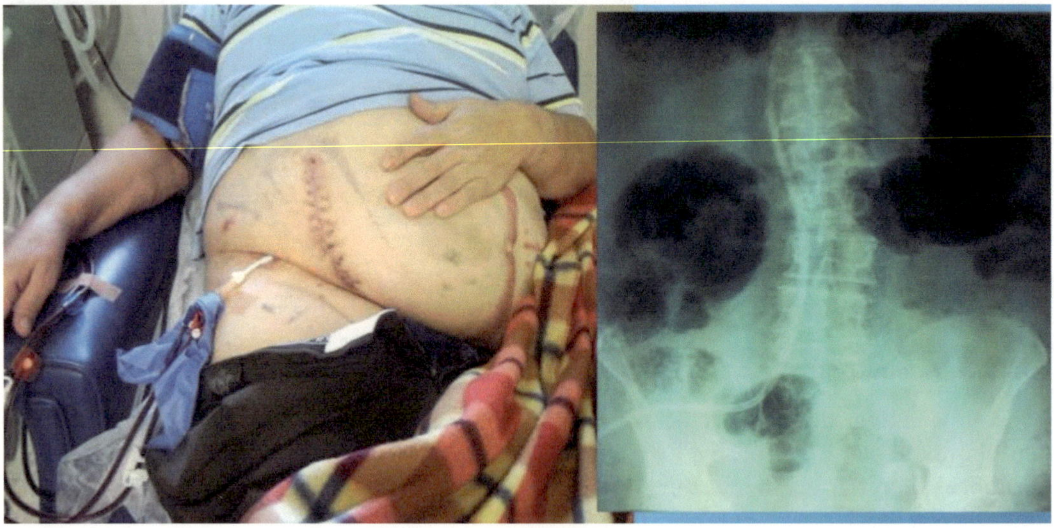

Fig. 13. Tunneled iliac catheter and radiological control.

We then proceed to channel the **inferior vena cava**; we perform this procedure using fluoroscopy or angiography. First we implant a transient catheter in femoral vein, then place the patient in left lateral position with knees flexed and produce a lumbar puncture at the level of the iliac crest, 10 cm from the midline in an upward direction, close to the vertebral body to avoid puncturing the ureter (Figure 14).

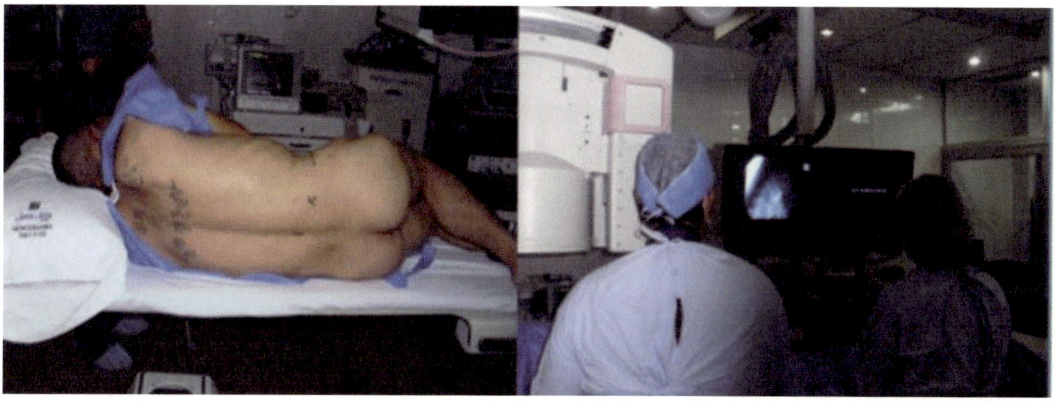

Fig. 14. Position of patient for implantation ideal of catheter in inferior vena cava, and angiography guide.

It is necessary to use a needle with a minimum length of 18 cm. The infusion of contrast medium allows the inferior vena cava location, then directing the needle toward her, and once punctured proceed to catheter implantation in technique like any tunneled catheter. (Figure 15 and 16).

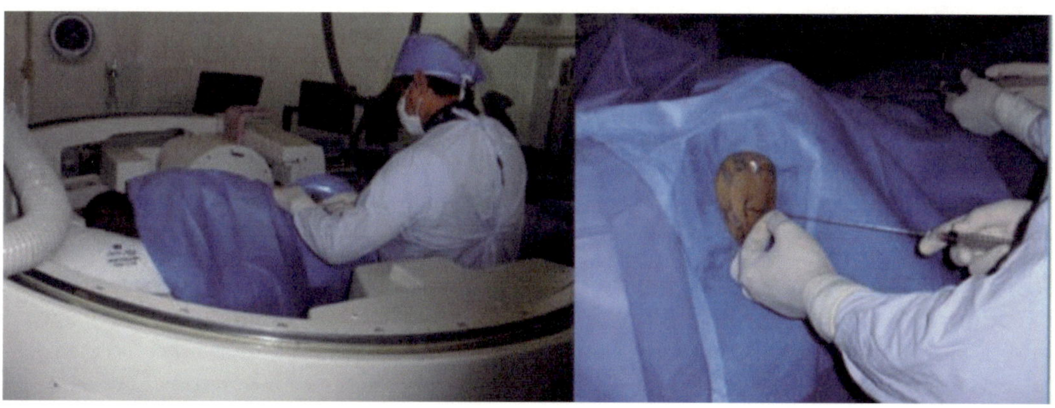

Fig. 15. Angiography guide, and needle with a minimum length of 18 cm. Procedure performed by the author of the chapter.

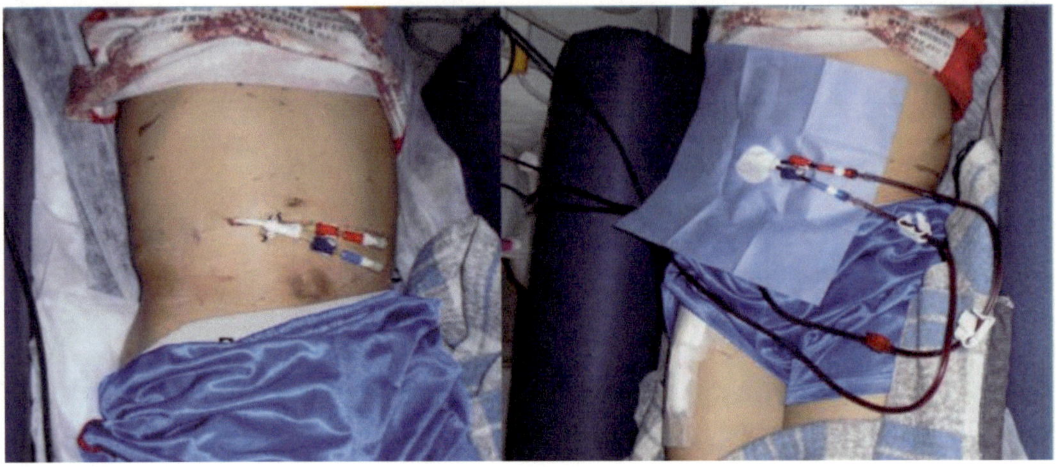

Fig. 16. Tunneled inferior vena cava catheter in use.

Other vascular access used by other groups, and with which we have not experience is transhepatic access.

## 3. Preventive antibiotic intervention before the implantation of catheters

For many years the recommended procedure for every patient scheduled for the implantation of a central venous catheter was to receive antibiotics that covered both Gram (+) and Gram (-) bacteria 30 minutes before the procedure.

In the year 2007 we presented our work in this subject. We performed two periods of experimentation. First, we administered the combination of first generation cephalosporin and amino glycoside 30 minutes before the catheter's implantation and second we suspended the antibiotics and practiced universal techniques for avoiding infection.

Our results showed that in the first period, 1,93% of 156 procedures had infectious complications. In the second period 2,29% of 304 procedures had complications, concluding then that the practices of preventive antibiotics don´t have any benefices and was abandoned in our unit. (9) (Figure 17).

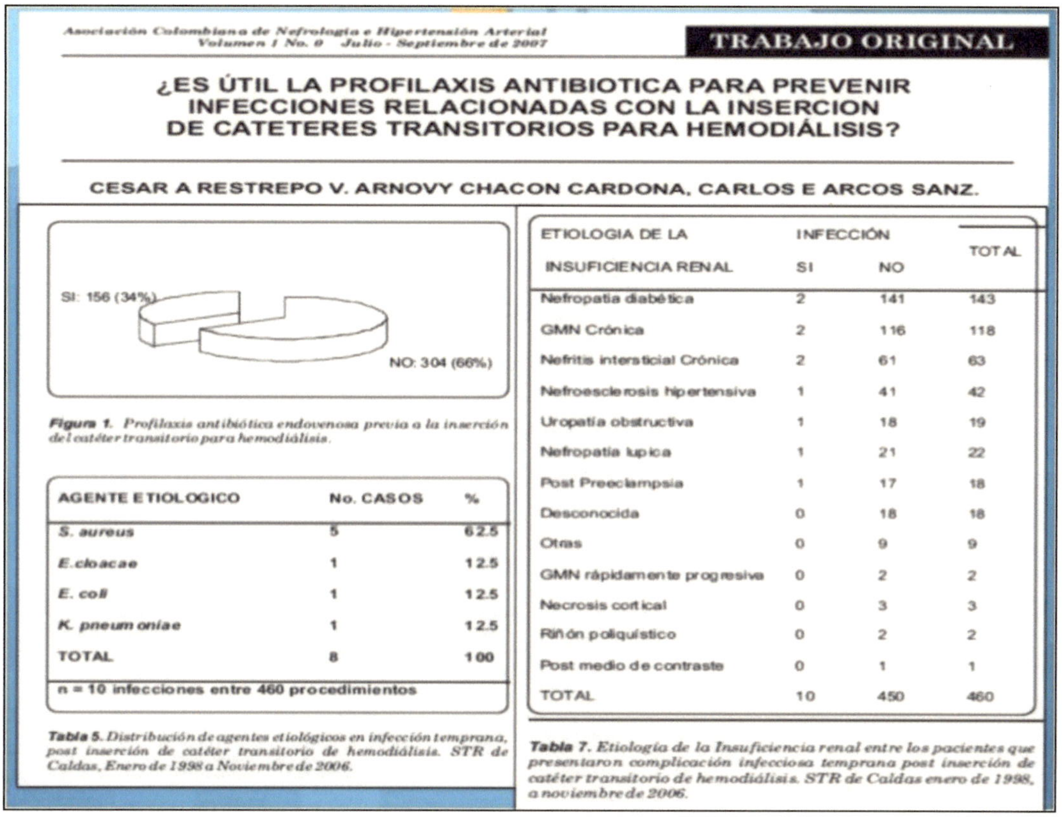

Asociación Colombiana de Nefrologia e Hipertensión Arterial
Volumen 1 No. 0 Julio - Septiembre de 2007

TRABAJO ORIGINAL

¿ES ÚTIL LA PROFILAXIS ANTIBIOTICA PARA PREVENIR INFECCIONES RELACIONADAS CON LA INSERCION DE CATETERES TRANSITORIOS PARA HEMODIÁLISIS?

CESAR A RESTREPO V. ARNOVY CHACON CARDONA, CARLOS E ARCOS SANZ.



**Figura 1.** *Profilaxis antibiótica endovenosa previa a la inserción del catéter transitorio para hemodiálisis.*

| AGENTE ETIOLOGICO | No. CASOS | % |
|---|---|---|
| *S. aureus* | 5 | 62.5 |
| *E.cloacae* | 1 | 12.5 |
| *E. coli* | 1 | 12.5 |
| *K. pneumoniae* | 1 | 12.5 |
| TOTAL | 8 | 100 |
| n = 10 infecciones entre 460 procedimientos | | |

**Tabla 5.** *Distribución de agentes etiológicos en infección temprana, post inserción de catéter transitorio de hemodiálisis. STR de Caldas, Enero de 1998 a Noviembre de 2006.*

| ETIOLOGIA DE LA INSUFICIENCIA RENAL | INFECCIÓN SI | INFECCIÓN NO | TOTAL |
|---|---|---|---|
| Nefropatia diabética | 2 | 141 | 143 |
| GMN Crónica | 2 | 116 | 118 |
| Nefritis intersticial Crónica | 2 | 61 | 63 |
| Nefroesclerosis hipertensiva | 1 | 41 | 42 |
| Uropatía obstructiva | 1 | 18 | 19 |
| Nefropatia lupica | 1 | 21 | 22 |
| Post Preeclampsia | 1 | 17 | 18 |
| Desconocida | 0 | 18 | 18 |
| Otras | 0 | 9 | 9 |
| GMN rápidamente progresiva | 0 | 2 | 2 |
| Necrosis cortical | 0 | 3 | 3 |
| Riñón poliquístico | 0 | 2 | 2 |
| Post medio de contraste | 0 | 1 | 1 |
| TOTAL | 10 | 450 | 460 |

**Tabla 7.** *Etiología de la Insuficiencia renal entre los pacientes que presentaron complicación infecciosa temprana post inserción de catéter transitorio de hemodiálisis. STR de Caldas enero de 1998, a noviembre de 2006.*

Fig. 17. No benefit with antibiotic prophylaxis for prevention of central venous catheters infections.

## 4. Radiological control after the implantation of jugular catheters

It has been suggested that every patient with a central venous catheter implanted on his or her superior hemithorax, must have PA chest radiography before actually using the catheter to confirm a correct placement. In occasions it is necessary to take the patient to hemodialysis therapy immediately after implanting the catheter and the radiological control can delay this process. In the year 2008 we published our experience with 245 jugular catheters implanted in the past years, all of them had PA chest radiography performed after the implantation. Only 4 cases (1,6%) had a significant complication (10). Based on this and if the implantation of the catheter was easy, we avoid soliciting the radiography and immediately proceed to the hemodialysis practice. (Figure 18).

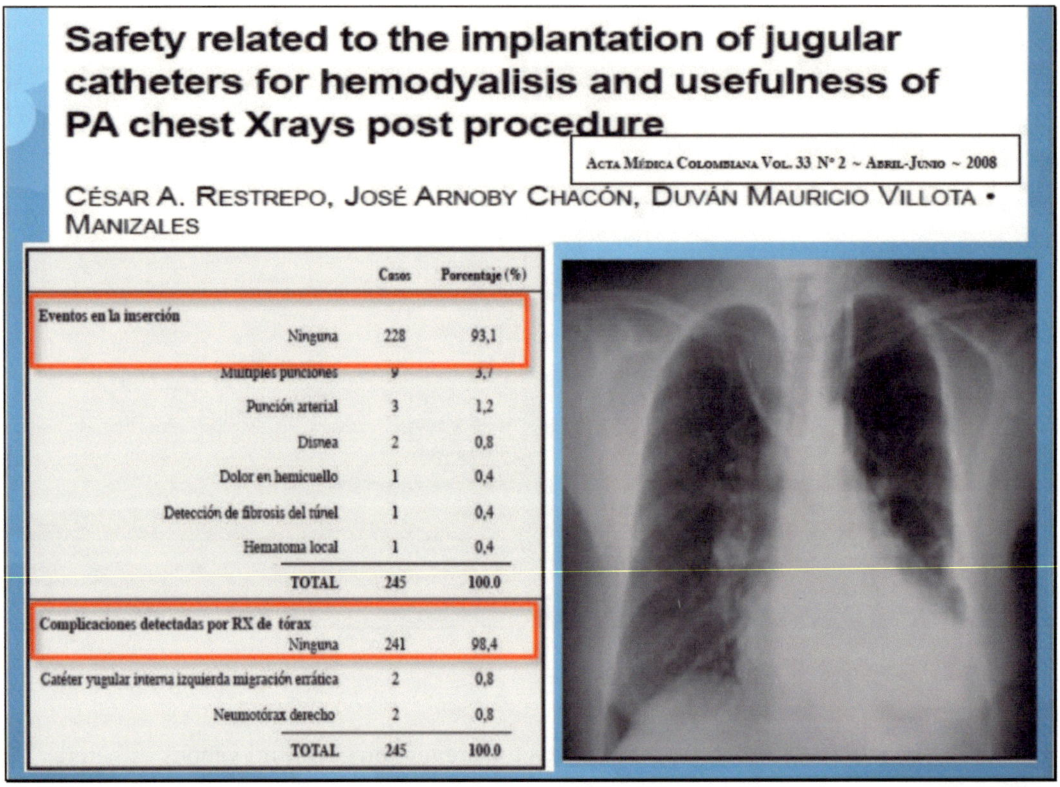


Fig. 18. PA chest radiograph post insertion of central catheter is unnecessary.

Interestingly in 4 patients with insertion of catheters in left jugular vein we observed abnormal catheter course, corresponding to persistent left superior vena cava, anatomical abnormality confirmed by radiological or echocardiographic studies. (11) (Figure 19).

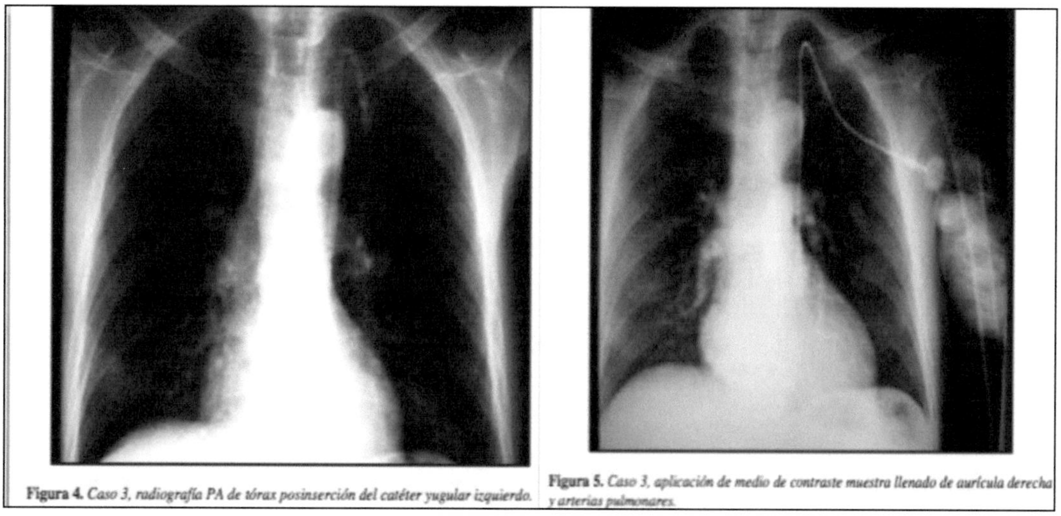


Fig. 19. Catheter in left persistent superior vena cava, confirm by Radiological studies.

## 5. References

Polkinghorne K R, McDonald S P, Atkins R C, Kerr P G. Vascular Access and all-cause mortality: A propensity score analysis. J Am Soc Nephrol 2004; 15: 477-486.

Rayner HC, Besarab A, Brown WW, Disney A, Salto A, Pisoni RL. Vascular access results from the Dialysis Outcome and Practice Patterns Study (DOPPS): performance against Kidney Disease Outcomes Quality Initiative (K/DOQI) clinical practice guidelines. Am J Kidney Dis 2004;44(Suppl2):S22-S26.

Restrepo Valencia C A, Buritica Barragan C M. Axillary catheter for hemodialysis, an alternative vascular Access. Nefrologia 2008; 28: 77-81.

Andel H, Rab M, Felfernig M, Andel D, Koller R, Kamolz L-P, Zimpfer M. The axillary vein central venous catheter in severely burned patients. Burns 25: 753-756, 1999.

Taylor BL, Yellowlees I. Central venous cannulation using the infraclavicular axillary vein. Anesthesiology 72: 55-58, 1990.

Restrepo Valencia C A, Buritica Barragan C M. Placement of vascular access catheters for haemodialysis in the innominate vein: a little-used approach. Nefrologia 2009; 29: 354-357.

Agrawal S, Alaly J R, Misra M. Intracardiac access for hemodialysis: A case series. Hemodialysis Int 2009;13:S18-S23

Restrepo Valencia C A, Buritica Barragan C M, Arango A. Catheter in the superior vena cava for hemodialysis as a last resort in superior hemithorax. Nefrologia 2010; 30: 463-466.

Restrepo V C A, Chacon A C, Arcos Sanz C E. Es útil la profilaxis antibiótica para prevenir infecciones relacionada con la inserción de catéteres transitorios para hemodiálisis?. Revista Asocolnef 2007; 1: 4-9.

Restrepo C A, Chacon J A, Villota D M. Safety related to the implantation of jugular catheters for hemodyalisis and usefulness of PA chest X rays postprocedure. Acta Med Colomb 2008; 33: 68-74.

Cruz J, Restrepo C A. Accidental implantation of hemodialysis catheter in persistent left superior vena cava. Acta Med Colomb 2007; 32: 227-230.

# 20

# The Role of Nephron-Sparing Surgery (NSS) for Renal Tumours >4 cm

Amélie Parisel, Frederic Baekelandt, Hein Van Poppel and Steven Joniau
*University Hospitals Leuven*
*Belgium*

## 1. Introduction

For many years, radical nephrectomy (RN) has been the gold standard treatment for renal tumours. However, at present the available evidence supports elective nephron-sparing surgery (NSS) as the standard surgical treatment for renal cortical tumours ≤4 cm (clinical stage T1a). Furthermore, an increasing body of evidence demonstrates that even a minor loss of renal function can increase cardiovascular morbidity and consequently reduce life expectancy (Go et al., 2004). Thus, surgeons have the responsibility to preserve as much renal parenchyma as possible.

International guidelines at present recommend NSS for small renal tumours up to 4 cm. However, the role of NSS for larger renal tumours (stage T1b: 4.1 - 7 cm, stage T2: >7 cm) remains controversial. During the last couple of years, data has emerged which demonstrates that NSS can be safely performed with acceptable complication rates compared to RN (Van Poppel et al., 2010). The advantage of NSS lies in avoiding the development of end-stage renal disease and the need for haemodialysis, while maintaining quality of life (Lesage et al., 2007).

The size of the tumour is no longer considered to be a limiting factor for NSS and some now advocate NSS whenever possible and feasible (Becker et al., 2009).

## 2. Open partial nephrectomy

### 2.1 Oncologic control

#### 2.1.1 Positive Surgical Margins (PSM): Incidence, clinical relevance

NSS aims to preserve renal function without lacking its primary goal: eradicate the tumour. One of the challenges of NSS is to achieve negative surgical margins (NSM). It means that there are no cancer cells seen at the outer edge of the resection piece. This is marked with ink.

In general, the incidence of PSM in T1b tumours is between 0 % (Patel et al., 2009) and 16.7% (Lee et al., 2010). Lee showed that the difference in recurrence rate for patients with PSM compared to NSM was not significant.

Coffin et al (Coffin et al., 2011) found that an imperative indication for NSS had an impact on PSM rates (p=0.03). However, he also noticed that the median tumour size was significantly larger in the imperative indication group, compared to the elective indication group (p=0.03).

| Publication | TNM | Single vs multi-institution | n= | PSM % |
|---|---|---|---|---|
| Roos pT1b (J Urol 2010) | pT1b | Single | 73 | 7.6 * |
| Coffin (2011) | all sizes | Single | 155 | 9.7 |
| Joniau (2008) | pT1b | Single | 67 | 5.8 |
| Porpiglia (2010) World J Urol | pT1b | Multi | 63 | 6.5 |
| Porpiglia (2010) BJU | pT1b | Single | 33 | 0 |
| Patel (2009) | pT1b | Single | 15 | 0 |
| Coffin (2011) | all sizes | Single | 155 | 9.7 |

* There were 12/158 Positive frozen section, therefore a RN was performed.

Table 1. PSM rates.

Nevertheless, he noticed that tumour size was not a significant predictor of recurrence, while multifocality was associated with recurrence. These findings demonstrate that the clinical impact of PSM is not as important as previously thought. To evaluate the impact of PSM, Bensalah et al. (Bensalah et al., 2010) collected 111 cases with PSM from an international multicentre database. Tumours were stage T1, T2 or T3 without nodal invasion or distant metastasis. He compared those with a population of 664 patients who had NSM at resection: groups were matched for age, indication, tumour size and grade. With comparable follow up (PSM 37 versus NSM 35.4 months), the recurrence rate was higher in PSM group than NSM group (10.1% versus 2.2%). However, Overall Survival (OS) and cancer specific survival (CSS) were not significantly different. He also compared 101 PSM with 102 NSM matched for surgical indication (elective versus imperative), tumour size and Fuhrman grade and also found a higher rate of tumour recurrence (10.9% vs. 2.9%), however OS and CSS were again similar.

Russo (Russo 2010) commented the study of Bensalah (Bensalah 2010): in his experience he has more PSM for small renal tumours than for larger, particularly when they are endophytic.

Yossepowitch (Yossepowitch et al., 2008) analysed a cohort of 1344 patients who had undergone partial nephrectomy: there were 77 cases of PSM. Surprisingly, the larger the tumour, the lower the incidence of PSM was. He could not show an association between PSM and a higher risk of recurrence or metastatic progression.

These observations suggest that the presence of PSM is a risk factor for recurrence but does not impact on OS and CSS. These facts also argue for a closer follow up in the first post-operative years.

Most patients with PSM will not experience local recurrence (Van Poppel et al., 2007). Positive margins detected at frozen section or at final histology should not be considered an indication for RN.

### 2.1.2 Overall survival, cancer-specific survival, progression free survival

We reviewed 98 patients operated at our institution between 1997 and 2009 for a renal tumour larger than 4 cm. All patients underwent an open partial nephrectomy. Mean diameter was 5.32 cm. At final histopathology, three quarters of the tumours were malignant and 2.7% were staged pT3a. 53.4% of the renal cell cancers (RCC) showed a low grade (Furhman grade 1-2) versus 46.6% high grade (Furhman grade 3-4). The 5-year OS and CSS rates were 77.9% and 98%, respectively. We observed 5 local reccurences (5.1%) and 7 metastatic recurrences (7.1%). (Joniau et al., 2011)

Roos and Brenner (Roos et al., 2010) compared 73 patients who had undergone elective NSS for T1b or greater tumours with a pair-matched cohort of 100 radical nephrectomies: the OS rates were comparable for NSS vs. RN. The 5, 10 and 15-year CSS rates after NSS (95%, 91% and 82%, respectively) were comparable with RN (97%, 95 and 88%, respectively).The 5, 10 and 15-year PFS rate after NSS (89%, 85% and 76%, respectively) were similar to RN (92%, 89% and 77%, respectively). In a retrospective study by Antonelli (Antonelli et al., 2008), there was no significant difference in progression and survival rates between NSS and RN both for tumours ≤ 4 cm as for those >4 cm. Interestingly, even when not significant, the group of patients with the larger tumours treated with radical surgery experienced a progression rate which was double compared to those who underwent NSS. In the same study, when operated by NSS, the patients with a T1a tumours had a higher risk of local recurrence in the operated kidney, as well as in the contralateral kidney. T1b tumours showed a higher risk of metastatic and local recurrence. Cytonuclear grading was correlated with higher risk of recurrence in tumours larger than 4 cm. However, even in large tumours with high cytonuclear grade, the type of surgery had no significant influence on oncologic outcomes: nor on progression rate nor on disease free survival rate at 5 years.

Nemr (Nemr et al., 2007) described similar oncologic outcomes for NSS and RN in T1b renal tumours: Mean follow up was 45 months and there was no significant difference in recurrence free survival with 100% for PN vs. 89.3% for RN.

Margulis (Margulis et al., 2007) retrospectively compared RN (576) with NSS (34) for tumours >4 cm: recurrence occurred in 4 patients (12%) who underwent NSS vs. 164 patients (28.9%) who underwent RN at a median follow-up of 24.2 and 13.2 months, respectively. 5-year RFS was higher for NSS but CSS was similar. 27% of NSS were performed for elective indications; the remainders had solitary kidneys (29%) or chronic kidney disease (CKD) (44%). The indication does not seem to impact 5-year RFS and CSS. However, this was a retrospective comparison of a small group of NSS versus a large group of RN cases, with a selection bias resulting in an imbalance for smaller tumour size and more pT3a in the NSS group compared to the RN group.

Coffin et al (Coffin et al., 2011) tried to determine the impact of an imperative indication for NSS on the oncologic outcomes. The study counted 155 patients who underwent NSS: 96 elective indications and 59 imperative indications. 62.7% (37 patients) with imperative indications were staged pT1B or higher versus 22% (22 patients) with elective indications. NSS was applied whenever possible: the usual limitations were tumour size and location. Imperative cases were associated with lower 5- and 10-year OS rates. Tumour size was also a significant prognostic factor for 5- and 10-year Overall Survival.

Becker (Becker et al., 2006) evaluated the oncologic outcomes of NSS in tumours larger than 4 cm with mean follow up of 6.2 years. There were 10% of deaths but none was cancer related. The Cancer specific survival was 100% after 5, 10 and 15 years. Of the 69 patients, 5.8% experienced disease recurrence. 5-, 10- and 15-year overall survival rates were 94.9%, 86.7% and 86.7%, respectively.

In carefully selected patients with tumours >4 cm, NSS appears to obtain equivalent oncologic outcomes compared to those achieved with RN. Although higher morbidity rates were seen after NSS, the complication type and severity were acceptable.

| Publication | TNM | Single vs multi-institution | n= | DFS 5 years % | Local Reccurence % | Distant Metastase % | Median FU months | mean diam cm |
|---|---|---|---|---|---|---|---|---|
| Margulis (2007) | pT2-pT3b | single | 34 | 82 | 0 | 12 | 62.1 | 5.2 |
| Antonelli (2008) | pT1b | Single | 52 | 93 | 1.9 | 5.3 | 54.3 | 4.8 |
| Roos (J Urol 2010) | pT1b | Single | 73 | 95 | 1.3 | 9.6 | 55.2 | 5.0 |
| Coffin (2011) | all sizes | Single | 155 | 81.8 | * | * | 95 | 3.7 |
| Coffin (2011) | pT1b | Single | 59 | 74 | * | * | 95 | ? |
| Joniau (2008) | pT1b | Single | 67 | 84 | 4 | 6 | 40.2 | 4.5 |
| Patard (2004) | pT1b | multi | 65 | 93.8 | 3.6 | 7.1 | 51 | 5.3 |
| Becker (2006) | pT1b | Single | 69 | 100 | 5.8 | 5.8 | 70 | 5.3 |
| Leibovitch (2004) | pT1b | Single | 91 | 98 | 5.4 | 4.4 | 64 | 4.9 |
| Hafez (1999) | | | 175 | 86 | 0.8 | ? | 47 | |

Table 2. Oncologic outcomes.

### 2.2 Complications

#### 2.2.1 Complication rates of NNS vs. RN

Haemorrhage is the most common intra-operative complication (1.2 -4.5%). Post-operative complications are urinary fistula formation (1.4-17%), acute renal failure (0.7-26%), post-operative bleeding (0-4.5%), wound infection (1.2-5.9%), perinephric abscess (0.6-3.2%), chronic renal insufficiency (3.2-12%) and urinary retention (Lesage et al., 2007). Non-urological complications include pulmonary and cardiac complications, and also delirium.

We have recently published results of an uncontrolled and retrospective study of 67 patients who underwent NSS for T1b RCC at our institution. A rate of 3% of post-operative haemorrhage requiring embolization was observed, and none developed a urinary fistula. Four patients (6%) had positive resection margins; none of these developed tumour recurrence. After a median (range) follow-up of 40.1 (1-98.3) months, 10 patients (15%) had died, of whom only one death was related to NSS (postoperative hypovolemic shock). The recurrence rate was 10%: 3 patients (4%) developed a local recurrence and 4 (6%) loco-regional or distant disease but all of these patients were alive at last follow-up (Joniau et al., 2009).

In our recently updated series of 98 open partial nephrectomies for cT1b tumours, two patients died in the peri-operative period, but both had extensive cardiac histories. We encountered 7 post-operative acute kidney haemorrhages: of those, 3 required a reoperation,

2 were embolized and 2 were treated conservatively. There was one urinary fistula which was successfully managed by placing a double-J stent. Thus, major complication rate (Dindo score ≥3) was 9.2%.

Coffin (Coffin et al., 2011) encountered a higher complication rate in NSS compared to RN. Total complication rate was 37.7% (of 69 patients) versus 24.5%, respectively. Rates of pulmonary complications and delirium were comparable in both techniques (9.4% versus 9.6% and 3.1% versus 1.1%, respectively) while cardiac complications were more frequent after RN (20.2% versus 1.5% after NSS). Urinary fistula rate was 5.8%. Transfusion rate was higher in NSS (23.2%) versus RN (13.8%). Spleen damage was not encountered during NSS but occurred three times during RN. Contrary to most studies, NSS did not require surgical revision but one patient was re-operated after a RN. (Roos et al., 2010)

| Publication | Approach | Single vs multi-institution | N = | C % | SR % | RN % | CR % | I % | II % | IIIa % | IIIb % | IV % | V |
|---|---|---|---|---|---|---|---|---|---|---|---|---|---|
| Porpiglia (2010) | Lap | multi | 41 | 7.3 | 7.3 | 2.4 | 26 | 4.8 | 7.3 | 7.3 | 7.3 | | 0 |
| *Porpiglia (2010) | Lap | one | 33 | 0 | 6 | 3 | 27 | 9 | 3 | 9 | 6 | | 0 |
| Becker (2006) | open | one | 69 | - | | | 13 | | | 10 | 3 | | 0 |
| Patel (2009) | Robot | one | 15 | 0 | 6 | | 26.6 | 0 | 6.6 | 13.2 | 0 | 6.6 | 0 |
| Joniau (2011) | open | one | 98 | - | 3 | 0 | 27,5 | 8.16 | 11.2 | 0 | 5.1 | 2 | 1 |

C= Conversion
SR = Surgical Revision
RN = Radical Nephrectomy
CR = Complication rate
I, II, III, IV, V = Complication rate according to the Dindo-Clavien classification

Table 3. Complication Rate.

NSS has a higher rate of complications, however this remains acceptable. Most complications can be managed in a conservative or minimally invasive fashion and therefore in none of the reports, an impact on the length of hospital stay or the hospital costs was found.

### 2.2.2 Risk factors for complications

#### 2.2.2.1 Imperative indications

Is there an impact of imperative indications for NSS on peri-operative complications? In a study by Cofin, no significant difference was seen between elective and imperative indications regarding operating time, but the elective group had better surgical outcomes: less blood loss and better control of post-operative creatinin level (Coffin 2011). For oncologic outcomes, Antonelli (Antonelli et al., 2008) found a lower recurrence rate and a higher disease free survival rate at 5 years in elective indications compared with imperative indications.

#### 2.2.2.2 Elderly

Being older than 65 years does not seem to be a significant prognostic factor for having surgical as well as medical complications after partial nephrectomy. The difference was statistically significant for cardiac complications only (Roos et al., 2010).

## 2.3 Renal function

### 2.3.1 Renal function deterioration after NSS vs. RN

Acute reduction in functional renal mass leads the remnant glomeruli to maintain the renal function by several mechanisms: adaptive glomerular hypertrophy, hyperperfusion, hypertension and hyperfiltration. These phenomena result in proteinuria.

NSS aims to achieve two goals: a complete excision of the tumour but at the same time guarantee an optimal preservation of renal function. With less excision of healthy renal tissue with NSS, we can expect less glomerulosclerosis and renal failure (Van Poppel et al., 2003). Therefore, NSS seems to be the best way to prevent Chronic Kidney Disease (CKD).

In one of our studies on OPN for T1b renal tumours (Joniau et al., 2009), 10% of patients developed de novo renal insufficiency. Six of those seven patients had imperative indication. Serum creatinin levels dropped significantly in imperative indication, while this was not seen in elective and relative indications.

In our last study of 98 open partial nephrectomies for T1b, estimated Glomerular Filtration Rate (eGFR) deteriorated postoperatively on average by 1.74 $ml/min/1.73m^2$.

10.2% of patients developed CKD post-operatively, but 20.4% patients had an improved CKD stage after surgery.

In his study, Roos (Roos & Brenner, 2010) also observed a significant difference in eGFR at last follow up and in e GFR difference (calculated as e GFR preoperative - eGFR at last follow up). After NSS, 14.5% of patients (10) had reached an eGRF < $60ml/min/1.73m^2$ versus 44.7% (42) after RN.

In a retrospective study (Lane et al., 2010) Lane studied 2402 patients with a normal preoperative kidney function (serum creatinin less or equal to 1.4 mg/dl) and compared: 1833 PN versus 569 RN. Tumour stage was pT1b or more in 31% of PN and 64% of RN. NSS even - with a warm ischemia time of longer than 31 minutes - demonstrated better renal outcomes, however patients in the RN group were older, had more co-morbidities and were affected by larger and more aggressive tumours.

A solitary kidney is not a contra-indication for NSS. Lee (Lee 2010) reports 38 patients with solitary kidney who underwent partial nephrectomy: 53. 1% of them had a tumour larger than 4 cm and 76.3 % had post operatively a GFR more than 30 $ml/min/1.73m^2$. He noticed an acceptable complication rate: 7.9% Clavien I, 18.4% for Clavien II and 5.3% Clavien III. One patient required immediate post-operative haemodialysis and another one long term haemodialysis for a mean follow up of 20 months.

Partial nephrectomy offers minimal reduction of renal function, but on the other hand unfortunately exposes the patient to higher peri-operative risk.

### 2.3.2 Surgical aspects influencing renal function preservation

For small tumours, clamping the renal artery is sometimes not necessary. Resection without clamping can provide adequate oncologic surgery with a lower peri-operative complication rate and limited renal function deterioration. In the case of larger renal tumours, surgery requires in most cases an interruption of renal blood flow through pedicle clamping.

Clamping is necessary to resect the tumour in a bloodless field, to minimise intra-operative blood loss, to contribute to a better vision during dissection and to facilitate renorraphy. Ischemia induces endothelial lesions which lead via multi-inflammatory response to vasoconstriction and vasospasms and thus ischemia. The low renal blood flow induces renal cell lesions and subsequent release of angiotensin II and eicosanoids. During ischemia, there is a failure of oxidative phosphorylation and depletion in adenosine triphosphate (ATP). It causes cellular swelling by passive diffusion of water into cells. Cell swelling prevents reperfusion when unclamping (no reflow phenomenon) and ATP degradation produces free radicals which cause further cell damage (reperfusion injury).

#### 2.3.2.1 Impact of clamping time

For warm ischemia, maximal clamping time to preserve renal function was previously thought to be less than 31 minutes. Later it was suggested to try to limit warm ischemia time to less than 20 minutes (Becker et al., 2009). But Thompson goes further and states that "every minute counts". In his retrospective study, he analysed 362 patients with solitary kidneys and demonstrated that 25 minutes is the best cut-off for clamping time to make the distinction of patients at risk for acute renal failure, a GFR < 15ml /min per 1.73 $m^2$ and new-onset stage IV chronic kidney disease during follow up. Each additional minute increased this risk. The same cut off for irreversible renal damage was found in a prospective study (Funahashi 2009).

Thus we should consider 20-25 minutes to be the best cut-off to avoid adverse renal consequences, keeping in mind the shorter the clamping time the better. We should not forget that even with extended ischemia, partial nephrectomy still offers better renal function outcomes compared to RN (Lane et al., 2010).

#### 2.3.2.2 Impact of clamping technique

Regarding clamping technique, Coffin did not observed a difference in postoperative renal function between mechanical and digital clamping of the pedicle.

There is no consensus for type of clamping: arterial or "en bloc" arterial and venous clamping. It is also not known whether intermittent clamping is better than continuous.

#### 2.3.2.3 Cooling

Kidney cooling prior to clamping can prevent cell damage. The optimal temperature to achieve this seems to be 15°C (Becker 2009).

When ischemia time is estimated to be probably more than 25 minutes, cold ischemia is a good option. The principle is to cool the kidney with ice slush for 10 minutes, after which the hilum should be clamped. Nevertheless, also cold ischemia time must be limited to the minimum. A maximum of 35 minutes has been proposed by several authors (Thompson et al 2007).

#### 2.3.2.4 Pharmacologic strategies

In order to reduce the impact of ischemia, it is advised to provide preoperative hydration to facilitate renal perfusion and stimulate urine production. Therefore, furosemide administered intra-operatively is useful. Intravenous mannitol at a dose of 1 ml/kg has also been proven to be beneficial for optimal reperfusion (Becker et al., 2006). Weizer and his

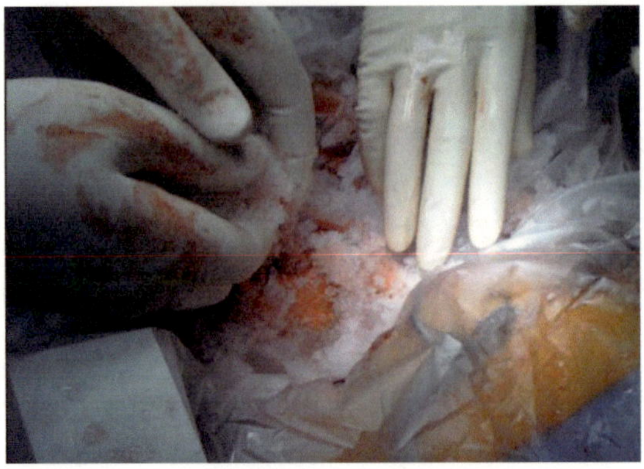

Fig. 1. Cooling.

team use the following schema: 12,5 g mannitol are administered ten minutes before resection and the same additional dose is given at removal of the clamp (Weizer et al., 2011). The use of an angiotensin-converting enzyme inhibitor such as enalapril has also been proposed. This should theoretically prevent vasospasm and induce vasodilatation. To prevent thrombosis, administration of heparin intravenously has been proposed but its benefit has not been proved.

Other important points are to maintain a normal blood pressure and hemodynamic stability in the peri-operative and postoperative period.

## 3. Alternative surgical techniques

### 3.1 Simple enucleation

#### 3.1.1 Definition, surgical technique

Urologic surgeons are increasingly proposing careful, pure enucleation consisting of an incision of the renal parenchyma within a few millimetres of the tumour, followed by a blunt dissection following a plane between the pseudo-capsule and the healthy renal parenchyma, thereby minimizing loss of nephrons.

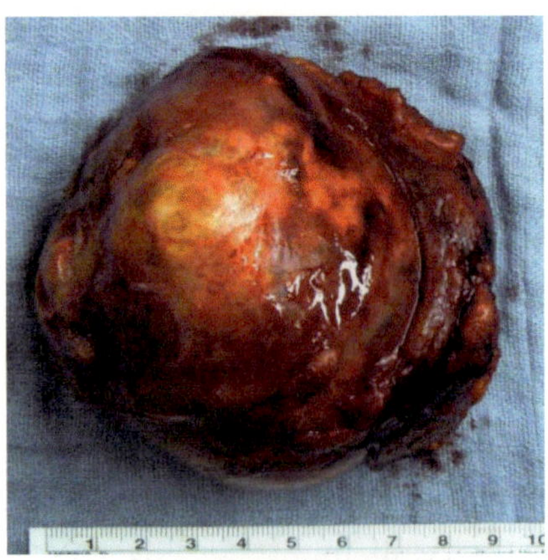

Fig. 2. Enucleation.

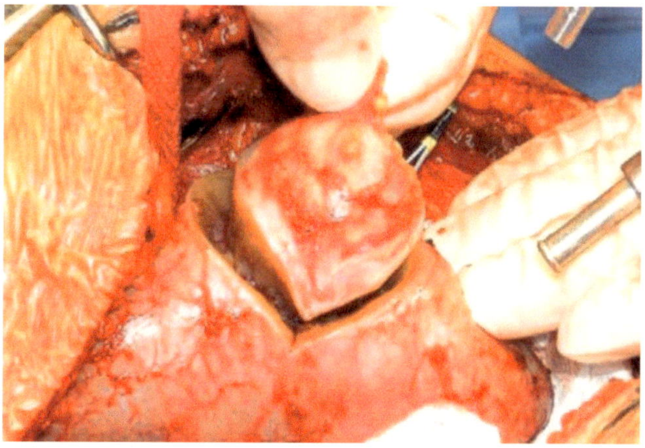

Fig. 3. Wedge Resection.

### 3.1.2 Simple enucleation versus standard partial nephrectomy

#### 3.1.2.1 Positive surgical margin rate

Minervini (Minervini et al., 2011) retrospectively analysed 1519 patients operated for renal cell carcinoma to determine the impact of simple enucleation on oncologic outcomes: 982 underwent a standard partial nephrectomy versus simple enucleation in 537 cases. 25.9% of patients belonging to the standard partial nephrectomy group versus 21.3% of patients in the simple enucleation group had a renal cell carcinoma larger than 4 cm. PSM rate was significantly lower in the simple enucleation group (0.2%) versus the standard partial nephrectomy group (3.4%) ($p<0.001$).

#### 3.1.2.2 Cancer-specific survival rate

For tumours smaller than 4 cm, pure enucleation provides long-term cancer-specific survival rates similar to RN and is not associated with a greater risk of local recurrence compared to partial nephrectomy (Carini 2006). Minervini (Minervini 2011) compared standard partial nephrectomy with simple enucleation: he could not find any significant difference between those 2 techniques after adjusting for cancer-specific survival probabilities: age at surgery (younger or older than 65 years), tumour stage (pT1a, pT1b or pT3a) and Fuhrman nuclear grades (1-2 versus 3). Patients who underwent a simple enucleation and had a Fuhrman nuclear grade 4 showed a significantly worse cancer-specific survival compared to patients who were treated with standard partial nephrectomy.

In another publication (Carini et al., 2006), Carini and Minervini reviewed 71 simple enucleations for renal cell carcinoma with diameter 4 to 7 cm. Median follow up was 74 months. There was no peri-operative mortality and no major complications requiring reintervention. Oncologic outcomes were acceptable: 5- and 8-year cancer-specific survival rates were 85.1% and 81.6%, respectively. Tumour stage had an impact on cancer-specific survival: 5-year cancer-specific survival rate was 95.1% for tumours of 4 cm, 83.3% for stage pT1b and 58.3% for stage pT3a tumours. He reported 10 patients (14.1%) with progressive disease but only 4.2% with local recurrence.

Simple enucleation can be performed for tumours larger than 4 cm. Long-term outcomes are comparable to standard NSS.

### 3.2 Laparoscopic partial nephrectomy

Laparoscopic partial nephrectomy (LPN) offers the benefits of a minimal invasive approach together with the benefits of preserving renal function.

### 3.2.1 Surgical aspects

#### 3.2.1.1 Transperitoneal versus retroperitoneal approach

62% of the tumours were operated transperitoneally in the study of Patel (Patel et al., 2010). Porpiglia (Popiglia et al., 2010) observed a higher rate of the transperitoneal approach for tumors larger than 4 cm, with no higher rate of conversion to open surgery.

#### 3.2.1.2 Resection technique

Most surgeons performing laparoscopic NSS prefer an enucleo- resection: excision of the tumour with a thin layer peritumoral healthy parenchyma (Porpiglia et al., 2010). In several studies, a laparoscopic ultrasound probe was used to identify the lesion intraoperatively (Porpiglia et al., 2010; Patel et al., 2010), even when it concerned large renal tumours (> 4 cm).

#### 3.2.1.3 Impact of clamping technique and time on renal function

In all the centres of the study by Porpiglia, the renal artery was clamped alone (Porpiglia et al., 2010).

Patel described clamping of both, the artery and the vein in case of large, endophytic and central tumors. On the other hand, the artery alone is clamped for small, peripheral or cortical tumors (Patel et al., 2010).

To prevent vascular injury, bulldog clamps are preferred to a Satinsky clamp, even though the true benefit of this approach remains to be proven (Weizer et al., 2011). Some surgeons use vessel loops with a hem-o–lock as clamp in order to prevent pedicle lesions.

To prevent renal function loss, Shao (Shao et al, 2011) proposed another technique consisting in selective clamping of the feeding segmental renal artery. This technique demands a larger dissection to expose 2-3 arterial branches for selective clamping. The demarcation line of the parenchymal ischemia is observed to ensure the resection area is clamped. In case the ischemic area does not encompass the tumour, multiple segmental arteries are clamped. Patients with tumours larger than 4 cm were included if their resection was estimated feasible. There were 11 cT1b tumours operated: respectively 5 operated with main renal artery clamping and 6 with selective clamping. Of, the latter group, half of them had to be converted to main renal artery clamping. There was a significant increase in operative time, blood loss and warm ischemia time in the selective clamping. 3 months post-operatively, GFR was estimated with a camera-based method measuring the renal uptake of technetium 99m diethylenetriamine-pentaacetic acid. The GFR reduction of the affected side was significantly less with selective clamping. Half of the tumours larger than 3.5 cm tumours required clamping of 2 or more segmental arteries. Complication rate was acceptable. This technique seems not really appropriate for large tumours given the high conversion rate.

A critique to the laparoscopic approach remains that ischemia time is usually longer than in open procedure. In a European survey (Porpiglia et al., 2010), mean warm ischemia time was 25.7 minutes with a range 15-46 minutes. Cooling techniques in laparoscopy are time consuming. Clamping usually lasts from the beginning of the resection to the end of parenchymal suture. In order to reduce warm ischemia time, Nguyen (Nguyen et al., 2008) proposed to remove the clamp after the first layer of parenchymal suture. The remaining renorrhaphy is thus performed in the revascularized kidney. This technique decreases warm ischemia time by over 50%. There was a trend towards improved outcomes: less overall complications (16% vs. 22%), less postoperative renal haemorrhage (2% vs. 4%) and a decreased re-intervention rate (6% vs. 16%). However, those differences were not statistically significant. No patient had a positive resection margin, required open conversion or showed renal dysfunction.

#### 3.2.1.4 Impact of parenchymal suture on renal function

The goal of efficient renorraphy is to reduce warm ischemia time. The type of suture (running of interrupted) is not correlated with longer warm ischemia time.

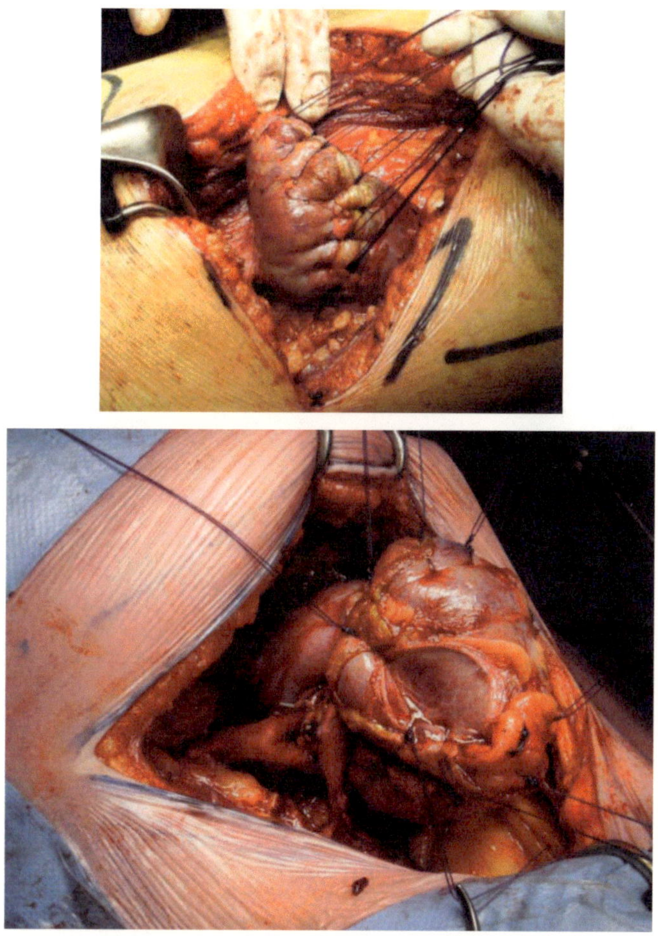

Fig. 4-5. Examples of interrupted suture in open surgery.

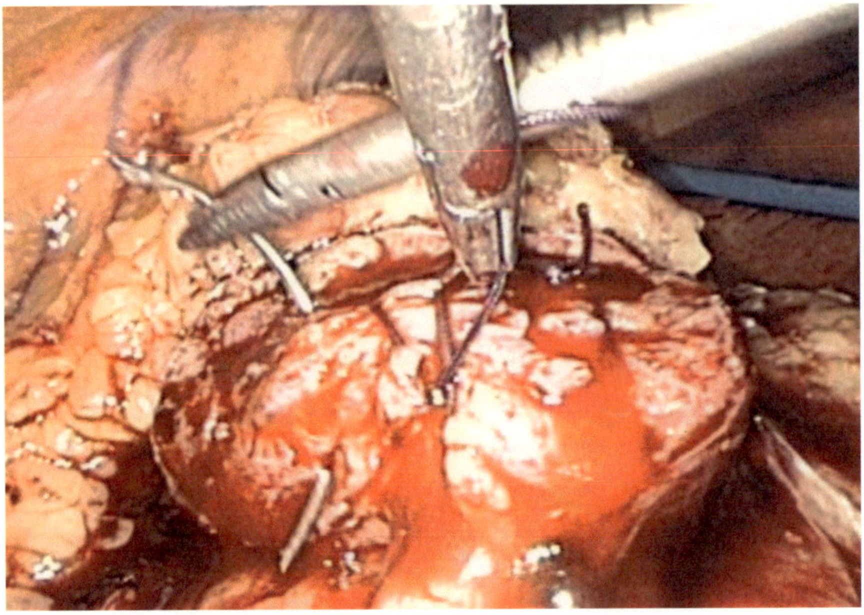

Fig. 6. Laparoscopic running suture.

Likewise, the use of haemostatic sealant had no significant impact on warm ischemia time (Porpiglia et al., 2010).

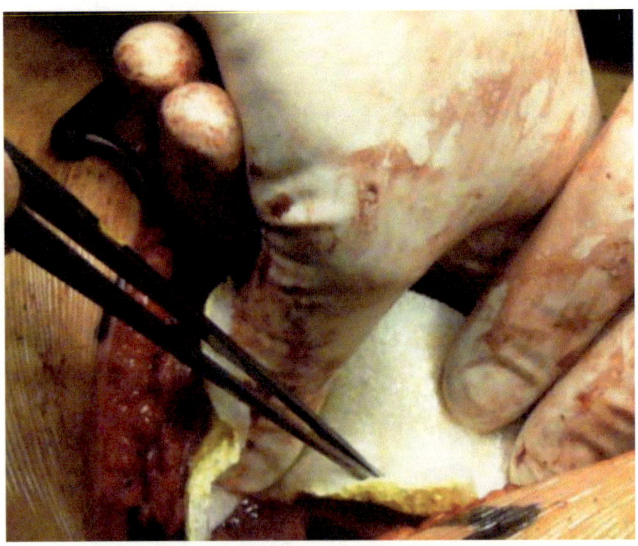

Fig. 7. Hemostatic sealant application.

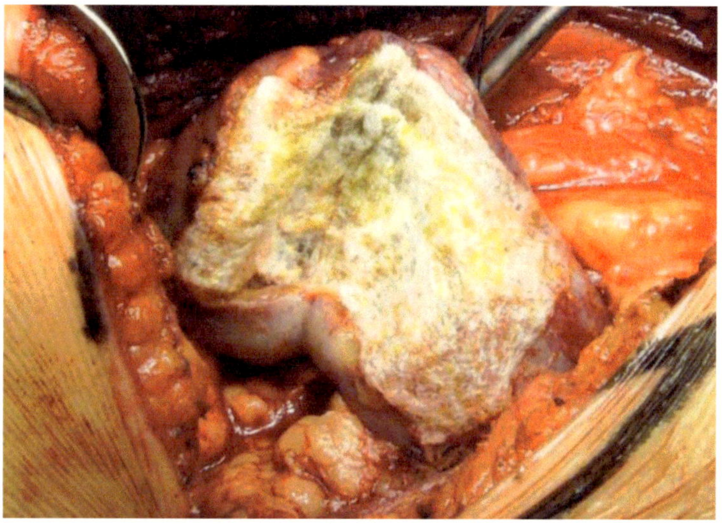

Fig. 8. Tumor bed after hemostatic sealant application.

### 3.2.2 Complications: Open versus Laparoscopy

Open NSS is well established in T1a tumours and is becoming increasingly accepted in T1b tumours. In the last few years, a tendency to apply a laparoscopic approach for T1a renal tumours has been observed. In some centres this is already the standard of care. Indeed, in experienced hands, the laparoscopic approach achieves intermediate-term oncological and renal function outcomes comparable to open surgery.

In a multicenter study (Porpiglia et al., 2010), 63 patients underwent a laparoscopic partial nephrectomy by enucleo-resection with intraoperative ultrasound. The conversion rate was 7.3%: always for bleeding but without requiring RN. Postoperative complication rate was 26%: acute hemorrhage, urinary fistula, fever, chyluria and retroperitoneal hematoma. Acute hemorrhage was the most frequent (9.7%). Half of them were treated with embolization, the other half with reoperation. One patient required a RN. Urinary fistulas (4.4%) required a double J placement and one patient necessitated a re-operation. 6.5% of patients had PSM. There was no correlation between PSM status and tumour size or location.

### 3.2.3 Impact of tumour size

#### 3.2.3.1 Impact of tumour size on peri-operative and post-operative complications

Porpiglia (Porpiglia et al., 2010) reviewed 100 consecutive laparoscopic partial nephrectomies. A third of these procedures concerned tumours larger than 4 cm. Intraoperatively, the latter required more often a transperitoneal approach and pelvicalyceal repair. Also, warm ischemia time was longer and they were associated with greater blood loss, however no significant bleeding or conversion occurred. Complication rates were similar in the small versus large tumour groups respectively: fever (6% vs. 3%), acute hemorrhage (4.5% vs. 15.1%, p=0.06), retroperitoneal hematoma (1.5% vs. 6%). One case of pneumonia was seen in the small tumour group and one urinary fistula in large tumours group.

The sole significant risk factor for overall complications was the cortico-medullar location of the tumour (Porpiglia et al., 2010).

#### 3.2.3.2 Impact of tumour size on renal function

In the same study of Porpiglia (Porpiglia et al., 2010), small and large tumours groups had comparable preoperative serum creatinin and estimated GFR. On the 5th post-operative day, elevation of serum creatinin level was not significantly higher in the large tumour group, but deterioration of eGFR was statistically significant ($p > 0.004$).

The size of the tumour had no significant impact on the warm ischemia time (Porpiglia et al., 2010).

In large tumours, they recorded 4 cases (12%) with CKD progression, but these could not be explained by a longer warm ischemia time.

#### 3.2.3.3 Impact of tumour size on oncologic outcome

Comparable to Russo in open partial nephrectomy, Porpiglia (Porpiglia et al., 2010) had a higher PSM rate in small tumours. Thus it appears that, as seen in open NSS, tumour size does not impact on PSM risk in the laparoscopic approach.

## 3.3 Robot-assisted laparoscopic partial nephrectomy

Laparoscopy causes less morbidity than a flank incision. Robotic assistance is useful for suturing and tying (Weizer et al., 2011). This technique combines the minimally invasive approach of laparoscopy with the freedom of movement and dexterity acquired with the robot. Preliminary results with robotic NSS are comparable to results obtained with LPN (Van Poppel, 2010). With similar oncologic outcomes, the robotic approach seems to have a shorter learning curve compared to laparoscopic approach. It offers other benefits: lower intra-operative blood loss, reduced hospital stay and shorter warm ischemia time (Benway et al., 2010).

### 3.3.1 Surgical aspects

#### 3.3.1.1 Retroperitoneal or transperitoneal approach

The retroperitoneal access has the advantage of reducing the risk of intraperitoneal urine leak, intestinal lesions and future adhesions. Robot-assisted Retroperitoneal Partial Nephrectomy (RRPN) is indicated for posterior, interpolar or lower pole tumours. Morbid obesity and previous intra-abdominal surgery are no contra-indications. One major disadvantage of the retroperitoneal approach is the smaller working space, requiring a good coordination and more help from the assistant. Weizer (Weizer et al., 2011) described 2 conversions in 16 RRPN : one to conventional laparoscopy (difficulty of positioning robot's arms) and one to a transperitoneal approach because of peritoneal perforation. Six complications occurred: musculo-skeletal pain in one, 2 pneumonias, one urinary retention, one urinary fistula, one atrial fibrillation. In this study, all tumours were smaller than 3.5 cm. A retroperitoneal approach does not seem indicated for T1b tumours. The transperitoneal approach is preferred for tumours larger than 4 cm and upper pole tumours.

#### 3.3.2 Complications in Robot assisted laparoscopic partial nephrectomy

The complication rate in a series of 183 Robot-assisted Partial Nephrectomy (RAPN) was 9.8%: 8.2% were major complications and 1.6% minor (Benway et al., 2010).

#### 3.3.3 Impact of tumour size

Patel (Patel et al., 2010) described 71 transperitoneal robotic partial nephrectomies. On preoperative imaging, 15 were larger than 4 cm.

Peri-operatively, warm ischemia time was significantly longer in larger tumours. (p=0.011). He noted no intra-operative complications. The other peri-operative parameters: operative time, need to repair the collecting system, estimated blood loss, elective conversions were not significantly different between the smaller and the larger tumour groups. Post-operative complication rate was similar. There were also no differences in post-operative variables: length of stay and change of haemoglobine. Tumour size between 4 and 7.9 cm was not a risk factor for increased peri- and post-operative complications in patients undergoing robotic partial nephrectomy.

#### 3.3.4 PSM

Benway (Benway et al., 2010) compared 118 LPN and 129 RAPN: the PSM rates were 0.8% and 3.9%, respectively. The PSM rate was higher in RAPN, however this was not significant (p=0.11). Wang (Wang & Bhayani, 2010) reviewed 100 LPN versus 100 RAPN and also noted no significant differences in PSM rate. Benway (Benway et al., 2010), in a review of 183 RAPN, described 3.8% PSM. Gill (Gill et al., 2007) reported a PSM rate of 2.85% in LPN versus 1.26% in open procedures. Kural (Kural et al., 2009) reported no PSM but his study contained only 10 RAPN. On his 71 RAPN, Patel (Patel et al., 2010) had no PSM in 15 tumours larger than 4 cm and 3 PSM on 56 smaller tumours. To our knowledge, no study showed an increased PSM rate in tumours measuring between 4 and 7 cm.

#### 3.3.5 Renal function

Having a tumour larger than 4 cm was not significantly predictive of an increased risk of kidney function loss at the first post- operative day or at 1-3 month follow-up. However, only 9 tumours larger than 4 cm and 28 smaller tumours were included (Patel et al., 2010)

#### 3.3.6 Oncologic outcomes

Robot-assisted partial nephrectomy is still a young technique. Follow up is yet too limited to evaluate recurrence-free survival and cancer-specific survival rates.

## 4. Conclusion

Our latest study showed excellent surgical feasibility and cancer-specific survival for NSS in T1b RCC (Joniau et al., 2008). Local cancer control was achieved in the large majority of patients, with preservation of renal function in those with elective indications. NSS is at present the gold standard treatment for renal tumours less than 4 cm. Other studies confirmed the feasibility of NSS for tumours of 4 to 7 cm, achieving good oncologic outcomes and preserving kidney function.

The presence of PSM seemed to not have an impact on survival.

Warm ischemia time (WIT) remains a key point. It has to be reduced or avoided as much as possible. If the procedure is suspected to be laborious and WIT lasts more than 25 min, several techniques are useful to help preserve renal function: use of mannitol, cooling …

A laparoscopic approach avoids a painful flank incision but is associated with a longer WIT. Robot assistance joins the minimally invasiveness of the laparoscopic approach with the dexterity of the open NSS. We need longer follow-up before final conclusions can be drawn on oncologic outcomes and renal function preservation of robot-assisted NSS.

In the future, NSS is going to be used for an increasing number of indications. Tumor size does not seems to be a limiting factor anymore. Becker (Becker et al., 2011) already showed the feasibility of NSS even for tumours larger than 7 cm.

## 5. References


Antonelli A., Cozzoli A. &Nicolai M. (2008).Nephron-sparing surgery versus radical nephrectomy in the treatment of intracapsular renal cell carcinoma up to 7 cm, *Eur Urol*, Vol. 53 (April 2008), pp. 803-809

Becker F., Siemer S. &Hack M. (2006). Excellent Long-term Cancer Control with Elective Nephron-Sparing Surgery for selected Renal Cell Carcinomas Measuring more than 4 cm, *Eur Urol,* Vol. 49, (March 2006), pp. 1058-64

Becker F., Van Poppel H. & Hakenberg O W. (2009). Assessing the impact of ischemia time during partial nephrectomy, *EurUrol,*Vol. 56, (Octobre2009),pp. 625-35

Becker F., Roos F. &Janssen M. (2011). Short-term functional and oncologic outcomes of nephron-sparing surgery for renal tumours larger than 7 cm, *EurUrol*, Vol. 29, (June 2011),pp. 931-937

BensalahK., PantuckAJ. &Rioux-Leclercq N. (2010). Positive Surgical Margin Appears to have negligible Impact on Survival of Renal Cell Carcinomas treated by Nephron-Sparing Surgery, *Eur Urol*, Vol. 57, (March 2010), pp.466-473

Benway BM., Bhayan S. & Rogers CG. (2009). Robot-assisted Partial Nephrectomy for renal tumors: a multi-institutionalanalysis of perioperative outcomes, *J Urol,* Vol. 182, (September 2009), pp.866-872

BenwayBM., Bhayani CB. & Rogers CG, (2010). Robot-assisted partial nephrectomy: an international experience, *Eur Urol*, Vol. 57, (May 2010), pp. 815-820.

Carini M., Minervini A. & Masieri L. (2006). Simple enucleation for the treatment of PT1a Renal Cell Carcinoma: our 20-year experience, Vol. 50, (December 2006), pp. 1263-68

Carini M., Minervini A. & Lapini A. (2006). Simple enucleation for the treatment of renal cell carcinoma between 4 and 7 cm in greatest dimension: progression and long-term survival, *J Urol* , Vol. 175 , No.6, ( June 2006) pp.2022-2206

Coffin G., Hupertan V. & Taskin L. (2011). Impact of Elective versus Imperative Indications on Oncologic Outcomes After Open Nephron-Sparing Surgery for the treatment of Sporadic Renal Cell Carcinoma, *Ann Surg Onco,*Vol.18 (April 2011), pp. 1151-57

Funahashi Y., Hattori R. & Yamamoto T. (2009). Ischemic renal damage after Nephron Sparing Surgery in Patients with Normal Contralateral Kidney, *Eur Urol,*,Vol. 55, No. 1, (January 2009), pp. 209-216

Gill I., Kavoussi L.,& Lane B. (2007). Comparison of 1800 laparoscopic and open partial nephrectomies for single renal tumors, *J Urol*, Vol. 178, No. 1, (July 2007), pp. 41-46

Go A., Chertow G. & Fan D. Chronic kidney disease and the risks of death, cardiovascular events and hospitalization, N Engl J Med , Vol.135, No.13 (September 2004), pp.1296-305

Joniau S, Vander Eeckt K & Srirangam S. (2008) Outcome of nephron-sparing surgery for T1b renal cell carcinoma, *BJU Int*, Vol. 103, No.10 (May 2009), pp.1344-8.

Joniau S., Baekelandt F. & Simmons M. (2011) Comparing open versus laparoscopic partial nephrctomy for renal tumors of stage cT1c, in press

Kural A., Atug F. &Tufek I. (2009). Robot Assisted partial Nephrectomy versus laparoscopic Nephrectomy: comparison of Outcomes, *J Endourology*, Vol. 23,No.9 (September 2009), pp. 1491-97

Lane B., Fergany A. & Weight C. (2010). Renal functional outcomes after Partial Nephrectomy With Extended Ischemic Intervals are better than after Radical Nephrectomy, *J Urol, Vol.* 184, No.4, (October 2010), pp. 1286-1290

Lee D., Hruby G. & Benson M. (2010). Renal function and oncologic outcomes in nephron sparing surgery for renal masses in solitary kidneys, *World J Urol*, Vol. 29, No.3, (June 2011), pp.343-348

LeibovitchB., Blute M. &ChevilleJ. (2004).Nephron Sparing Surgery for appropriately selected renal cell Carcinoma between 4 and 7 cm, results in outcome similar to radical nephrectomy, *J Urol*, Vol. 171, No.3, ( March 2004), pp. 1066-1070

Lesage K., Joniau S. & Francis K., (2007).Comparison between open partial and radical nephrectomy for renal tumours: perioperative outcome and health-related quality of life, *Eur Urol*, Vol. 51, No.3, (March 2007), pp. 614-620

Minervini A., Ficarra V. & Antonelli A.(2011).Simple enucleation is equivalent to Partial Nephrectomy for renal cell carcinoma : Results of a nonrandomized, retrospective, Comparative Study, *J Urol*, Vol. 185, No.5,(May 2011), pp. 1604-1610

Margulis V., Tamboli P.&Jacobsohn K., (2007).Oncological efficacy and safety of nephron-sparing surgery for selected patients with locally advanced renal cell carcinoma, *BJU* , Vol.100, No.6, (December 2007), pp.1235-1239

Nemr E, Azar G, Fakih F, et al (2007).Partial Nephrectomy for renal cancers larger than 4 cm, *ProgUrol*, Vol.17, No.4, (June 2007), pp. 810-814

Nguyen M. & Gill I., (2008). Halving Ischemia Time During Laparoscopic Partial Nephrectomy, *J Urol*, Vol. 179, No.2 (Februari 2008), pp. 627-632

Patel M., Krane S. & Bhandari A. (2010).Robotic Partial Nephrectomy for Renal Tumors Larger Than 4 cm. *Eur Urol*, Vol. 57 No.2, ( Februari 2010), pp. 310-316

Porpiglia F., Volpe A. &Bilia M. (2006). Assessment of risks factors for complications of laparoscopic partial nephrectomy, *Eur Urol*, Vol.53, No.3 (March 2008) pp. 590-3

Porpiglia F., Fiori C. &Piechaud T. (2010).Laparoscopic partial nephrectomy for large renal masses : results of European survey, *World J Urol*,Vol.28, No.4, ( August 2010), pp. 525-529

PorpigliaF, Fiori Ch. &Bertolo R., (2010). Does tumor size really affect the safety of laparoscopic partial, nephrectomy, *BJUInt*, Vol.108, No.2, (July 2011), pp. 268-273

Roos F., Brenner W. & Jager W, (2010). Perioperative morbidity and renal function in young and elderly patients undergoing elective nephron-sparing surgery or radical nephrectomy for renal tumors larger than 4 cm, *BJU Int*, Vol.107, No.4, (February 2011), pp. 554-561

Russo P (2010) Editorial comment on: Positive Surgical Margin Appears to have negligible Impact on Survival of Renal Cell Carcinomas treated by Nephron-Sparing Surgery, *Eur Urol*, Vol.57, No.3, (March 2010), pp. 466-473

Shao P., Qin C. & Yin C. (2011). Laparoscopic Partial Nephrectomy with segmental renal artery clamping : technique and clinical outcomes, *Eur Urol*, Vol. 59,No.5, (May 2011), pp.849-855

Thompson R.,Frank I. & al (2007). The impact of ischemia time during open nephron sparing surgey on solitary kidney : a multi-institutional study, *J Urol*, Vol 177, No.2, (Sept 2007), pp 471-476

Van Poppel H (2003) Open surgical Treatment of Localised Renal Cell Cancer, EAU Updates Serie1 :pp. 220-225

Van Poppel H. &Joniau S. (2007) How important are surgical margins in Nephron Sparing Surgery, *Eur Urol Suppl* ,Vol.6, pp. 533-539

Van PoppelH. (2010). Efficacy and safety of nephron sparing surgery, *Int J Urol*,Vol.17, No.4,(April 2010), pp.314-26

Van Poppel H., Da Pozzo L. & Albrecht W. (2010) .A prospective, Randomised EORTC Intergroup Phase 3 Study Comparing the Oncologic Outcome of Elective Nephron-Sparing Surgery and Radical Nephrectomy for Low-Stage Renal Cell Carcinoma, *Eur Urol*, Vol.59, No.4, (April 2011), pp. 543-552

Wang AJ, Bhayani CB (2009) Robotic partial nephrectomy versus laparoscopic partial nephrectomy for renal cell carcinoma: single surgeon analysis of > 100 consecutive procedures, *Urology*, Vol.73, No.2, (Februari 2009), pp.306-310

Weizer AZ., Patella GV.& Montgomery JS. (2011). Robot-assisted Retroperitoneal Partial Nephrectomy: Technique and Perioperative Results , *J Endourol,* Vol 25 , No.4 (April 2011),pp. 553-557

Yossepowitch O., Thompson R. & Leibovich B. (2008). Positive Surgical Margins at partial nephrectomy: predictors and oncologic outcomes. *J Urol*, Vol. 179, No.6, (June 2008), pp. 2158-63

# 21

# Benign Prostate Hyperplasia and Chronic Kidney Disease

Ricardo Leão, Bruno Jorge Pereira and Hugo Coelho
*Urology Department, Centro Hospitalar de Coimbra*
*Portugal*

## 1. Introduction

Benign Prostate Hyperplasia (BPH) is a common disease in adult men and its incidence is age related. On the basis of clinical criteria, the Baltimore Longitudinal Study of Aging found that the prevalence of BPH is approximately 25% in men aged 40 to 49 years, 50% in men aged 50 to 59 years, and 80% in men aged 70 to 79 years (Arrighi, Metter et al. 1991).

BHP is theoretically the detection of prostatic hyperplasia, which is the benign proliferation of the stroma and epithelium, by histological study. However histological studies for all men are unfeasible in clinical practice, so BHP usually refers to the palpable enlargement of the prostate, which can be detected by clinical or ultrasonographic examination, or presence of urinary symptoms loosely defined as lower urinary tract symptoms (LUTS), which are usually classified as obstructive or irritative (Levy and Samraj 2007).

Chronic kidney disease (CKD) encompasses a spectrum of different pathophysiologic processes associated with abnormal kidney function, and a progressive decline in glomerular filtration rate (GFR). *Chronic renal failure* (CRF) applies to the process of continuing significant irreversible reduction in nephron number, *end-stage renal disease* (ESRD) represents a stage of CKD where the accumulation of toxins, fluid, and electrolytes normally excreted by the kidneys results in the *uremic syndrome*. This syndrome leads to death unless the toxins are removed by renal replacement therapy, using dialysis or kidney transplantation (Fauci 2007). The prevalence of CRF using the Modification of Diet in Renal Disease equation is 26% in adults who are 70 years and older. Men are at 67% greater risk for advanced chronic renal failure and at 44% greater risk for end stage renal disease than women (Rule, Lieber et al. 2005).

Despite the many possible causes of obstructive uropathy, in studies of elderly patients with acute renal failure, the most common cause among all patients was BPH (Kumar, Hill et al. 1973; Tseng and Stoller 2009). Kumar et al., showed in their studies that acute renal failure in patients with obstructive uropathy were due to BPH (38%), neurogenic bladder (19%), obstructive pyelonephritis (15%).

Attending to high prevalence of BPH in older men with CKD it is invaluable to take into consideration the relationship between these two clinical entities. However, despite the high prevalence of CKD and BPH in elderly men, there is limited knowledge on the association between these two conditions.

The purpose of this chapter is to discuss the relationship between BPH and CKD, bearing in mind the epidemiology, pathophysiology, the clinical and imagiologic presentation of BPH and how it can contribute to CKD.

## 2. Epidemiology – Benign prostatic hyperplasia and chronic kidney disease

Benign prostatic hyperplasia is characterized by the nonmalignant overgrowth of prostatic tissue surrounding the urethra, ultimately constricting the urethral opening and giving rise to associated lower urinary tract symptoms (McVary 2006; Wei, Calhoun et al. 2008).

Diagnosis of BPH is made based on histologic examination of a prostatic tissue (biopsy, surgery or autopsy), however surrogate measures, namely lower urinary symptoms, bladder outlet obstruction and prostate enlargement are often used to define BPH as a clinical syndrome (Emberton, Andriole et al. 2003). For this reason, many consequences of BPH are not studied for it is impractical. This factgives us limited insight into the incidence and progression of the disease (Jacobsen, Girman et al. 2001). The prevalence of BPH thus can be calculated on the basis of histologic criteria (autopsy prevalence) or clinical criteria (clinical prevalence) (Wein 2007).

The 1984 milestone study by Berry and colleagues summarized the data from five studies demonstrating that no men younger than 30 had evidence of BPH and the prevalence rose with each age group, peaking at 88% in men in their 80s (Berry, Coffey et al. 1984).

BPH is considered a disease of aging male and can have a familial inheritance, especially if large prostate volumes and surgical intervention at a young age are seen in the pedigree (Wein 2007).

Definitions of BPH, have undergone several changes in the past decade, and, at present, no single criterion can be applied. In the past, the term "prostatism" was used, incorrectly referring to the prostate as the sole source of the typical LUTS (lower urinary tract symptoms) found in aging men. It has been pointed out that there are at least three interrelated phenomena that can be assessed independently, namely the symptoms (Wein 2007), enlargement of the prostate gland and presence of obstruction (Nielsen, Nordling et al. 1994). In a given patient, all three, two of the three, or only one of the three entities might be present. Paul Abrams was the investigator that changed the earlier and inappropriate term (prostatism) to lower urinary tract symptoms (LUTS) (Nielsen, Nordling et al. 1994; Abrams 1999)

BPH (histologically) is present in about 8% of men aged 31 to 40 years, and this prevalence increases markedly with age to about 90% by ninth decade(Berry, Coffey et al. 1984; Rosen, Altwein et al. 2003; McVary 2006). Studies in United States, England, Austria, Norway, Denmark, China, Japan, and India showed that the prevalence of BPH increases rapidly in the fourth decade of life, reaching nearly 100% in the ninth decade (Harbitz and Haugen 1972; Carter and Coffey 1990; Wein 2007) (Pradhan and Chandra 1975). It is striking that the age-specific autopsy prevalence is remarkably similar in all populations studied regardless of ethnic and geographic origin (Berry, Coffey et al. 1984).

However, we must take into account the aging population and increasing number of patients who need medical care for symptoms (LUTS) or consequences of BPH. Number of consultations for BPH and urinary symptoms constitute the largest share of visits in our department and in urology departments worldwide. In 1989, there were approximately 1,3 million office visits to physician for BPH (Schappert 1993), and in 1992 approximately 170.000 prostatectomies were performed among inpatients in the United States (Xia, Roberts et al. 1999; Wei, Calhoun et al. 2008). Agency for Health Care Policy and Research Diagnostic and Treatment for BPH showed that from 22.5 million white men aged 50 to 79 years in the United States, in 1990, approximately 5.6 million needed medical consultation and treatment for BPH, demonstrating this disease is a prevalent health problem (Wei, Calhoun et al. 2008).

Although BPH is not a life-threatening condition, the impact of BPH on quality of life (QoL) can be significant and should not be underestimated (McVary 2006). According to the World Health Organization although the death rate attributable to BPH is negligible, the estimated DALY's (The sum of years of potential life lost due to premature mortality and the years of productive life lost due to disability) due to BHP is quite considerable. Most of the disability is probably due to severe clinical symptoms and/or late complications of BPH like CKD (Organization 2011).

Chronic kidney disease is a serious condition associated with premature mortality, decreased quality of life, and increased health-care expenditures. Untreated CKD can result in end-stage renal disease requiring dialysis or kidney transplantation.

The 1999-2004 National Health and Nutrition Examination Survey (NHANES) determined that 16.8% of the U.S. population aged >20 years had CKD (according to 1999-2004 data), compared with 14.5% from the 1988-1994 NHANES, an increase of 15.9% based on crude estimates of prevalence (Saydah 2007) which reflects the increasing needs for health care policy for CKD.

## 3. The relationship between benign prostatic hyperplasia and chronic kidney disease – A consequence of urinary outflow obstruction?

Although the exact etiology of BPH is not known it seems (from recent studies and daily clinical practice) that the natural history and evolution of benign prostatic enlargement ends up in urinary obstruction causing degradation of renal function over time.

Both diseases are extremely common among aging male, leading some to suggest that it is a natural concomitant of aging (Wu, Li et al. 2006).

In his 1989 retrospective study of 19 patients who were admitted to renal dialysis units for end-stage renal disease caused by BPH, authors (Sacks, Aparicio et al. 1989) raised awareness of BPH as a cause for CKD and suggested a more adequate screening of renal function in men with untreated LUTS. More recently a cross-sectional survey in Spain of 2,000 randomly sampled men who were 50 years or older showed a 2.4% prevalence of self-reported renal failure related to a prostate condition (9% reported renal failure from any cause) (Hunter, Berra-Unamuno et al. 1996; Rule, Lieber et al. 2005). The main limitation of this study was that it relied on the self report of CKD, and no distinction between Acute Renal Failure (ARF) or CKD was made. Nonetheless it remains one largest studies that reveals a connection between CKD and BPH (Hunter, Berra-Unamuno et al. 1996). Another study (Hill, Philpott et al. 1993) showed that men presenting for prostate surgery had a 7,7% prevalence of renal failure compared to a 3,7% prevalence in age matched men presenting for nonprostate surgery. This proves that renal failure in men with advanced BPH does not only reflect older age. Other statistical study revealed that men presented to urologist for BPH treatment showed an average of 13,6% of renal failure(McConnell, Barry et al. 1994).

The Rochester Epidemiology Project found a significant association between signs and symptoms of BPH and CKD in their population-based sample of 476 white men (Rule, Jacobson et al. 2005; Rule, Lieber et al. 2005). There was a significant association between CKD and moderate/ severe LUTS and peak flow rate of <15 mL/s. In conclusion there was a cross-sectional association between signs and symptoms of bladder outlet obstruction and chronic kidney disease in community-dwelling men (Rule, Lieber et al. 2005).

In contrast, a population-based study from Austria did not find LUTS to be an independent risk factor for impaired kidney function in men. A total of 2.469 men entered the cross-sectional study and 439 with CKD were assessed in longitudinal analysis. LUTS was assessed using the IPSS (International Prostate Symptom Score) questionnaire. There was no significant association between degree of LUTS and GFR after adjusting for age in this cross-sectional study (Ponholzer, Temml et al. 2006).

Furthermore a 30,466 men study from the HUNT II (Second Health Study in Nord-Trøndelag; 1995-1997) failed to show a connection between LUTS and CKD (Hallan, Kwong et al. 2010). Results have shown that men with moderate to severe LUTS, indicating BPH, did not have increased risk of future kidney failure after adjusting for age, and inclusion of men with such symptoms did not improve the effectiveness of a CKD screening strategy using kidney failure as the main outcome (Hallan, Kwong et al. 2010; Hallan and Orth 2010).

Nonetheless quite recently evidence of association between BPH and CKD has arisen in two different studies. In a recent study by Yamasaki *et* al, the Post-Void Residue (PVR) of the patients with CKD was significantly greater than that of the patients without CKD and the presence of post-void residual urine was independently associated with CKD, indicating a close association between CKD and residual urine. In this study the PVR is used as a surrogate measure of Bladder Outlet Obstruction (BOO) and thus of urodinamically relevant BPH (Yamasaki 2010). Authors reported a higher prevalence (31,8%) of CKD among BPH patients (Yamasaki 2010). In another study by Hong et al (Hong, Lee et al. 2010), the results showed that a decreased Qmax (Peak flow rate), with a history of hypertension and/or diabetes, were significantly associated with CKD in men seeking management for LUTS caused by BPH of various severity. Although the prevalence of CKD can be considered relatively low among men with BPH, the possibility of CKD should be considered in those who have a low Qmax, obstructive urinary symptoms, or have comorbidities such as hypertension and DM (Hong, Lee et al. 2010). In this study the authors report 494 patients from a group of 2741 BPH patients that were classified as having CKD (eGFR < 60 mL/min/1,73 $m^2$).

The 1994 Agency for Health Care Policy and Research created BPH clinical guidelines that recommended serum creatinine screening in men presenting with lower urinary tract symptoms, however a 2003 update discontinued the serum creatinine measurements (Rule, Lieber et al. 2005). These different approaches to BPH patients may lead to a significant amount of patients underdiagnosed for CKD.

As we take all this data into account, one should bear in mind that BPH is an almost ubiquitous condition in the old man. The low occurrence of CKD in BPH clinical trials should not be used to infer a weak association between the two disease processes. However it is clear that not all expressions of BPH are associated with CKD: Prostate volume, PSA (Prostate Specific Antigen) and even LUTS do not share a strong association with CKD (Rule, Jacobson et al. 2005; Ponholzer, Temml et al. 2006; Hallan, Kwong et al. 2010).

Bladder outlet obstruction signs and symptoms (QMax, PVR, Obstructive LUTS) are significant predictors of CKD (Rule, Jacobson et al. 2005; Yamasaki 2010), bladder outlet obstruction probably makes the bridge between CKD and BPH (Hong, Lee et al. 2010). This is probably a reflection of the etiology of CKD secondary to BPH.

We should also never forget that CKD is a multifactorial process, and it becomes difficult to separate the contribution of BHP from all the other renal insults. This also takes its toll on the design of the studies as many men with concomitant disease are excluded, and thus making it harder for investigators to take into account the true influence of BPH on CKD.

## 4. BPH physiopathology, disease progression and renal failure

The exact etiology of BPH is unknown, however the similarity between BPH and the embryonic morphogenesis of the prostate has led to hypothesis that BPH may result from a reawakening of embryonic induction process in adulthood (Oesterling 1996; McVary 2006).

The most common renal pathology finding in men with obstructive nephropathy due to BPH is chronic interstitial nephritis (Coroneos, Assouad et al. 1997; Rule, Lieber et al. 2005) and 30% of cases have been attributed to obstructive uropathy.

Late or end stage renal failure secondary to prostatic or bladder outflow obstruction should be amenable to prevention if cases are recognised early, however it still difficult to recognise which men with BPH are at risk of renal failure and need close investigation. For this reason we truly believe that is important to recognize factors that can be measured and are important bases or risk factors for the evaluation and treatment of BPH.

To assess BPH as risk factor for chronic kidney disease or renal failure it is important to understand the surrogate measures often used to diagnose BPH. These factors are essentially clinical, anatomical and physiological.

### 4.1 Benign prostate enlargement

BPH/BPE first develops in the periurethral *transition zone* of the prostate. The transition zone consists of two separate glands immediately external to the preprostatic sphincter. Prostate enlargement also involves an increase in the number of glands, particularly the periuretheral glands, and increase in smooth muscle and connective tissue in the periuretheral region of the prostate (McNeal 1978; Rule, Lieber et al. 2005; Wein 2007). Prostate size can be estimated by digital rectal examination (DRE) (underestimate true prostate size) but reliability across observers is in general considered poor (Wein 2007), for these reasons in all cross-sectional studies prostate volume is assessed by TRUS (trans-rectal ultrasound).

In the physiological point of view, as the prostate enlarges, it compresses the urethra, preventing the outflow of urine and contributing to the common lower urinary tract symptoms.

Previous studies which examined the association between prostate size and renal function gave conflicting results (Rule, Lieber et al. 2005), some showing a strict relation between prostate size and GFR (Olbrich, Woodford-Williams et al. 1957) but other studies did not (Terris, Afzal et al. 1998)

Other authors, like Shapiro *et* al. emphasize the role of prostatic smooth muscle in pathophysiology of BPH (Shapiro, Hartanto et al. 1992). These authors advocated that the amount of muscle in prostate size and its contractile properties are an important factor in BPH. Smooth muscle cells in are not optimal for force generation. They present a downregulation of smooth muscle myosin heavy chain and a significant upregulation of nonmuscle myosin heavy chain, suggesting either proliferation or loss of normal modulation pathways (Lin, Robertson et al. 2000). Factors that determine passive tone in prostate remain to be elucidated (Wein 2007). However it is known that active muscle tone in human prostate is regulated by adrenergic nervous system (Schwinn 1994). Adrenergic neurotransmitters have been involved in prostate smooth muscle regulation as well as contraction, and α-adrenergic blockade leads to a significant downregulation of normal protein gene expression, specifically smooth muscle myosin heavy chain (Boesch, Dobler et al. 2000; Wein 2007).

Recent studies were made to relate prostate size and LUTS in BPH. Hassanzadeh *et.* al, found a significant correlation between urgency and prostate size (Hassanzadeh, Yavari-kia et al. 2010), which can be considered as predictive factor for the disease and probably a strong link between BPE and CKD.

So, prostate and its enlargement can contribute for outflow obstruction not only by is static component (periurehral compression caused by stromal component) but also dynamic component (smooth muscle cells and adrenergic pathway). Prostate growth is only one of the components of LUTS in aging men.

### 4.2 Lower Urinary Tract Symptoms (LUTS)

Lower urinary tract symptoms (LUTS) are clinical criteria to define a man with urinary problems. Most of the men with BPH have voiding dysfunction, complaining with nocturia, urgency, week urinary stream, increased urinary frequency and sense of incomplete bladder emptying after micturition.

Many studies were done to achieve a scientific relation between LUTS and CKD, however until recent years there was no palpable evidence connecting these two entities. Hill et al. in a retrospective study did not find any relation between duration of symptoms and serum creatinine levels (Hill, Philpott et al. 1993). Likewise Gerber *et* al. did not achieve any success in linking serum creatinine levels and LUTS (Gerber, Goldfischer et al. 1997). Hong *et* al., reported that although there was no significant association between overall symptoms (IPSS score) with CKD, individual obstructive symptoms such as hesitancy and/or weak stream was significantly associated with CKD status (Hong, Lee et al. 2010)

Our clinical practice shows us that many men with LUTS do not value their symptoms, and do not seek medical care. Those older men often tolerate and disregard their lower urinary tract symptoms. In our opinion under reported symptoms can induce a significant bias in most of studies already done.

Although many patients who do not value their symptoms, mainly the older ones, the frequency of symptoms and its interference with quality of live (QoL) is the principal factor that drive men to consult a physician (Hong, Rayford et al. 2005).

Patient perceptions are receiving greater emphasis as part of clinical decision-making (Jacobsen, Guess et al. 1993; Roberts, Rhodes et al. 1994). The variability of relationships between symptom severity and the likelihood that the symptoms relate with CKD requires further investigations. However one must take into account that the absence of lower urinary tract symptoms in older man does not necessarily exclude BPH with urinary outlet obstruction. Moreover, whether symptoms can be graded according to severity (International Prostate Symtpoms Score - IPSS) this does not predict the degree of obstruction to urinary flow. However, when men with complete chronic urinary retention and severe symptoms needing surgical intervention were evaluated, the authors found as much as 30% of men with renal insufficiency (Sacks, Aparicio et al. 1989).

### 4.3 Post-voiding residual urine volume – Chronic urinary retention

Chronic urinary retention is thought to be the dominant mechanism by which BPH can cause chronic renal failure (Rule, Lieber et al. 2005). Rule *et* al, defined chronic urinary retention (CUR) as a post-void residual urine (PVR) higher than 100 mL, and reported that CUR was significantly associated in CKD in community-dwelling men. For years it has been well described that large volumes (»300 mL) affect renal function in advanced BPH (Styles, Neal et al. 1988; Rule, Lieber et al. 2005; Yamasaki 2010).

Recent studies, however, demonstrate that the volume of residual urine (post void) necessary to impair renal function is not that elevated. Yamasaki et al, verified in their study a cut-off of 12 ml for PVR (Yamasaki 2010), confirming PVR as a significant and independent risk factor for CKD. This study showed for the first time that patients with BPH can develop impaired renal function with small amounts of post-void urine (PVR< 100 ml). Furthermore, these findings indicated a higher prevalence of CKD in patients with BPH, acknowledging it as a risk factor for CKD. However, the mechanism by which small PVR influence renal function remains unknown.

Although, as Yamasaki et al. demonstrated low post-void residual urine can cause deterioration of renal function it is scientifically accepted that large residual pos-void urine are in line more severe cases of renal function deterioration (Yamasaki 2010).

#### 4.3.1 Acute urinary retention

Acute urinary retention (AUR) is defined as an acute complication of benign prostatic hyperplasia, patients suffers from an acute, sudden and painful inability to micturate. AUR represents an immediate indication for intervention or even surgery. Between 25% and 30% of men who underwent transurethral resection of prostate (TURP) had AUR as their main indication (Wein 2007). This complication is not exclusive for patients suffering from BPH, other causes can trigger acute urinary retention, like surgery, anaesthesia, trauma, medications, medical examination and urinary tract infections (mainly prostatitis).

In 2002 the self-reported rate of AUR in a cross sectional study in Spanish men was 5.1% (Hunter, Berra-Unamuno et al. 1996).

Acute urinary retention is not common in men under sixty years, and may be responsible for the majority of acute renal failure cases due to obstructive uropathy (Prakash, Saxena et al. 2001). Men in whom acute urinary retention is promptly relieved by bladder catheterization acute renal failure does not develop but long-term tubular dysfunction may still occur (Rule, Lieber et al. 2005). It is believed that acute urinary retention without prior history of chronic urinary retention do not lead to chronic renal failure. High bladder compliance allows men to maintain a normal GFR, however renal tubular dysfunction may persist after the acute urinary retention episode and probably result in progressive renal disease.

### 4.4 Bladder remodelling – Bladder response to urinary obstruction

The bladder has a central role in pathophysiology of BPH and its complications.

Current evidence suggests that the bladder´s response to obstruction is largely an adaptative one, although it is only a partially adptative one. It is also clear for many authors and physicians that LUTS in men with BPH or prostate enlargement are more closely related to obstruction-induced changes in bladder function than to the outflow obstruction directly.

There are of two types of bladder changes. First, changes that lead to detrusor instability (clinically associated with symptoms of frequency and urgency). Second, changes associated with decreased detrusor contractility (emptying symptoms - low urinary stream, hesitancy, intermittency, increased residual urine) and detrusor failure (Wein 2007).

The development of bladder wall thickening (easily measurable by ultrasound) and trabeculation due to smooth muscle hypertrophy and connective tissue permeation is responsible for increased bladder pressure in patients with high pressure chronic retention (Jones, Ellis et al. 1991; Rule, Lieber et al. 2005). Gosling *et* al, were some of the first authors who established endoscopically that major detrusor changes and trabeculation were due to an increase in detrusor collagen (Gosling and Dixon 1980). Severe trabeculation is related to significant residual urine, suggesting that increased collagen in the bladder wall is probably responsible for incomplete bladder emptying to rather than impaired muscle function (Wein 2007). Detrusor hypertrophy is one of the first modifications in the bladder and, as in animal models, the initial response is the development of smooth muscle hypertrophy (Gosling, Kung et al. 2000; Levin, Haugaard et al. 2000). This is an adaptative response associated with intra and extracellular changes in the smooth muscle cells that leads to detrusor instability. Obstruction also induces changes in smooth muscle cells contractile protein expression, impairing cell-to-cell communication (Levin, Haugaard et al. 2000), with changes in myosin heavy chain isoform expression (Lin, Robertson et al. 2000) that lead to detrusor instability and in some cases to impaired contractility (Wein 2007).

Cellular and physiological changes in bladder muscle and collagen, contribute to a high pressure bladder that perpetuates itself with worsening ability to empty and causing kidney lesions.

These mechanisms of bladder remodelling develop in a hypofunctional bladder, with low compliance. Comiter *et* al. reported that in a series of men with symptomatic BPH, 78% of patients with low bladder compliance had renal failure (Comiter, Sullivan et al. 1997). Low bladder compliance and detrusor instability may be causal mechanisms for renal failure in men in chronic urinary retention (Rule, Lieber et al. 2005).

In other studies (animal experimental studies) in addition to obstruction-induced changes in the smooth muscle cell and collagen of the bladder wall, there was clear evidence that obstruction may modulate neural-detrusor responses, causing reduced bladder contractility and altered sensation (Chai, Andersson et al. 2000)

Bladder remodelling is a response to continued bladder obstruction, and detrusor smooth muscle cell is a key contributor to the complex symptoms associated with prostatic obstruction (Christ and Liebert 2005), namely in BPH/BPE (benign prostatic enlargement).

### 4.5 Ureterovesical junction and upper tract dilation

In general, ureterovesical junction obstruction caused by bladder remodelling in chronic urinary retention is a contributing mechanism for renal failure in BPH (Rule, Lieber et al. 2005). Upper tract dilation occurs as a consequence of a continuum bladder outlet obstruction and remodelling (detrusor hypertrophy and scarring) leading to anatomical ureterovesical junction obstruction (Jones, Ellis et al. 1991). Upper urinary tract dilation or hydronephrosis is consistent with chronic renal failure from obstructive uropathy. In men with BPH and increased serum creatinine, hydronephrosis is common (one third), and is found in 90% of men with BPH who are hospitalized for uremic symptoms (Sacks, Aparicio et al. 1989). In ultrasound evaluation it is common among patients with bilateral hydroureteronephrosis to observe compressing and thinning of renal cortex, with obvious impact in renal function. A history of enuresis, painless chronic retention, and palpable bladder should suggest a diagnosis of high pressure chronic retention with its attendant risk of hydroureteronephrosis (Sacks, Aparicio et al. 1989).

### 4.6 Other causes

Recurrent urinary tract infections in men with chronic urinary retention due to BPH may also contribute to chronic renal failure (Rule, Lieber et al. 2005).

Secondary hypertension due to chronic urinary retention is also a described complication of BPH, leading to hypertensive kidney disease (Ghose and Harindra 1989).

Nephrogenic diabetes insipidus caused by partial or chronic urinary obstruction can result in renal failure (Klahr 2001).

Other clinical entities like diabetes and hypertension are independent factors that can lead to CKD (Gerber, Goldfischer et al. 1997). Patients with BPH are probable carriers of these pathologies that are likely to seriously aggravate renal function and must be taken into account as sombre conditioners of renal disease.

## 5. Clinical presentation

BPH is a chronic and progressive condition (Jacobsen, Girman et al. 2001) patients generally have a history of lower urinary tract symptoms and indolent obstructive uropathy.

Clinical presentation of BPH/obstructive uropathy varies and reflects the source and duration of obstruction. In BPH, symptoms results from the direct bladder outlet obstruction (BOO) from enlarged tissue (static component) and the increased smooth muscle tone and resistance within the enlarged gland (dynamic component). This physiologic issues reflect in voiding dysfunctions, that significantly affects the health and quality of life of many older men.

Most of the patients have characteristic symptoms. Patients' complaints are usually nocturia, urgency (imperious will to hold urine, some with complaints of incontinence), weak urinary stream (with decreased flow rate, low values in Qmax and Qaverage), a sense of incomplete bladder emptying, straining during micturition, increased micturition frequency and dribbling during or after urination (Rule, Lieber et al. 2005). Physical examination consists in a digital rectal examination (evaluating prostate characteristics and volume) and lower abdominal percussion and palpation to assess for bladder distension.

Recurrent or persistent urinary tract infections (UTI) are associated with prolonged urinary stasis of lower urinary tract obstruction, dysuria, frequency, urgency and hematuria are common complaints among men with UTI.

Chronic urinary retention as consequence of BPH has been defined as a palpable bladder that corresponds to a high PVR (Neal 1990), and most of the patients with chronic urinary retention have an indolent and progressive disease, with worsening of urinary symptoms and the majority of these patients just seek for medical care in bad health conditions with sharp renal insufficiency. It is always necessary to investigate symptoms and signs of chronic renal failure - nausea, vomiting, lethargy, edema and hypertension, that occur at late stage, usually with irreversible renal damage (Sacks, Aparicio et al. 1989), principally in older patients with other comorbidities (mainly diabetes and hypertension). In rare cases patients who resort to the emergency room because of anuria, require interventional procedures like indwelling catheter, nephrostomy (uni or bilateral) and sometimes (depending the level of renal function) hemodialysis.

Although signs and symptoms of BPH are normally present, there are a significant number of patients that are relatively asymptomatic (Tseng and Stoller 2009) (without significant voiding dysfunction), but can present primarily clinical sequel of renal insufficiency - uremia; with nausea, vomiting and mental status changes - and analytical changes - electrolyte disturbances (hypercaliemia and nonanion gap acidosis).

Older patients with voiding dysfunctions caused by chronic urinary obstruction, might present hypertension due to hypervolemia in the case of bilateral obstruction or increased renin release (Tseng and Stoller 2009). Hypertension, on other hand can be itself the sole cause of renal failure.

The development and validation (for different languages) of the standardized, self-administered symptom index (International Prostate Symptom Score [IPSS]) has been a critical event in the clinical research on LUTS and BPH (Cockett, Barry et al. 1992; Wein 2007). This diagnostic and follow-up tool is extraordinary, and the availability of validated translations in many common languages allows cross-cultural comparisons among man with BPH or LUTS from other causes.

In addition the enumeration of symptoms by frequency and time of occurrence, the bother associated with the symptoms, interference with activities of daily living, and the impact the symptoms have on quality of life are important in distinguishing characteristics that we must take into account in evaluation of BPH patients. (Wein 2007).

Left untreated, BPH can cause serious complications including renal failure can occur, as acute renal failure (discussed above), urinary tract infections, bladder stones, hematuria, incontinence and mortality related with BPH.

### 5.1 Other complications of benign prostatic hyperplasia

#### 5.1.1 Mortality

La Vecchia et al, reported that in the early 1980s, overall mortality from BPH ranged between 0,5 and 1,5/100 000 in most western European countries (La Vecchia, Levi et al. 1995). Between the early 1950s and the late 1990s, the overall mortality from BPH in the European Union (EU) fell from 5.9 to 3.5 per million, and the decline since the late 1950s was over 96%. Comparable falls were observed in the USA and Japan, and BPH mortality rates in the late 1990s were lower than in the EU (1.8/10(6) in the USA, 1.4 in Japan). BPH mortality trends were downwards also in the Eastern Europe, although rates in the late 1990s were about fourfold higher than in the EU (Levi, Lucchini et al. 2003).

Recent works have proven decreasing mortality rates related with BPH. The fall in BPH mortality, evident in statistics on underlying cause, was confirmed by statistics on all certified causes of death. In England, underlying-cause mortality reduced from 9.2 deaths per million in 1995 to 4.5 deaths per million in 2006 (Duncan and Goldacre 2011). The fall is remarkable in scale, likely to be attributable to clinical care, and could be regarded as an indicator of improving standards of care (Duncan and Goldacre 2011).

It is important to remember that patients in renal failure have an increased risk for complications following TURP compared with patients with normal renal function (25% versus 17%) (Holtgrewe, Mebust et al. 1989) and the mortality increases up to sixfold (Holtgrewe and Valk 1962; Melchior, Valk et al. 1974).

#### 5.1.2 Bladder stones

In a large autopsy study the prevalence of bladder stones was eight times higher in men with a histological diagnosis of BPH (3.4%) than in control subjects (0.4%), but no increased incidence of ureteral or kidney stones was found (Grosse 1990). Bladder stones are in line with urinary retention, stasis and urinary infection, factors that propitiate ion aggregation and stone nucleation.

#### 5.1.3 Urinary tract infections

In previous surgical series, urinary tract infections (UTIs) constitute the main indication for surgical intervention (12% of patients) (Holtgrewe, Mebust et al. 1989). Urinary tract infections are generally due to chronic urinary obstruction caused by increased amounts of residual urine, that predispose to UTIs (Mebust, Holtgrewe et al. 1989).

#### 5.1.4 Urinary incontinence

Incontinence is one of the most feared complications from surgical intervention for BPH (McConnell, Barry et al. 1994), although it may be the result of BPH secondary to overdistention of the bladder (overflow incontinence) or to detrusor instability. It is estimated to affect up to one half or more of all obstructed patients (urge incontinence) (McConnell, Barry et al. 1994; McConnell, Bruskewitz et al. 1998; Wein 2007).

### 5.1.5 Hematuria

Gross hematuria with clots with no other identifiable cause is common among BPH patients. Faubert *et* al, showed more than 30% of patients with microscopic or gross hematuria (Faubert 1998). Evidence suggests that in the patients predisposed to hematuria the micro-vessel density in prostate is higher than in controls (Wein 2007), suggesting that vascular lesions can be the cause of hematuria.

## 6. Diagnostic tests

Although nowadays it is increasingly rare to find a patient with chronic renal failure from chronic urinary retention due to BPH, about 13,6% (range from 0,3 to 30%) of men with BPH may present with CKD defined by a baseline serum creatinine of more than 133 mmol/L (1,5 mg/dL). This is particularly true in older patients with cognitive deterioration and autonomy impairment. In order to diagnose and monitor the impact of a bladder outlet obstruction due to BPH in the upper urinary tract, some laboratory and imaging tests should be considered: standardized questionnaires, serum creatinine levels or estimated glomerular filtration rate (eGFR), urinalysis, serum prostatic specific antigen (PSA) levels, uroflowmetry with peak flow rate determination, renal ultrasonography, bladder ultrasonography with detrusor thickness evaluation, transrectal prostate ultrasonography, pre and post-void residual urinary volume, cystometry, other urodynamic studies and urethrocystoscopy.

### 6.1 Symptom assessment by standardized questionnaires

BPH Impact Index (BII) is a questionnaire that assesses the effect of symptoms on everyday life and their interference with daily activities, and thus aimes to capture the impact of the condition. This questionnaire can be administered in conjunction with the IPSS and provides useful additional information (AUA 2010).

Symptom quantification is useful for diagnosis, determination of disease severity and monitoring of BPH. IPSS has become the international standard. It is derived from the American Urological Association Symptom Index (AUA-7 or AUA SI) described by Barry and colleagues in 1992 (Barry, Fowler et al. 1992; Barry, Fowler et al. 1992).

A recent multivariate analysis conducted by Hong *et* al., found associations of individual symptoms from the IPSS questionnaire and CKD status – obstruction-related symptoms, e.g. weak stream and hesitancy were significantly associated with CKD in age and comorbidity-adjusted analyses (Hong, Oh et al. 2010). Irritative symptoms, on the other hand, had no positive correlation with CKD. According to a subsample from the Olmsted County Study, moderate to severe LUTS (IPSS > 7) were positively correlated with CKD (Rule, Lieber et al. 2005). Kidney failure risks were 2.60 (CI 95%, 1.47-4.58) and 4.08 (CI 95%, 1.74-9.53) times higher for men with moderate and severe LUTS compared with men with no or mild LUTS, respectively (p<0,001) (Hallan, Kwong et al. 2010). However, after adjusting for age and

| | Not at all | Less than 1 time in 5 | Less than half the time | About half the time | More than half the time | Almost always |
|---|---|---|---|---|---|---|
| **Incomplete emptying** Over the past month, how often have you had a sensation of not emptying your bladder completely after you finish urinating? | 0 | 1 | 2 | 3 | 4 | 5 |
| **Frequency** Over the past month, how often have you had to urinate again less than two hours after you finished urinating? | 0 | 1 | 2 | 3 | 4 | 5 |
| **Intermittency** Over the past month, how often have you found you stopped and started again several times when you urinated? | 0 | 1 | 2 | 3 | 4 | 5 |
| **Urgency** Over the last month, how difficult have you found it to postpone urination? | 0 | 1 | 2 | 3 | 4 | 5 |
| **Weak stream** Over the past month, how often have you had a weak urinary stream? | 0 | 1 | 2 | 3 | 4 | 5 |
| **Straining** Over the past month, how often have you had to push or strain to begin urination? | 0 | 1 | 2 | 3 | 4 | 5 |
| | None | 1 time | 2 times | 3 times | 4 times | 5 times or more |
| **Nocturia** Over the past month, many times did you most typically get up to urinate from the time you went to bed until the time you got up in the morning? | 0 | 1 | 2 | 3 | 4 | 5 |
| **Total IPSS Score** | | | | | | |

Table 1. International Prostate Symptom Score (IPSS).

Additional Question:

| | Delighted | Pleased | Mostly satisfied | About equally satisfied and dissatisfied | Mostly dissatisfied | Unhappy | Terrible |
|---|---|---|---|---|---|---|---|
| **Quality of life due to urinary symptoms** If you were to spend the rest of your life with your urinary condition the way it is now, how would you feel about that? | 0 | 1 | 2 | 3 | 4 | 5 | 6 |

Table 2. Additional Question evaluating quality of life.

**Total score:**
0-7 Mildly symptomatic
8-19 Moderately symptomatic
20-35 Severely symptomatic

therefore in isolation, IPSS is not a basis for kidney failure screening (Hallan, Kwong et al. 2010). Kidney function decreases with age and age significantly correlates with LUTS. Ponholzer A. *et* al also concluded that LUTS was not associated with increased loss of kidney function (Ponholzer, Temml et al. 2006).

Even though symptom score assessment do not directly correlates with CKD or can't be used to establish the diagnosis of BPH, it may serve as a basis for symptom severity and management approach to patients with LUTS. Further testing should be considered in patients with an IPSS score ≥ 8.

### 6.2 Serum creatinine

For decades, medical textbooks have stated that patients with BPH should have serum creatinine measured (Humes 2000; Goldman 2008). Clinical practice guidelines disagree on serum creatinine screening among men being evaluated for LUTS. The routine measurement of serum creatinine levels is not indicated in the initial evaluation according to the AUA Guideline Management of BPH (AUA 2010). This recommendation is based on the conclusion that baseline renal insufficiency appears to be no more common in men with BPH than in men of the same age group in the general population. On the other hand, the EAU Guidelines on BPH (2004) and the nephrology-focused NICE (National Institute for Health and Clinical Excellence) guidelines for the United Kingdom advocate that it is probably cost effective to measure serum creatinine levels in all patients. This is based on the fact that bladder outlet obstruction due to BPH might cause hydronephrosis and renal failure (Sacks, Aparicio et al. 1989).

Patients with BPH and renal insufficiency have much higher postoperative complications (25% complication rate compared with 17% for patients without the condition) and mortality (up to sixfold) than those with normal renal function (Holtgrewe and Valk 1962; Melchior, Valk et al. 1974; Mebust, Holtgrewe et al. 2002). Most studies have found that the incidence of azotaemia in men with BPH varies from 15-30% (Mukamel, Nissenkorn et al. 1979). The Agency for Health Care Policy and Research (AHCPR) and the Fourth International Consultation on BPH highly recommends serum creatinine evaluation (McConnell, Barry et al. 1994). MTOPS data suggest that creatinine measurement is not necessary if voiding is normal. Estimated glomerular filtration rate (eGFR) is a more reliable measure to define CKD and is preferred over simple creatinine measurement (Roehrborn 2008).

### 6.3 Urinalysis

Urinalysis is a simple and inexpensive test that is recommended for the primary evaluation of a patient with suspected BPH. It is used to rule out urinary tract infection and hematuria. On the other hand, the finding of proteinuria/microalbuminuria may be indicative of renal failure.

### 6.4 Total PSA

Total PSA should be offered to patients with more than 10 years of life expectancy and in whom the PSA measurement may change the management of the symptoms (AUA 2010). In conjunction with digital rectal examination (DRE), total PSA measurement is the cornerstone of prostatic basic screening. PSA and prostatic volume can be used to evaluate the risks of either needing surgery or developing acute urinary retention.

### 6.5 Uroflowmetry / Peak urinary flow rate

Uroflowmetry is a simple and noninvasive urodynamic test that allows an objective evaluation of the patient micturition. Even though uroflowmetry is an unspecific evaluation, the micturition graphic may show some recognizable patterns (e.g. meatal stenosis, urethral stricture, BPH) and represent a reproducible way to quantify the strength of the urinary stream. It is a useful preoperative test. Peak urinary flow rate (PFR), or Qmax, appears to predict surgical outcome - patients with a preoperative Qmax > 15 mL/s have poorer outcomes than patients with preoperative Qmax < 15 mL/s do. PFR is an independent predictor for CKD rather than reported LUTS by standardized questionnaires (Hong, Lee et al. 2010). A study conducted by Rule *et* al. in community-dwelling men showed that men with CKD were more likely to have a slow urinary stream (Qmax < 15 mL/s) considering CKD as serum creatinine > 133 µmol/L or as eGFR < 60 mL/min/1,73 m$^2$. (Rule, Jacobson et al. 2005).

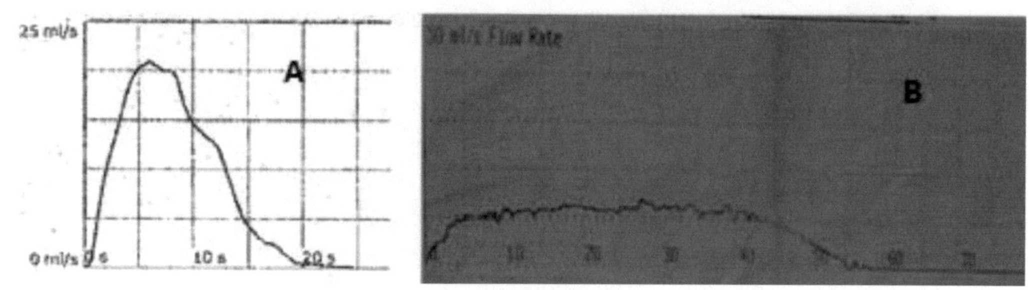


Fig. 1. Uroflowmetry. A) Normal patient; B) BPH patient.

### 6.6 Renal ultrasonography

Koch *et* al., performed renal ultrasound scans in a consecutive series of 556 elderly men with LUTS. 14 (2.5%) had hydronephrosis and serum creatinine levels appeared to be correlated with dilatation of the renal pelvis. The authors concluded that renal ultrasound is only indicated in patients with an elevated serum creatinine level and/or post-void residual urine volume (Koch, Ezz el Din et al. 1996). Renal ultrasonography has many advantages over intravenous urography (IVU) for upper urinary tract imaging: simultaneous evaluation of the bladder, post-void residual urine volume and prostate, better characterization of eventual renal masses, no radiation, no side-effects and lower cost.

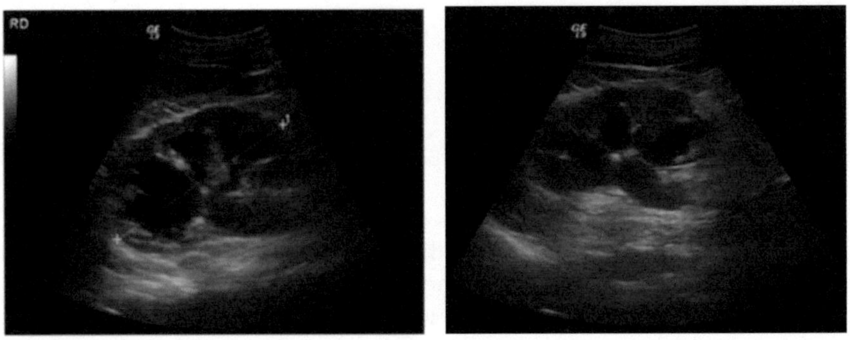


Fig. 2. Renal Ultrassound. Two ultrasound scans in BPH patient showing bilateral (right and left kidney respectively) ureterohydronephrosis.

### 6.7 Bladder ultrasonography

Chronic urinary retention leads to bladder wall thickening with trabeculations via smooth muscle hypertrophy and connective tissue infiltrates (Jones, Gilpin et al. 1991). This can lead in to a decline in bladder compliance with consequent functional or mechanical obstruction at the ureterovesical junction (Sutaria and Staskin 2000). More recently, the measurement of bladder wall thickness by transabdominal ultrasound has gained considerable interest as a non-invasive tool to assess bladder outflow obstruction (Kojima, Inui et al. 1997). Ultrasonic measurement of detrusor wall thickness at the anterior wall of bladders filled with ≥ 250 mL can securely detect bladder outlet obstruction if the value is ≥ 2 mm (Gabuev and Oelke 2011).

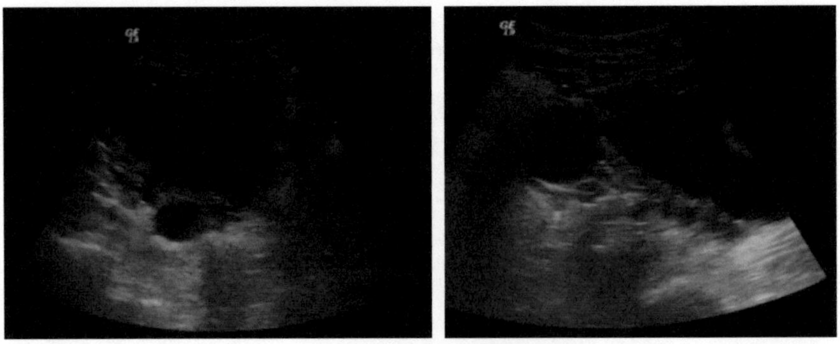

Fig. 3. Bladder Ultrassound. Two ultrasound scans in BPH patient. It is possible to observe the trabecullation, bladder wall thickening and diverticulum.

Manieri *et* al. concluded that bladder wall thickness appeared to be a useful predictor of bladder outlet obstruction, with a value exceeding that of uroflowmetry (Manieri, Carter et al. 1998). However, measurement of bladder wall thickness is currently not part of the recommended diagnostic work-up of patients with LUTS because reliable data on inter- and intra-observer variability, as well as reproducibility, are still lacking.

### 6.8 Post-void residual urine evaluation

Post-void residual urine volume can be measured with sufficient accuracy noninvasively by transabdominal ultrasonography. The measurement variation caused by the method is less than the biologic range of PVR variation (McConnell, Barry et al. 1994). It may also be measured by invasive methods (catheterization).

It has been well described that large residual urine volumes (>300 mL) affect renal function in advanced BPH (Neal, Styles et al. 1987; Rule, Jacobson et al. 2005). A PVR of more than 100 mL is defined as chronic urinary retention which is significantly associated with CKD in community-dwelling men (Rule, Jacobson et al. 2005). Nevertheless, small residual urine volumes (<100 mL) may also affect renal function as the presence of PVR relates with renal function regardless of the quantity of PVR (Yamasaki, Naganuma et al. 2011). Thus ultrasonographic evaluation of post-void residual is a useful test in the prevention of CKD secondary to BPH. Chronic urinary retention is related with CKD (Rule, Jacobson et al. 2005).

### 6.9 Prostate TRUS

Prostate transrectal ultrasonography (TRUS) is performed to assess prostate size and shape, tissue characterization and occult carcinoma. There is no relationship between prostatic enlargement measures and CKD (Rule, Jacobson et al. 2005).

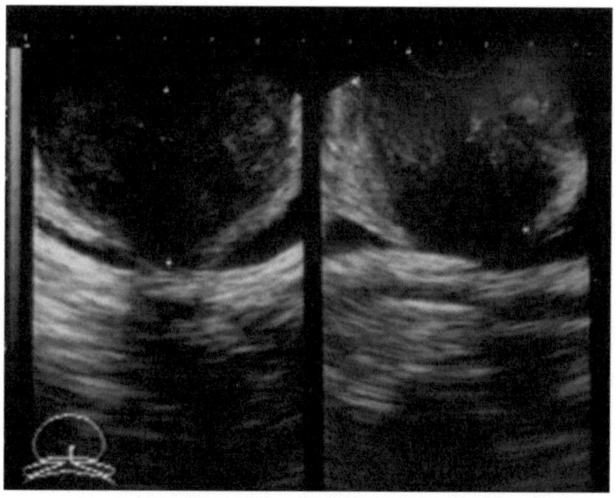

Fig. 4. Prostate Ultrassound. Prostate transrectal ultrasonography (sagital view).

### 6.10 Cystometry

It is not a routine exam for BPH evaluation. However, cystometry can help to identify high bladder pressure, low bladder compliance and detrusor instability that considerably affects renal function (Rule, Lieber et al. 2005; Yamasaki, Naganuma et al. 2011).

### 6.11 Pressure-flow studies

Pressure-flow studies can differentiate between patients with a low Qmax secondary to obstruction and those whose low Qmax is caused by a decompensated or neurogenic bladder. They are most useful for distinguishing between bladder outlet obstruction and impaired detrusor contractility.

### 6.12 Urethrocystoscopy

Urethrocystoscopy should not be done routinely but is optional during later evaluation if invasive treatment is strongly considered (McConnell, Barry et al. 1994). Nevertheless, it is a useful preoperative procedure to plan the most appropriate approach. This investigation can confirm causes of outflow obstruction while eliminating intravesical abnormalities.

## 7. Treatment

Patients with mild symptoms are most appropriately managed by watchful waiting, patients with moderate symptoms should receive pharmacotherapy and patients with severe bother most benefit from surgical management. A man with preoperative IPSS $\geq$ 17 has an 87% chance of experiencing a substantial symptom reduction (Meigs, Mohr et al. 2001).

A group of patients at increased risk of progression can be identified on the basis of specific risk factors (e.g. age, symptoms, PSA level, Qmax, prostate volume and post-void residual urine). It might be appropriate to identify these patients at risk of progression and initiate early preventative treatment (Emberton et al., 2003)(Gabuev and Oelke 2011). For example, a higher frequency of kidney failure in patients presenting for prostate surgery than for nonprostate surgery has been shown, and several studies have shown improvement in kidney function after prostatectomy (Hill et al., 1993).

### 7.1 Acute treatment

Patients who present to the emergency department with bladder outlet obstruction and high serum creatinine should receive a urethral catheter and subsequently evaluated in order to distinguish between acute and chronic renal failure. Hospitalization is often required in these cases. If ureterohydronephrosis and azotaemia persists despite bladder desobstruction, an ureterovesical junction obstruction should be considered and bilateral percutaneous nephrostomy or bilateral ureteric stents (if feasible) are advisable for temporarily drainage. Patients may need urgent and transitory dialysis.

Neoureterocystostomy after a prostate ablative procedure may be adequate for definite ureterovesical junction obstruction resolution.

### 7.2 Watchful waiting

Watchful waiting (WW) is an appropriate strategy for men who are not bothered by their symptoms and have not developed BPH related complications.

This option should include education, reassurance, periodic monitoring and lifestyle advice to the patient. Lifestyle counseling include: reduction of fluid intake during specific times for control of urinary frequency (e.g. at night or when going out in public) but not of the total amount of daily fluid (above 1500 mL per day), avoidance of alcohol and caffeine because they have diuretic and irritant effect, bladder retraining to increase its capacity and constipation treatment. Watchful waiting is based on the notion that some symptoms may spontaneously improve whilst others may remain stable for years. The PSA level and the prostate volume may be helpful in predicting the risk of acute urinary retention, although they should not be used as a sole determinant for active therapy (Levy and Samraj 2007). Approximately 85% of men will be stable on WW at 1 year, deteriorating progressively to 65% at 5 years (Wasson, Reda et al. 1995; Netto, de Lima et al. 1999). This approach is not suitable for men with installed CKD due to bladder outlet obstruction.

### 7.3 Medical treatment

Medical approaches are not used to treat BPH complications (in which CKD is included). They are used for LUTS relief and for prevention of BPH progression (especially 5 alpha reductase inhibitors - 5-ARI).

#### 7.3.1 Alpha-blockers

Alpha-blockers address the dynamic component of prostatic obstruction by antagonizing the adrenergic receptors responsible for smooth muscle tone within the stroma, prostate capsule and bladder neck, providing the most rapid symptom relief. They include: terazosin, doxazosin, alfuzosin, tamsulosin and silodosin. These drugs have similar efficacy but different patterns of side-effects:

| Alpha-Blocker | Dosage | Side-effects |
|---|---|---|
| **Terazosin** | 1 mg once a day<br>May increase up to 20 mg a day | Asthenia, hypotension, dizziness, somnolence |
| **Doxazosin** | 1 mg once a day<br>May increase up to 8 mg once daily | Orthostatic hypotension, fatigue and dyspnea |
| **Alfuzosin** | 10 mg once a day | Fatigue, edema, rhinitis, headache, upper respiratory tract infection |
| **Tamsulosin** | 0,4 mg once a day | Dizziness, rhinitis, abnormal ejaculation |
| **Silodosin** | 8 mg once a day<br>4 mg once a day for men with moderate kidney dysfunction | Diarrhea, headache and commons cold symptoms, nasal congestion, retrograde ejaculation (the most common) |

Table 3. Alpha blockers used, dosage and side-effects.

The older, less costly, generic alpha blockers remain reasonable choices. However, these require dose titration and blood pressure monitoring. Alpha-blockers are the most prescribed medications for BPH as long as they have a rapid (symptoms may improve in 48 hours) and significant improvement on LUTS.

#### 7.3.2 5-alpha-reductase inhibitors

5-Alpha-Reductase Inhibitors (5-ARI) are anti-androgenic hormonal agents that address the static component of BPH by reducing the prostate volume (up to 20-30%). They include finasteride and dutasteride and are more effective in prostates larger than 40 mL (Boyle, Gould et al. 1996). According to some trials, finasteride significantly reduced acute urinary retention and the need for surgical treatment in men with BPH.

5-ARIs are the only pharmacologic treatment that may be used to prevent progression of LUTS secondary to BPH and to reduce the risk of urinary retention and future prostate-related surgery. Therefore, indirectly, it may be useful in preventing BPH complications such as chronic kidney failure. However, they can't revert CKD related to BPH after installed.

| 5-Alpha-Reductase Inhibitor | Dosage | Side-effects |
|---|---|---|
| Finasteride | 5 mg once a day | Erectile dysfunction, decreased libido, decreased serum PSA, gynecomastia |
| Dutasteride | 1 mg once a day<br>May increase up to 8 mg once daily | |

Table 4. 5 alpha-reductase inhibitors used, dosage and side-effects.

Finasteride inhibits exclusively the 5-AR type II isoenzyme, while dutasteride inhibits both types I and II. This difference in activity leads to a reduction in serum levels of dihydroxytestosterone (DHT) by approximately 70% with finasteride compared to approximately 95% with dutasteride (Clark, Hermann et al. 2004).

Finasteride (and probably dutasteride) is an appropriate and effective treatment alternative in men with refractory hematuria presumably due to prostatic bleeding (Foley, Soloman et al. 2000; Kearney, Bingham et al. 2002; Perimenis, Gyftopoulos et al. 2002).

### 7.3.3 Combination therapy

The Medical Therapy of Prostate Symptoms (MTOPS) Study demonstrated that in the long term, among men with larger prostates, combination therapy is superior to either alpha-blocker or 5-ARI therapy in preventing progression and improving symptoms (McConnell, Roehrborn et al. 2003).

### 7.3.4 Phytotherapy

The use of plant-derived agents (*Serenoa repens* or Saw palmetto, *Pygeum africanum*) on LUTS and BPH has been popular in Europe for many years and has recently spread in the USA. Their mechanism of action is still unclear. However they seem to improve urinary symptoms without important side effects. In some studies the efficacy of these compounds was found to be equivalent to 5-ARIs and alpha-blockers (Lowe 2001; Debruyne, Koch et al. 2002). The most widely studied and used, *Serenoa repens*, has no effect on prostate volume or the PSA test, but slightly decreases the prostate epithelium. It does not cause erectile dysfunction, but the herb may aggravate chronic gastrointestinal disease such as peptic ulcer (Bent, Kane et al. 2006).

## 7.4 Surgical treatment

Men who develop serious complications from BPH should be treated surgically in most of the cases. Both Agency for Health Care Policy and Research and International Consensus

Guidelines recommend surgery if the patient has refractory or recurrent urinary retention (failing at least one attempt of catheter removal) or any of the following conditions clearly secondary to BPH: recurrent UTI, recurrent gross hematuria, bladder stones, renal insufficiency, or large bladder diverticula (McConnell, Barry et al. 1994) (Denis et al., 1998). Studies suggest that dialysis dependent patients may recover renal function up to a year after prostatic surgery. In this setting, efforts should be made to identify and treat BPH in patients under dialysis.

Surgeries are associated with postoperative risks such as erectile dysfunction (4% to 10% incidence) and urinary incontinence (0.5% to 1.5%) (Flanigan, Reda et al. 1998) (McConnell, Bruskewitz et al. 1998). The 5-year recurrence rate of BPH following surgery is 2% to 10%(Flanigan, Reda et al. 1998). Proper therapy can be offered to the right men and the costs of long-term renal damage and post-surgical complications can be avoided.

### 7.5 Standard surgical procedures

TURP (transurethral resection of the prostate) is the hallmark of the urologist, the one against which other therapeutic measures are compared. It takes 20 to 30 minutes to resects an average gland weighing of 30 g and carry risks complications like bleeding, infections, retrograde-ejaculation, hospital stay, impotence and incontinence.

In patients presenting with renal failure due to bladder outflow obstruction, TURP restores normal voiding pattern in many cases. However renal failure due to bladder outflow obstruction tends to be more refractory and 57% of patients in Thomas *et* al. study were dialysis dependent after surgery. Only 3 of 14 patients experienced return to normal renal function post TURP (Thomas, Thomas et al. 2009).

Mortality following prostatectomy has decreased significantly within the past two decades and is less than < 0.25% in contemporary series (Holman, Wisniewski et al. 1999; Hahn, Farahmand et al. 2000). The risk of a TUR-syndrome (fluid intoxication, serum Na+<130 nmol/L) is in the range of 2%. Risk factors for the development of the TUR-syndrome are excessive bleeding with opening of venous sinuses, prolonged operation time, large glands and past or present smoking.

Open prostatectomy is the treatment of choice for large glands (>80-100 mL), bladder stones or if resection of bladder diverticula is indicated. Open prostatectomy involves the surgical removal (enucleation) of the inner portion of the prostate via a suprapubic or retropubic prostatectomy.

### 7.6 Minimally invasive surgical therapies

Standard operations are *TURP* in small (≤80-100mL) or open prostatectomy in large prostates (>80-100mL). Minimally invasive, alternative surgeries may be considered in selected men and offer advantages regarding risk of bleeding, duration of catheterization, or maintenance of sexual function. (Gabuev and Oelke 2011).

*Transurethral incision of the pro*state (TUIP) or bladder neck incision is recommended for smaller gland (weigh <25g) and has been found to be less invasive than TURP (Orandi 1990). TUIP has several advantages over TURP, such as a lower incidence of complications, minimal risk of bleeding and blood transfusion, decreased risk of retrograde ejaculation, shorter operating time and hospital stay, and an importantly higher long-term failure rate.

*Transurethral electrovaporiz*ation (TUVP) is a modification of TURP and TUIP, employing high electrical current to vaporize and coagulate the obstructive prostate tissue. Long-term efficacy is comparable with TURP, but high number of patients has been found to experience irritative side effects (Desautel, Burney et al. 1998).

*Transurethral needle ablation* (TUNA) is a simple and relatively inexpensive procedure which uses a needle to deliver high-frequency radio waves to destroy the enlarged prostatic tissue. TUNA is a successful treatment for small-sized gland and it poses a low or no risk for incontinence and erectile dysfunction (Ramon, Lynch et al. 1997).

*Transurethral microwave thermother*apy (TUMT) heats the prostate using a microwave antennae mounted on a urethral catheter (Thorpe and Neal 2003). TUMT has been found to be safe and cost effective, with reasonable improvement in urine flow rate and minimal impairment on sexual function (Richter, Rotbard et al. 1993).

*Transurethral ethanol ablation of the prostate* (TEAP) has been recently introduced as a minimally invasive alternative treatment for patients with BPH. TEAP produces necrotic effect on prostatic tissues, leading to fibrosis and shrinkage. It is an effective minimally invasive treatment option for medically high-risk symptomatic patients with BPH that can be performed as an outpatient procedure under regional anesthesia (El-Husseiny and Buchholz 2011).

*Laser prostatectomy*: four types of lasers have been used to treat LUTS, namely neodymium: yttrium-aluminum-garnet (Nd: YAG) laser, holmium YAG laser (Ho:YAG), potassium titanyl phosphate (KTP), and diode laser. It has been found to be safe and effective technique, with significant improvement in urinary flow rates and symptoms. Short surgery time, shorter catheter use, minimal blood loss and fluid absorption, decreased hospital stay, low erectile dysfunction rates, and bladder neck contractures are few of the advantages of laser prostatectomy over the TURP and other conventional techniques (Donovan, Peters et al. 2000; Bent, Kane et al. 2006). Laser surgery is specially indicated in patients receiving anticoagulant therapy that want to maintain ejaculation or are unfit for TURP.

*Transrectal HIFU* (high intensity focus ultrasonography) therapy is the only technique that provides non-invasive tissue ablation; however, general anesthesia or at least heavy intravenous sedation is required. Long-term efficacy is limited, with a treatment failure rate of approximately 10% per year.Significant increase in uroflow and a decrease in postvoid residual volume have been observed, but the cost is three times higher than that of TURP (Madersbacher, Kratzik et al. 1993).

## 8. Future approaches to BPH

Increasing average life expectancy, especially due to better health care and better education of the population, make us believe that soon we shall have, seek for medical care, a greater number of people suffering from elderly diseases. The health burden of disorders such as BPH will be a major dome for research in the future.

Recent investigation is underway in this field, some basic and translational research is being done, in an attempt to better understand and treat this prevalent disease.

Recently Woo *et.* al reported the use of a Prostatic Urethral Lift (PUL) procedure, which is a novel, minimally invasive treatment for symptomatic benign prostatic hyperplasia (BPH). PUL aims to mechanically open the prostatic urethra without ablation or resection, with patients reporting sustained symptom relief for 12 months with minimal morbidity (Woo, Chin et al. 2011).

Tadalafil and other phosphodiesterase type 5 (PDE5) inhibitors have demonstrated beneficial effects on smooth muscle relaxation, smooth muscle and endothelial cell proliferation, nerve activity, and tissue perfusion that may impact LUTS (Andersson, de Groat et al. 2011). Consistent evidence of improvements in LUTS has been shown with PDE5-Is, either alone or in combination with α-blockers (Martinez-Salamanca, Carballido et al. 2011). However, urodynamic results or objective measures of urinary flow are lacking (Martinez-Salamanca, Carballido et al. 2011).

De Souza *et* al, investigated the effects of *Orbignya speciosa*, a nanoparticle extract, newly developed phytotheraphy that can be safely used on the management of BPH (de Souza, Palumbo et al. 2011).

In our country (Portugal) a recent study led by Pisco *et.* al, aimed to evaluate whether prostatic arterial embolization could be a feasible way to treat lower urinary tract symptoms associated with benign prostatic hyperplasia. Their preliminary results and short-term follow-up suggest good symptom control without sexual dysfunction associated with a reduction in prostate volume (Pisco, Pinheiro et al. 2011).

Rick *et* al, in recent times used growth hormone-releasing hormone (GHRH) in animal models. They concluded that GHRH antagonists can lower prostate weight in experimental BPH with significant reductions in protein levels of IL-1β, NF-κβ/p65, and cyclooxygenase-2 (COX-2), suggesting that GHRH antagonists should be considered for further investigation as therapy for BPH (Rick, Schally et al. 2011)

It is important in a near future to characterize a *clinical phenotype* of BPH; measure disease severity and outcomes; design clinical trials; study concepts for drug therapy, behavioral and lifestyle interventions and additional intervention therapies (AUA 2010).

## 9. Conclusion

Benign prostatic hyperplasia and chronic kidney disease are two common and prevalent entities in elderly men. It has been reported in several studies that threads of evidence suggest that BPH is a risk factor for chronic kidney disease. An average of 13,6% patients presenting to urologic clinics for the treatment of BPH had renal failure. The low occurrence of CKD in BPH clinical trials should not be used to infer a weak association between these two disease processes (Rule et al., 2005). From our own experience we deem that the average of patients with BPH and some degree of renal disease can be higher, mostly because older men most of the times ignore their micturition problems and seek for clinical help just in a later degree of BPH.

Although BPH is not a life-threatening condition, the impact BPH on quality of life (QoL) can be significant and should not be underestimated. On the other hand CKD is an important medical problem that can even be critical (Fox, Larson et al. 2004)

It has been well documented that bladder outlet obstruction by an enlarging prostate can lead to renal insufficiency. Relationship between symptoms severity and elevated serum creatinine in men with BPH have not been well defined. Recent data make us believe that combination of all these factors leading to chronic and progressive urinary retention, high bladder pressure, ureterohydronephrosis work together causing progressive renal injury. Obstructive process root cellular and physiological changes in bladder muscle and collagen, contribute to a high pressure bladder that perpetuates itself with worsening ability to empty and causing kidney lesions leading to renal failure.

The advent of medical treatment has obviated the need for surgery in many patients with BPH. Men in acute urinary retention or those with urinary tract infection and other BPH-complications, may benefit from more aggressive BPH treatment to prevent renal failure, especially if the conditions are recurrent.

Other kidney risk factors such as diabetes mellitus, cardiovascular disease, hypertension, obesity and dyslipidemia may also be considered in the patient with BPH. Etiology of CKD is often multifactorial and BPH may accelerate the progression of CKD in other disease processes.

Older men with BPH often tolerate and ignore lower urinary tract symptoms and may not present for medical consultation until they develop uremic syndrome. Thus, these patients should have prostatic obstruction considered during evaluation and treatment as this diagnosis can be easily missed in unreported LUTS. Close follow-up is mandatory.

We emphasize that CKD secondary to BPH is a preventable disease, and if early detected can prevent costs of CKD treatment (including hemodialysis) with considerable saves (economic, health care, social).

Findings that we mentioned in this chapter suggest that progressive nephropathy caused by prostatic/bladder outflow obstruction - urinary outflow obstruction - might be averted by more adequate screening of renal function in men with untreated BPH.

## 10. References

Abrams, P. (1999). "LUTS, BPH, BPE, BPO: A Plea for the Logical Use of Correct Terms." *Rev Urol* 1(2): 65.

Andersson, K. E., W. C. de Groat, et al. (2011). "Tadalafil for the treatment of lower urinary tract symptoms secondary to benign prostatic hyperplasia: pathophysiology and mechanism(s) of action." *Neurourol Urodyn* 30(3): 292-301.

Arrighi, H. M., E. J. Metter, et al. (1991). "Natural history of benign prostatic hyperplasia and risk of prostatectomy. The Baltimore Longitudinal Study of Aging." *Urology* 38(1 Suppl): 4-8.

AUA, Ed. (2010). *Guideline on the Management of Benign Prostatic Hyperplasia (BPH).*

Barry, M. J., F. J. Fowler, Jr., et al. (1992). "Correlation of the American Urological Association symptom index with self-administered versions of the Madsen-Iversen, Boyarsky and Maine Medical Assessment Program symptom indexes. Measurement Committee of the American Urological Association." *J Urol* 148(5): 1558-1563; discussion 1564.

Barry, M. J., F. J. Fowler, Jr., et al. (1992). "The American Urological Association symptom index for benign prostatic hyperplasia. The Measurement Committee of the American Urological Association." *J Urol* 148(5): 1549-1557; discussion 1564.

Bent, S., C. Kane, et al. (2006). "Saw palmetto for benign prostatic hyperplasia." *N Engl J Med* 354(6): 557-566.

Berry, S. J., D. S. Coffey, et al. (1984). "The development of human benign prostatic hyperplasia with age." *J Urol* 132(3): 474-479.

Boesch, S. T., G. Dobler, et al. (2000). "Effects of alpha1-adrenoceptor antagonists on cultured prostatic smooth muscle cells." *Prostate Suppl* 9: 34-41.

Boyle, P., A. L. Gould, et al. (1996). "Prostate volume predicts outcome of treatment of benign prostatic hyperplasia with finasteride: meta-analysis of randomized clinical trials." *Urology* 48(3): 398-405.

Carter, H. B. and D. S. Coffey (1990). "The prostate: an increasing medical problem." *Prostate* 16(1): 39-48.

Chai, T. C., K. E. Andersson, et al. (2000). "Altered neural control of micturition in the aged F344 rat." *Urol Res* 28(5): 348-354.

Christ, G. J. and M. Liebert (2005). "Proceedings of the Baltimore smooth muscle meeting: identifying research frontiers and priorities for the lower urinary tract." *J Urol* 173(4): 1406-1409.

Clark, R. V., D. J. Hermann, et al. (2004). "Marked suppression of dihydrotestosterone in men with benign prostatic hyperplasia by dutasteride, a dual 5alpha-reductase inhibitor." *J Clin Endocrinol Metab* 89(5): 2179-2184.

Cockett, A. T., M. J. Barry, et al. (1992). "Indications for treatment of benign prostatic hyperplasia. The American Urological Association Study." *Cancer* 70(1 Suppl): 280-283.

Comiter, C. V., M. P. Sullivan, et al. (1997). "Urodynamic risk factors for renal dysfunction in men with obstructive and nonobstructive voiding dysfunction." *J Urol* 158(1): 181-185.

Coroneos, E., M. Assouad, et al. (1997). "Urinary obstruction causes irreversible renal failure by inducing chronic tubulointerstitial nephritis." *Clin Nephrol* 48(2): 125-128.

de Souza, P. A., A. Palumbo, Jr., et al. (2011). "Effects of a nanocomposite containing Orbignya speciosa lipophilic extract on Benign Prostatic Hyperplasia." *J Ethnopharmacol* 135(1): 135-146.

Debruyne, F., G. Koch, et al. (2002). "Comparison of a phytotherapeutic agent (Permixon) with an alpha-blocker (Tamsulosin) in the treatment of benign prostatic hyperplasia: a 1-year randomized international study." *Eur Urol* 41(5): 497-506; discussion 506-497.

Desautel, M. G., T. L. Burney, et al. (1998). "Outcome of vaportrode transurethral vaporization of the prostate using pressure-flow urodynamic criteria." *Urology* 51(6): 1013-1017.

Donovan, J. L., T. J. Peters, et al. (2000). "A randomized trial comparing transurethral resection of the prostate, laser therapy and conservative treatment of men with symptoms associated with benign prostatic enlargement: The CLasP study." *J Urol* 164(1): 65-70.

Duncan, M. E. and M. J. Goldacre (2011). "Mortality trends for benign prostatic hyperplasia and prostate cancer in English populations 1979-2006." *BJU Int* 107(1): 40-45.

El-Husseiny, T. and N. Buchholz (2011). "Transurethral ethanol ablation of the prostate for symptomatic benign prostatic hyperplasia: long-term follow-up." *J Endourol* 25(3): 477-480.

Emberton, M., G. L. Andriole, et al. (2003). "Benign prostatic hyperplasia: a progressive disease of aging men." *Urology* 61(2): 267-273.

Faubert, P. F., Porush, J.G., Ed. (1998). *Renal disease in the elderly* New York Marcel Dekker

Fauci, B., Kasper, Hauser, Longo, Jameson, Loscalzo, Ed. (2007). *Harrison's Principles of Internal Medicine*. 17th, Mc Graw Hill

Flanigan, R. C., D. J. Reda, et al. (1998). "5-year outcome of surgical resection and watchful waiting for men with moderately symptomatic benign prostatic hyperplasia: a Department of Veterans Affairs cooperative study." *J Urol* 160(1): 12-16; discussion 16-17.

Foley, S. J., L. Z. Soloman, et al. (2000). "A prospective study of the natural history of hematuria associated with benign prostatic hyperplasia and the effect of finasteride." *J Urol* 163(2): 496-498.

Fox, C. S., M. G. Larson, et al. (2004). "Predictors of new-onset kidney disease in a community-based population." *JAMA* 291(7): 844-850.

Gabuev, A. and M. Oelke (2011). "[Latest Trends and Recommendations on Epidemiology, Diagnosis, and Treatment of Benign Prostatic Hyperplasia (BPH).]." *Aktuelle Urol* 42(3): 167-178.

Gerber, G. S., E. R. Goldfischer, et al. (1997). "Serum creatinine measurements in men with lower urinary tract symptoms secondary to benign prostatic hyperplasia." *Urology* 49(5): 697-702.

Ghose, R. R. and V. Harindra (1989). "Unrecognised high pressure chronic retention of urine presenting with systemic arterial hypertension." *BMJ* 298(6688): 1626-1628.

Goldman, L., Ausiello, D.A., Ed. (2008). *Cecil Medicine*. Philadelphia, Saunders Elsevier.

Gosling, J. A. and J. S. Dixon (1980). "Structure of trabeculated detrusor smooth muscle in cases of prostatic hypertrophy." *Urol Int* 35(5): 351-355.

Gosling, J. A., L. S. Kung, et al. (2000). "Correlation between the structure and function of the rabbit urinary bladder following partial outlet obstruction." *J Urol* 163(4): 1349-1356.

Grosse, H. (1990). "[Frequency, localization and associated disorders in urinary calculi. Analysis of 1671 autopsies in urolithiasis]." *Z Urol Nephrol* 83(9): 469-474.

Hahn, R. G., B. Y. Farahmand, et al. (2000). "Incidence of acute myocardial infarction and cause-specific mortality after transurethral treatments of prostatic hypertrophy." *Urology* 55(2): 236-240.

Hallan, S. I., D. Kwong, et al. (2010). "Use of a prostate symptom score to identify men at risk of future kidney failure: insights from the HUNT II Study." *Am J Kidney Dis* 56(3): 477-485.

Hallan, S. I. and S. R. Orth (2010). "The KDOQI 2002 classification of chronic kidney disease: for whom the bell tolls." *Nephrol Dial Transplant* 25(9): 2832-2836.

Harbitz, T. B. and O. A. Haugen (1972). "Histology of the prostate in elderly men. A study in an autopsy series." *Acta Pathol Microbiol Scand A* 80(6): 756-768.

Hassanzadeh, K., P. Yavari-kia, et al. (2010). "Non-obstructive lower urinary tract symptoms versus prostate volume in benign prostatic hyperplasia." *Pak J Biol Sci* 13(23): 1129-1134.

Hill, A. M., N. Philpott, et al. (1993). "Prevalence and outcome of renal impairment at prostatectomy." *Br J Urol* 71(4): 464-468.

Holman, C. D., Z. S. Wisniewski, et al. (1999). "Mortality and prostate cancer risk in 19,598 men after surgery for benign prostatic hyperplasia." *BJU Int* 84(1): 37-42.

Holtgrewe, H. L., W. K. Mebust, et al. (1989). "Transurethral prostatectomy: practice aspects of the dominant operation in American urology." *J Urol* 141(2): 248-253.

Holtgrewe, H. L. and W. L. Valk (1962). "Factors influencing the mortality and morbidity of transurethral prostatectomy: a study of 2,015 cases." *J Urol* 87: 450-459.

Hong, S. J., W. Rayford, et al. (2005). "The importance of patient perception in the clinical assessment of benign prostatic hyperplasia and its management." *BJU Int* 95(1): 15-19.

Hong, S. K., S. T. Lee, et al. (2010). "Chronic kidney disease among men with lower urinary tract symptoms due to benign prostatic hyperplasia." *BJU Int* 105(10): 1424-1428.

Hong, S. K., J. J. Oh, et al. (2010). "Prediction of outcomes after radical prostatectomy in patients diagnosed with prostate cancer of biopsy gleason score >/= 8 via contemporary multi (>/=12)-core prostate biopsy." *BJU Int*.

Humes, H. D., Ed. (2000). *Kelley's Textbook of Internal Medicine*. Philadelphia, Lippincott Williams & Wilkins.

Hunter, D. J., A. Berra-Unamuno, et al. (1996). "Prevalence of urinary symptoms and other urological conditions in Spanish men 50 years old or older." *J Urol* 155(6): 1965-1970.

Jacobsen, S. J., C. J. Girman, et al. (2001). "Natural history of benign prostatic hyperplasia." *Urology* 58(6 Suppl 1): 5-16; discussion 16.

Jacobsen, S. J., H. A. Guess, et al. (1993). "A population-based study of health care-seeking behavior for treatment of urinary symptoms. The Olmsted County Study of Urinary Symptoms and Health Status Among Men." *Arch Fam Med* 2(7): 729-735.

Jones, D. A., S. A. Gilpin, et al. (1991). "Relationship between bladder morphology and long-term outcome of treatment in patients with high pressure chronic retention of urine." *Br J Urol* 67(3): 280-285.

Jones, S. A., J. R. Ellis, et al. (1991). "The relationship between visual stimulation, behaviour and continuous release of protein in the substantia nigra." *Brain Res* 560(1-2): 163-166.

Kearney, M. C., J. B. Bingham, et al. (2002). "Clinical predictors in the use of finasteride for control of gross hematuria due to benign prostatic hyperplasia." *J Urol* 167(6): 2489-2491.

Klahr, S. (2001). "Urinary tract obstruction." *Semin Nephrol* 21(2): 133-145.

Koch, W. F., K. Ezz el Din, et al. (1996). "The outcome of renal ultrasound in the assessment of 556 consecutive patients with benign prostatic hyperplasia." *J Urol* 155(1): 186-189.

Kojima, M., E. Inui, et al. (1997). "Noninvasive quantitative estimation of infravesical obstruction using ultrasonic measurement of bladder weight." *J Urol* 157(2): 476-479.

Kumar, R., C. M. Hill, et al. (1973). "Acute renal failure in the elderly." *Lancet* 1(7794): 90-91.

La Vecchia, C., F. Levi, et al. (1995). "Mortality from benign prostatic hyperplasia: worldwide trends 1950-92." *J Epidemiol Community Health* 49(4): 379-384.

Levi, F., F. Lucchini, et al. (2003). "Recent trends in mortality from benign prostatic hyperplasia." *Prostate* 56(3): 207-211.

Levin, R. M., N. Haugaard, et al. (2000). "Obstructive response of human bladder to BPH vs. rabbit bladder response to partial outlet obstruction: a direct comparison." *Neurourol Urodyn* 19(5): 609-629.

Levy, A. and G. P. Samraj (2007). "Benign prostatic hyperplasia: when to 'watch and wait,' when and how to treat." *Cleve Clin J Med* 74 Suppl 3: S15-20.

Lin, V. K., J. B. Robertson, et al. (2000). "Smooth muscle myosin heavy chains are developmentally regulated in the rabbit bladder." *J Urol* 164(4): 1376-1380.

Lowe, F. C. (2001). "Phytotherapy in the management of benign prostatic hyperplasia." *Urology* 58(6 Suppl 1): 71-76; discussion 76-77.

Madersbacher, S., C. Kratzik, et al. (1993). "Tissue ablation in benign prostatic hyperplasia with high-intensity focused ultrasound." *Eur Urol* 23 Suppl 1: 39-43.

Manieri, C., S. S. Carter, et al. (1998). "The diagnosis of bladder outlet obstruction in men by ultrasound measurement of bladder wall thickness." *J Urol* 159(3): 761-765.

Martinez-Salamanca, J. I., J. Carballido, et al. (2011). "Phosphodiesterase Type 5 Inhibitors in the Management of Non-neurogenic Male Lower Urinary Tract Symptoms: Critical Analysis of Current Evidence." *Eur Urol.*

McConnell, J. D., M. J. Barry, et al. (1994). "Benign prostatic hyperplasia: diagnosis and treatment. Agency for Health Care Policy and Research." *Clin Pract Guidel Quick Ref Guide Clin*(8): 1-17.

McConnell, J. D., R. Bruskewitz, et al. (1998). "The effect of finasteride on the risk of acute urinary retention and the need for surgical treatment among men with benign prostatic hyperplasia. Finasteride Long-Term Efficacy and Safety Study Group." *N Engl J Med* 338(9): 557-563.

McConnell, J. D., C. G. Roehrborn, et al. (2003). "The long-term effect of doxazosin, finasteride, and combination therapy on the clinical progression of benign prostatic hyperplasia." *N Engl J Med* 349(25): 2387-2398.

McNeal, J. E. (1978). "Origin and evolution of benign prostatic enlargement." *Invest Urol* 15(4): 340-345.

McVary, K. T. (2006). "BPH: epidemiology and comorbidities." *Am J Manag Care* 12(5 Suppl): S122-128.

Mebust, W. K., H. L. Holtgrewe, et al. (1989). "Transurethral prostatectomy: immediate and postoperative complications. A cooperative study of 13 participating institutions evaluating 3,885 patients." *J Urol* 141(2): 243-247.

Mebust, W. K., H. L. Holtgrewe, et al. (2002). "Transurethral prostatectomy: immediate and postoperative complications. Cooperative study of 13 participating institutions evaluating 3,885 patients. J Urol, 141: 243-247, 1989." *J Urol* 167(1): 5-9.

Meigs, J. B., B. Mohr, et al. (2001). "Risk factors for clinical benign prostatic hyperplasia in a community-based population of healthy aging men." *J Clin Epidemiol* 54(9): 935-944.

Melchior, J., W. L. Valk, et al. (1974). "Transurethral prostatectomy in the azotemic patient." *J Urol* 112(5): 643-646.

Mukamel, E., I. Nissenkorn, et al. (1979). "Occult progressive renal damage in the elderly male due to benign prostatic hypertrophy." *J Am Geriatr Soc* 27(9): 403-406.

Neal, D. E. (1990). "Irreversible renal failure in men with outflow obstruction: is it a preventable disease?" *Postgrad Med J* 66(782): 996-999.

Neal, D. E., R. A. Styles, et al. (1987). "Relationship between detrusor function and residual urine in men undergoing prostatectomy." *Br J Urol* 60(6): 560-566.

Netto, N. R., Jr., M. L. de Lima, et al. (1999). "Evaluation of patients with bladder outlet obstruction and mild international prostate symptom score followed up by watchful waiting." *Urology* 53(2): 314-316.

Nielsen, K. K., J. Nordling, et al. (1994). "Critical review of the diagnosis of prostatic obstruction." *Neurourol Urodyn* 13(3): 201-217.

Oesterling, J. E. (1996). "Benign prostatic hyperplasia: a review of its histogenesis and natural history." *Prostate Suppl* 6: 67-73.

Olbrich, O., E. Woodford-Williams, et al. (1957). "Renal function in prostatism." *Lancet* 272(6983): 1322-1324.

Orandi, A. (1990). "Transurethral resection versus transurethral incision of the prostate." *Urol Clin North Am* 17(3): 601-612.

Organization, W. H. (2011). "Global Burden Disease." from http://www.who.int/healthinfo/global_burden_disease/estimates_country/en/index.html.

Perimenis, P., K. Gyftopoulos, et al. (2002). "Effects of finasteride and cyproterone acetate on hematuria associated with benign prostatic hyperplasia: a prospective, randomized, controlled study." *Urology* 59(3): 373-377.

Pisco, J. M., L. C. Pinheiro, et al. (2011). "Prostatic arterial embolization to treat benign prostatic hyperplasia." *J Vasc Interv Radiol* 22(1): 11-19; quiz 20.

Ponholzer, A., C. Temml, et al. (2006). "The association between lower urinary tract symptoms and renal function in men: a cross-sectional and 5-year longitudinal analysis." *J Urol* 175(4): 1398-1402.

Pradhan, B. K. and K. Chandra (1975). "Morphogenesis of nodular hyperplasia--prostate." *J Urol* 113(2): 210-213.

Prakash, J., R. K. Saxena, et al. (2001). "Spectrum of renal diseases in the elderly: single center experience from a developing country." *Int Urol Nephrol* 33(2): 227-233.

Ramon, J., T. H. Lynch, et al. (1997). "Transurethral needle ablation of the prostate for the treatment of benign prostatic hyperplasia: a collaborative multicentre study." *Br J Urol* 80(1): 128-134; discussion 134-125.

Richter, S., M. Rotbard, et al. (1993). "Efficacy of transurethral hyperthermia in benign prostatic hyperplasia." *Urology* 41(5): 412-416.

Rick, F. G., A. V. Schally, et al. (2011). "Antagonists of growth hormone-releasing hormone (GHRH) reduce prostate size in experimental benign prostatic hyperplasia." *Proc Natl Acad Sci U S A* 108(9): 3755-3760.

Roberts, R. O., T. Rhodes, et al. (1994). "Natural history of prostatism: worry and embarrassment from urinary symptoms and health care-seeking behavior." *Urology* 43(5): 621-628.

Roehrborn, C. G. (2008). "BPH progression: concept and key learning from MTOPS, ALTESS, COMBAT, and ALF-ONE." *BJU Int* 101 Suppl 3: 17-21.

Rosen, R., J. Altwein, et al. (2003). "Lower urinary tract symptoms and male sexual dysfunction: the multinational survey of the aging male (MSAM-7)." *Eur Urol* 44(6): 637-649.

Rule, A. D., D. J. Jacobson, et al. (2005). "The association between benign prostatic hyperplasia and chronic kidney disease in community-dwelling men." *Kidney Int* 67(6): 2376-2382.

Rule, A. D., M. M. Lieber, et al. (2005). "Is benign prostatic hyperplasia a risk factor for chronic renal failure?" *J Urol* 173(3): 691-696.

Sacks, S. H., S. A. Aparicio, et al. (1989). "Late renal failure due to prostatic outflow obstruction: a preventable disease." *BMJ* 298(6667): 156-159.

Saydah, S., Eberhardt, M., Rios-Burrows, N., Williams, M., Geiss, L. (2007) "Prevalence of Chronic Kidney Disease and Associated Risk Factors --- United States, 1999--2004."

Schappert, S. M. (1993). "National Ambulatory Medical Care Survey: 1991 summary." *Adv Data*(230): 1-16.

Schwinn, D. A. (1994). "Adrenergic receptors: unique localization in human tissues." *Adv Pharmacol* 31: 333-341.

Shapiro, E., V. Hartanto, et al. (1992). "The response to alpha blockade in benign prostatic hyperplasia is related to the percent area density of prostate smooth muscle." *Prostate* 21(4): 297-307.

Styles, R. A., D. E. Neal, et al. (1988). "Long-term monitoring of bladder pressure in chronic retention of urine: the relationship between detrusor activity and upper tract dilatation." *J Urol* 140(2): 330-334.

Sutaria, P. M. and D. R. Staskin (2000). "Hydronephrosis and renal deterioration in the elderly due to abnormalities of the lower urinary tract and ureterovesical junction." *Int Urol Nephrol* 32(1): 119-126.

Terris, M. K., N. Afzal, et al. (1998). "Correlation of transrectal ultrasound measurements of prostate and transition zone size with symptom score, bother score, urinary flow rate, and post-void residual volume." *Urology* 52(3): 462-466.

Thomas, A. Z., A. A. Thomas, et al. (2009). "Benign prostatic hyperplasia presenting with renal failure--what is the role for transurethral resection of the prostate (TURP)?" *Ir Med J* 102(2): 43-44.

Thorpe, A. and D. Neal (2003). "Benign prostatic hyperplasia." *Lancet* 361(9366): 1359-1367.

Tseng, T. Y. and M. L. Stoller (2009). "Obstructive uropathy." *Clin Geriatr Med* 25(3): 437-443.

Wasson, J. H., D. J. Reda, et al. (1995). "A comparison of transurethral surgery with watchful waiting for moderate symptoms of benign prostatic hyperplasia. The Veterans Affairs Cooperative Study Group on Transurethral Resection of the Prostate." *N Engl J Med* 332(2): 75-79.

Wei, J. T., E. Calhoun, et al. (2008). "Urologic diseases in america project: benign prostatic hyperplasia." *J Urol* 179(5 Suppl): S75-80.

Wein, A. J., Kavoussi, L.R., Novick, A.C., Partin, A.W., Peters, C.A., Ed. (2007). *Campbell-Walsh Urology*, Saunders Elsevier

Woo, H. H., P. T. Chin, et al. (2011). "Safety and feasibility of the prostatic urethral lift: a novel, minimally invasive treatment for lower urinary tract symptoms (LUTS) secondary to benign prostatic hyperplasia (BPH)." *BJU Int* 108(1): 82-88.

Wu, S. L., N. C. Li, et al. (2006). "Natural history of benign prostate hyperplasia." *Chin Med J (Engl)* 119(24): 2085-2089.

Xia, Z., R. O. Roberts, et al. (1999). "Trends in prostatectomy for benign prostatic hyperplasia among black and white men in the United States: 1980 to 1994." *Urology* 53(6): 1154-1159.

Yamasaki, T., T. Naganuma, et al. (2011). "Association between chronic kidney disease and small residual urine volumes in patients with benign prostatic hyperplasia." *Nephrology (Carlton)* 16(3): 335-339.

Yamasaki, T., Naganuma, T., Iguchi, T., Kuroki, Y., Kuwabara, N., Takemoto, Y., Shoji, T., Nakatani, T. (2010). "Association between chronic kidney disease and small residual urine volumes in patients with benign prostatic hyperplasia." *Nephrology (Carlton)* 16(3): 5.

# 22

# Asymptomatic Bacteriuria (ASB), Renal Function and Hypertension

Suzanne Geerlings
*Infectious Disease specialist,*
*Department of Internal Medicine, Division of Infectious Diseases,*
*Tropical Medicine and AIDS Center for Infection and Immunity Amsterdam (CINIMA)*
*Academic Medical Center, Amsterdam*
*The Netherlands*

## 1. Introduction

Chronic kidney disease is an increasing public health problem. In the United States, the prevalence is estimated to be approximately 11% of the adult population. Chronic kidney disease may progress to end-stage renal failure, a condition associated with high morbidity and mortality. Diabetes mellitus (DM) is one of the main causes of kidney disease and end-stage renal failure. In the United States, DM is the primary diagnosis in 44% of all new cases of renal replacement therapy. Vascular complications are the most common cause of diabetic nephropathy, but it is possible that urinary tract infections (UTIs) also contribute to renal insufficiency in patients with DM.

The urinary tract is normally sterile. However, asymptomatic bacteriuria (ASB), which is defined as the presence of a positive urine culture with at least 10e5 cfu/ml collected from a patient without symptoms of a UTI, is a common phenomenon, especially in women. Different studies report a prevalence of approximately 1-5% among healthy young women, increasing to over 20% in the elderly and 12-26% in women with DM. A Swedish study among 1,462 adult women showed that women with bacteriuria at study entry had an increased risk of having bacteriuria six and twelve years later, compared to women without bacteriuria (Odds Ratio (OR) 6.9 and 3.1, after six and twelve years, respectively). Another Swedish study among 116 schoolgirls with ASB showed that at baseline renal parenchymal reduction was found in 10.3%, while reflux was found in 20.7%, but only 30% of the 116 patients had a history referable to an earlier UTI. A 3-year follow-up of these 116 schoolgirls with ASB (treated or untreated) showed that the risk of developing renal damage as a result of ASB in a schoolgirl with a roentgenographically normal urinary tract seemed to be small.

*Escherichia coli* is the most prevalent causative microorganism in both symptomatic and asymptomatic bacteriuria, accounting for more than 80% of uncomplicated UTIs. Previous studies have demonstrated that patients with renal scarring due to pyelonephritis are at increased risk for the development of hypertension and chronic kidney disease. Results from previous in vitro and in vivo studies indicate that a UTI with *E. coli* can lead to renal damage, either by the microorganism itself or by the following host response. For instance, it has been shown that type 1 fimbriae (the adhesive organelles at the outer surface of the bacterial membrane) can cause scarring in the renal parenchyma of rats, with large foci of inflammation. This might be due to the activation of polymorphonuclear leukocytes by type 1 fimbriated-strains, which leads to the release of tissue destroying enzymes. Mice models have shown that although neutrophils are important in bacterial clearance, they can also cause renal damage.

In a clinical study, renal scarring was detected in 29 of 63 adult women ten to twenty years after hospitalization for pyelonephritis. In contrast, no study has convincingly shown that ASB can lead to a clinically relevant decline in renal function in otherwise healthy women. Several authors in the first half of the twentieth century have suggested a role of bacteriuria in the etiology of hypertension, but the pathogenesis is not understood.

## 2. ASB and renal function decline in healthy women

### 2.1 Study population, baseline cohort

Between 1974 and 1986 all women, born between 1911 and 1945, who lived in the city of Utrecht and surroundings, the Netherlands, were invited for a breast-cancer-screening program, with a participation rate of 68 to 72%. A total number of 38,994 women, aged 39 to 68 years old at intake, participated (the baseline cohort). Baseline measurements, performed between 1974 and 1986, included extensive questionnaires, a short medical examination, and the collection of a midstream morning urine sample. Data obtained through the questionnaires included age, marital status, smoking habits, parity, menopausal age, diet and drug use. During the medical examination weight and height were measured. Approximately 200 ml urine was stored in plastic polypropylene jars, without preserving agents, and stored at -20°C for future analyses. All women gave oral consent to use their data and urine samples for future scientific research.

### 2.2 Study population, follow-up cohort

From 1993 to 1997, 50,313 women living in Utrecht and surroundings who were scheduled for breast cancer screening during this period received an invitation by mail to join an additional study to assess the relation between nutrition and cancer and other chronic diseases, the Prospect-EPIC study (the follow-up cohort). A total of 17,357 women (participation rate 34.5%) agreed to take part . Participants were between 49 and 70 years old at enrolment. Information was collected on the basis of two self-administered questionnaires and a medical examination including blood pressure. Non-fasting blood samples were successfully drawn from 97.5% of the women, and stored under liquid nitrogen at -196°C. Approximately 88% of the women signed a detailed informed consent, enabling the researchers to use their blood samples for future analysis, and to obtain information on future morbidity and mortality.

To address the relation between *E. coli* bacteriuria and renal function development, we performed a full cohort analysis for women who participated in both the baseline cohort and the follow-up cohort. *E. coli* bacteriuria was diagnosed by a real-time Polymerase Chain Reaction in this urine sample. Participants were between 49 and 70 years old at enrolment. The mean duration of follow-up was 11.5 ± 1.7 years, ranging from 8.1 to 18.6 years from baseline until participation in the follow-up study. Forty-eight of 490 women (10%) were classified with *E. coli* bacteriuria at baseline. At study endpoint, the mean creatinine clearance for women with baseline bacteriuria was 87 ± 21 ml and without baseline bacteriuria 85 ± 18 ml per minute, respectively (Figure 1). *E. coli* bacteriuria at baseline was not associated with creatinine levels at follow-up, adjusted for age and weight and the distribution in stages of renal function was not different for women with bacteriuria compared to women without bacteriuria.

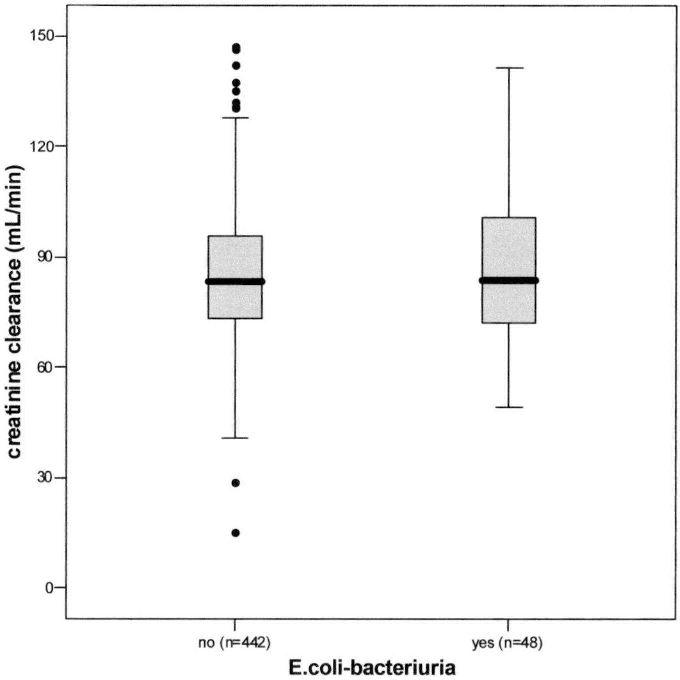


Fig. 1. Differences in creatinine clearance between women WITHOUT DM with and without ASB. (Meiland R, Stolk RP, Geerlings SE, Peeters PH, Grobbee DE, Coenjaerts FE, Brouwer EC, Hoepelman AI. Association between *Escherichia coli* bacteriuria and renal function in women: long-term follow-up. Arch Intern Med. 2007 Feb 12;167(3):253-7.)

### 2.3 Nested case-control study population

To obtain follow-up information on end-stage renal failure, we obtained data from the Renal Replacement Registry Netherlands (RENINE) that were available May 2002. RENINE is a foundation in which all Dutch nephrologists participate and where patients are registered who at one time have used kidney replacing therapy (hemodialysis or renal transplantation), with a coverage rate throughout the years of nearly 100%. Data from the baseline cohort and RENINE were matched on (maiden and married) name combined with date of birth to select the cases. A group consisting of four times the number of cases was randomly selected from the baseline cohort to form the control group. Four women participated in the follow-up cohort and were also selected as one of the cases who received kidney replacing therapy during follow-up; one woman underwent kidney transplantation before blood withdrawal (and was excluded for the cohort analysis), three women developed end-stage renal failure thereafter (and were included in both analyses). After excluding four individuals with a missing urine sample 49 cases and 206 controls were included. Among the cases, the mean duration until the date of kidney replacing therapy was 13.8 ± 7.4 years, with a minimum and maximum duration of 1.6 and 25.5 years, respectively. In the control group, the mean follow-up (i.e. the time from participation in the baseline cohort until study-endpoint in May 2002) was 27.0 ± 0.2 years.

No difference in duration until kidney replacing therapy was found between bacteriuric and non-bacteriuric individuals (14.6 versus 13.7 years, p = 0.80). Seven of 49 women who developed renal failure had *E. coli* bacteriuria at baseline, compared to 29 of 206 women in the control group (both 14%). The OR for the development of renal failure in the presence of *E. coli* bacteriuria, corrected for age, was 1.1 (95% CI 0.4–2.8, p = 0.86).

In a Swedish study the prevalence of ASB in women was 4%. After 15 years a reinvestigation was carried out, 40 cases (with ASB) and 40 age-matched healthy controls participated. Nobody had developed progressive renal disease. The age-dependent decrease after 15 years was the same in both groups.

The results of these longitudinal findings give strong support to the absence of an association between ASB and renal function decline in healthy women. As an explanation, Svanborg et al. found that certain *E. coli* strains stop expressing adherence factors like type 1 and P fimbriae once they have established bacteriuria. Therefore, these strains can remain present in the bladder without triggering an inflammatory response from the host and without side effects.

In conclusion, no relation between ASB and renal function decline has been demonstrated in healthy women. It has been recommended in American and European guidelines not to screen or to treat ASB in premenopausal non-pregnant women and older persons living in the community. The results of these studies confirm these recommendations.

## 3. ASB and hypertension in healthy women

Several authors in the first half of the twentieth century have suggested a role of bacteriuria in the etiology of hypertension. For instance, Kass showed small differences in blood pressure between bacteriuric and non-bacteriuric women aged 15 to 64 years old.

The association between ASB and hypertension was investigated in a cohort study of 444 women who were followed for the development of hypertension in relation to *E. coli* bacteriuria at baseline. Hypertension was defined as the (previous) use of antihypertensive medication and/or a measured systolic blood pressure of at least 160 mm Hg or a diastolic blood pressure of 95 mm Hg or higher. A history of having had a heart attack or stroke was assessed at follow-up by the two additional questions: "Have you ever had a heart attack / stroke?". Mean age at baseline was 45.0 ± 3.2 years and 48 women (10%) had *E. coli* bacteriuria. After 11.5 years women who had *E. coli* bacteriuria at baseline had a mean blood pressure at study endpoint of 133 ± 20 mmHg systolic and 78 ± 11 mmHg diastolic, and women without bacteriuria had values of 129 ± 20 and 78 ± 11 mmHg, respectively (p-value for difference 0.33 and 0.88). Interestingly, although *E. coli* bacteriuria was not associated with the blood pressure as a continuous variable, it was associated with the development of hypertension during follow-up (OR 2.8, 95% CI 1.4–5.5). This was mainly due to more bacteriuric women that started antihypertensive drugs when compared to non-bacteriuric participants. This association remained statistically significant after correction for age, weight and creatinine. Eight of the 45 women (18%) who had to be excluded because of the use of antihypertensive medication at baseline, had *E. coli* bacteriuria, which was higher than the percentage of 9% of the final study group without antihypertensive drugs at baseline (p = 0.06). However, no association between ASB and renal function decline was demonstrated. The incidence of heart attacks or strokes was not increased among women with bacteriuria at baseline. These results suggest that bacteriuria increase also the chance to develop hypertension.

Although more recent studies also found a correlation, only one prospective study has shown that bacteriuria is associated with the development of hypertension. In the above mentioned cohort study, a higher prevalence of hypertension in the bacteriuric group after 12 years of follow-up was found. However, the underlying mechanism of this finding is not clear. Hypertension is a lasting increase in blood pressure with a heterogeneous etiology consisting of both genetic and environmental factors. Patients share the inability to excrete sodium at a normal arterial pressure. If bacteriuria would lead to hypertension, the most attractive explanation would be that hypertension arises secondary to renal scarring caused by the (type 1 fimbriae of the) uropathogens. In the multivariate analysis, correction for creatinine did not change the results, but hypertension can occur before the reduction in creatinine clearance becomes apparent. An alternative explanation is that both bacteriuria and hypertension are found more frequently among individuals with comorbidity or that they share a same (currently unknown) cause. This is supported by the higher prevalence of bacteriuria among women who used antihypertensive drugs at baseline. Given the importance of hypertension the nature of this correlation needs to be studied in future studies.

## 4. ASB and renal function decline and hypertension in patients with DM

Women with DM have an increased prevalence of ASB, but also an increased risk on symptomatic UTI's and developing complications of UTI's such as renal abscesses. It was also shown that at short term follow-up treatment of ASB in women with DM did not appear to reduce complications. *E. coli* is the leading uropathogen in non-diabetic as well as in diabetic patients. Ninety percent of *E. coli* possesses type 1 fimbriae, the adhesive organelles found at the outer bacterial membrane. We have shown in vitro that type 1-fimbriated *E. coli* have an increased adherence to uroepithelial cells voided by women with DM. Others demonstrated that UTI's with type 1-fimbriated *E. coli* can lead to scar formation in the renal parenchyma of infected rats.At present, conclusive and prospective data with a long follow-up period directly relating ASB (with *E. coli*) to long-term risk of renal failure in diabetic patients are lacking. Taken together, we hypothesized that ASB in women with DM could lead to a faster decline in renal function, and decided to enlarge our cohort of diabetic women and to prolong the follow-up period. Besides the effects on renal function, we also studied the influence of ASB on the development of hypertension.

The association between ASB and renal function decline (and hypertension) in patients with DM was investigated in a prospective study with women with DM type 1 (n=296) and type 2 (n=348). All patients were interviewed and their medical records were reviewed at baseline and at study closure to collect all relevant information. All patients were asked to provide 1 or 2 midstream urine specimens. The women were followed up for a mean (SD) duration of 6.1 (1.9) years. Women with DM type 1 were younger, but had a longer duration of DM, than women with DM type 2. At baseline, 201 women with DM type 2 (58%) were treated with insulin only, 97 (28%) with oral hypoglycemic medication only, 41 (12%) with a combination of both, and five women (2%) were on a diet only (data were incomplete for 4 women). Because the Cockcroft-Gault formula for the estimation of the creatinine clearance includes age, adjusting for age in a multivariate model is not possible. Therefore patients were stratified into 3 age strata to assess the impact of age on the association between ASB and the (relative increase in the) creatinine clearance (respectively 18 to 36, 37 to 55, and 56 to 75 years old). All analyses were performed on the entire study population and on women with DM type 1 and DM type 2 separately.The prevalence of ASB was 17% in the study population, lower in women with type 1 DM (12%) compared to women with type 2 DM (21%), but multivariate analysis revealed that this was due to the difference in age. *E. coli* was cultured in 74 (67%) of the 110 women with ASB. Other isolated microorganisms included *enterococci (9%), group B streptococci (8%), Klebsiella pneumoniae (6%), Staphylococcus aureus (3%), Proteus mirabilis (2%), Enterobacter* species (2%). The prevalence of leukocyturia (5 or more leukocytes per high-power field) was 15% in women with ASB, suggesting that bacteria were present without resulting into an inflammatory response. The creatinine clearance decreased from 87 at baseline to 76 mL/min at study endpoint in diabetic women with ASB, and from 97 mL/min to 88 mL/min in those without ASB (Figure 2). In the univariate analysis, ASB was associated with a higher relative decrease in creatinine clearance (14 ± 22% and 9 ± 23% in women with versus women without ASB, respectively, p = 0.03), but not with the absolute decrease in creatinine clearance (12 ± 19 and 9 ± 20 mL/min, respectively, p = 0.12). Using univariate analysis, age, the length of follow-up, the duration of DM and microalbuminuria were identified as possible confounding factors when studying the influence of ASB on renal function development. Therefore, a multivariate analysis was done, according to age strata, and including the length of follow-up, duration of DM, and microalbuminuria at baseline. In the multivariate analysis no association was found between ASB and the relative or the absolute decrease in creatinine clearance. Also when women with DM type 1 and those with DM type 2 were analyzed separately, no association was found (data not shown). Finally, also no association with a faster decline in renal function was found when only the urines with *E. coli* as the cultured microorganism were included in the analysis

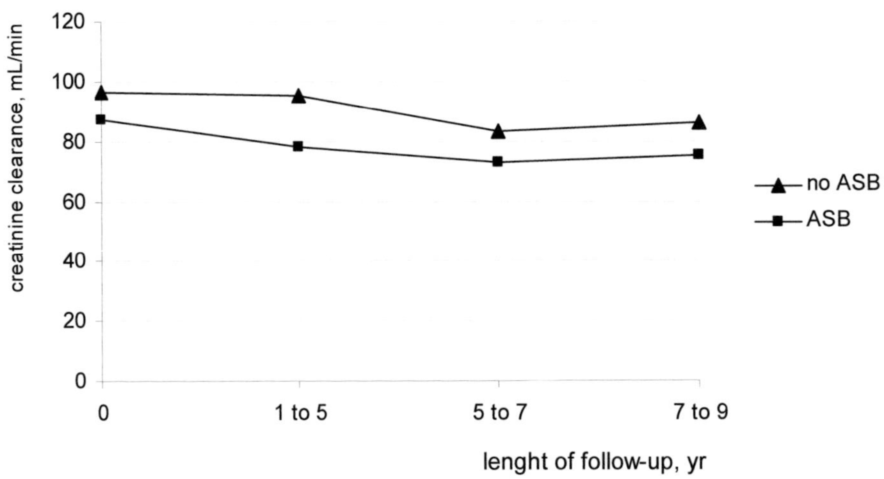


Fig. 2. Differences in creatinine clearance between women WITH DM with and without ASB. (Meiland R, Geerlings SE, Stolk RP, Netten PM, Schneeberger PM, Hoepelman AIM. Asymptomatic bacteriuria in women with diabetes mellitus. Arch Intern Med 2006; 166: 2222-7.)

Diabetic women with ASB developed hypertension more often than women without ASB (54% vs 37%; p=.045). However, in the multivariate analysis, including age, duration of DM, and length of follow-up, the association between ASB and hypertension disappeared (p>.20); a higher age was the strongest predictor for hypertension. In conclusion, in this prospective study after 6 years of follow-up, no association was found between ASB and a decline in renal function or the development of hypertension in women with type 1 DM or type 2 DM. As shown, women with ASB at baseline had a lower creatinine clearance at study end point, a faster relative decrease in creatinine clearance, and hypertension more often when compared univariately with women without ASB. However, the differences were mainly explained by differences in age and duration of DM, and all differences disappeared in the multivariate analyses.

Comparable results were found in a small Polish study (25 patients with DM, including both men and women), in which no differences in the incidence of hypertension and renal function decline were demonstrated between patients with and those without ASB after 14 years.

In a recent Canadian study it was investigated whether successive isolates of urinary *E. coli* from the same diabetic woman were genetically similar. It was shown that untreated diabetic women with ASB may carry a genetically unique *E. coli* strain for up to 13 months. Women who received treatment for ASB had bacteriuria for a shorter duration and carried a single strain of *E. coli* for a shorter period compared with women who did not receive treatment. However, treatment was followed by recurrent infections for most women, usually with a new strain of *E. coli*. The ASB-causing *E. coli* from diabetic women did not have virulence characteristics typical of UTI-causing strains. This non-virulent microorganism might be an explanation of the low number of patients who have also leukocyturia, as a result of the absence of a host response to this.

Because in the above mentioned prospective study no evidence was found that ASB in itself can lead to a decline in renal function, either in women with type 1 DM or in women with type 2 DM, it is not likely that treatment of ASB will lead to a decrease in the incidence of diabetic nephropathy. This is in accordance with a recent study of women with DM with ASB in which a comparison was made between women who received antibiotic therapy and women who received placebo. In that study, no difference was seen in serum creatinine levels after a mean follow-up of 2 years.

In conclusion, the hypothesis that ASB will lead to renal function deterioration in women with DM can be rejected because no difference in renal function development, in either women with type 1 DM or those with type 2 DM were found. Also, the incidence of hypertension was not increased when comparing women with ASB versus women without ASB. Therefore, at this time, screening and subsequent treatment for ASB are not indicated in patients with DM.

## 5. ASB in renal transplant recipients

It has been found that up to 50% of renal transplant recipients have ASB and UTIs. Many risk factors contribute to the high incidence of UTIs and ASB, which can undermine graft function and survival. In a retrospective study the impact of ASB on renal transplant outcome was analysed in 189 renal transplant recipients. Screening resulted into 298 episodes of ASB in 96 recipients (follow-up 36 months). Significant risk factors included female gender, glomerulonephritis as the disease that led to transplantation, and double renal transplant. There were no differences in serum creatinine, creatinine clearance, or proteinuria between patients with and without bacteriuria. The incidence of pyelonephritis in these patients was 7.6 episodes per 100 patient-years compared with 1.1 in those without ASB. A total of 2-5 ASB episodes were independent factors associated with pyelonephritis whereas more than 5 episodes was a factor associated with rejection. Studies show contradictory results whether antibiotic treatment results into a lower prevalence of ASB in these patients.

## 6. Conclusions

*E. coli* bacteriuria is not associated with a decline in renal function or the development of end-stage renal failure in a population of generally healthy adult women. However, *E. coli* bacteriuria may increase the risk of future hypertension, but the pathogenesis is not understood.

Women with DM (type 1 or type 2) with ASB do not have an increased risk for a faster decline in renal function or the development of hypertension. Therefore, screening and treatment of ASB in diabetic women is not warranted.

Since nearly all studies are performed in women, it is not possible to make conclusions about the association between ASB, renal function and hypertension in men.

No differences in renal function prognosis between patients with and without ASB following kidney transplantation were demonstrated. However, the incidence of pyelonephritis was much higher in the group of patients with ASB. Therefore, screening protocols may be beneficial in this group of patients.

## 7. References

Lindberg U, Claesson I, Hanson LA, Jodal U. Asymptomatic bacteriuria in schoolgirls. VIII. Clinical course during a 3-year follow-up. J Pediatr. 1978 Feb;92(2):194-9.

Meiland R, Stolk RP, Geerlings SE, Peeters PH, Grobbee DE, Coenjaerts FE, Brouwer EC, Hoepelman AI. Association between *Escherichia coli* bacteriuria and renal function in women: long-term follow-up. Arch Intern Med. 2007 Feb 12;167(3):253-7.

R Meiland, SE Geerlings, RP Stolk,.IM. Hoepelman, PHM Peeters, FEJ Coenjaerts, DE Grobbee. *Escherichia coli* bacteriuria in female adults is associated with the development of hypertension. International Journal of Infectious Diseases. 2010 April 14(4): e304-307.

Tencer J. Asymptomatic bacteriuria--a long-term study. Scand J Urol Nephrol. 1988;22(1):31-4.

Meiland R, Geerlings SE, Stolk RP, Netten PM, Schneeberger PM, Hoepelman AIM. Asymptomatic bacteriuria in women with diabetes mellitus. Arch Intern Med 2006;166:2222-7.

Semetkowska-Jurkiewicz E, Horoszek-Maziarz S, Galiński J, Manitius A, Krupa-Wojciechowska B. The clinical course of untreated asymptomatic bacteriuria in diabetic patients--14-year follow-up. Mater Med Pol. 1995 Jul-Sep;27(3):91-5.

Nicolle LE, Bradley S, Colgan R, Rice JC, Schaeffer A, Hooton TM. Infectious Diseases Society of America guidelines for the diagnosis and treatment of asymptomatic bacteriuria in adults. Clin Infect Dis. 2005;40(5):643-54.

Harding GK, Zhanel GG, Nicolle LE, Cheang M; Manitoba Diabetes Urinary Tract Infection Study Group. Antimicrobial treatment in diabetic women with asymptomatic bacteriuria. N Engl J Med. 2002 Nov 14;347(20):1576-83.

Dalal S, Nicolle L, Marrs CF, Zhang L, Harding G, Foxman B. Long-term *Escherichia coli* asymptomatic bacteriuria among women with diabetes mellitus. Clin Infect Dis. 2009 Aug 15;49(4):491-7.

Fiorante S, López-Medrano F, Lizasoain M, Lalueza A, Juan RS, Andrés A, Otero JR, Morales JM, Aguado JM. Systematic screening and treatment of asymptomatic bacteriuria in renal transplant recipients. Kidney Int. 2010 Oct;78(8):774-81. Epub 2010 Aug 18.

# 23

# Sleep Disorders Associated with Chronic Kidney Disease

Robert L. Benz[1], Mark R. Pressman[2] and Iqbal Masood[1]
[1]*Department of Nephrology*
[2]*Department of Sleep Medicine*
*Lankenau Medical Center and Lankenau Institute for Medical Research, Wynnewood, USA*

## 1. Introduction

Twenty-six million American adults have Chronic Kidney Disease (CKD). Chronic Kidney Disease is defined as kidney damage for 3 or more months with or without decreased GFR. Chronic Kidney Disease is divided into five stages, from Stage 1 to Stage 5. End-Stage renal disease is the 5$^{th}$ stage of CKD when dialysis is needed to sustain life. Sleep disorders are common and under recognized in advanced stages of Chronic Kidney Disease. Sleep disorders affect the quality of life and may also increase cardiovascular morbidity and mortality.

Subjective sleep complaints are reported by more than 50% of patients on Hemodialysis (HD) (1). Common organic sleep disorders in patients with CKD include Sleep Apnea Syndrome (SAS), Periodic Limb Movement Disorder (PLMD) and Restless Leg Syndrome (RLS). These disorders are more common in the dialysis population than in the general population. When dialysis patients with a sleep disorders were studied objectively in sleep laboratory, 53% to 75% were found to have sleep apnea, which is higher than general population (2-4%) (2). Sleep disorders in CKD patients have been linked to increased incidences of cardiovascular disease including coronary artery disease, left ventricular hypertrophy and hypertension. (3, 4, 5, 6). Heart disease is the major cause of death in patients with CKD (www.kidney.org). In fact most patients who have advanced CKD and are not on dialysis are more likely to die from heart disease before they start dialysis.

Daytime somnolence resulting from sleep disorders may lead to diminished quality of life and cognition (7, 8).PLMD is associated with increased mortality in patients with ESRD. (49). Early diagnosis and treatment may improve quality of life.

## 2. Subjective complaints in dialysis patients

Subjective sleep complaints are common in dialysis patients and include difficulty initiating and maintaining sleep, problems with restless, jerking legs, and/or day time sleepiness. Sleep disorders are very inconvenient for the patients and affect their activities of daily living. Most patients believe that relief of these symptoms would improve subjective quality of life. A large number of dialysis patients take sleep-inducing medications. Sleep complaints are more common in elderly patients on dialysis than in younger patients and male patients are more likely to have sleep complaints than women (10). Caucasian patients have a higher prevalence of restless legs syndrome than African American (1, 10). Subjective complaints are also high in patients with increased caffeine intake, pruritis, bone pain, cigarette use, and premature discontinuation of dialysis (1). As in general population, increased stress, anxiety, depression, and worry are also associated with poor subjective sleep quality in dialysis patients (10-12).

## 3. Factors contributing to sleep disturbances (Figure 1)

No consistent relationship has been detected between subjective sleep complaints of poor sleep and Blood Urea Nitrogen (BUN), Creatinine, or Kt/V (see glossary) (1, 11, & 13). Anemia has been associated with complaints of poor sleep with improvement after treatment with recombinant erythropoietin (14). Mild hypercalecmia has also been associated with increased frequency of subjective insomnia (15). Frequent napping during day time dialysis may also be a factor which contributes to fragmented sleep at night.

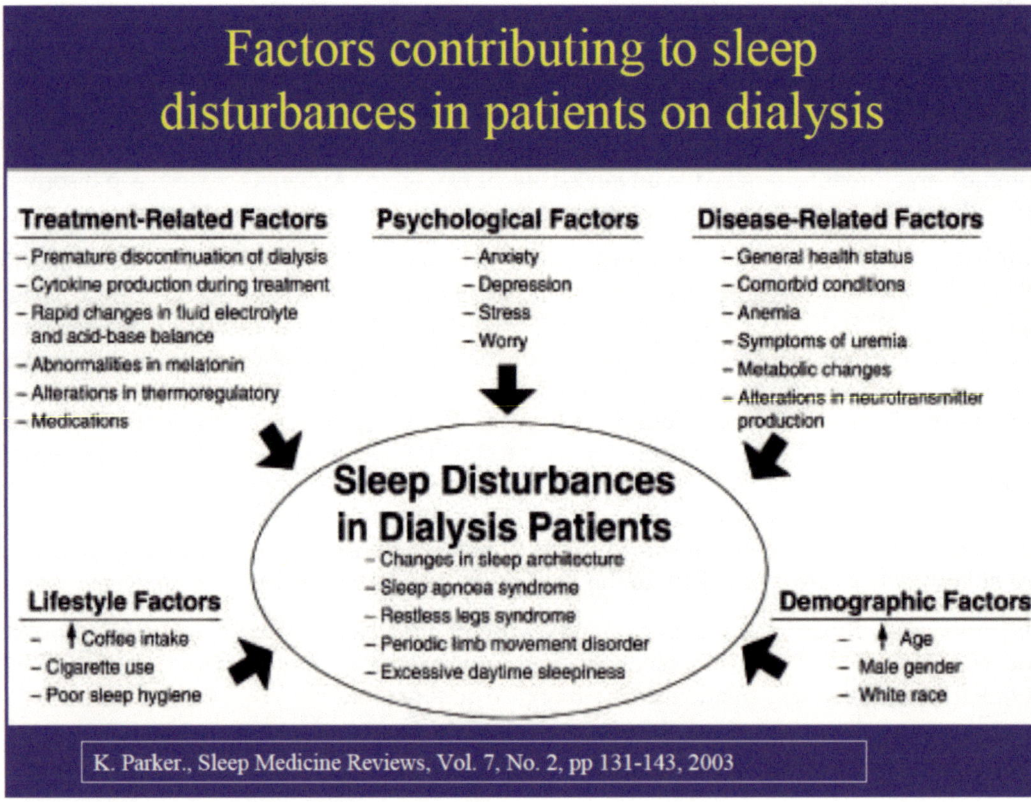


Fig. 1. Factors associated with sleep disturbances.

Nocturia, one of the earliest symptoms of kidney disease may also lead to reduced sleep due to frequent awakening. Untreated sleep apnea has also been linked to nocturia. Most of the awakenings attributed to nocturia by patients are attributable to sleep disorders, particularly sleep apnea (63).

## 4. Changes in sleep architecture

Nocturnal sleep of patients on dialysis is short and fragmented with total sleep time ranging between 260 and 360 minutes. Sleep efficiency is between 66% and 85% with a large amount of wakeful time (77-135 min), and numerous arousals (25-30/h of sleep) (16-18). Patients have increased patterns of Stage I and Stage II sleep, decreased slow wave (deep sleep), and REM sleep (17, 18). Thus dialysis patients have both reduced quantity and quality of sleep. Changes in sleep patterns in advanced CKD patients who are not on dialysis are similar to patients on dialysis (21)

## 5. Sleep Apnea Syndrome (SAS)

Sleep apnea is classified as obstructive (OSA) due to intermittent closure of the upper airway or central due to intermittent loss of respiratory drive or both (mixed). More than 50% of patients with ESRD have sleep apnea (7, 19). Prevalence appears to be similar in advanced CKD patients who are not on dialysis and those treated with peritoneal or hemodialysis (7, 20). Sleep Disordered Breathing (SDB) is observed with similar frequency in dialysis dependent and dialysis independent CKD patients. Sleep apnea in CKD patients is more frequently obstructive (21).

## 6. Pathogenesis-figure 2

Sleep apnea in patients with ESRD is mostly obstructive but several observers have reported features of both obstructive and central sleep apnea (16,31). Sleep apnea is caused by both impaired central ventilatory control and upper air way occlusion during sleep. Enhanced ventilatory sensitivity to hypercapnea correlates with apnea severity (22). Conversion from conventional Hemodialysis (CHD) to nocturnal Hemodialysis (NHD) has been associated with reduced severity of sleep apnea due to reduction in ventilatory sensitivity to hypercapnea(31). Upper airway occlusion can be caused by fluid overload and interstitial edema in the upper air way (23). Displacement of fluids from the lower limbs increases neck circumference and pharyngeal resistance and reduces upper air way cross sectional area, contributing to the pathogenesis of obstructive sleep apnea (OSA). Pharyngeal cross sectional area in patients on CHD was smaller than the control, suggesting that this may predispose to upper airway occlusion during sleep (22). Conversion from CHD to NHD is associated with an increase in pharyngeal cross sectional area, possibly due to improve fluid removal(31). Conversion from continuous ambulatory peritoneal dialysis (CAPD) to nocturnal peritoneal dialysis has been shown to reduce the frequency of sleep apnea (24). Upper airway dilator muscle dysfunction due to neuropathy or myopathy associated with chronic uremia or the underlying cause of renal disease such as diabetes mellitus can cause narrowing of pharyngeal muscles (31). There could also be some role for oxidative stress, inflammatory cytokines and middle molecules, all elevated in ESRD in the development of ventilatory instability and or upper airway occlusion, but this has not been established (66).

The apnea -hypopnea index (AHI) is an index used to assess the severity of sleep apnea based on the total number of complete cessations (apnea) and partial obstructions (hypopnea) of breathing occurring per hour of sleep found during polysomnography. Patients with advanced CKD not on dialysis who are non-diabetic are predisposed to more severe AHI as compared to patients with less advanced CKD (25). In patients with diabetes no such association was found probably due to the fact that diabetes itself may be an

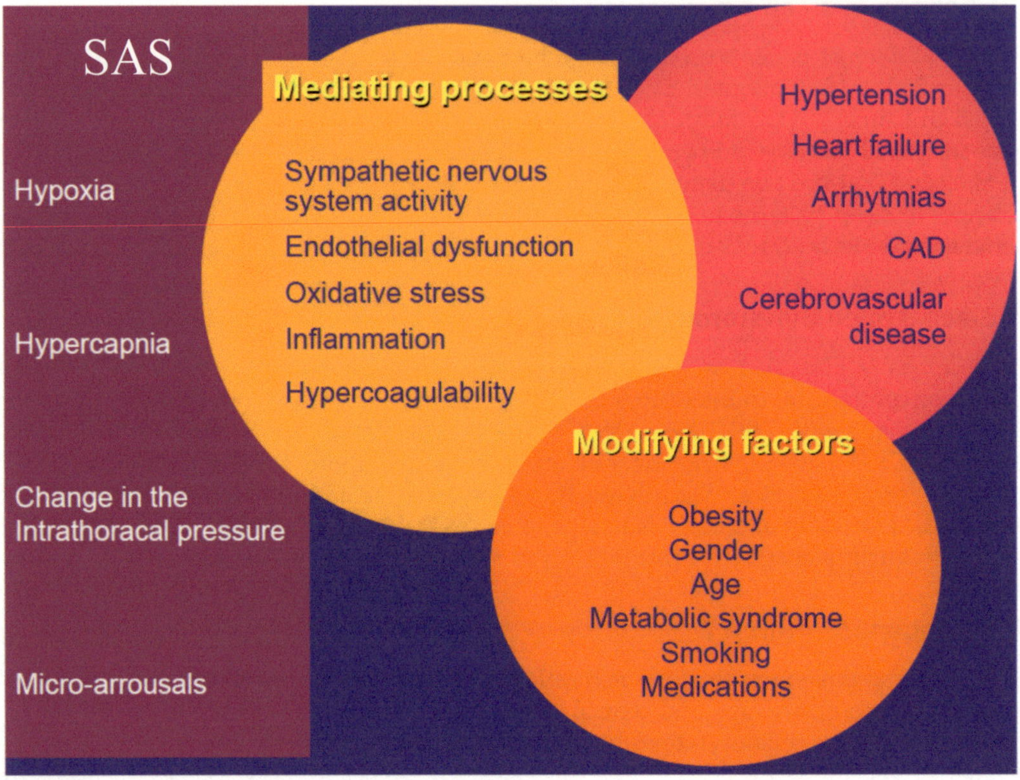


Fig. 2. Pathogenesis of sleep Apnea Syndrome (SAS).

overriding factor for the development of sleep apnea (25). It was also found that AHI index correlated weakly with urea level in all patients, but not with creatinine clearance.

Obesity is not required for ESRD patients to develop sleep apnea. Snoring is less intense in patients with CKD who have sleep apnea than in patients with sleep apnea with normal renal function (67).

## 7. Clinical significance

Sleep apnea worsens the symptoms of CKD such as daytime fatigue, sleepiness, and impaired neurocognitive function. Hypoxemia during sleep is associated with nocturnal hypertension, left ventricular hypertrophy, impaired sympathovagal balance, and increased risk of cardiovascular complications including death (68-69). Sleep apnea may exacerbate the infectious complications common in ESRD patients because sleep disruption and deprivation degrade immune function (26). Severe sleep apnea is an independent predictor of graft loss among female kidney transplant patients (27).

## 8. Diagnosis

Subjective sleepiness can be assessed with a number of simple scales, such as the Epworth Sleepiness Scale (ESS) or the Stanford Sleepiness Scale. The ESS is a self-administered questionnaire with 8 questions and is more commonly used. It provides a measure of a person's general level of daytime sleepiness, or their average sleep propensity in daily life .The ESS asks people to rate, on a 4-point scale (0 – 3), their usual chances of dozing off or falling asleep in 8 different situations or activities that most people engage in as part of their daily lives. The total ESS score is the sum of 8 item-scores and can range between 0 and 24.The higher the score, the higher the person's level of daytime sleepiness. Most people can answer the ESS, without assistance, in 2 or 3 minutes. (www.sleepfoundation.org).

Although the characteristic features of sleep apnea may be absent, a history of snoring, witnessed apnea during sleep, and day time sleepiness are suggestive of sleep apnea. Objective diagnostic testing includes home ambulatory monitoring which records air flow, snoring, respiratory movement, oxygen saturation, and heart rate.

Polysomnography (PSG), also known as a sleep study is a nocturnal, laboratory- test used in the diagnosis of Sleep Apnea Syndrome (SAS). It is often considered the standard for diagnosing OSAS, determining the severity of the disease, and evaluating various other sleep disorders that can exist with or without OSAS. PSG consists of a simultaneous recording of multiple physiologic parameters related to sleep and wakefulness. It generally includes monitoring of the patient's airflow through the nose and mouth, blood pressure, heartbeat as measured by an electrocardiograph, blood oxygen level,EEG wave patterns, eye movements(EOG), and the movements of respiratory muscles and limbs(EMG).

Polysomnography can be performed in a sleep laboratory or center and includes comprehensive monitoring of respiration, sleep stages and leg movements. Polysomnography is used to quantify the Apnea-Hypopnea Index (AHI). AHI is an index used to assess the severity of sleep apnea based on the total number of complete cessations (apnea) and partial obstructions (hypopnea) of breathing occurring per hour of sleep. These pauses in breathing must last for at least 10 seconds and be associated with a 3% or greater decrease in oxygenation of the blood. To determine AHI, add the total number of apnea events, plus hypopnea events and divide by the total number of minutes of actual sleep time, then multiply by 60.For example:

Apnea + Hypopnea divided by actual sleep time, then multiply by 60
200 apneas, 200 Hypopneas (400 Total Events)
420 Minutes Actual Sleep Time (7 hours x 60)
Divide 400 by 420 = .95 x 60 = 57 AHI (Severe OSA)

In general, the AHI can be used to classify the severity of disease (mild 5-15, moderate 16-30, and severe greater than 30).

Multiple Sleep Latency Test (MSLT) and the Maintenance of Wakefulness Test (MWT) can be considered for the evaluation of day time sleepiness. MSLT is used to measure the time elapsed from the start of a daytime nap period to the first signs of sleep, called sleep latency. The test is based on the idea that the sleepier people are, the faster they will fall asleep. The MWT is a daytime polysomnographic procedure which quantifies wake tendency by measuring the ability to remain awake during sleep conducive circumstances. The test isolates a person from factors that can influence sleep such as temperature, light, and noise. Furthermore, the patient is also advised to not take any hypnotics, drink alcohol, or smoke before or during the test. After allowing the patient to lie down on the bed, the time between lying down and falling asleep is measured and used to determine one's daytime sleepiness.

## 9. Treatment

Sleep apnea should be treated if the patient has symptoms such as fragmented sleep and day time sleepiness or significant oxygen desaturation. In patients without sleep related symptoms who have PSG suggestive of severe sleep apnea, consideration should be given to treat patients with severe disease (Apnea/hypopnea index >30), since sleep apnea of this severity has been associated with increased cardiovascular morbidity and mortality. Sleep apnea should also be treated if it is exacerbating co-existing medical condition such as hypertension, myocardial ischemia, and respiratory failure or nocturnal hypoxemia.

Management of sleep apnea includes treatment of any underlying medical conditions such as obesity or hypothyroidism, correction of aggravating factors such as use of alcohol or sedatives close to the bedtime. Continuous Positive Airway Pressure (CPAP) is a method of respiratory ventilation used primarily in the treatment of sleep apnea . The CPAP machine delivers a stream of compressed air via a hose to a nose mask, full-face mask, or hybrid, splinting the airway (keeping it open under air pressure) so that unobstructed breathing becomes possible, therefore reducing and/or preventing apneas and hypopnea. Pressman and Benz first reported in 1993 that CPAP improves both OSA and central apnea in ESRD patients, suggesting that CPAP eliminates the repetitive cyclical pattern of apnea followed by deep breathing, then followed by another central apnea.(28) The degree of hypopnea following apnea may be a function of the magnitude of respiratory drive necessary to overcome upper air way occlusion at the end of apnea. By preventing air way collapse, CPAP probably eliminates the deep breathing that results in hyperventilation and then lowered respiratory drive, thus setting the stage for next central sleep apnea. Also high levels of CPAP are successful in treatment of central sleep apnea due to the fact that central sleep apnea probably occurred following passive airway closure, which in turn caused stimulation of mucosal sensory receptors and reflex apnea. (28)

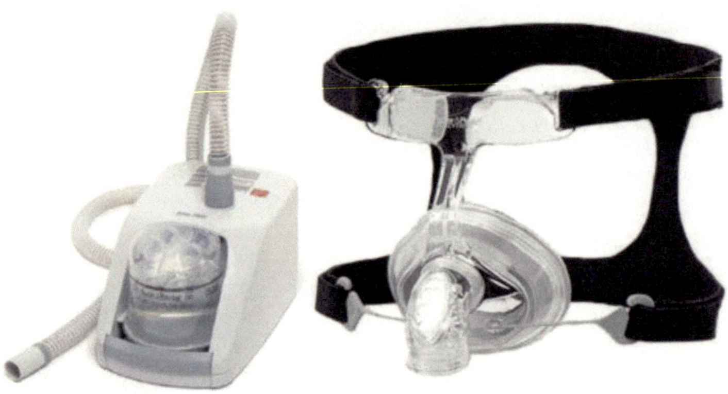

Fig. 3. CPAP Machine and Mask.

Sleep apnea is not corrected by conventional hemodialysis or peritoneal dialysis. Apnea frequency has been reduced by the use of bicarbonate rather than acetate based dialysate (29). Intensive daily dialysis has been shown to resolve sleep apnea in one critically ill patient (30). Nocturnal Hemodialysis(see glossary) that enables patients to receive hemodialysis 6-8 hours per night for 6 nights has been shown to improve sleep apnea (31). (Figure 4) Improvements are usually more significant in patients with more severe sleep apnea.

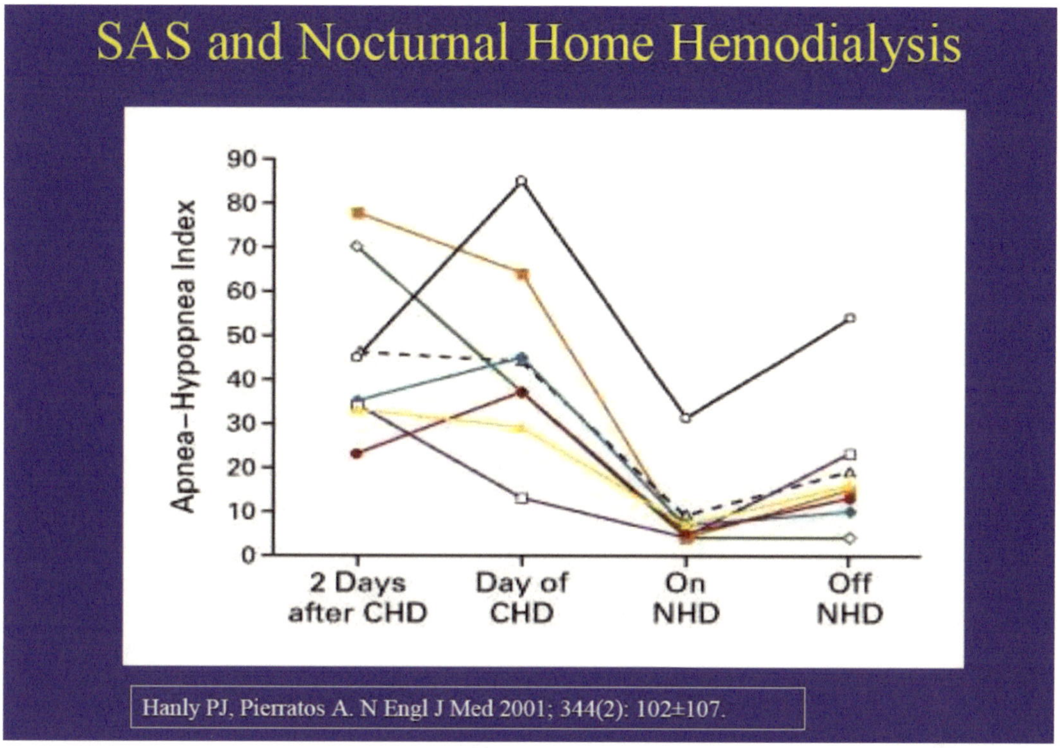


Fig. 4. Improvement of Sleep Apnea with Nocturnal Hemodialysis.

Although case reports have indicated correction of sleep apnea after successful kidney transplantation (32), preliminary results from case series suggest that sleep apnea resolves only in a minority of patients after kidney transplantation (33). The administration of branched chain amino acids has shown improvement in apnea index in one patient, although the mechanism and implications are not understood. (34).

## 10. Restless leg syndrome and periodic limb movement disorder

Restless leg syndrome (RLS) is a disorder characterized by sensation that usually occurs prior to sleep onset and causes an almost irresistible urge to move the legs, resulting in delayed sleep onset and disrupted sleep (35). RLS may be idiopathic or secondary to other conditions such as pregnancy, rheumatoid arthritis or uremia. Almost 80% of patients with RLS also have periodic limb movement disorder (PLMD), a condition characterized by episodic limb movements associated with nocturnal awakening and disrupted sleep.

RLS has been reported in 14-23% in patient on CHD and 20-57% in CKD patients (21, 36). The prevalence of PLMD is greater than 50% in CHD and CAPD(see glossary) population (1, 2, 35-38). RLS has also been reported to be 4.5% in transplanted patients. The prevalence of RLS is significantly lower in transplant patients than in patients on maintenance dialysis. Declining renal function is associated with increasing prevalence of RLS.

RLS and PMLD may be equally important as sleep apnea in patients with CKD. RLS severity score has been correlated to self perceived sleep problems, nocturnal awakening, delayed sleep onset latency, decreased total sleep time, increased use of sleep medications and self reported nocturnal leg movements (36). Polysomnographic studies of dialysis patients with RLS and or PLMD showed increase in sleep latency, Stage 1 and Stage 2 sleep, and decreased total sleep time and efficiency (38-41).

## 11. Pathophysiology

The pathophysiological mechanisms involved in RLS and PLMD are not very clear. Anemia, iron, and vitamin deficiencies, disturbance in peripheral and central nervous system (CNS) functioning and musculoskeletal abnormalities have all been proposed. It is likely that alteration of dopamine activity in the nervous system plays a role (42-43).

Correction of anemia by treatment with erythropoietin has been associated with reduction in the frequency of PLMD, improvement in sleep quality and day time alertness (44).Iron deficiency probably plays a dual role in that it causes anemia and is also a co-factor in the metabolism of dopamine in the brain. Treatment with intravenous iron is associated with a significant improvement in RLS and PLMD(45).Peripheral neuropathy, secondary to uremia or the underlying cause of renal disease such as diabetes may also predispose to develop RLS and or PLMD. Data regarding the clinical and laboratory correlation of RLS and PLMD is inconsistent. Higher predialysis urea and creatinine levels have been associated with increase RLS complaints in one study (1) but no relationship was detected in others (36, 41). Higher intact parathyroid hormone(PTH) levels has been found in dialysis patients with PLMD vs. those without the disorder(46), but lower levels have been noted in uremic patient with RLS in comparison without symptoms(47).

## 12. Diagnosis/Clinical significance

RLS is diagnosed clinically. PLMD is diagnosed objectively with polysomnography, which reveals periodic, involuntary movements of the legs during sleep.

PLMD can be identified on a polysomnogram by examining spiked activity coming from the electromyogram (EMG), which measures muscle movement during sleep. Specifically, anterior tibialis recording is usually sufficient in detecting the periodic limb movement episodes. Periodic limb movements typically last 0.5-5 seconds in duration and usually occurs approximately every 20-40seconds. The severity is described in terms of leg movement per hour of sleep (periodic limb movement index, PLMI). PLMI >5 is considered abnormal. Additionally, the examination of EEG test results will indicate micro-arousals, which can also lead to a diagnosis. PLMD can occur independently of RLS, and is more common with advancing age (35). RLS is almost always associated with PLMD, but PLMD can occur in the absence of RLS.

RLS is associated with difficulty initiating sleep, poor sleep quality, and impaired health quality of life (48) (FIGURE-5). RLS has been associated with depression. PLMD has been associated with increased mortality in patient with ESRD (49).

## 13. Treatment

General treatment measures include reducing potential exacerbating factors such as excess caffeine, alcohol, nicotine, medical conditions (anemia, iron deficiency), and medications

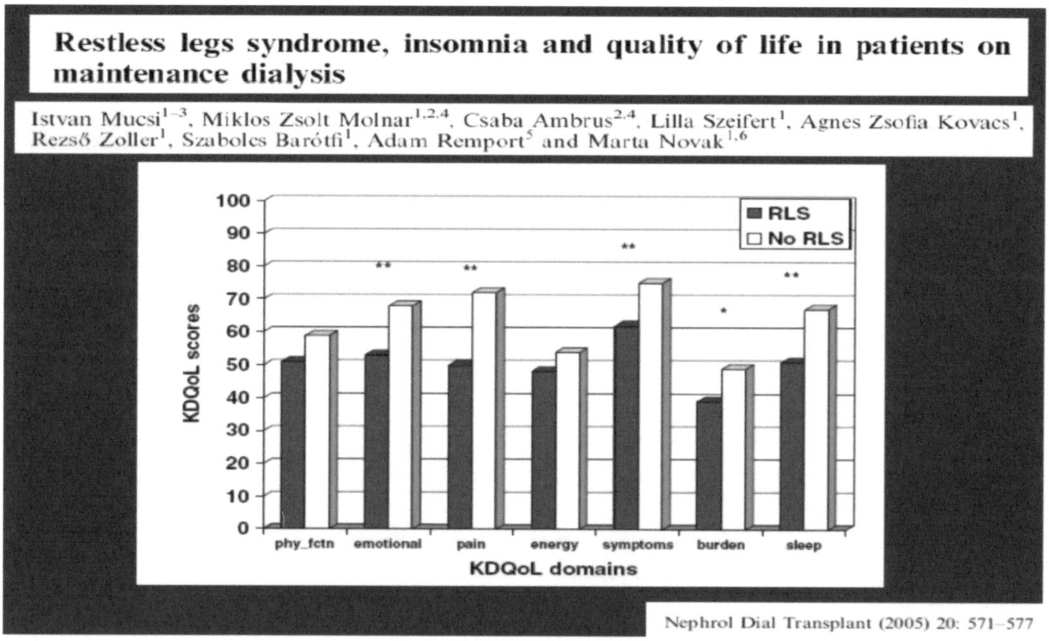


Fig. 5. RLS, Insomnia and quality of life in patients on maintenance dialysis.

(tricylcic antidepressants, Serotonin reuptake inhibitors, dopamine antagonists). Medical therapy includes L-Dopa and dopamine agonists such as pramipexole and ropirinole (64). These medications are favored over benzodiazepines. Gabapentin can also be used as alternative. The frequency of PLMD is not affected by switching from CHD to NHD (28). Kidney transplantation has been associated with an improvement in both RLS and PLMD in several small studies (50, 51).

## 14. Excessive day time sleepiness

Excessive day time sleepiness (EDS) has been described in dialysis patients. Seventy-seven percent of patients on CAPD reported taking day time naps and 51% reported falling asleep unintentionally (46). The **Multiple Sleep Latency Test** (MSLT) is a sleep disorder diagnostic tool. It is used to measure the time elapsed from the start of a daytime nap period to the first signs of sleep, called **sleep latency**. The test is based on the idea that the sleepier people are, the faster they will fall asleep. The test consists of four or five 20-minute nap opportunities that are scheduled about two hours apart. The test is often performed after an overnight sleep study. During the test, data such as the patient's, EEG, muscle activity, and eye movements are monitored and recorded. The entire test normally takes about 7 hours.In one study, 44 HD patients were studied. Potential subjects with other major chronic conditions or those with medications known to have CNS effects were excluded from the study. In addition, to exclude those with obvious causes of EDS, subjects with a history suggestive of SAS, RLS and PLMD were also excluded. All subjects underwent polysomnography along with MSLT. One third of patients of the subjects had MSLT scores consistent with abnormal sleepiness (mean sleep latency <8min). High AHI was significantly associated with lower MSLT score, but explained only 10% of the variance in MSLT score, suggesting that additional factors play an important role in the expression of day time sleepiness in this group (65).

Benz etal reported the effects of hematocrit normalization with recombinant erythropoietin on the sleep of 10 HD patients (44). All subjects underwent an initial nocturnal polysomnogram, with seven completing a 40 minutes MWT the next day. Tests were repeated after normalization of hematocrit. Treatment resulted in a significant reduction of nocturnal periodic limb movements and improvement on the MWT.

SAS, RLS and PLMD are prevalent in patients with advanced kidney disease and could explain EDS, but some studies suggested that other factors related to renal disease or its treatment may contribute to EDS (52, 53).

Mild elevations of BUN and creatinine in renal failure patients have been associated with increased slow wave activity in the waking EEG and abnormalities in cognitive function, which may explain the susceptibility of patients with advanced renal disease to sleepiness (54). Elevation of parathyroid hormone has been associated with increased waking EEG slow wave activity in uremic animals and stable dialysis patient (55). The metabolites of creatinine may inhibit GABA responses (in mouse neurons) and may interfere with neurotransmissions necessary for sleep to occur. These changes may destabilize the wakeful state by increasing day time sleepiness propensity and decreasing nocturnal sleep (56).

Treatment with dialysis may also predispose patients to sleepiness. Abnormal production of interleukin-1, TNF-alpha, factor S can increase somnolence (57, 58). Rapid removal of these sleep inducing substances has also been postulated as the cause for fragmented nocturnal sleep and resulting day time sleepiness and fatigue in one study on patients on CAPD (59). Dialysis also results in rapid change in electrolytes, acid base balance and serum osmolarity which may decrease arousal and alertness (60). Treatment with dialysis may also disrupt the circadian pattern sleepiness due to inappropriately timed elevation of serum melatonin in response to the hemoconcentration (61) or from change in rhythm of body temperature (62). Medications such as antihypertensive and antidepressants may also contribute to the EDS in CKD patients.

## 15. Summary

- Sleep complaints and disorders are common in patients with CKD whether on dialysis or not and are characterized by difficulty in initiating and maintaining sleep, restless/jerking legs, and daytime sleepiness.
- Polysomnographic studies have demonstrated that dialysis patients have overall decreased quantity and quality of sleep, suggesting that behavioral interventions such as sleep hygiene and the appropriate use of medications may be helpful.
- Most common sleep disorders in CKD patients include SAS, RLS, and PLMD.
- SAS has been effectively treated with CPAP in patients with chronic kidney disease and ESRD. Switching from CHD to NHD may also be useful.
- RLS and PLMD are also very common and are associated increased mortality in patients on dialysis. Treatments include correcting anemia, iron deficiency and dopamine agonists.

- Day time sleepiness is common in patients with ESRD and patients with CKD not on dialysis.
- Sleep disorders have negative impacts on overall quality of life in patients with kidney diseases and may affect rehabilitative potential of treatment.

## 16. Glossary of dialysis-related terms

**Blood Urea Nitrogen** (BUN) is the blood test used to measure nitrogen in the form of Urea, which is the by product from protein metabolism produced in liver and removed by kidney

**Dialysate**-the fluid used in dialysis, typically with a lower solute concentration than the blood, into which metabolic waste and excess electrolytes diffuse.

**Hemodialysis**(HD)-a process of removal of fluid and solutes through a semi-permeable membrane into dialysate by passing the blood through an artificial kidney. Hemodialysis is most commonly delivered to patients three times a week for three to four hours (Conventional Hemodialysis-CHD), but may also be given more slowly across the day or night (Nocturnal Hemodialysis-NHD).

**Nocturnal Hemodialysis** (NHD). Nocturnal hemodialysis or nightly hemodialysis is a form of hemodialysis which is done at home by the patient or a family member when the patient is sleeping at night. Most patients dialyze five to seven nights a week, anywhere from six to12 hours, on average for eight hours.

**Peritoneal Dialysis** (PD)-the process of removal of fluid and wastes from the body using the semi-permeable membrane of the peritoneum for the diffusion and osmosis,

**Continuous Ambulatory Peritoneal Dialysis** (CAPD)-continuous dialysis process that involves infusion of fluid into peritoneum, a prolonged dwell period for dialysis and drainage. The procedure typically involves four exchanges of fluid daily.

**Kt/V** is a way of measuring dialysis adequacy. Kt/V is defined as the dialyzer clearance of urea (**K**, obtained from the manufacturer in mL/min, and periodically measured and verified by the dialysis team) multiplied by the duration of the dialysis treatment (**t**, in minutes) divided by the volume of distribution of urea in the body (**V**, in mL), which is approximately equal to the total body water.

## 17. References

[1] Walker S, Fine A, Kryger MH. Sleep complaints are common in a dialysis unit. Am J Kidney Dis 1995; 26(5): 751±756

[2] Pressman MR, Benz RL. High incidence of sleep disorders in end stage renal disease. Sleep Research 1995; 24: 417.

[3] Jung, HH, Han, H & Lee, JH: sleep apnea, Coronary artery disease, and antioxidant status in hemodialysis patients, Am J kidney Dis, 45:875-82, 2005

[4] Zoccali, C, Mallamci, F, Tripepi, G & Benedetto, FA: Autonomic neuropathy is linked to nocturnal hypoxemia and to concentric hypertrophy and remodelling in dialysis patients, Nephrol Dial Transplant, 16:70-7, 200

[5] Zoccali, C, benedetto, FA, Tripepi, G, Cambareri, F, Panuccio, V, Candela, V, Mallamaci, F, Enia, G, labate, C& Tassone, F: Nocturnal hypoxemia, night day arterial pressure changes and left ventricular geometry in dialysis patients, Kidney Int, 53:1078-84, 1998

[6] Row, BW: Intermittent hypoxia and cognitive function: implication from chronic animal models. Adv Exp med Biol, 618:51-67, 2007

[7] Kimmel, PL, Miller, G & mendelson, WB:sleep apnea syndrome in chronic renal disease, Am J Med, 86:308-14, 1989

[8] Shayamsunder, AK, Patel, SS, Jain, V, peterson, RA & Kimmel, PL: Sleepiness, sleeplessness, and pain in end stage renal disease: distressing symptoms for patients, Semin Dial, 18:109-18, 2005

[9] Holley JL, Nespor S, rault R, Characterizing sleep disorders in chronic hemodialysis patients. ASAIO Trans 1991:37(3):M456-M457

[10] Kutner NG, Bliwise DL, Brogan D, Zhang R. Race and restless sleep complaint in older chronic dialysis patients and nondialysis community controls. J Gerontol B Psychol Sci Soc Sci 2001; 56(3): 170±175

[11] Holley JL, Nespor S, Rault R. A comparison of reported sleep disorders in patients on chronic hemodialysis and continuous peritoneal dialysis. Am J Kidney Dis 1992; 19(2): 156±161.

[12] Parker K. Dream content and subjective sleep quality in stable patients on chronic dialysis. ANNA J 1996; 23(2): 201±210.

[13] Puntriano M. The relationship between dialysis adequacies and sleep problems in hemodialysis patients. Anna J 1999;26(4): 405±407.

[14] Evans RW, Rader B, Manninen DL. The quality of life of hemodialysis recipients treated with recombinant human erythropoietin. Cooperative Multicenter EPO Clinical Trial Group [see comments]. JAMA 1990; 263(6): 825±830.

[15] Virga G, Stanic L, Mastrosimone S, Gastaldon F, da Porto A, Bonadonna A. Hypercalcemia and insomnia in hemodialysis patients. Nephron 2000; 85(1): 94±95

[16] Mendelson WB, Wadhwa NK, Greenberg HE, Gujavarty K, Bergofsky E. Effects of hemodialysis on sleep apnoea syndrome in end-stage renal disease. Clin Nephrol 1990; 33(5): 247±251.

[17] Wadhwa NK, Seliger M, Greenberg HE, Bergofsky E, Mendelson WB. Sleep related respiratory disorders in end-stage renal disease patients on peritoneal dialysis. Perit Dial Int 1992; 12(1): 51±56

[18] Hallett MD, Burden S, Stewart D, Mahony J, Farrell PC. Sleep apnoea in ESRD patients on HD and CAPD. Perit Dial Int 1996; 16 (Suppl. 1): S429±S433.

[19] Unruh MI, Sanders MH, Redline S, Piraino BM, Umans JG, Hammond TC, Sharief I, Punjabi NM, Newman AB:Sleep apnea in patient on conventional thrice -weekly hemodialysis comparison with matched controls from the sleep heart health Study, J Am Soc Nephrol 2006:17:3503-3509

[20] Wadhwa NK, Mendelson WB. A comparison of sleep-disordered respiration in ESRD patients receiving hemodialysis and peritoneal dialysis. Adv Perit Dial 1992;8:195–8.

[21] Nikolaos Markou, Maria Kanakaki, Pavlos Myrianthefs, Dimitrios Hadjiyanakos, Dimosthenis Vlassopoulos, Anastasios Damianos, Konstantinos Siamopoulos, Miltiadis Vasiliou and Stavros Konstantopoulos. Sleep-Disordered Breathing in Nondialyzed Patients with Chronic Renal Failure.Lung 2006;184:43-49
[22] Beecroft J, Duffin J, Pierratos A, et al. Enhanced chemo-responsiveness in patients with sleep apnoea and end-stage renal disease. Eur Respir J 2006;28:151–8.
[23] Anastassov GE, Trieger N. Edema in the upper airway in patients with obstructive sleep apnea syndrome. Oral Surg Oral Med Oral Pathol Oral Radiol Endod 1998;86:644–7.
[24] Tang SC, lam B, Lai AS, Pang CB, Tso WK, Khong PL, Ip MS, Lai KN:Alleviation of sleep apnea during nocturnal peritoneal dialysis is associated with reduced air way congestion and better uremic clearance. Clin J Am Soc Nephrol 2009;4:410-418
[25] Nicolaos M, Maria K etal. Sleep-Disordered Breathing in Nondialyzed Patients with ChronicRenal Failure: Lung (2006) 184:43–49
[26] Benca RM, Quintas J. Sleep and host defenses: a review. Sleep 1997;20:1027–37.
[27] Szentkiralyi A, Czira ME, Molnar MZ, Kovesdy CP etal. High risk of obstructive sleep apnea is a risk factor of death censored graft loss in kidney transplant recipients: an observational cohort study: Sleep Med. 2011 Mar;12(3):267-73. Epub 2011 Feb 2
[28] Pressman MR; Benz RL; Schleifer CR; Peterson DD: Sleep disordered breathing in ESRD: acute benfecial effects of treatment with nasal continous positive airway pressure. Kidney Int 1993 May;43(5):1134-9
[29] Jean G, Piperno D, Francois B, et al. Sleep apnea incidence in maintenance hemodialysis patients: influence of dialysate buffer. Nephron 1995;71: 138–42.
[30] Fein AM, Niederman MS, Imbriano L, et al. Reversal of sleep apnea in uremia by dialysis. Arch Intern Med 1987;147:1355–6.
[31] Hanly PJ, Pierratos A. Improvement of sleep apnea in patients with chronic renal failure who undergo nocturnal hemodialysis. N Engl J Med 2001;344(2):102–7.
[32] Langevin B, Fouque D, Leger P, et al. Sleep apnea syndrome and end-stage renal disease. Cure after renal transplantation. Chest 1993;103:1330–5
[33] Beecroft J, Zaltzman J, Prasad R, et al. Evaluation of sleep apnea in patients with chronic renal failure treated with kidney transplantation. Proc Am Thorac Soc 2006;3:A568.
[34] Soreide E, Skeie B, Kirvela O, Lynn R, Ginsberg N, Manner T et al. Branched-chain amino acid in chronic renal failure patients: respiratory and sleep effects. Kidney Int 1991; 40(3): 539±543.
[35] Sloand JA, Shelly MA, Feigin A, et al. A doubleblind, placebo-controlled trial of intravenous iron dextran therapy in patients with ESRD and restless legs syndrome. Am J Kidney Dis 2004; 43:663–70.
[36] Winkelman JW, Chertow GM, Lazarus JM. Restless legs syndrome in end-stage renal disease. Am J Kidney Dis 1996;28:372–8.
[37] Huiqi Q, Shan L, Mingcai Q. Restless legs syndrome (RLS) in uremic patients is related to the frequency of hemodialysis sessions. Nephron 2000;86:540.

[38] Miranda M, Araya F, Castillo JL, et al. Restless legs syndrome: a clinical study in adult general population and in uremic patients. Rev Med Chil 2001;129:179–86.

[39] Benz RL, Pressman MR, Hovick ET, et al. Potential novel predictors of mortality in end-stage renal disease patients with sleep disorders. Am J Kidney Dis 2000;35:1052–60

[40] Walker SL, Fine A, Kryger MH. L-DOPA/carbidopa for nocturnal movement disorders in uremia. Sleep 1996;19:214–8.

[41] Trenkwalder C, Stiasny K, Pollmacher T, et al. L-dopa therapy of uremic and idiopathic restless legs syndrome: a double-blind, crossover trial. Sleep 1995;18:681–8.

[42] Sateia MJ, editor. The international classification of sleep disorders. 2nd edition (Diagnostic andcoding manual). Westchester (PA): American Academy of Sleep Medicine; 2005. p. 178–82.

[43] Gigli GL, Adorati M, Dolso P, et al. Restless legs syndrome in end-stage renal disease. Sleep Med 2004;5:309–15

[44] Benz RL, Pressman MR, Hovick ET, et al. A preliminary study of the effects of correction of anemia with recombinant human erythropoietin therapy on sleep, sleep disorders, and daytime sleepiness in hemodialysis patients (The SLEEPO study). Am J Kidney Dis 1999;34:1089–95.

[45] Sloand JA, Shelly MA, Feigin A, et al. A doubleblind, placebo-controlled trial of intravenous iron dextran therapy in patients with ESRD and restless legs syndrome. Am J Kidney Dis 2004; 43:663–70.

[46] Stepanski E, Faber M, Zorick F, Basner R, Roth T. Sleep disorders in patients on continuous ambulatory peritoneal dialysis. J Am Soc Nephrol 1995; 6(2): 192±197

[47] Collado-Seidel V, Kohnen R, Samtleben W, Hillebrand GF, Oertel WH, Trenkwalder C. Clinical and biochemical findings in uremic patients with and without restless legs syndrome. Am J Kidney Dis 1998; 31(2): 324±328.

[48] Unruh ML, Levey AS, D'Ambrosio C, et al. Restless legs symptoms among incident dialysis patients: association with lower quality of life and shorter survival. Am J Kidney Dis 2004;43:900–9.

[49] Benz RL, Pressman MR, Hovick ET, et al. Potential novel predictors of mortality in end-stage renal disease patients with sleep disorders. Am J Kidney Dis 2000;35:1052–60

[50] Molnar MZ, Novak M, Ambrus C, et al. Restless legs syndrome in patients after renal transplantation. Am J Kidney Dis 2005;45:388–96.

[51] Winkelmann J, Stautner A, Samtleben W, et al. Long-term course of restless legs syndrome in dialysis patients after kidney transplantation. Mov Disord 2002;17:1072–6.

[52] Berry RB, Gleeson K. Respiratory arousal from sleep: mechanisms and significance. Sleep 1997; 20(8): 654±675.

[53] MacFarlane JG, Shahal B, Mously C, Moldofsky H. Periodic K-alpha sleep EEG activity and periodic limb movements during sleep: comparisons of clinical features and sleep parameters. Sleep 1996; 19(3): 200±204.

[54] Teschan PE, Bourne JR, Reed RB, Ward JW. Electrophysiological and neurobehavioral responses to therapy: the National Cooperative Dialysis Study. Kidney Int Suppl 1983(13): S58±S65.

[55] Goldstein DA, Feinstein EI, Chui LA, Pattabhiraman R, Massry SG. The relationship between the abnormalities in electroencephalogram and blood levels of parathyroid hormone in dialysis patients. J Clin Endocrinol Metab 1980; 51(1): 130±134.

[56] De Deyn PP, Macdonald RL. Guanidino compounds that are increased in cerebrospinal fluid and brain of uremic patients inhibit GABA and glycine responses on mouse neurons in cell culture [see comments]. Ann Neurol 1990; 28(5): 627±633.

[57] Lai KN, Lai KB, Lam CW, Chan TM, Li FK, Leung JC. Changes of cytokine profiles during peritonitis in patients on continuous ambulatory peritoneal dialysis. Am J Kidney Dis 2000; 35(4): 644±652.

[58] Rousseau Y, Haeffner-Cavaillon N, Poignet JL, Meyrier A, Carreno MP. In vivo intracellular cytokine production by leukocytes during haemodialysis. Cytokine 2000; 12(5): 506±517.

[59] Moldofsky H, Krueger JM, Walter J, Dinarello CA, Lue FA, Quance G et al. Sleep-promoting material extracted from peritoneal dialysate of patients with end-stage renal disease and insomnia. Peritoneal Dialysis Bulletin 1985 (July±September): 189±193.

[60] Plum F, Posner JB. Multifocal, diffuse, and metabolic brain diseases causing stupor or come. In: Plum FP, Posner JB, eds. The Diagnosis of Stupor and Coma. Philadelphia: F.A. Davis; 1985. pp. 177±303.

[61] Vaziri ND, Oveisi F, Reyes GA, Zhou XJ. Dysregulation of melatonin metabolism in chronic renal insuficiency: role of erythropoietin-deficiency anemia. Kidney Int 1996; 50(2): 653±656.

[62] Parker K, Bliwise D, Rye D. Hemodialysis disrupts basic sleep regulation: Hypothesis building. Nursing Research 2000; 49(6): 327±332.

[63] Pressman MR, Fiqueroa WG, etal. Nocturia. A rarely recognized symptom of sleep apnea and other occult sleep disorders: Arch Intern Med. 1996 Mar 11;156(5):545-50.

[64] R Allen et al. Ropinirole decreases periodic leg movements and improves sleep parameters in patients with restless legs syndrome. Sleep 2004 27: 907-914.

[65] Parker KP, Bliwise DL, Bailey JL, Rye DB, . Day time sleepiness in stable hemodialysis patients. Am J of Kid Dis 2003.41:394-402

[66] Patrick Hanley:Sleep Disorders and End-Stage Renal Disease.Sleep Med Clin 2(2007) 59-66

[67] Parker KP, Bliwise DL, Clinical comparison of hemodialysis and sleep apnea patients with excessive day time sleepiness.ANNA J 1997:24:663-665

[68] Zoccali C, Mallamaci F, Tripepi G& Benedetto FA:Autonomic neuropathy is linked to nocturnal hypoxemia and to concentric hypertrophy and remodelling in dialysis patients.Nephrol Dial Transplant 16:70-7, 2007

[69] Zoccali C, Benedetto FA, Tripepi G, Cambareri F etal.Nocturnal Hypoxemia, night-day arterial pressure changes and left ventricular geometry in dialysis patient.Kidney Int, 53:1078-84, 1998

# 24

# The Allo-Immunological Injury in Chronic Allograft Nephropathy

I. Enver Khan, Rubin Zhang, Eric E. Simon and L. Lee Hamm

*Tulane University School of Medicine, New Orleans, LA, USA*

## 1. Introduction

Progressive loss of renal allograft function after the first year of kidney transplant is often referred to as chronic rejection, transplant nephropathy, transplant glomerulopathy or chronic allograft nephropathy (CAN) and the use of these terms is often interchangeable. Clinically, it is usually diagnosed by a slowly rising serum creatinine level, increasing proteinuria and worsening hypertension (Zhang et al., 2004). CAN is the second most common cause of graft loss after the leading cause, death with a functioning graft (DWFG) (Zhang et al., 2004). According to estimates, 25-30% of patients currently awaiting kidney transplant have received a transplant before.

With the widespread usage of induction agents and the advancements in immunosuppressive medications, the first year outcomes after kidney transplant have shown steady improvement. In the United States, the incidence of acute rejection (AR) in the first year is below 10% (United States Renal Data System [USRDS]) while the unadjusted graft survival is 96%, 92% and 85% for living, deceased and extended criteria deceased donors respectively (Organ Procurement and Transplant Network/Scientific Registry of Transplant Recipients [OPTN/SRTR], 2008).

In the long term though, the survival of grafts has shown very little improvement over the past decade. The 5 year graft survival is reported at 81%, 71% and 55% for living, deceased and extended criteria deceased donors in the time interval of year 2000-2005. This, in comparison, is hardly different from the 79%, 68% and 51% reported in the interval of 1994-1999 (OPTN/SRTR, 2008). The median graft survival years for all kidney transplants, according to a report published in 2004 has changed little when comparing transplants performed in the years 1988 through 1995, ranging between 7.5 to 8.0 years. (Meier-Kriesche et al, 2004)

An overall shortage of organs and the high cost of providing any form of renal replacement therapy inclusive of a kidney transplant, calls for attention into making efforts for kidney transplants to last longer. This would entail looking into the pathological processes that result in the eventual failure of grafts, delineating as far as possible one process from the other, and examining immunological and non-immunological determinants that may be targeted with the eventual goal of adopting strategies that may help in prolonging the survival of renal allografts (Zhang et al, 2004). The non-immunological factors may include poor graft quality, ischemia and reperfusion injury, delayed graft function, recurrent or de novo kidney disease, hypertension, diabetes, obstruction, infection, renal artery stenosis and calcineurin inhibitor toxicity. It has been recently suggested that the autoimmunity may also contribute to the post-transplant allograft injury (Dinavahi et al., 2011; Porcheray et al., 2010; Vendrame et al.,2010). Here, we will focus our discussion on the allo-immunological injury, as this mechanism has been well established and its importance has been increasingly recognized in the pathogenesis of CAN.

## 2. Pathological classification

The 8th Banff Conference on Allograft Pathology, held in 2005 (Solez et al, 2007) focused on removing the term CAN as a pathological entity. This term was first used in 1991 when it replaced the term 'chronic rejection'. While it was successful in removing the notion that an immunologically mediated mechanism was in all instances the reason for the graft to slowly deteriorate, its use as a generic term came in the way of ascertaining a specific diagnosis and identification of the actual pathological process at play.

While the pathological findings of 'interstitial fibrosis and tubular atrophy' (IF/TA) are common in most instances of chronic allograft injury, other features can sometimes point towards the actual disease process. For example, arterial fibrointimal thickening with duplication of internal elastica (fibroelastosis), arteriolar and small artery hyalinosis, glomerulosclerosis, along with IF/TA can be a manifestation of chronic hypertension (Olson et al, 1998); hyaline arteriolar changes, sometimes with peripheral hyaline nodules, and IF/TA either in 'striped' ischemic or diffuse form can be secondary to calcineurin inhibitor (CNI) toxicity (Morozumi et al, 2004, Basauschina et al, 2004 and Mihatsch et al, 1995); IF/TA with relative glomerular sparing, dilated tubules, atubular glomeruli and intratubular Tamm-Horsfall protein casts with extravasation into the interstitium may suggest chronic obstruction (Klahr et al, 2003); IF/TA with chronic inflammation, intranuclear inclusions highlighted on immunostaining for the SV40 large T antigen can be due to BK virus infection (Drachenberg et al, 2005), a polyoma virus that may infect the tubular cells in immune suppressed patients. In other instances, recurrent or de novo vascular or glomerular diseases may lead to glomerulosclerosis along with IF/TA.

This leads to a new category of "interstitial fibrosis and tubular atrophy, no evidence of any specific etiology" to replace "CAN". There is further sub-categorization within the category of "IF/TA, no evidence of any specific etiology" and this is based on amount of interstitial fibrosis, and the degree of atrophy and loss of tubules. It is described as mild (Grade I), moderate (Grade II) and severe (Grade III) determined by <25%, 25-50% and >50% of the cortical area involved respectively (Salez et al, 2007). The pitfall to this classification is that the degree of IF/TA in a renal graft is yet to be shown to correlate with the prognosis and overall graft survival. This is therefore an area where protocol biopsies done at previously determined time intervals, and the correlation of these results with graft survival in the long term, will provide invaluable prognostic information.

In the same revision of the Banff criteria, there was also the introduction of the subcategories of 'chronic active antibody mediated rejection' and 'chronic active T-cell mediated rejection' within the categories of antibody mediated rejection (AMR) and T-cell mediated rejection respectively. These were introduced to highlight the features of arterial and capillary changes, believed to be pathognomonic of an immunologically mediated chronic allograft injury which would also have IF/TA, in other words identifying true chronic rejection. The need for introducing the subcategory of chronic antibody mediated rejection (CAMR) was based on the abundantly available literature that highlighted the presence of complement fragments (C4d) positivity (explained in more detail in Role of B cells and DSA) and the presence of anti-HLA antibodies in transplant patients correlating with the chronic failing of the allografts. When these are seen in the presence of pathological changes specific to an active process of AMR taking place, that subset of patients could be safely assumed to be undergoing an immunologically mediated, in specific humorally mediated reaction. The diagnostic criteria therefore for 'CAMR' are as follows;

Morphological features of duplication or 'double contours' in glomerular basement membranes, and/or peri-tubular capillary basement membrane multi-layering (PTCBMML) and/or IF/TA with or without PTC loss, and/or fibrous intimal thickening in arteries without duplication of the internal elastica

1. C4d deposition in the peri-tubular capillaries (PTC)
2. The presence of donor specific antibodies (DSA)

The pathological significance of these findings and their role in causing deterioration in graft function will be highlighted in the section "Role of B-cells and DSA" below. Transplant glomerulopathy of membrano-proliferative glomerular nephritis (MPGN) pattern should be distinguished from the immune complex-mediated MPGN that is frequently associated with hepatitis C infection or due to recurrent or de novo glomerular disease. They appear similar (MPGN) on light microscopy, but their distinction can be made by electron microscopy, as transplant glomerulopathy does not have immune-complex deposits on the glomerular basement membrane.

'Chronic active T-cell mediated rejection' is described as a subcategory of "T-cell mediated rejection" and it denotes the presence of chronic allograft arteriopathy with arterial intimal fibrosis along with mononuclear cell infiltration and fibrosis and the formation of neo-intima. These changes and their role will also be described in more detail in the section "Role of T-cell" below.

## 3. Role of T cells

The introduction of an "allograft" into an immunocompetent individual would typically result in a process of recognizing the graft tissue as foreign "allorecognition" and the initiation of what is known as an "alloresponse", invariably resulting in tissue inflammation, architectural distortion and infiltration by T-cells that are responsive to the graft resulting in loss of function and eventual failure of the graft, a process we call acute cellular rejection. This occurs after a number of steps taking place at the molecular and cellular level, steps that have been recognized and become the target of therapy in order to prevent rejection.

Allorecognition can occur by three well-described mechanisms referred to as direct, indirect and the semi direct pathways. (Safinia et al, 2010). In the direct pathway recipient T cells recognize intact allogeneic major histocompatibility complex or MHC-peptide complexes expressed by foreign cells, while in the indirect pathway T cells recognize peptides derived from allogeneic MHC proteins presented by antigen-presenting cell and finally the semi direct pathway where recipient dendritic cells acquire intact allogeneic MHC-peptide complexes from donor cells and present them to recipient T cells. (Harrera et al., 2004; Lechlar and Batchelar, 1982; Warrens et al., 1994). In the context of transplantation, while the direct and the indirect pathways are well recognized and understood, the semi-direct pathway is not known to be of clinical importance in allograft rejection. (Figure 1)

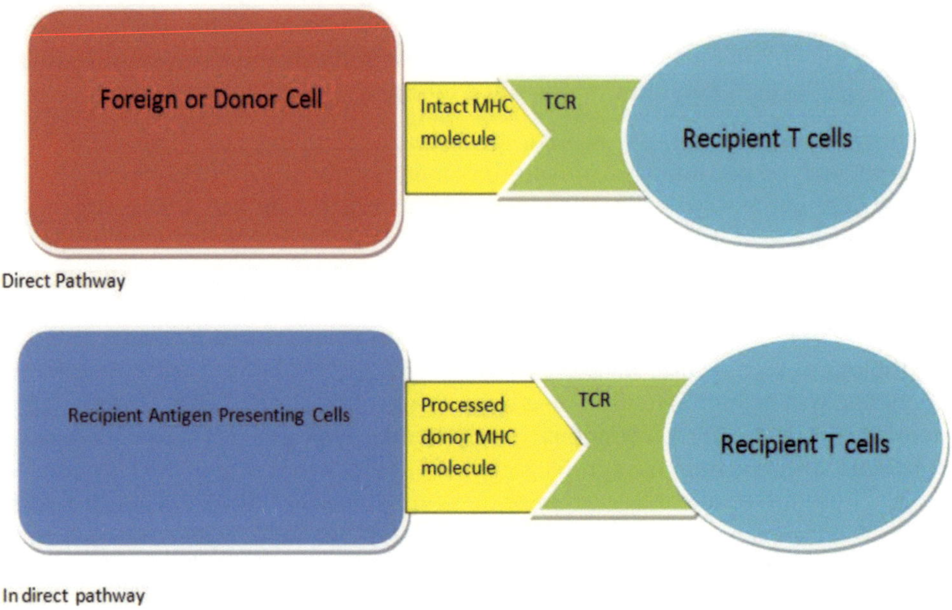


Fig. 1. Mechanism of antigen presentation in the direct and indirect pathways.

As far as the direct pathway is concerned, if the immunological milieu is left unaltered, a strong and effective alloresponse would follow primarily due to the very high number of recipient T-cells that will recognize the transplant tissue as foreign. Due to the nature of this mechanism, this pathway is of primary importance in the immediate post transplant period. T-cell depletion using various immunosuppressive regimens, including induction protocols, severely compromises this process. Another phenomenon observed is depletion of donor derived dendritic cells through apoptosis and elimination by recipient immune reactivity. This is also accompanied by a decline in the number of recipient T cells with direct antidonor allospecificity with time, most pronounced in the CD4+ CD45RO+ (memory) subset (Hornick et al, 1998). However, this decline in direct pathway responses with time is as pronounced in patients with chronic rejection as in those with stable graft function and this supports the view that the direct pathway of allorecognition is of little importance in the context of chronic graft failure.

As the direct pathway declines with time, recipient dendritic and other antigen presenting cells travel through the graft, picking up soluble MHC alloantigens or antigens derived from donor cells and present them to T-cells activating CD4 + and CD 8+ cells (the indirect pathway) (Auchincloss et al. , 1993; Kievits et al.,1991). The predominant antigen presentation is done through MHC-Class II cells which have an affinity towards the CD4+

T-cell subtype. The indirect alloresponse, while less rapid compared with the direct pathway, dominates reactivity to transplanted antigens in the long term. This is the main reason why, despite tolerance afforded by the direct pathway, immune suppression is required for as long as the graft remains viable. Any inflammation induces the expression of MHC class II molecules on endothelial and epithelial cells in the graft, conferring the ability to present antigen to CD4+ T cells (Bal et al., 1990).

Clinically, the activity of T-cells in renal allografts is represented by cellular rejection. The diagnosis is made by detecting tubulitis, interstitial infiltration and edema, and sometimes intimal arteritis. A grade is assigned depending on the severity of these lesions. The inflammatory activity of T-cells results in renal injury resulting in architectural distortion of the renal parenchyma. The Banff Classification for T-cell mediated rejection along with histological description of each category and sub category is described below.

### 3.1 T-cell mediated rejection

Acute T-cell mediated rejection (Type/Grade)

i. Significant tubular and interstitial infiltration (Figure 2)
ii. Intimal arteritis (vascular rejection) (Figure 3)
iii. Transmural arteritis and/or arterial fibrinoid change and necrosis of medial smooth muscle cells with accompanying lymphocytic inflammation (Figure 4)

Chronic T-cell mediated rejection

'Chronic allograft arteriopathy' (arterial intimal fibrosis with mononuclear cell infiltration in fibrosis, formation of neo-intima)

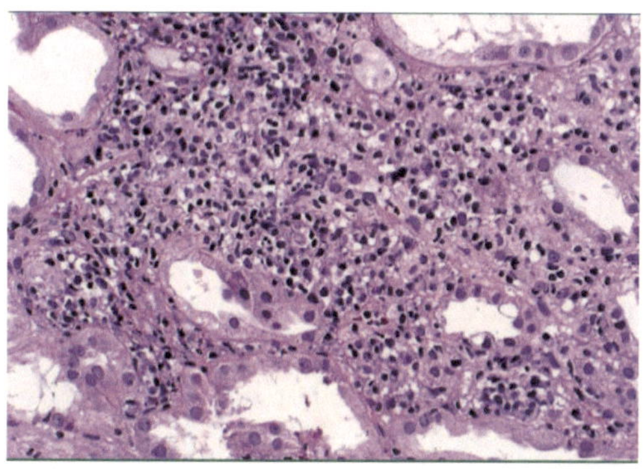

Fig. 2. Infiltration of tubules and interstitium with T cells (*Courtesy of Suzanne Meleg-Smith, MD.*)

## 4. Role of B cells and DSA

Based on the principles of immunology, B cells are known to play vital roles, from antigen presentation, immune regulation, to their most characteristic role of differentiating into plasma cells that secrete antibodies. The secretion of antibodies and their role in the pathogenesis of CAN is what makes B cells of great clinical significance in the long term survival of the renal graft.

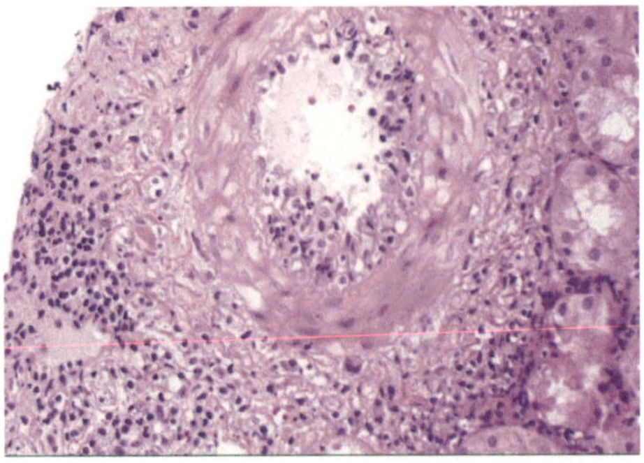

Fig. 3. Infiltration of arterial intima with T cells (*Courtesy of Suzanne Meleg-Smith, MD.*)

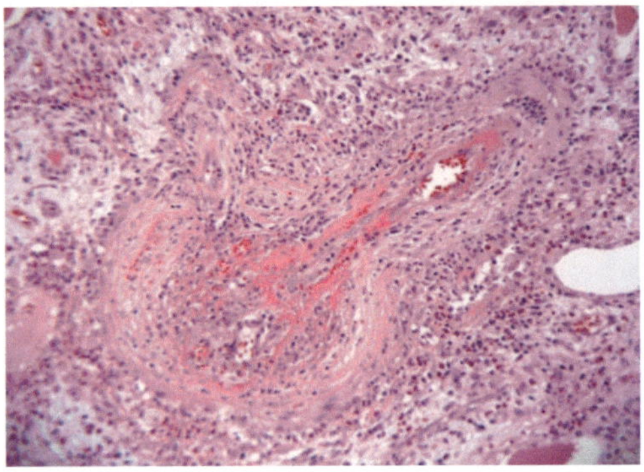

Fig. 4. Fibrinoid necrosis of arterial wall and transmural infiltration of T cells (*Courtesy of Suzanne Meleg-Smith, MD.*)

The association between graft dysfunction with antibodies produced against donor human leukocyte antigens (HLA) has long been recognized (Jeannet et al., 1970; Terasaki et al. 2007). Their role in acute AMR is well defined and they have been popularly referred to as DSA. Their pathogenesis became evident with the discovery of deposition of complement fragments (C4d) along peritubular capillaries (PTC) in grafts of patients suffering from graft dysfunction and known to have circulating DSAs (Feuch et al., 1991). (Figure 5)

In the context of CAN, arteriopathy or glomerulopathy in the transplanted kidney is also linked to C4d deposition in the PTCs and to DSAs (Mauiyyedi et al., 2001). The pattern of renal injury in these circumstances was further elaborated with the evidence that when chronic failure occurs in the renal allograft and circulating DSAs are present along with C4d deposition in the PTCs, capillaritis and basement membrane multi-lamination was seen (Regele et al.,2002). Other features described and attributed to this pathology include duplication of the glomerular basement membrane, mononuclear cell infiltration in the glomeruli and the PTCs along with loss of normal glomerular capillary endothelial fenestrations (Colvin et al. 2006). With well-described morphological features, along with association of DSA and C4d deposition, "chronic antibody mediated rejection (CAMR)" gained its place in the revision of the BANFF classification in 2005 (Solez et al., 2007). The presence of proteinuria is not pathognomonic but can be seen and graft function may seem quite stable for years. While the pathogenesis is strongly linked to circulating DSAs, prior sensitization or an episode of acute AMR are not essential pre-requisites. Instead, DSAs may develop slowly and sub clinically, and eventually lead to the dysfunction of the allograft mediated by a slow inflammatory process.

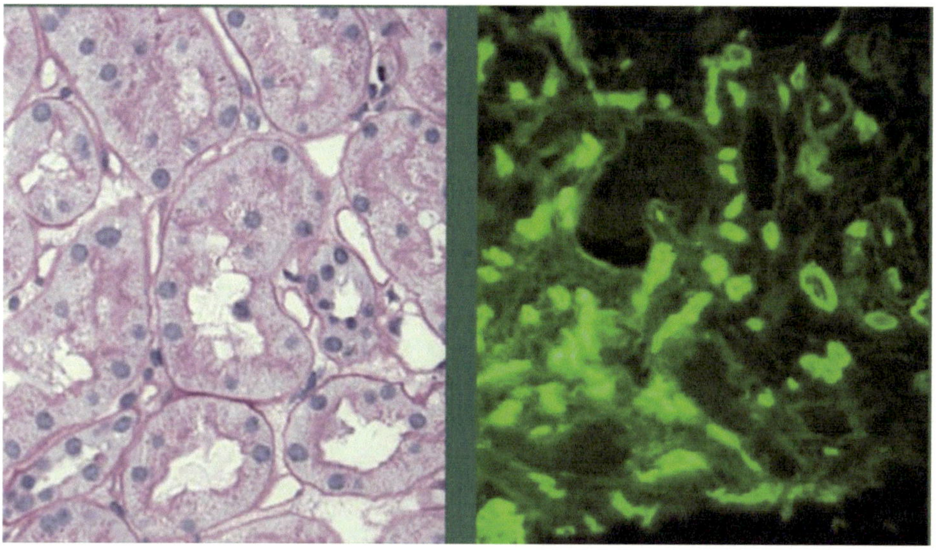

Fig. 5. Peritubular capillary deposition of C4d (right) in acute antibody mediated rejection.(*Courtesy of Suzanne Meleg-Smith, MD.*)

With the development of a diagnostic criterion for CAMR, many of the pathological findings that had known to exist have been tied in and explain the underlying mechanism of renal injury. However, there are few caveats that still make the accurate recognition of this clinical entity challenging.

One factor is that under certain circumstances, C4d deposition might not be seen. This could happen when the DSAs induce damage via a non-complement fixing mechanism (Collins et al., 2008). Further, in advanced stages of CAMR, when tubular atrophy has already developed, it may well be hard to recognize positive C4d staining. Conversely, when typical changes such as PTC multi-lamination are seen in the absence of C4d deposition and circulating DSA, there could be a possibility of another diagnosis such as chronic or resolving thrombotic micro-angiopathy or these lesions could be assumed to be from a previous episode of acute antibody-mediated injury.Laboratory studies have demonstrated that complement, although relied on in order to make a clinical diagnosis, is not necessary in the pathogenesis of CAMR. Induction of DSAs that are non-complement fixing can have the same pathological changes as DSA that fix complement. Also, in animals that are selectively deficient in C3 (RAG1 -/-), introduction of complement fixing antibodies results in similar pathological changes and poor outcomes of the graft (Jin et al. 2005). What has been found to have a more pronounced role in the development of allograft arteriopathy characteristic of CAMR, is a host of changes in the endothelium brought about by the infiltration of natural killer (NK) cells that express FcγRIII, which is a receptor for the Fc (Fragment crystallizable) or the constant region of antibodies. Hence it is believed that in the pathogenesis of CAN mediated by circulating DSAs, NK cells have much more of a role than complement (Hirohasha et al., 2008).

Yet another phenomenon observed in the context of circulating antibodies is that sometimes, there may be no evidence of graft destruction at all, even with varying degree of C4d deposition. This process, termed accommodation, has been the focus of research in recent years, with a wealth of insight provided by transplantation of organs across the barrier of ABO incompatibility. Though anti-A or B isoagglutinin reappear after transplant, they can co-exist without precipitating rejection (Gonzalez-Strawinski et al., 2008). Interestingly, C4d deposition can be observed but, compatible with other observations, does not necessarily mean that CAMR is taking place. Understanding the mechanism by which the graft attains this ability to remain "non-reactive" despite the presence of antibodies circulating against it is of great interest as it can be therapeutically mimicked when DSAs are known to exist that would otherwise lead to an immunologically mediated rejection of the graft. Accommodated grafts have been found to have changes in the cells of the endothelium and that are believed to help in the adaptation to the presence of antibodies. These changes include increased expression of bcl-xL, (Salama et al. 2001), increased muc-1 expression (Park et al. 2003) and increase in the expression of indolamine-2,3-dioxygenase (Minnei et al., 2008) in the glomerular and PTC endothelium.

In conclusion, CAMR occurs slowly, with the first step being the development of DSA, followed by an immunological reaction that *may* result in the deposition of C4d, the resultant development of visible pathological changes characteristic of CAMR and then eventual graft loss. The speed at which these events occur is variable and the challenge is not just limited to the difficulty in diagnosis, but also in terms of therapy. In the future, the main strategies to counteract the risk for CAMR will be focused on screening for the development of new DSA, following the titers of known DSAs and correlating them with the function of the transplanted kidney. Also, as we learn more about the adaptive capabilities that lead to accommodation, strategies will likely be developed to mimic them in vivo to prolong the renal graft survival.

## 5. Acute and sub-acute rejection

Many studies have pointed out that the long term outcomes of transplanted kidneys that underwent episodes of AR are inferior compared to those that did not. The long term outcomes are even worse if the episodes of rejection have been multiple or if the acute rejection occurs late, usually meaning more than 6 months after the transplant. The obvious correlation here is that many times, non-compliance with immunosuppressive medications would be a confounding factor. What is also an obvious factor is that each episode of rejection leaves the transplanted organ with progressively increasing amounts of interstitial fibrosis and tubular atrophy with a cumulative effect of functional decline, eventually resulting in organ failure.

However, the incidence of AR has markedly declined, with the actual incidence within the first year being less than 10% (USRDS, 2008). This decrease has not translated into an improvement in the overall graft survival or the median survival time of renal allografts. An explanation to this phenomenon may be that even when there is no acute allograft dysfunction in terms of worsening creatinine clearance, proteinuria or hypertension, there is an ongoing inflammatory infiltration that leads to structural damage and eventual scarring of the renal parenchyma, termed as subclinical rejection. This entity is usually discovered by protocol biopsies, which are not performed in a cross-sectional manner. This means that an inflammatory response, which is not very severe, but in most cases chronic does occur and over time results in graft loss. There has been a clear demonstration that subclinical rejection leads to an early development of CAN and graft loss particularly if there is coexisting interstitial fibrosis and tubular atrophy (Cosio et al, 2005; Nankivell et al., 2004, Moreso et al., 2006; Shishido et al., 2003; Veronese et al. 2004). It is also important to stress that while there may not be a significant functional deterioration at the time sub-clinical rejection is diagnosed, many times the actual injury as demonstrated by protocol biopsies may be of high grade. One study categorized the results of a cohort of protocol biopsies and revealed that 1 out of 3 of these cases has interstitial acute rejection Grade 1 and 2 out of 3 were classified as borderline changes (Nankivell et al., 2004). There has also been a repeated demonstration that the degree of infiltration seen in protocol biopsies revealing subclinical rejection has correlated to the degree of HLA incompatibility further proving that this infiltration is driven by an immunological phenomenon. There are instances when there is clear histological demonstration of infiltration in the renal parenchyma with no rise in serum creatinine implying that there is no functional decline. This further elaborates the unreliability and underestimation of renal dysfunction offered by measuring serum creatinine level (Kaplan et al., 2003; Levey et al., 1999).

This raises the question of whether protocol biopsies should be performed on a regular interval. While some studies have demonstrated a clear benefit in terms of a decreased incidence of AR and lower serum creatinine at two years after the kidney transplant (Rush et al., 1998), there have been other studies that indicate that treatment of subclinical infiltration on the basis of a protocol biopsy may not have significant improvement in the long term and may further expose the patient to increased amounts of immunosuppression and further the risk of CNI toxicity. Therefore, with the currently existing data, most centers do not perform protocol biopsies on all patients; however, experts do recommend performing protocol biopsies on at least some of the patients that are considered high risk where an inflammatory infiltrate likely means a clinical rejection. If left untreated, it will likely result in an accelerated course towards CAN and the eventual loss of function of the allograft.

## 6. Degree of HLA mismatch

Three pairs of human leukocyte antigens (HLA) loci A, B and DR are traditionally used for organ allocation. They exist on chromosome 6 with both alleles inherited from either parent are co-expressed, resulting in any individual having 6 antigens. There is tremendous amount of variation in the actual antigen that is coded by each of these loci among individuals as this gene exhibits what is known as polymorphism. With advances in molecular biology more than 230 polymorphisms have been identified for HLA-A, more than 470 for HLA-B and more than 380 for HLA-DR. Their relevance stems from the fact that these antigens are expressed on the surface of all cells and are the major barrier to transplantation. Because of the way our immunological system is designed, the recognition of self versus foreign antigens is mediated through these HLA antigens. Hence when foreign tissue is introduced to the immune system of a host and it is recognized as foreign, it is due to lack of tolerance that the host has developed towards its own variety of HLA antigens.

As these antigens are carried on fixed loci, their inheritance follows a Mendelian pattern, and a combination of HLA-A, B and DR is inherited by an individual from both parents.

Hence, when identical twins or siblings, who have the same HLA antigens donate to each other, the survival is superior compared to randomly matched cadaveric donors, with an intermediate level of graft survival seen when parents or genetically non-identical siblings donate where one of the haplotypes are matched. In population based programs, which rely predominantly on cadaveric donation, finding single or double haplotype match is obviously not very common. The goal is to find a donor and recipient combination that has zero to minimum mismatches, meaning the least amount of HLA antigens expressed on the surface of donor cells that are not present in the recipient. There has also been recognition of the fact that there are some HLA mismatches that are more significant than others, for example having a DR mismatch is now known to be much more detrimental to graft survival than having a mismatch of the A and B antigens (Coupel et al., 2003; Opelz 1985).

In the earlier years of transplantation, having HLA mismatches led to a high incidence of early rejection and eventual graft failure. With the modern and more potent immunosuppressive agents used today, such episodes are rare in the first year. However, despite the immune suppression and the low incidence of AR in the first year, the long term survival of grafts from well matched (6 antigen match or zero mismatch) donors have a longer survival than from those who are not as well matched and according to recent analysis of the national database in the United States (OPTN/SRTR, 2008) this effect is seen in living donors and deceased donors of both extended and non-extended criteria. Despite the above stated evidence pointing towards better survival among well matched organ allocation, only 13% of the organs allocated in the US are well matched. (Takemoto et al., 2000). The main reasons are that despite the large numbers of people on the waiting list, well matched organs are difficult to find. When they are found, the absolute match may be in a different part of the country. If organ allocation is done by HLA only, not considering geographical location, the cold-ischemia time increases as the organ is transported. As the cold-ischemia time increases, chances of delayed graft function increase and overall it negatively affects outcomes and costs. According to an analysis, the added advantage of a zero mismatch is lost once the cold-ischemia time exceeds 36 hours (Lee et al., 2000).

Exposure to foreign antigens whether in the form of organ donation, blood transfusion and in the case of women, through child birth, leads to development of antibodies that are reactive towards these antigens, a process referred to as "sensitization". A measure known as the Panel Reactive Antibodies (PRA) estimates the degree of sensitization that a potential recipient has and this reflects the likelihood of having difficulty finding an organ to which the recipient does not have preformed antibodies against. Pre-existing DSA or developing de-novo DSA in the post-transplant period predisposes the recipient to develop AMR. Even if there is no overt episode of AMR clinically, the graft survival is still poor, which is explained by development of transplant glomerulopathy from CAMR.

Strategies to prevent CAN due to HLA incompatibility include matching donors and recipients with minimal mismatches, cross matching to ensure that there is no DSA. If DSA are present, various desensitization protocols utilizing intravenous immunoglobulin and plasmapheresis can be used to decrease the likelihood of AMR. In the post transplant period, a watchful evaluation of kidney function with close monitoring of serum markers as well as urinalysis should be kept to recognize early development of AMR and CAMR. The threshold to evaluate renal dysfunction with kidney biopsy should be low in patients at increased risk of rejection due to HLA incompatibility. In the outset, patients who are likely to be in need of kidney transplantation should be transfused with caution during their course of CKD as well as when they are on renal replacement therapy to keep sensitization at minimum.

## 7. Gender

Due to lack of the Y chromosome in women, antigens coded for by the Y chromosome are recognized as foreign when organ transplantation occurs from a male donor to a female recipient (McGee et al., 2010, 2011). While this does not manifest immunologically as strongly as HLA incompatibility, it does have an effect of having shorter graft survival when an organ is taken from a male donor and transplanted to a female recipient (McGee et al., 2010). This effect is more strongly noted among bone marrow transplants, but is also present to some degree in solid organ transplants such as the kidney (Gratwohl et al., 2008). The decreased survival of male to female donation compared to female to male donation is seen despite the fact that in most instances a higher nephron mass of a male donor kidney is transplanted into a smaller body of a female recipient.

## 8. Summary

The significant improvement in the short-term graft survival has not transformed into a much better long-term graft survival. CAN is an important cause of graft loss and it represents a complex process culminating immunological and non-immunological injuries. The occurrences of overt acute rejections, either cellular, humoral or both, in the early stage driven by allo-immunity can have an important bearing on the long term immunological milieu that prevails and hence influences the graft survival. Sub-clinical rejection and/ or chronic rejection from inadequate immunosuppression are frequently undiagnosed and untreated. Persistent DSA or de novo development of DSA after kidney transplant is increasingly recognized as an independent and detrimental factor for transplant glomerulopathy. Other than allo-reactivity, there are emerging data suggesting that the pre-existing or de novo developing autoimmunity, mediated by either auto-antibodies and/or autoreactive T cells, may also cause post-transplant allograft injury (Dinavahi et al., 2011; Porcheray et al., 2010; Vendrame et al.,2010). Therefore, to appropriately identify and address the actual disease process, knowledge of the ongoing pathogenesis is needed in order to improve the long-term graft survival. From allo-immunological standpoint, it may include optimizing HLA match, avoiding sensitization, timely detecting and treating AR episodes, and maintaining adequate levels of immunosuppression to prevent the development of DSA, sub clinical rejection and chronic rejection of allografts.

## 9. References

Auchincloss H, Lee R, Shea S et al. (1993). The role of 'indirect' recognition in initiating rejection of skin grafts from major histocompatibility complex class II-deficient mice. *ProcNatlAcadSci USA*; Vol. 90, pp. 3373–3377

Bal V, McIndoe A, Denton G et al. (1990). Antigen presentation by keratinocytes induces tolerance in human T cells. *Eur J Immunol*; Vol. 20, pp. 1893–1897

Busauschina A, Schnuelle P, van der Woude FJ. (2004) Cyclosporine nephrotoxicity. *Transplant Proc*; Vol. 36 (Suppl 2S), pp. 229S–233S

Collins AB, Farris AB, Smith RN et al. (2008). Pitfalls in the diagnosis of chronic antibody mediated rejection: loss of peritubular capillaries, wide spectrum and transient nature of C4d deposition. *Am J Transplant*; Vol. 86 (Suppl), pp. 188–189

Colvin RB, Nickeleit V. (2006).Renal transplant pathology, In: *Heptinstall's Pathology of the Kidney, 6thedn, vol. 2.*Jennette JC, Olson JL, Schwartz MM, Silva FG (eds). pp 1347-1490,Lippincott-Raven, Philadelphia

Cosio FG, Grande JP, Wadei H et al.(2005). Predicting subsequent decline in kidney allograft function from early surveillance biopsies. *Am J Transplant*; Vol. 5, pp. 2464–2472

Coupel S, Giral-Classe M, Karam G, et al. (2003) Ten-year survival of second kidney transplants: impact of immunologic factors and renal function at 12 months. *Kidney Int*; Vol. 64, pp. 674-680

Dinavahi R, George A, Tretin A, et al. (2011). Antibodies reactive to non-HLA antigens in transplant glomerulopathy. *Journal of the American Society of Nephrology*;Vol. 22, pp. 1168-78

Drachenberg CB, Hirsch HH, Papadimitriou JC. (2005) Polyoma virus disease in renal transplantation: Review of pathological findings and diagnostic methods. *Hum Pathol*; Vol. 36, pp. 1245–1255

Feucht HE, Felber E, Gokel MJ et al. (1991). Vascular deposition of complement split products in kidney allografts with cell-mediated rejection. *CliniExpImmunol*; Vol. 86, pp. 464–470

Gonzalez-Stawinski GV, Tan CD, Smedira NG et al. (2008). Decay-accelerating factor expression may provide immunoprotection against antibody mediated cardiac allograft rejection. *J Heart Lung Transplant*; Vol. 27, pp. 357–361

Gratwohl A, Döhler B, Stern M, Opelz G. (2008). H-Y as a minor histocompatibility antigen in kidney transplantation: a retrospective cohort study. *Lancet*; Vol. 372, pp. 49-53

Herrera OB, Golshayan D, Tibbott R et al. (2004) A novel pathway of alloantigen presentation by dendritic cells. *J Immunol*; Vol. 173, pp. 4828–4837

Hirohashi T, Uehara S, Chase C et al. (2008). One possible mechanism of antibody mediated, complement independent transplant arteriopathy in mice. *Am J Transplant*; Vol. 86(Suppl), pp. 112–113

Hornick PI, Mason PD, Yacoub MH et al. (1998) Assessment of the contribution that direct allorecognition makes to the progression of chronic cardiac transplant rejection in humans. *Circulation*; Vol. 97, pp. 1257–1263.

Jeannet M, Pinn VW, Flax MH et al. (1970). Humoral antibodies in renal allotransplantation in man. *N Engl J Med*; Vol. 282, pp. 111–117.

Jin YP, Jindra PT, Gong KW et al. (2005). Anti-HLA class I antibodies activate endothelial cells and promote chronic rejection. Transplantation 2005; Vol. 79, pp. S19–S21

Kaplan B, Schold J, Meier-Kriesche HU. (2003). Poor predictive value of serum creatinine for renal allograft loss. *Am J Transplant*; Vol. 3, pp. 1560–1565

Kievits F, Ivanyi P. (1991). A subpopulation of mouse cytotoxic T lymphocytes recognizes allogeneic H-2 class I antigens in the context of other H-2 class I molecules. *J Exp Med*; Vol. 174, pp. 15–19

Klahr S, Morrissey J. (2003). Obstructive nephropathy and renal fibrosis: The role of bone morphogenic protein-7 and hepatocyte growth factor. *Kidney IntSuppl*; Vol.87, pp. S105–S112

Lechler RI, Batchelor JR. (1982). Restoration of immunogenicity to passenger cell-depleted kidney allografts by the addition of donor strain dendritic cells. *J Exp Med*; Vol. 155, pp. 31–41

Lee CM, Carter JT, Alfrey EJ, et al. (2000). Prolonged cold ischemia time obviates the benefits of 0 HLA mismatches in renal transplantation. *Arch Surg*; Vol. 135, pp. 1016-1019

Levey AS, Bosch JP, Lewis JB et al. (1999). A more accurate method to estimate glomerular filtration rate from serum creatinine: a new prediction equation. Modification of Diet in Renal Disease Study Group. *Ann Intern Med*; Vol. 130: pp. 461–470

Mauiyyedi S, Pelle PD, Saidman S et al. (2001). Chronic humoral rejection: identification of antibody-mediated chronic renal allograft rejection by C4d deposits in peritubular capillaries. *J Am SocNephrol*; Vol. 12,pp. 574–582

McGee J, Magnus JH, Zhang R,et al (2011). Race and Gender are not Independent Risk Factors of Allograft Loss after Kidney Transplantation. American Journal of Surgery; Vol .201, pp.463-467.

McGee J, Magnus JH, Islam T, et al (2010). Donor-Recipient Gender and Size Mismatch Impacts Graft Success after Kidney Transplantation. *Journal of American College of Surgeon*; Vol. 210, pp. 718-25

Meier-Kriesche HU, Schold JD, Kaplan B. (2004) Long-term renal allograft survival: Have we made significant progress or is it time to rethink our analytic and therapeutic strategies? *A J Transplant*; Vol.4, pp. 1289-1295

Mihatsch MJ, Ryffel B, Gudat F. (1995). The differential diagnosis between rejection and cyclosporine toxicity. *Kidney Int*; Vol.48 (Suppl 52) pp. S63–S69

Moreso F, Ibernon M, Goma M et al. (2006). Subclinical rejection associated with chronic allograft nephropathy in protocol biopsies as a risk factor for late graft loss. *Am J Transplant*; Vol.6, pp. 747–752.

Morozumi K, Taheda A, Uchida K, Mihatsch MJ. (2004). Cyclosporine nephrotoxicity: How does it affect renal allograft function and transplant morphology? *Transplant Proc*; Vol. 36 (Suppl 2S), pp.251S–256S

Nankivell BJ, Borrows RJ, Fung CL et al. (2004). Natural history, risk factors, and impact of subclinical rejection in kidney transplantation. *Transplantation*; Vol. 78,pp.242–249.

Olson JL. (1998). Hypertension: Essential and secondary forms. In: *Heptinstall's Pathology of the Kidney, 5th Ed.*Jennette JC, Olson JL, Schwartz MM, Silva FG, eds. pp. 943–1002, Lippincott-Raven, Philadelphia

Opelz G. (1985). Correlation of HLA matching with kidney graft survival in patients with or without cyclosporine treatment. *Transplantation*; Vol. 40, pp. 240-243

OPTN/SRTR Annual Report 2008

Park WD, Grande JP, Ninova D et al. (2003). Accommodation in ABO incompatible kidney allografts, a novel mechanism of self-protection against antibody-mediated injury. *Am J Transplant*; Vol 3, pp. 952–960

Porcheray F, DeVito J, Yeap BY, et al. (2010). Chronic humoral rejection of human kidney allografts associates with broad autoantibody responses. *Transplantation*; 89:1239-46.

Regele H, Bohmig GA, Habicht A et al. (2002). Capillary deposition of complement split product C4d in renal allografts is associated with basement membrane injury in peritubular and glomerular capillaries: a contribution of humoral immunity to chronic allograft rejection. *J Am SocNephrol*; Vol. 13, pp. 2371–2380

Rush D, Nickerson P, Gough J et al. (1998). Beneficial effects of treatment of early subclinical rejection: a randomized study. *J Am SocNephrol*; Vol. 9, pp. 2129–2134

Safinia N, Afzali B, Atalar K, Lombardi G, Lechler RI. (2010). T-cell alloimmunity and chronic allograft dysfunction. *Kidney Int;* Vol. 78 (Suppl 119) pp. S2–S12

Salama AD, Delikouras A, Pusey CD et al. (2001). Transplantaccommodation in highly sensitized patients: a potential role for Bcl-xL and alloantibody. *Am J Transplant;* Vol. 1, pp. 260–269

Shishido S, Asanuma H, Nakai H et al. (2003). The impact of repeated subclinical acute rejection on the progression of chronic allograft nephropathy. *J Am SocNephrol;* Vol. 14, pp. 1046–1052

Solez, K, Colvin, RB, Racusen, LC, et al. (2007). Banff '05 Meeting Report: differential diagnosis of chronic allograft injury and elimination of chronic allograft nephropathy ('CAN'). *Am J Transplant;* Vol. 7, pp. 518-526

Takemoto SK, Terasaki PI, Gjertson DW, Cecka JM. (2000). Twelve years' experience with national sharing of HLA-matched cadaveric kidneys for transplantation. *N Engl J Med;* Vol. 343, pp. 1078-1084

Terasaki PI, Ozawa M, Castro R. (2007). Four-year follow-up of a prospective trial of HLA and MICA antibodies on kidney graft survival. *Am J Transplant;* Vol. 7, pp. 408–415

Vendrame F, Pileggi A, Laughlin E, et al. (2010). Recurrence of type 1 diabetes after simultaneous pancreas-kidney transplantation, despite immunosuppression, is associated with autoantibodies and pathogenic autoreactive CD4 T-cells. *Diabetes;*Vol. 59, pp. 947-57

Veronese FV, Noronha IL, Manfro RC et al. (2004). Prevalence and immunohistochemical findings of subclinical kidney allograft rejection and its association with graft outcome.*Clin Transplant;* Vol. 18, pp. 357–364

Warrens AN, Lombardi G, Lechler RI. (1994). Presentation and recognition of major and minor histocompatibility antigens. *TranspIImmunol;* Vol. 2, pp. 103–107

www.USRDS.com(Accessed June 15, 2011)

Zhang R, Kumar P, Ramcharan T, et al. (2004). Kidney Transplantation: the evolving challenges. *American Journal of Medical Sciences;* Vol. 328, pp. 156-61.

# 25

# Prevention and Regression of Chronic Kidney Disease and Hypertension

Hiroyuki Sasamura
*Department of Internal Medicine, School of Medicine, Keio University*
*Japan*

## 1. Introduction

Chronic kidney disease (CKD) is a disease which is characterized by the presence of renal damage or decreased GFR for at least 3 months. The prevalence of CKD in the US has been reported to be 3.3% (stage 1), 3.0% (stage 2), 4.3% (stage 3), 0.2% (stage 4), and 0.1% (stage 5) (Levey et al., 2003; 2002). Because of the increasing elderly population in industrial countries, the development of new strategies for the prevention and regression of CKD is important.

Clinical studies have suggested that renin-angiotensin system (RAS) inhibitors can exert a renoprotective effect independent of blood pressure, and attenuate the progression of renal dysfunction (Bakris, 2010; Berl, 2009; Stojiljkovic et al., 2007). Recent studies have suggested that the use of RAS inhibitors, when combined with other treatment modalities such as aggressive blood pressure control, lowering of blood lipids, tight glucose control for diabetics, and lifestyle changes may cause remission of albuminuria, and stablization or even reversal of the decline in GFR, i.e. regression of CKD in some patients (Aros et al., 2002; Macconi, ; Ruggenenti et al., 2008).

These early clinical findings are important, because they suggest that appropriate interventions may be effective for causing an improvement in renal function, which raises the hope that a 'cure' for CKD may eventually be found in the future. In our laboratory, we have been examining the molecular mechanisms involved in the pathogenesis of CKD and hypertension. Our underlying concept is that both these diseases are highly related, and share common pathophysiological mechanisms, including the abnormal accumulation of extracellular matrix proteins in the kidney. The result is glomerulosclerosis, when the matrix accumulates in the renal glomeruli, and renal arteriolosclerosis, when the matrix is deposited in the renal arterioles and small vessels. In this chapter, we will review the evidence from our and other laboratories that these processes may be reversed in animal models, and possibly in humans.

### 2.1 Studies on CKD prevention

Regardless of the initial injury, most causes of CKD (including diabetic nephropathy, and chronic glomerulonephritis) share several common pathological features, one of which is the development of glomerular scarring or glomerulosclerosis.

| Stage | Description | GFR |
|---|---|---|
| 1 | Kidney damage with normal or ↑GFR | ≧ 90 |
| 2 | Kidney damage with mild ↓GFR | 60-89 |
| 3 | Moderate ↓GFR | 30-59 |
| 4 | Severe ↓GFR | 15-29 |
| 5 | Kidney failure | <15 or dialysis |

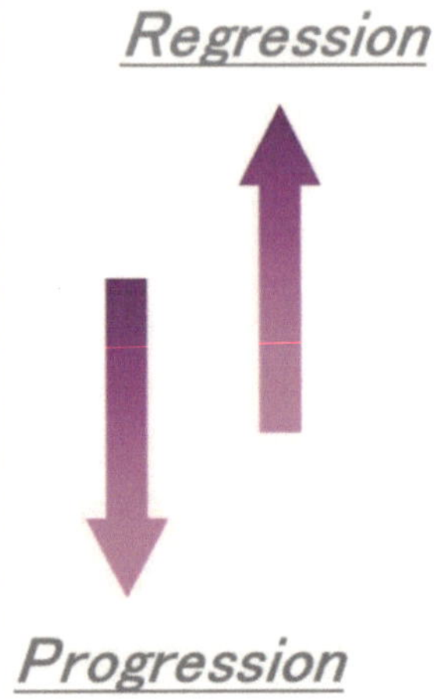


Fig. 1. Relationship between progression and regression of chronic kidney disease.

Glomerulosclerosis occurs because of the excessive deposition of components of the extracellular matrix (ECM) in the glomeruli, resulting in changes in glomerular integrity and albuminuria. This process is triggered by increased synthesis of ECM components, and decreased degradation of ECM components, resulting in net accumulation of ECM (Ma et al., 2007). It is thought that, once renal function declines below a 'point of no return', the decline in glomerular function continues inexorably due to the continuous accumulation of ECM and progression of glomerulosclerosis. Glomerular hypertension has been suggested to play an important role in this process, because the decrease in glomerular filtration leads to a compensatory increase in glomerular hypertension, resulting in a vicious cycle which causes progression of glomerular injury and loss of renal function (Neuringer et al., 1992).

Because of the progressive nature of CKD, one of the optimum strategies for reducing CKD would be to find interventions to prevent new-onset CKD. Multiple clinical studies have shown that the use of RAS inhibitors in patients with and without diabetes can cause a decline in the progression of CKD, which may be mediated, at least in part, by a blood pressure-independent mechanism (Bakris, 2010; Berl, 2009; Stojiljkovic et al., 2007). More recently, several studies have suggested that the use of RAS inhibitors may also be effective in preventing new-onset CKD, especially in patients with diabetes. In particular, Ruggenenti et al. showed in the BENEDICT trial that, in hypertensive patients with type 2 diabetes and no microalbuminuria at baseline, the angiotensin-converting enzyme (ACE) inhibitor trandolapril significantly decreased the risk of developing microalbuminuria compared with conventional therapy (Ruggenenti et al., 2008) . Similarly, in the recent ROADMAP study, the use of the ARB olmesartan was associated with a delayed onset of microalbuminuria (Haller et al.) . These results are important, because they suggest that diabetic nephropathy can be prevented or at least delayed by appropriate intervention (Remuzzi et al., 2006).

At present, it is unclear from clinical studies whether these measures may be effective for prevention of new-onset CKD in non-diabetic patients. However, the data from animal studies are encouraging, and suggest that early intervention with a RAS inhibitor may be effective for the prevention of renal injury due to hypertension (Ishiguro et al., 2007; Nakaya et al., 2001), salt-loading (Nakaya et al., 2002), or irradiation (Moulder et al., 1996).

### 2.2 Studies on CKD regression

Although it has been widely accepted that established sclerosis is irreversible, recent studies have emerged to challenge this concept and to focus on developing new therapies to cause regression or reversal of established glomerulosclerosis (Ma et al., 2007), (Ruggenenti et al., 2001). In particular, studies have suggested that treatment with high-dose RAS inhibitor may be effective in causing regression of glomerular lesions in animal models (Ma et al., 2005), (Teles et al., 2009), (Macconi et al., 2009).

Recently, we reported that transient treatment with an angiotensin receptor blocker (ARB) at a 50-100 times the normal dose in rodents causes regression of glomerulosclerosis in mice (Hayashi et al., 2010). In this study, the effects of treatment with different doses of ARB on established lesions of glomerulosclerosis were examined in the adriamycin nephropathy model, with a focus on whether the regression was sustained after cessation of the ARB treatment. Furthermore, the involvement of matrix metalloproteinase (MMP)-2 in the mechanism of glomerulosclerosis regression were examined both in vitro and in vivo, using a non-specific MMP inhibitor (doxycycline), and knockout (KO) mice with targeted deletion of MMP-2.

The principal findings of the study are shown in Fig. 2. and Fig. 3. It was found that transient treatment for two weeks with the ARB candesartan caused a regression of established glomerulosclerosis, which was clearly evident with the high doses of ARB and was sustained 6 months after cessation of all treatments. Moreover, the ARB treatment

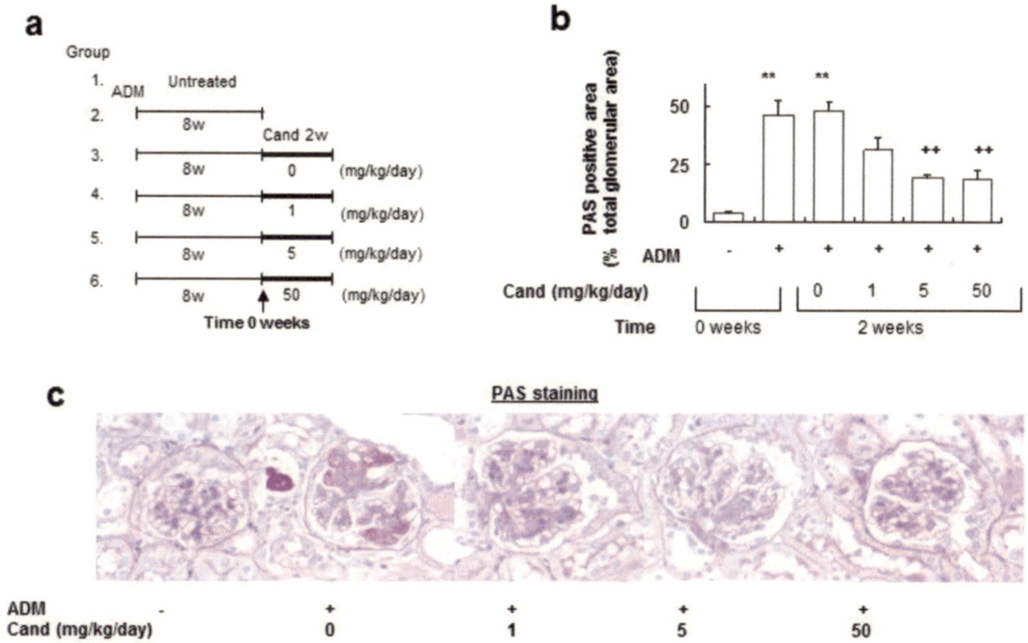


Fig. 2. Effects of different doses of ARB (candesartan) on regression of glomerulosclerosis in the adriamycin-nephropathy model. (a) Experimental protocol (b) Effects on glomerular sclerosis (c) Representative photomicrographs. Reproduced with permission from Hayashi et al. Kidney Int 78:69-78, 2010.

caused a dose-dependent increase in glomerular MMP-2 activity and decrease in type IV collagen accumulation. The ARB-induced regression of glomerulosclerosis was attenuated by pretreatment with the MMP inhibitor doxycycline, as well as in mice with targeted deletion of the MMP-2 gene, suggesting the possibility that increased expression of MMP-2 may contribute to the regression of glomerulosclerosis and type IV collagen deposition seen in the high-dose ARB-treated groups.

The MMP family constitutes a multigene family of zinc- and calcium-dependent endopeptidases which play a major role in the degradation of collagen and other ECM components (Woessner, 1991), (Baramova et al., 1995), (Sasamura et al., 2005). MMP-2 (also known as gelatinase A) is a MMP which is found in the conditioned media of cultured fibroblasts, and is involved in the cleavage of multiple ECM proteins including type IV collagen (Woessner, 1991), (Baramova et al., 1995). In contrast to gelatinase B (MMP-9), MMP-2 is not highly expressed in normal or diseased glomeruli (Urushihara et al., 2002). However, it has been shown that renal MMP-2 expression and activity are upregulated by ACE inhibitors in rats with diabetes (McLennan et al., 2002), (Sun et al., 2006). Moreover, Turkay et al reported that the ACE inhibitor enalapril also increased hepatic MMP-2 expression in rats with experimental hepatic fibrogenesis (Turkay et al., 2008), while Westermann et al. showed that the ARB irbesartan increased MMP-2 activity in the hearts of mice with cardiomyopathy (Westermann et al., 2007), suggesting that the RAS plays a key role in regulation of MMP-2 expression in the kidney and other tissues.

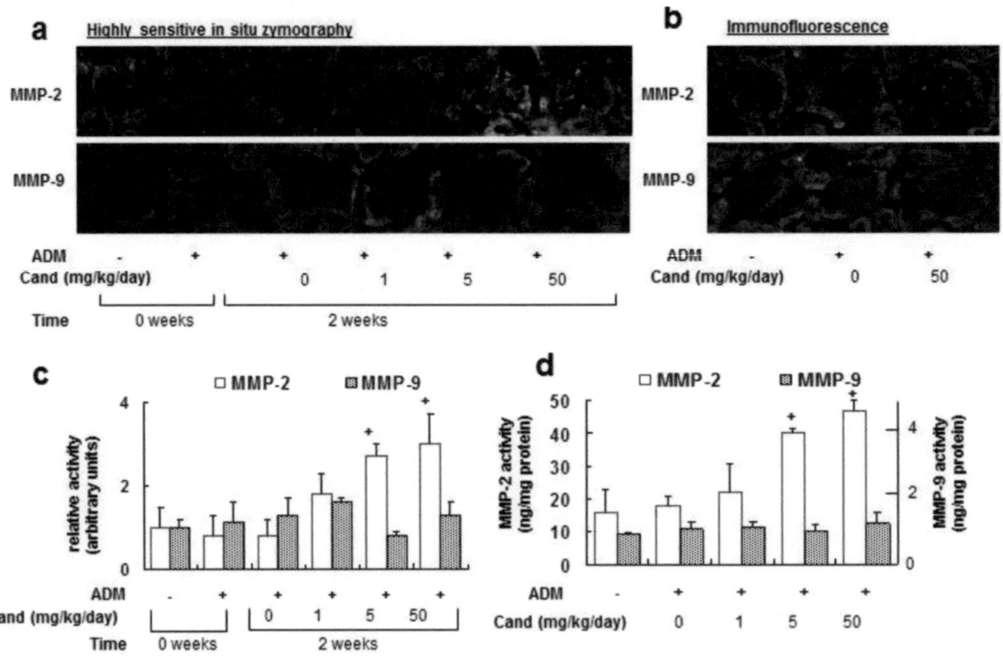


Fig. 3. Effects of different doses of ARB (candesartan) on glomerular MMP-2 and MMP-9 activity and expression in the adriamycin-nephropathy model. Representative results of (a) highly-sensitive in situ zymography (b) immunofluorescence. Quantification of glomerular MMP activity by (c) in situ zymography (d) ELISA. Reproduced with permission from Hayashi et al. Kidney Int 78:69-78, 2010.

As shown in Fig. 3, the results of highly-sensitive in situ zymography and immunofluorescence suggested that MMP-2 might be upregulated in glomerular podocytes, but this could not be determined accurately because of the relatively low expression of MMP-2 protein. Therefore, to further characterize the mechanisms of the ARB-induced increase in glomerular MMP-2 activity, we examined the effects of ARB treatment in cultured podocytes. These experiments revealed that ARB treatment of podocytes resulted in a dose-dependent increase in MMP-2 activity in the supernatant. Podocytes are known to express components of the RAS, including renin, angiotensinogen, angiotensin-converting enzyme, and AT1 and AT2 receptors (Durvasula et al., 2006), (Durvasula et al., 2008), (Liebau et al., 2006). Morever, functional expression of the renin-angiotensin system has been documented in both mouse and human podocytes (Durvasula et al., 2008), (Liebau et al., 2006). To examine the possibility that the effects of ARB were mediated through inhibition of the RAS, further studies were performed using an ACE inhibitor, and a non-peptide Ang II antagonist (Saralasin). The use of these different RAS inhibitors yielded similar results, suggesting that the effects of ARB were mediated by inhibition of the intrinsic RAS in podocytes.

Moreover, it was observed in vitro that the increase in MMP-2 activity was greatest at the high doses of candesartan (greater than 0.1 umol/L), whereas maximum plasma concentrations in humans administered a standard dose of candesartan are below the nanomolar range (Pfister et al., 1999). Assuming that local (glomerular) concentrations of ARB will be greatest with the high-doses of ARB, these in vitro results are consistent with the in vivo observation that the glomerulosclerosis regression was maximal with the high doses of ARB.

In humans, it is known that MMP-1 (collagenase-1) also plays a major role in the breakdown of collagens, in particular type I and type III collagen. It has been reported that rodents lack the human MMP-1 gene, and MMP-13 (collagenase-3) is the main collagenase in mice (Henriet et al., 1992), (Parks et al., 2000.). When the possibility that MMP-13 may also contribute to the observed changes was examined, it was found that ARB treatment did not increase glomerular MMP-13 activity, but rather decreased the activity, suggesting that increased MMP-13 activity did not contribute to the observed regression of glomerulosclerosis in the adriamycin nephropathy model (Hayashi et al., 2010).

We also examined whether the effects of ARB could be attenuated by pretreating the mice with doxycycline, or by performing studies on mice with a deletion of the MMP-2 gene. It was found that neither inhibition of MMP nor deletion of MMP-2 completely abolished the effects of high-dose ARB, suggesting that other mechanisms may be involved, including the involvement of other proteases such as the serine protease plasminogen activator inhibitor-1 (PAI-1) (Ma et al., 2005). Other studies have suggested that regeneration of glomerular podocyte function may also play a role in the regression of glomerulosclerosis by RAS inhibitors (Macconi et al., 2009).

It should be noted that the effects of ARB on regression may differ widely in different animal models. In particular, the effects of ARB on regression were less marked in the 5/6 nephrectomy model (Ma et al., 2005). This may be because the adriamycin model relies on a single (acute) injury to the glomeruli, whereas the injury in the 5/6 nephrectomy model is a continuous process. In the studies on the adriamycin nephropathy model, it was found that

MMP-2 activity decreased to baseline after the ARB treatment was discontinued. The transient increase in MMP-2 was probably sufficient to permanently reverse the glomerulosclerosis in that model, but its effect in other disease states is unclear.

Interestingly, clinical studies using different ARBs (Rossing et al., 2005), (Hollenberg et al., 2007), (Burgess et al., 2009) also suggest that high-dose ARB treatment may have a greater beneficial effect on the kidney compared to standard doses. One potential reason may be that standard doses of ARB do not fully suppress the RAS in the kidneys. Another possibility is that mechanisms unrelated to RAS inhibition may be involved, for example an antioxidant action independent of AT1 receptor blockade (Chen et al., 2008). Currently, we are performing further studies to examine why high-dose ARB is particularly effective in ameliorating glomerular injury.

### 2.3 Clinical studies of CKD regression

The clearest clinical demonstration of glomerulosclerosis regression was provided by Fioretto et al., who showed that pancreas transplantation in patient with type 1 diabetes caused regression of established lesions of glomerulosclerosis in patients with type 1 diabetes (Fioretto et al., 1998).

There are also several studies which examined the effect of RAS inhibition on structural changes in diabetic and non-diabetic CKD. In the study on type 1 diabetic patients with microalbuminuria, treatment with enalapril, perindopril, or metoprolol resulted in a decrease in glomerular basement membrane thickness after 3-4 years of follow-up (Nankervis et al., 1998) (Rudberg et al., 1999). Other studies have suggested that glomerular volumes may be reduced by RAS inhibition, however the contribution of changes in blood pressure is unclear (Perrin et al., 2008). On the other hand, a recent study by Mauer et al. did not detect a statistical difference in mesangial fractional volume in patients treated with placebo, ARB, or ACEI (Mauer et al., 2009). In the ESPRIT study, 3-year treatment with enalapril or nifedipine did not cause a significant change in renal structural abnormalities (2001).

In the case of type 2 diabetes, the study by the Diabiopsies group suggested that treatment with perindopril resulted in stabilization of the percentage of sclerosed glomeruli, but this could not be confirmed by electron microscopy (Cordonnier et al., 1999). In the case of non-diabetic CKD, Ohtake et al. reported that treatment of 15 patients with mild to moderate IgA and non-IgA mesangial proliferative glomerulonephritis with an ARB for an average of 28 months caused a decrease in mesangial matrix expansion and interstitial fibrosis (Ohtake et al., 2008). In summary, although there is encouraging evidence that RAS inhibition can cause regression of glomerular structural changes in humans, the clinical data are not as clear as the data from animal experiments, possibly because the human studies have not focused on the use of high-dose RAS inhibitors.

### 2.4 The search for clinical biomarkers of disease regression

One of the reasons that there are relative few large-scale studies on CKD regression is that demonstration of resolution of glomerular lesions requires repeat kidney biopsies, which may not be feasible in large populations. One potential way to overcome this problem is to find surrogate biomarkers of disease regression in the serum and urine of patients with early (stage 1-2) CKD, using the new science of metabolomics (Hayashi et al., 2011).

Metabolomics is a discipline dedicated to the global study of metabolites, their dynamics, composition, interactions, and responses to interventions or to changes in their environment (Oresic, 2009), and the recent development of metabolome analysis technology allows the global 'metabolome' to be assessed comprehensively in individual patients. An important advantage of metabolome analysis is the potential to identify new and unidentified metabolites which could have important pathophysiological functions. In a recent study, we obtained serum and urine samples from 15 patients and 7 healthy volunteers, and compared the metabolome profiles of the two groups. Serum or urine samples (100 ul) were added to methanol (900 ul) containing internal standards, deproteinised, and subjected to anionic and cationic capillary electrophoresis time-of-flight mass spectrometry (CE-TOFMS) analysis

The results of our metabolome analysis suggested that serum and urine levels of several amino acid, nucleic acid, and carbohydrate metabolites were altered in patients from an early stage of CKD (Hayashi et al., 2011). We also found evidence for the presence of several novel metabolites which were markedly increased or decreased in the patients with CKD compared to controls. We are performing further studies to examine the structure of these unidentified products, with the final aim to find new biomarkers of disease regression which may be utilized in clinical studies.

### 3.1 Prevention of hypertension

It has been recognized that the kidney plays an important role in the control of systemic blood pressure, and is involved in the pathogenesis of hypertension, which is a major risk factor for cardiovascular disorders such as stroke, heart failure, vascular disease, and end-stage renal disease, and an important cause of morbidity and mortality. Similar to CKD, the development of hypertension appears to be progressive: the systolic blood pressure of an individual patient rises progressively over time, so that median values of systolic blood pressure in the population increases at every age (Qureshi et al., 2005).

In our laboratory, we have been studying the use of RAS inhibitors to prevent the development of hypertension, using the spontaneously hypertensive rat (SHR) and other animal models of hypertension. Previous studies by Harrap et al. demonstrated that treatment of SHR from age 6 to 10 weeks with an angiotensin-converting enzyme (ACE) inhibitor resulted in the sustained suppression of hypertension at age 25 weeks (Harrap et al., 1986), (Harrap et al., 1990). Studies from the group of Berecek et al. suggested that these results could result from a decrease in arginine vasopressin (AVP) levels (Lee et al., 1991), (Zhang et al., 1996). Similar findings have been reported by other laboratories, using both ACE inhibitors (Giudicelli et al., 1980), (Christensen et al., 1989) and ARBs (Morton et al., 1992), (Gillies et al., 1997).

In our laboratory, it was found that treatment of stroke-prone SHR (SHRSP) with an ACE inhibitor from age 3 to 10 weeks resulted in a sustained suppression of blood pressure, whereas such an effect was not found with the vasodilator hydralazine (Nakaya et al., 2001). The same results were found with an ARB, suggesting that this effect could be explained by the inhibitory actions of ACE inhibitors and ARB on the RAS. Importantly, it was also found that the development of renal injury was also suppressed in this model.

To examine if the effects of RAS inhibitors to suppress the development of hypertension was specific to the SHR and its related strains, studies were performed on the Dahl salt-sensitive rat, which is a model of salt-sensitive hypertension with a low renin profile (Nakaya et al., 2002). These studies revealed that treatment of Dahl salt-sensitive rats with an ARB during the same 'critical period' (age 3 to 10 weeks) prevented the later development of salt-induced hypertension in this model even when the ARB treatment had been discontinued, and also a partial attenuation of renal injury induced by salt loading.

To examine the mechanisms of these long-lasting effects of RAS blockade, further studies were performed using the SHR/L-NAME model, which is a model of accelerated hypertension characterized by marked renal injury (Ishiguro et al., 2007). SHR were treated with a RAS inhibitor (ACE inhibitor or ARB), or a vasodilator (hydralazine), or a calcium chanel blocker (CCB, nitrendipine) during the 'critical period' from age 3 to 10 weeks. Medications were discontinued at age 10 weeks, and the rats observed without treatment for two months. At age 18 weeks, the rats were administered the NO synthase inhibitor L-NAME in the drinking water for 3 weeks to induce renal injury, and sacrificed at age 21 weeks. Interestingly, the rats treated with a RAS inhibitor had reduced vascular injury (arterial hypertrophy, endothelial thickening, and lumen narrowing) compared to vasodilator- or CCB-treated rats, and reduced renin mRNA, probably due to attenuation of the intrarenal vascular injury and renal ischemia induced by L-NAME. To explain all these experimental findings, we proposed a 'reno-vascular amplifier' mechanism for the development of hypertension and renal injury in this model (Fig. 4). High blood pressure is known to cause vascular hypertrophy in the resistance vessels, which consists predominantly of inward 'eutrophic' remodeling. When this remodeling is accentuated, as in the SHR/L-NAME model, glomerular perfusion decreases, which results in increased synthesis of renin and activation of the RAS. These changes cause a further increase in the blood pressure, resulting in a vicious cycle which causes accelerated hypertension. RAS inhibitors can block this vicious cycle by attenuating both the increase in blood pressure, and importantly, by decreasing the vascular hypertrophy of the resistance arteries.

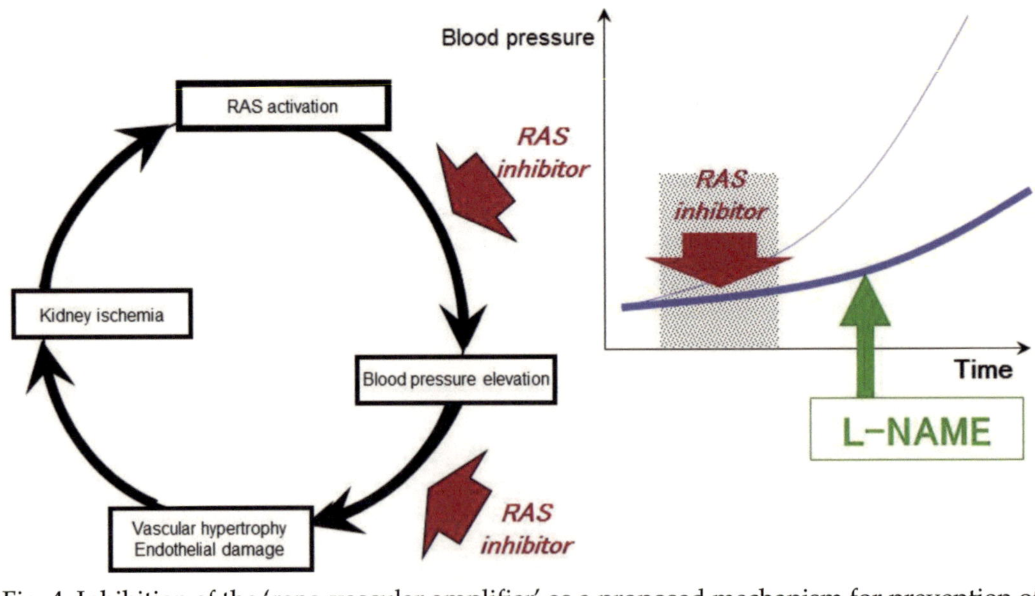


Fig. 4. Inhibition of the 'reno-vascular amplifier' as a proposed mechanism for prevention of hypertension in the SHR/L-NAME model.

This hypothesis was supported by experiments in which the agonist angiotensin II was administered during the 'critical period' from age 4 to 8 weeks, after which all treatments were discontinued. Rats which had been transiently exposed to angiotensin II during this period were found to have elevated values of blood pressure which were 10-20 mmHg higher than rats which had been exposed to saline vehicle. Morever these rats were more susceptible to the subsequent development of renal vascular injury, and increased renin synthesis at a later time point (age 18 weeks), and to have a much higher mortality after L-NAME administration (Ishiguro et al., 2007). Thus, the effects of angiotensin II administration were the opposite of the effects of ARB, and were found to cause an acceleration of the 'reno-vascular amplifier' in this model of accelerated hypertension and renal injury.

The results of animal studies on hypertension prevention have been supported clinically by the TROPHY study (Julius et al., 2006). In this prospective, randomized, multi-center study designed by Julius et al., patients with prehypertension and systolic blood pressure of 130-139 mmHg and/or diastolic blood pressure of 85-89 mmHg were randomized to placebo or the ARB candesartan cilexetil (16 mg/day) for two years, then both groups were switched to placebo for the next two years. The primary end-point was the development of hypertension. As in the animal studies, the treatment with ARB caused a suppression of the development of hypertension, not only during the active treatment period (first two years), but even after the active treatment had been discontinued. The absolute risk reduction at the end of two or four years was 26.8 % and 9.8 % respectively, whereas the corresponding values of relative risk reduction (when relative risk is defined as the frequency of events in the treated group divided by the events in the placebo group) were 66.3 % and 15.6 %, respectively. Changes in the systolic blood pressure at the end of the study were small (2 mmHg), but statistically significant.

### 3.2 Regression of hypertension

Hypertension is associated with increased peripheral arterial resistance, and most of the resistance develops in the resistance arteries of the microvasculature, which includes both arterioles and small arteries with diameters < 400 um. The importance of the microvasculature in the pathogenesis and maintenance of hypertension was originally proposed by Folkow, who pointed out that a vicious cycle exists between increased blood pressure and vascular hypertrophy (Folkow, 1990). According to this hypothesis, hypertension may be initiated by a specific fast-acting pressor mechanism (e.g. angiotensin II) that increases blood pressure and initiates a positive feedback loop that induces vascular hypertrophy and maintains the hypertension. The hypothesis was later refined by Lever and Harrap, who proposed further elements: an abnormal or 'reinforced' hypertrophic response to pressure, and an increase of a humoral agent that causes hypertrophy directly (Lever et al., 1992). Animal studies have provided evidence to support the hypothesis that arteriolar restructuring may act as a primary accelerator of hypertension and provide a driving force for the progression of hypertension (Feihl et al., 2006; Intengan et al., 2001; Skov et al., 2004)). In particular, increased renal vascular resistance has been well documented in the SHR model of hypertension (Dilley et al., 1984), and morphometric studies on the afferent arteriole of SHR and Wistar-Kyoto rats (WKY) have confirmed that afferent arteriolar diameters are smaller in SHR compared to WKY (Kimura et al., 1989) (Gattone et al., 1983). Importantly, these differences are already seen in the 4-week-old SHR, even before blood pressure is significantly increased compared to WKY controls (Kimura et al., 1989).

Moreover, when SHR and normotensive rats were crossbred to form second generation hybrids, a narrowed afferent arteriole lumen diameter at 7 weeks was found to be a predictor of the later development of hypertension (Skov et al., 2004).

In our laboratory, the morphological effects of treatment with an ARB or CCB during the 'critical period' on renal small artery structure were examined in SHR. SHR were treated with an ARB or CCB from age 3 to 10 weeks, and sacrificed at age 10 weeks. The arteriolar hypertrophy was significantly reduced in the ARB-treated rats compared to the CCB-treated rats, despite similar reductions in blood pressure. These results were consistent with reports from other groups using RAS inhibitors in both animal models (Freslon et al., 1983), (Christensen et al., 1989) and humans (Schiffrin et al., 1994), (Thybo et al., 1995).

Recently, we reported that treatment of SHR with established hypertension with high-dose ARB (at 50-100 times the normal dose in rodents) resulted in a sustained decrease in hypertension, suggesting that regression of hypertension is feasible in this model (Ishiguro et al., 2009). Similar results were reported previously by Smallegange et al. using an ACE inhibitor combined with a low-salt diet (Smallegange et al., 2004). Examination of the effects of transient high-dose ARB therapy on renal arteriolar structure revealed a remarkable reversal of the arteriolar hypertrophy found in SHR treated with ARB, whereas this effect was not seen with CCB (Fig. 5). Interestingly, these findings were particularly noticeable in the small arteries (diameter 30-100 um) and arterioles in the kidney, compared to small arteries from other vascular beds, such as the brain, heart, and mesentery.

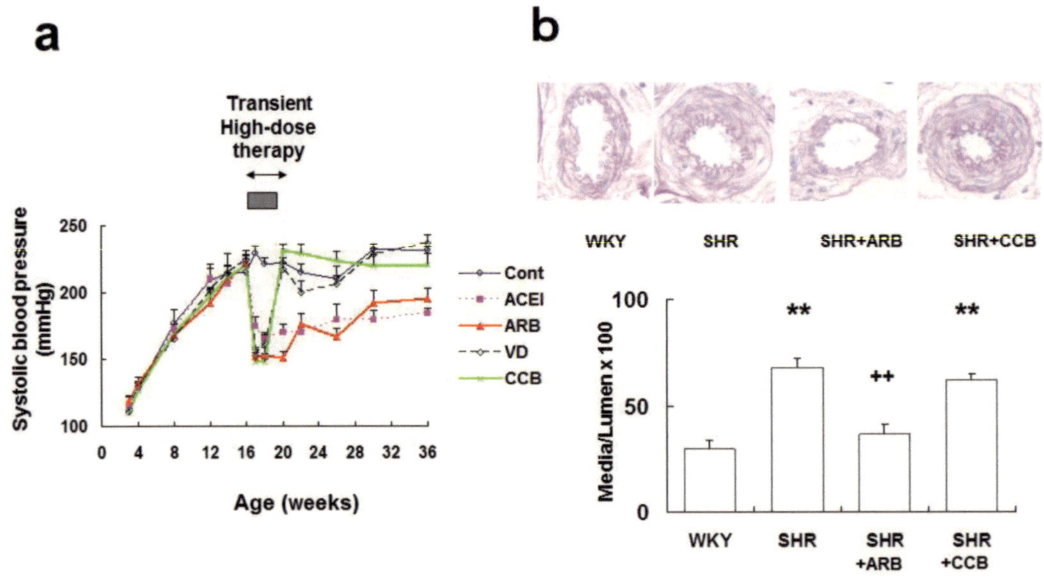


Fig. 5. Regression of hypertension in the SHR model by transient high-dose ARB treatment. (a) Effects on blood pressure (b) Effects on renal arteriolar media/lumen ratios. Reproduced with permission from Ishiguro/Hayashi et al. Hypertension 53:83-89, 2009.

To examine potential mechanisms of these changes, the gene expression profile of kidneys treated with ARB were compared with the kidneys treated with CCB. Using the Affymetrix rat 230 2.0 gene expression array, it was found that 1,345 genes were elevated in the ARB-treated rats compared to CCB-treated rats, while 5,671 were reduced. Several ECM-related genes were elevated in the ARB-treated rats, while MMP-9, TIMP-2, and TIMP-3 gene expressions were decreased in the ARB-treated group. These differences were also confirmed by real time RT-PCR. To examine if these changes in MMP expression could be involved in the observed reversal of renal arteriolar hypertrophy by ARB, the activities of different MMPs in the renal microvasculature were examined using a highly sensitive in situ zymography method. It was found that MMP-13 activity was markedly increased by ARB but not by CCB (Ishiguro et al., 2009). These results are compatible with a role for MMPs in the actions of ARB to cause reversal of renal arteriolar hypertrophy, and subsequent remodeling of the renal microvasculature (Fig.6).

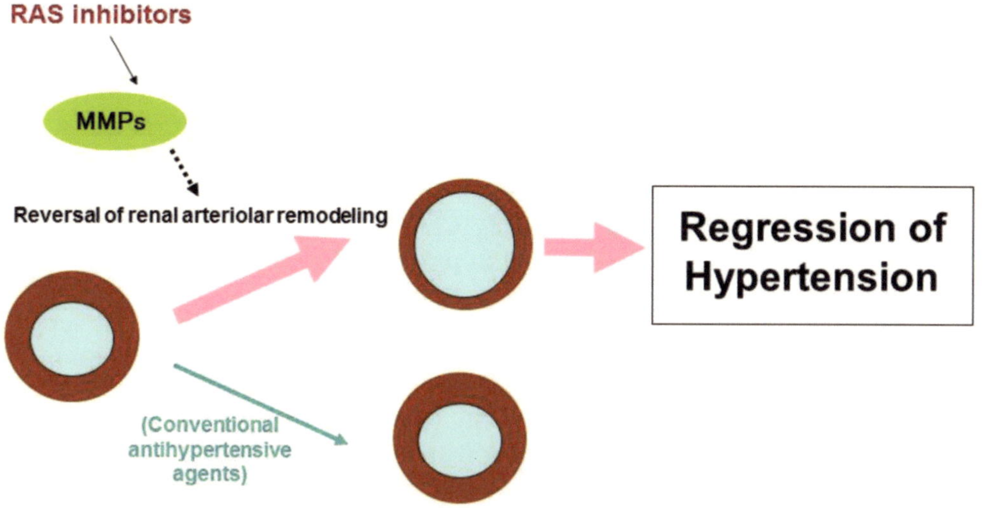


Fig. 6. Proposed hypothesis for the mechanism of regression of hypertension by high-dose renin-angiotensin inhibitors.

To our knowledge, there have been no clinical studies which were specifically designed to address the question whether regression of hypertension (i.e. reversal of Grade 1 hypertension to high-normal blood pressure) is feasible in humans. For this reason, we are currently performing a prospective, multi-center study (STAR CAST) study to examine the effects of one-year treatment with an ARB or CCB on regression of hypertension (Sasamura et al., 2008). In this study, patients aged 30-59 with newly diagnosed hypertension and a positive family history of hypertension are randomized to treatment for one year with either an ARB (candesartan) or CCB (nifedipine XL). After one year, the patient's antihypertensive drug dose will be reduced, then withdrawn. The antihypertensive drug withdrawal success rate will be compared between the two antihypertensive agents, as an index of the regression of hypertension in the two groups. Because of safety concerns, the patients' home blood pressure will be monitored in real time using a home blood pressure monitoring system (i-TECHO). Although this study is being performed using standard doses of ARB, it is hoped that this trial will provide information concerning whether RAS inhibitors are indeed different from other antihypertensive agents in terms of long-term effects on blood pressure. If the results are encouraging, we hope to perform further clinical studies on CKD and hypertension regression, using high or even ultrahigh doses of ARB.

## 4. Conclusion

The increasing evidence from laboratory and clinical studies on chronic kidney disease and hypertension suggest that effective interventions at an early stage may be beneficial in preventing the development of both these disorders. Because of the high prevalence of both chronic kidney disease and hypertension amongst the general population, further research on the development of methods to induce regression of these conditions may be expected to result in widespread health benefits.

## 5. References


Aros C, and Remuzzi G. (2002). The renin-angiotensin system in progression, remission and regression of chronic nephropathies. *J Hypertens Suppl* 20:S45-53.

Bakris G. (2010). Are there effects of renin-angiotensin system antagonists beyond blood pressure control? *Am J Cardiol* 105:21A-9A.

Baramova E, and Foidart JM. (1995). Matrix metalloproteinase family. *Cell Biol Int* 19:239-42.

Berl T. (2009). Review: renal protection by inhibition of the renin-angiotensin-aldosterone system. *J Renin Angiotensin Aldosterone Syst* 10:1-8.

Burgess E, Muirhead N, Rene de Cotret P, Chiu A, Pichette V, and Tobe S. (2009). Supramaximal dose of candesartan in proteinuric renal disease. *J Am Soc Nephrol* 20:893-900.

Chen S, Ge Y, Si J, Rifai A, Dworkin LD, and Gong R. (2008). Candesartan suppresses chronic renal inflammation by a novel antioxidant action independent of AT1R blockade. *Kidney Int* 74:1128-38.

Christensen KL, Jespersen LT, and Mulvany MJ. (1989). Development of blood pressure in spontaneously hypertensive rats after withdrawal of long-term treatment related to vascular structure. *J Hypertens* 7:83-90.

Cordonnier DJ, Pinel N, Barro C, Maynard M, Zaoui P, Halimi S, Hurault de Ligny B, Reznic Y, Simon D, and Bilous RW. (1999). Expansion of cortical interstitium is limited by converting enzyme inhibition in type 2 diabetic patients with glomerulosclerosis. The Diabiopsies Group. *J Am Soc Nephrol* 10:1253-63.

Dilley JR, Stier CT, Jr., and Arendshorst WJ. (1984). Abnormalities in glomerular function in rats developing spontaneous hypertension. *Am J Physiol* 246:F12-20.

Durvasula RV, and Shankland SJ. (2006). The renin-angiotensin system in glomerular podocytes: mediator of glomerulosclerosis and link to hypertensive nephropathy. *Curr Hypertens Rep* 8:132-8.

Durvasula RV, and Shankland SJ. (2008). Activation of a local renin angiotensin system in podocytes by glucose. *Am J Physiol Renal Physiol* 294:F830-9.

Feihl F, Liaudet L, Waeber B, and Levy BI. (2006). Hypertension: a disease of the microcirculation? *Hypertension* 48:1012-7.

Fioretto P, Steffes MW, Sutherland DE, Goetz FC, and Mauer M. (1998). Reversal of lesions of diabetic nephropathy after pancreas transplantation. *N Engl J Med* 339:69-75.

Folkow B. (1990). "Structural factor" in primary and secondary hypertension. *Hypertension* 16:89-101.

Freslon JL, and Giudicelli JF. (1983). Compared myocardial and vascular effects of captopril and dihydralazine during hypertension development in spontaneously hypertensive rats. *Br J Pharmacol* 80:533-43.

Gattone VH, 2nd, Evan AP, Willis LR, and Luft FC. (1983). Renal afferent arteriole in the spontaneously hypertensive rat. *Hypertension* 5:8-16.

Gillies LK, Lu M, Wang H, and Lee RM. (1997). AT1 receptor antagonist treatment caused persistent arterial functional changes in young spontaneously hypertensive rats. *Hypertension* 30:1471-8.

Giudicelli JF, Freslon JL, Glasson S, and Richer C. (1980). Captopril and hypertension development in the SHR. *Clin Exp Hypertens* 2:1083-96.

Haller H, Ito S, Izzo JL, Jr., Januszewicz A, Katayama S, Menne J, Mimran A, Rabelink TJ, Ritz E, Ruilope LM, Rump LC, and Viberti G. (2011). Olmesartan for the delay or prevention of microalbuminuria in type 2 diabetes. *N Engl J Med* 364:907-17.

Harrap SB, Nicolaci JA, and Doyle AE. (1986). Persistent effects on blood pressure and renal haemodynamics following chronic angiotensin converting enzyme inhibition with perindopril. *Clin Exp Pharmacol Physiol* 13:753-65.

Harrap SB, Van der Merwe WM, Griffin SA, Macpherson F, and Lever AF. (1990). Brief angiotensin converting enzyme inhibitor treatment in young spontaneously hypertensive rats reduces blood pressure long-term. *Hypertension* 16:603-14.

Hayashi K, Sasamura H, Ishiguro K, Sakamaki Y, Azegami T, and Itoh H. (2010). Regression of glomerulosclerosis in response to transient treatment with angiotensin II blockers is attenuated by blockade of matrix metalloproteinase-2. *Kidney Int* 78:69-78.

Hayashi K, Sasamura H, Hishiki T, Suematsu M, Ikeda S, Soga T, and Itoh H. (2011). Use of serum and urine metabolome analysis for the detection of metabolic changes in patients with stage 1-2 chronic kidney disease. *Nephro-Urol Mon* 3:164-171.

Henriet P, Rousseau GG, and Eeckhout Y. (1992). Cloning and sequencing of mouse collagenase cDNA. Divergence of mouse and rat collagenases from the other mammalian collagenases. *FEBS Lett* 310:175-8.

Hollenberg NK, Parving HH, Viberti G, Remuzzi G, Ritter S, Zelenkofske S, Kandra A, Daley WL, and Rocha R. (2007). Albuminuria response to very high-dose valsartan in type 2 diabetes mellitus. *J Hypertens* 25:1921-6.

Intengan HD, and Schiffrin EL. (2001). Vascular remodeling in hypertension: roles of apoptosis, inflammation, and fibrosis. *Hypertension* 38:581-7.

Ishiguro K, Sasamura H, Sakamaki Y, Itoh H, and Saruta T. (2007). Developmental activity of the renin-angiotensin system during the "critical period" modulates later L-NAME-induced hypertension and renal injury. *Hypertens Res* 30:63-75.

Ishiguro K, Hayashi K, Sasamura H, Sakamaki Y, and Itoh H. (2009). "Pulse" treatment with high-dose angiotensin blocker reverses renal arteriolar hypertrophy and regresses hypertension. *Hypertension* 53:83-9.

Julius S, Nesbitt SD, Egan BM, Weber MA, Michelson EL, Kaciroti N, Black HR, Grimm RH, Jr., Messerli FH, Oparil S, and Schork MA. (2006). Feasibility of treating prehypertension with an angiotensin-receptor blocker. *N Engl J Med* 354:1685-97.

Kimura K, Nanba S, Tojo A, Hirata Y, Matsuoka H, and Sugimoto T. (1989). Variations in arterioles in spontaneously hypertensive rats. Morphometric analysis of afferent and efferent arterioles. *Virchows Arch A Pathol Anat Histopathol* 415:565-9.

Lee RM, Berecek KH, Tsoporis J, McKenzie R, and Triggle CR. (1991). Prevention of hypertension and vascular changes by captopril treatment. *Hypertension* 17:141-50.

Lever AF, and Harrap SB. (1992). Essential hypertension: a disorder of growth with origins in childhood? *J Hypertens* 10:101-20.

Levey AS, Coresh J, Balk E, Kausz AT, Levin A, Steffes MW, Hogg RJ, Perrone RD, Lau J, and Eknoyan G. (2003). National Kidney Foundation practice guidelines for chronic kidney disease: evaluation, classification, and stratification. *Ann Intern Med* 139:137-47.

Liebau MC, Lang D, Bohm J, Endlich N, Bek MJ, Witherden I, Mathieson PW, Saleem MA, Pavenstadt H, and Fischer KG. (2006). Functional expression of the renin-angiotensin system in human podocytes. *Am J Physiol Renal Physiol* 290:F710-9.

Ma LJ, and Fogo AB. (2007). Modulation of glomerulosclerosis. *Semin Immunopathol* 29:385-95.

Ma LJ, Nakamura S, Aldigier JC, Rossini M, Yang H, Liang X, Nakamura I, Marcantoni C, and Fogo AB. (2005). Regression of glomerulosclerosis with high-dose angiotensin inhibition is linked to decreased plasminogen activator inhibitor-1. *J Am Soc Nephrol* 16:966-76.

Macconi D. (2010). Targeting the renin angiotensin system for remission/regression of chronic kidney disease. *Histol Histopathol* 25:655-68.

Macconi D, Sangalli F, Bonomelli M, Conti S, Condorelli L, Gagliardini E, Remuzzi G, and Remuzzi A. (2009). Podocyte repopulation contributes to regression of glomerular injury induced by ACE inhibition. *Am J Pathol* 174:797-807.

Mauer M, Zinman B, Gardiner R, Suissa S, Sinaiko A, Strand T, Drummond K, Donnelly S, Goodyer P, Gubler MC, and Klein R. (2009). Renal and retinal effects of enalapril and losartan in type 1 diabetes. *N Engl J Med* 361:40-51.

McLennan SV, Kelly DJ, Cox AJ, Cao Z, Lyons JG, Yue DK, and Gilbert RE. (2002). Decreased matrix degradation in diabetic nephropathy: effects of ACE inhibition on the expression and activities of matrix metalloproteinases. *Diabetologia* 45:268-75.

Morton JJ, Beattie EC, and MacPherson F. (1992). Angiotensin II receptor antagonist losartan has persistent effects on blood pressure in the young spontaneously hypertensive rat: lack of relation to vascular structure. *J Vasc Res* 29:264-9.

Moulder JE, Fish BL, Cohen EP, and Bonsib SM. (1996). Angiotensin II receptor antagonists in the prevention of radiation nephropathy. *Radiat Res* 146:106-10.

Nakaya H, Sasamura H, Hayashi M, and Saruta T. (2001). Temporary treatment of prepubescent rats with angiotensin inhibitors suppresses the development of hypertensive nephrosclerosis. *J Am Soc Nephrol* 12:659-66.

Nakaya H, Sasamura H, Mifune M, Shimizu-Hirota R, Kuroda M, Hayashi M, and Saruta T. (2002). Prepubertal treatment with angiotensin receptor blocker causes partial attenuation of hypertension and renal damage in adult Dahl salt-sensitive rats. *Nephron* 91:710-718.

Nankervis A, Nicholls K, Kilmartin G, Allen P, Ratnaike S, and Martin FI. (1998). Effects of perindopril on renal histomorphometry in diabetic subjects with microalbuminuria: a 3-year placebo-controlled biopsy study. *Metabolism* 47:12-5.

Neuringer JR, and Brenner BM. (1992). Glomerular hypertension: cause and consequence of renal injury. *J Hypertens Suppl* 10:S91-7.

Ohtake T, Oka M, Maesato K, Mano T, Ikee R, Moriya H, and Kobayashi S. (2008). Pathological regression by angiotensin II type 1 receptor blockade in patients with mesangial proliferative glomerulonephritis. *Hypertens Res* 31:387-94.

Oresic M. (2009). Metabolomics, a novel tool for studies of nutrition, metabolism and lipid dysfunction. *Nutr Metab Cardiovasc Dis* 19:816-24.

Parks WC, and Mecham RP. 2000. Matrix metalloproteinases Academic Press, Inc.: San Diego.

Perrin NE, Jaremko GA, and Berg UB. (2008). The effects of candesartan on diabetes glomerulopathy: a double-blind, placebo-controlled trial. *Pediatr Nephrol* 23:947-54.

Pfister M, Schaedeli F, Frey FJ, and Uehlinger DE. (1999). Pharmacokinetics and haemodynamics of candesartan cilexetil in hypertensive patients on regular haemodialysis. *Br J Clin Pharmacol* 47:645-51.

Qureshi AI, Suri MF, Kirmani JF, and Divani AA. (2005). Prevalence and trends of prehypertension and hypertension in United States: National Health and Nutrition Examination Surveys 1976 to 2000. *Med Sci Monit* 11:CR403-9.

Remuzzi G, Macia M, and Ruggenenti P. (2006). Prevention and treatment of diabetic renal disease in type 2 diabetes: the BENEDICT study. *J Am Soc Nephrol* 17:S90-7.

Rossing K, Schjoedt KJ, Jensen BR, Boomsma F, and Parving HH. (2005). Enhanced renoprotective effects of ultrahigh doses of irbesartan in patients with type 2 diabetes and microalbuminuria. *Kidney Int* 68:1190-8.

Rudberg S, Osterby R, Bangstad HJ, Dahlquist G, and Persson B. (1999). Effect of angiotensin converting enzyme inhibitor or beta blocker on glomerular structural changes in young microalbuminuric patients with Type I (insulin-dependent) diabetes mellitus. *Diabetologia* 42:589-95.

Ruggenenti P, Schieppati A, and Remuzzi G. (2001). Progression, remission, regression of chronic renal diseases. *Lancet* 357:1601-8.

Ruggenenti P, Perticucci E, Cravedi P, Gambara V, Costantini M, Sharma SK, Perna A, and Remuzzi G. (2008). Role of remission clinics in the longitudinal treatment of CKD. *J Am Soc Nephrol* 19:1213-24.

Sasamura H, Shimizu-Hirota R, and Saruta T. (2005). Extracellular matrix remodeling in hypertension. *Curr Hypertens Rev* 1:51-60.

Sasamura H, Nakaya H, Julius S, Takebayashi T, Sato Y, Uno H, Takeuchi M, Ishiguro K, Murakami M, Ryuzaki M, and Itoh H. (2008). Short treatment with the angiotensin receptor blocker candesartan surveyed by telemedicine (STAR CAST) study: rationale and study design. *Hypertens Res* 31:1851-1857.

Schiffrin EL, Deng LY, and Larochelle P. (1994). Effects of antihypertensive treatment on vascular remodeling in essential hypertensive patients. *J Cardiovasc Pharmacol* 24 Suppl 3:S51-6.

Skov K, and Mulvany MJ. (2004). Structure of renal afferent arterioles in the pathogenesis of hypertension. *Acta Physiol Scand* 181:397-405.

Smallegange C, Hale TM, Bushfield TL, and Adams MA. (2004). Persistent lowering of pressure by transplanting kidneys from adult spontaneously hypertensive rats treated with brief antihypertensive therapy. *Hypertension* 44:89-94.

Stojiljkovic L, and Behnia R. (2007). Role of renin angiotensin system inhibitors in cardiovascular and renal protection: a lesson from clinical trials. *Curr Pharm Des* 13:1335-45.

Sun SZ, Wang Y, Li Q, Tian YJ, Liu MH, and Yu YH. (2006). Effects of benazepril on renal function and kidney expression of matrix metalloproteinase-2 and tissue inhibitor of metalloproteinase-2 in diabetic rats. *Chin Med J (Engl)* 119:814-21.

Teles F, Machado FG, Ventura BH, Malheiros DM, Fujihara CK, Silva LF, and Zatz R. (2009). Regression of glomerular injury by losartan in experimental diabetic nephropathy. *Kidney Int* 75:72-9.

Thybo NK, Stephens N, Cooper A, Aalkjaer C, Heagerty AM, and Mulvany MJ. (1995). Effect of antihypertensive treatment on small arteries of patients with previously untreated essential hypertension. *Hypertension* 25:474-81.

Turkay C, Yonem O, Arici S, Koyuncu A, and Kanbay M. (2008). Effect of angiotensin-converting enzyme inhibition on experimental hepatic fibrogenesis. *Dig Dis Sci* 53:789-93.

Unstated A. (2001). Effect of 3 years of antihypertensive therapy on renal structure in type 1 diabetic patients with albuminuria: the European Study for the Prevention of Renal Disease in Type 1 Diabetes (ESPRIT). *Diabetes* 50:843-50.

Unstated A. (2002). K/DOQI clinical practice guidelines for chronic kidney disease: evaluation, classification, and stratification. *Am J Kidney Dis* 39:S1-266.

Urushihara M, Kagami S, Kuhara T, Tamaki T, and Kuroda Y. (2002). Glomerular distribution and gelatinolytic activity of matrix metalloproteinases in human glomerulonephritis. *Nephrol Dial Transplant* 17:1189-96.

Westermann D, Rutschow S, Jager S, Linderer A, Anker S, Riad A, Unger T, Schultheiss HP, Pauschinger M, and Tschope C. (2007). Contributions of inflammation and cardiac matrix metalloproteinase activity to cardiac failure in diabetic cardiomyopathy: the role of angiotensin type 1 receptor antagonism. *Diabetes* 56:641-6.

Woessner JF, Jr. (1991). Matrix metalloproteinases and their inhibitors in connective tissue remodeling. *Faseb J* 5:2145-54.

Zhang L, Edwards DG, and Berecek KH. (1996). Effects of early captopril treatment and its removal on plasma angiotensin converting enzyme (ACE) activity and arginine vasopressin in hypertensive rats (SHR) and normotensive rats (WKY). *Clin Exp Hypertens* 18:201-26.

# 26

# Health-Related Quality of Life in Chronic Renal Predialysis Patients Exposed to a Prevention Program – Medellín, 2007-2008

Carlos E. Yepes Delgado, Yanett M. Montoya Jaramillo,
Beatriz E. Orrego Orozco and Daniel C. Aguirre Acevedo
*School of Medicine, University of Antioquia, Pablo Tobón Uribe Hospital, Medellín, Colombia*

## 1. Introduction

Progressive transformation of disease profiles in the world can be partially explained by the existence of chronic diseases, as they are responsible for a large part of the worldwide morbidity and mortality rates, thus becoming pandemics. One of the diseases recognized as a public health problem is chronic renal failure (CRF) because of the negative impact it has on the health and health-related quality of life (HRQOL) of its sufferers (Atkins, 2005a, 2005b).

The concept of HRQOL is still inaccurate because it has been approached from a variety of disciplines such as philosophy, economics, medicine, sociology, public health, politics, ethics, etc. (Cardona & Agudelo, 2005).

According to the World Health Organization (WHO), HRQOL is the "individual's perception of their position in life in the context of the culture and value systems in which they live and in relation to their goals, expectations, standards and concerns." (WHO, 2002) This concept includes physical and psychological aspects as well as the degree of independence, social relationships, environment and spirituality (Cardona et al., 2003). The approximately four hundred instruments for measuring HRQOL (Cardona & Agudelo, 2005) can be grouped into four categories: the ones that measure HRQOL in terms of its global definition, the ones using component-oriented approaches, those which focus on one component, and the combinations of any of the above (Fleury & Lana Da Costa, 2004).

The relationship between HRQOL in CRF patients and the treatment after renal failure has been studied repeatedly (Amoedo et al., 2004; De Alvaro et al., 1997; García et al., 2003; Leanza et al., 2000; Pérez et al., 2007; Rebollo et al., 1999, 2000a, 2000b; Sanz et al., 2004). However, there are insufficient studies on the relationship between early progression of renal damage and well-being (National Kidney Foundation [NKF], 2007). The recommendations of the Institute of Medicine (IOM) Workshop "Assessing Health and health-related quality of life Outcomes in Dialysis" are recorded in the KDOQI guidelines and supported by scientific evidence. The IOM recommends assessing the aforementioned relationship with valid, reliable, and useful instruments such as the Medical Outcomes

Study 36-Item Short Form (SF-36). The version used in this study was adapted for the Colombian culture (Lugo et al., 2006).

To follow the WHO's recommendation (Tazeen, 2006), the Colombian Ministry of Social Protection proposed a CRF prevention and control program for Colombian healthcare providers (Martínez & Valencia, 2005). One of such institutions has been developing a renal protection program (RPP) since 2004. Besides patient uptake and follow-up, this program also assists patients in the early stages of the condition to prevent progression and renal damage, to delay the need for renal replacement therapies (RRT). The Renal Protection Program (RPP) is an interdisciplinary healthcare program. It is based on a protocol that establishes educational talks and regular medical appointments for conducting clinical examinations and laboratory tests. The program is geared toward CKD patients and welcomes them since the early stages of their condition. Likewise, the program actively searches for early-stage CKD patients and refers them to nephrologists. The professionals involved in this program are: general practitioners, internists, nutritionists, nurses, and nephrologists. Their degree of involvement varies depending on the patients' CKD stage. First, a follow-up is performed on the underlying condition. Afterwards, patients in the first and second stages of CKD are assigned to the program's first healthcare level, which offers medical appointments with internists and nutrition professionals once per year for stage 1 patients, and every semester for stage 2 patients. The second healthcare level of the program is for patients in stages 3 and 4, and offers medical appointments with internists, nephrologists, and nutritionists every three years for stage 3 patients and every two months for stage 4 patients.

In contrast, other Colombian healthcare providers offered conventional treatment (CT) in 2004. CT consists of providing healthcare through general medicine once the patients feel the need to request this service. Conventional treatment follows no healthcare guidelines, does not search for patients actively, and offers no laboratory tests or regular appointments.

This study compares changes in the HRQOL of two patient groups during the early stages of CRF (one group having been exposed to a RPP from 2007 to 2008). Its aim is to provide evidence of interventions that ease the burden this disease represents for patients, families and society.

## 2. Methods

A longitudinal study on two representative samples consisting of CRF patients in predialysis. The first group followed a renal protection program, and the other conventional treatment (CT). SF-36 questionnaire was applied twice for both groups, with an interval of one year. The RPP actively searches for patients and interdisciplinary standardized professional care, whereas CT consists of patient-requested medical care and follows no protocol.

The eligible population consisted of 5884 people complying with the following criteria: a. Having health insurance with either of the two healthcare promoting institutions during 2007; b. Having a CRF diagnosis that complies with the criteria established in the 2007 KDOQI guidelines (NKF,2007); c. Being older than 16, and d. Having received no dialysis or renal transplants. Exclusion criteria: being registered with both healthcare providers during the follow-up year.

A formula with repeated measurements proposed by Frison and Pocock in 1992 (Frison et al., 1992) was used to calculate the sample probabilistically. The criteria were: type 1 error: 0.05, type 2 error: 0.20 (Power: 80%), a difference of 10 in the average value of both groups, a standard deviation (SD) of 34 for both groups (the highest SD observed during the validation of the SF-36 domains (Lugo et al., 2006). The correlation between basal and follow-up measurements was fixed at 0.5.

The minimal sample size for each group was 137. There was a total of 274 patients. The researchers anticipated that locating patients would be difficult due to high mobility. Therefore, an oversampling of 50% was performed, obtaining a final sample of 411 patients, of which only 293 could be contacted. The sample for the healthcare provider offering the RPP consisted of 148 patients, and the sample for the healthcare provider offering conventional treatment consisted of 145 patients. This guaranteed the expected representativeness.

The SF-36 consists of eight domains that were calculated by transforming the ordinal scale of the form's items into the corresponding score from 0 to 100 (Lugo et al., 2006). This model has been used to define two summary scores, namely: the physical health summary score (PCS1) and the mental health summary score (MCS1). Each of these two components includes four SF-36 dimensions as follows: PCS1 includes physical functioning (PF), role-physical (RP), body pain (BP) and general health (GH); MCS1 includes: vitality (V), social functioning (SF), role-emotional (RE) and mental health (MH). Furthermore, summary scores for physical and mental health were calculated using the same method applied in a reproducibility study of the SF-36 summary scores in HRQOL assessments for Schizophrenia patients (Leese et al., 2008).

Physical functioning (PF) is measured by assessing the ability to perform different kinds of simple and strenuous activities. Role physical (RP) is measured based on how much patients can devote themselves to their jobs and other activities. Bodily pain (BP) is measured based on pain intensity and on how it hinders daily work. General Health (GH) refers to the patients' assessment of their own health. Vitality (V) is measured by assessing the perception of energy, exhaustion, or fatigue. Social functioning (SF) is measured by observing how much the patients' health problems affect their social activities. Role emotional (RE) is measured in terms of what activities the patients stop doing due to emotional problems. Mental health (MH) is measured by assessing how nervous, sad, calm, discouraged, or happy the patients feel. Change in health has a scale which is independent from the aforementioned domains and is used to assess the health state of patients. The current health state is compared with the one exhibited by the same individual one year prior to the measurement.

Upon receiving the patient's informed consent, the SF-36 was administered by qualified medicine students. Also, its correct administration was verified and double data entry was used to ensure reliability.

One year later the total number of patients surveyed with the SF-36 was 133 for the RPP and 130 for CT. For the second application of the SF-36, data analysis was carried out assigning zero to the domains of deceased patients and imputing the remaining missing values through multiple linear regression (Alisson, 2001).

After imputing the domains, summary scores were calculated and their distribution explored using the Kolmogorov-Smirnov test to verify the normality assumption. A comparison was made between the HRQOL values obtained in the two measurements for each group. For this purpose, the t-student test for independent samples or the Mann-Whitney U test were used. Likewise, the changes in HRQOL values within each group were compared using the t test for related samples or Wilcoxon's rank sum test. The report was generated by analyzing the means in order to establish comparisons between our results and the scientific literature.

For each summary score and dimension of the HRQOL perceived after one follow-up year, the adjusted mean was calculated to compare both interventions using an analysis of covariance model (ANCOVA) and a two-way analysis of variance adjusted for gender and history of hypertension, diabetes and dyslipidemia. The ANCOVA's covariables were: the HRQOL scores obtained at the start of the study, age, and stage of the condition. Furthermore, the effect size of HRQOL differences was calculated using Cohen's effect size index and its corresponding Hedges' bias correction formula (Cohen, 1988). All analyses were conducted using the program SPSS version 15.

## 3. Results

### 3.1 Demographic and clinical characteristics

The median (Md) age was 76 for CT and 65 for the RPP. The CT group was predominantly male. A significant difference (p=0.037) between the age of males (Md=63) and females

| Characteristic | RPP n=148 Md(Min-Max) | CT n=145 Md(Min-Max) | P value |
|---|---|---|---|
| Age | 65 (18-98) | 76 (31-97) | <0.001 |
| Hemoglobin | 13.6 (4.9-19.8) | 14.5 (10.2-17.5) | 0.001 |
| Glomerular Filtration Rate | 51 (2.1-147) | 47 (16.6-115.8) | 0.027 |
| Body Mass Index | 26.1 (18.2-46.5) | 25.3 (15.1-39.1) | 0.149 |
| Mean Arterial Pressure | 93.3 (75-123.3) | 93.3 (58.3-120.7) | 0.529 |
| | n (%) | n (%) | P value |
| Gender | | | |
| Male | 77 (52.0) | 119 (82.1) | <0.001 |
| Female | 71 (48) | 26 (27.9) | |
| Stage | | | |
| 1 and 2 | 44 (29.7) | 18 (12.4) | <0.001 |
| 3, 4 and 5 | 104 (70.3) | 127 (87.6) | |
| Comorbidities | | | |
| Arterial Hypertension | 141 (95.3) | 133 (91.7) | 0.218 |
| Diabetes | 60 (40.5) | 44 (30.3) | 0.068 |
| Dyslipidemia | 92 (62.2) | 106 (73.1) | 0.045 |

RPP: Renal Protection Program. CT: Conventional treatment; Md: Median. Min: minimum value. Max: maximum value.

Table 1. Distribution of demographic and clinical characteristics of predialysis patients with chronic renal failure. Medellin, 2007-2008.

(Md=68) was found in the RPP group. Clinical parameters such as arterial pressure, serum creatinine, and body mass index showed no significant differences between the study groups. For the CT group, serum hemoglobin values were significantly higher, and the glomerular filtration rate was lower. Most patients in both healthcare providing institutions had a history of arterial hypertension (90%) and dyslipidemia (60%). Distribution by stages showed that patients joined the Renal Protection Program at early stages of their condition (1 and 2=29.7 %), whereas CT patients requested treatment when their disease was at later stages (1 and 2=12.4%). See Table 1.

### 3.2 Perception of health-related quality of life

At the start of the study, the perception of HRQOL measured by the SF-36 showed no significant differences between the RPP and CT, except for MCS1 and role-emotional. However, the effect size (ES) was 0.08 and 0.13 respectively. The only domain exhibiting significant differences after one year was change in health, whose values favored the RPP with ES=0.11 (See Table 2).

As for the changes within each group after one year, the RPP patients showed a significant decrease only in physical functioning (p=0.038; ES=0.14), whereas CT patients showed a decrease in four domains: physical functioning (p=0.027; ES=0.14), general health (p=0.001; ES=0.29), social functioning (p=0.010; ES=0.22), and vitality (p=0.009; ES=0.22) and in MCS1 (p=0.044; ES=0.19).

| Domains and summary scores | Initial | | | 1 year | | |
|---|---|---|---|---|---|---|
| | RPP | CT: | t-Student | RPP | CT: | t-Student |
| | Mean (SD) | Mean (SD) | P value | Mean (SD) | Mean (SD) | P value |
| PCS1: | 60.9 (28.4) | 58.5 (27.6) | 0.470 | 58.9 (27.6) | 54.2 (28.7) | 0.160 |
| Physical Functioning | 70.0 (27.4) | 68.7 (26.4) | 0.662 | 65.8 (30.6) | 64.3 (31.1) | 0.684 |
| Role-Physical | 62.0 (41.4) | 63.3 (42.9) | 0.795 | 66.4 (42.3) | 59.7 (45.5) | 0.191 |
| Bodily Pain | 66.7 (28.6) | 67.8 (27.4) | 0.733 | 65.0 (28.3) | 64.2 (29.1) | 0.808 |
| General Health | 58.8 (23.6) | 60.4 (22.4) | 0.554 | 57.6 (23.5) | 53.1 (26.0) | 0.125 |
| MCS1: | 67.1 (33.2) | 75.1 (28.1) | 0.027 | 69.4 (27.6) | 69.7 (27.4) | 0.917 |
| Mental Health | 69.6 (26.8) | 73.3 (23.8) | 0.219 | 68.1 (24.5) | 69.8 (23.8) | 0.539 |
| Role-Emotional | 64.8 (43.1) | 76.0 (37.1) | 0.017 | 71.0 (40.9) | 70.1 (40.4) | 0.858 |
| Social Functioning | 76.3 (29.1) | 80.9 (27.0) | 0.160 | 77.3 (26.6) | 74.5 (28.5) | 0.390 |
| Vitality | 67.4 (27.0) | 67.8 (24.6) | 0.905 | 64.9 (24.9) | 61.9 (26.3) | 0.315 |
| Changes in Health | 66.1 (23.9) | 65.9 (21.1) | 0.955 | 68.5 (23.2) | 62.6 (22.9) | 0.029 |

RPP: Renal Protection Program. CT: Conventional treatment; PCS1: Physical health summary score. MCS1: Mental health summary score. SD: Standard deviation

Table 2. Distribution of HRQOL scores in patients with chronic renal failure in predialysis before and after an intervention. Medellín, 2007-2008.

| Domains and Summary Scores | Initial | | | 1 year | | |
|---|---|---|---|---|---|---|
| | Female | Male | t-Student | Female | Male | t-Student |
| | Mean (SD) | Mean (SD) | P value | Mean (SD) | Mean (SD) | P value |
| RPP | | | | | | |
| PCS1: | 54.6 (27.7) | 66.6 (28.0) | 0.010 | 53.0 (26.4) | 64.3 (27.8) | 0.013 |
| Physical Functioning | 61.5 (27.4) | 77.9 (25.1) | <0.001 | 57.3 (30.8) | 73.6 (28.3) | 0.001 |
| Role-Physical | 53.2 (41.8) | 70.1 (39.5) | 0.012 | 62.0 (44.7) | 70.5 (39.9) | 0.224 |
| Bodily Pain | 61.3 (28.5) | 71.7 (28.0) | 0.026 | 59.4 (27.3) | 70.2 (28.3) | 0.021 |
| General Health | 52.4 (22.2) | 64.7 (23.5) | 0.001 | 53.8 (22.6) | 61.1 (23.9) | 0.059 |
| MCS1: | 59.4 (36.1) | 74.3 (28.6) | 0.006 | 64.4 (28.7) | 74.0 (25.8) | 0.034 |
| Mental Health | 62.5 (29.1) | 76.2 (22.7) | 0.002 | 63.5 (23.5) | 72.3 (24.9) | 0.028 |
| Role-Emotional | 52.0 (45.0) | 76.5 (37.9) | <0.001 | 64.5 (43.1) | 77.0 (38.0) | 0.065 |
| Social Functioning | 74.0 (29.7) | 78.5 (28.6) | 0.354 | 73.7 (28.4) | 80.7 (24.6) | 0.109 |
| Vitality | 59.6 (27.5) | 74.6 (24.6) | 0.001 | 56.1 (23.9) | 73.0 (23.2) | <0.001* |
| CHANGES IN HEALTH | 65.1 (23.6) | 67.0 (24.2) | 0.622 | 66.2 (21.0) | 70.6 (25.0) | 0.245 |
| CT: | | | | | | |
| PCS1: | 51.3 (27.8) | 60.1 (27.4) | 0.142 | 47.6 (28.5) | 55.7 (28.7) | 0.198 |
| Physical Functioning | 61.5 (28.8) | 70.2 (25.7) | 0.130 | 55.6 (30.6) | 66.3 (31.0) | 0.112 |
| Role-Physical | 48.1 (43.0) | 66.6 (42.3) | 0.046 | 47.1 (44.9) | 62.4 (45.3) | 0.121 |
| Bodily Pain | 57.1 (29.0) | 70.1 (26.6) | 0.027 | 49.9 (25.7) | 67.3 (29.0) | 0.005+ |
| General Health | 61.9 (21.9) | 60.0 (22.6) | 0.700 | 59.6 (24.7) | 51.7 (26.2) | 0.162 |
| MCS1: | 65.9 (28.9) | 77.1 (27.6) | 0.065 | 61.4 (27.5) | 71.5 (27.1) | 0.086 |
| Mental Health | 61.5 (24.0) | 75.8 (23.1) | 0.005 | 64.5 (17.7) | 70.9 (24.8) | 0.213 |
| Role-Emotional | 66.6 (43.2) | 78.0 (35.4) | 0.216 | 52.5 (42.1) | 74.0 (39.2) | 0.013 |
| Social Functioning | 74.4 (30.2) | 82.4 (26.2) | 0.176 | 67.8 (21.5) | 76.0 (29.7) | 0.180 |
| Vitality | 58.5 (23.4) | 69.8 (24.5) | 0.033 | 56.9 (20.0) | 62.9 (27.5) | 0.292 |
| CHANGES IN HEALTH | 60.8 (21.5) | 67.1 (20.9) | 0.169 | 71.5 (18.9) | 60.7 (23.3) | 0.028 |

RPP: Renal Protection Program. CT: Conventional treatment PCS1: Physical health summary score. MCS1: Mental health summary score. SD: Standard deviation

*: Effect size =0.69 +: Effect size =0.61

Table 3. Distribution of HRQOL scores, by gender, in patients with chronic kidney disease in predialysis before and after an intervention. Medellín, 2007-2008.

### 3.3 Perception of health-related quality of life in terms of gender

In both groups HRQOL was lower for women both in the initial measurement and in the final measurement after one year. At the start of the study, the female patients of the RPP showed significant differences in most domains, and CT female patients showed these only in a few domains. One year later, the HRQOL difference between men and women in the RPP group remained unchanged for PCS1 (ES=0.40) and MCS1 (ES=0.34), and for the following domains: physical functioning (ES=0.53), bodily pain (ES=0.37), mental health (ES=0.35) and vitality (ES=0.69). For the CT group, the only significant differences were in bodily pain (ES=0.61), role-emotional (ES=0.51) and change in health (ES=0.48). See Table 3.

After one year, women within each group showed no changes in HRQOL measurements. Only the men following CT showed a significant decrease in general health (p=0.001 ES=0.33), social functioning (p=0.014 ES=0.15), vitality (p=0.007 ES=0.13), and change in health (p=0.012 ES=0.09).

### 3.4 Perception of health-related quality of life in terms of age

In both interventions, the physical component of HRQOL was more affected in patients older than 65 than in younger individuals. This was constant throughout the study. In the RPP group, these differences at the start of the study and one year later were statistically significant for PCS1 (p=0.001, ES start=0.08; p<0.001, ES year=0.06), for the physical functioning domain (p=0.001, ES start=0.30; p<0.001, ES year=0.03) and for bodily pain (p=0.009, ES start=0.02; p=0.025, ES year=0.10). In CT, however, the differences found between the age groups at the start were in PCS1 (p=0.025, ES start=0.44), in the physical functioning domain (p=0.001, ES start=0.61) and in role-physical (p=0.022, ES start=0.43). One year later, differences were found in physical functioning (p=0.022, ES year=0.57) and general health (p=0.021, ES year=0.45). See Table 4.

After analyzing changes within each group and for each age group, it was observed that the RPP patients who were 65 and older showed significant changes in physical functioning (p=0.006, ES=0.30) after one year. Patients younger than 65 showed no changes after this time. In CT, patients younger than 65 showed significant changes in MCS1 (p=0.044, ES=0.34) and in the social functioning domain (p=0.003, ES=0.53). Patients who were 65 and older showed changes after one year in physical functioning (p=0.050, ES=0.15), general health (p=0.001, ES=0.35) and vitality (p=0.044, ES=0.20) See Table 4.

### 3.5 Health-related quality of life adjusted for previous measurements, age, and gender

After adjusting the second measurement's raw HRQOL score (See Table 2) for the initial HRQOL score, significant differences were found between the RPP and the CT groups in the following domains: general health (a difference of 5.2 points favoring the RPP) and change in health (the difference of 5.9 points continues to favor the RPP). After adjusting it for gender, differences were found in PCS1 (a difference of 7.7 points favoring the RPP) and vitality (a difference of 6.9 points favoring the RPP). When the score was adjusted for age, differences were then found in physical functioning (a difference of 7.2 points favoring CT). No significant differences were found upon adjusting HRQOL for stage, hypertension, diabetes, and dyslipidemia (See Table 5).

| Domains and Summary Scores | Initial | | | 1 year | | |
|---|---|---|---|---|---|---|
| | 65 and older | Younger than 65 | t-Student | 65 and older | Younger than 65 | t-Student |
| | Mean (SD) | Mean (SD) | P value | Mean (SD) | Mean (SD) | P value |
| **RPP** | | | | | | |
| PCS1: | 53.3 (28.0) | 68.9 (26.8) | 0.001 | 51.0 (27.1) | 67.2 (25.9) | <0.001 |
| Physical Functioning | 62.7 (26.1) | 77.8 (26.9) | 0.001 | 53.8 (30.7) | 78.5 (24.9) | <0.001 |
| Role-Physical | 57.9 (42.5) | 66.3 (40.1) | 0.217 | 60.2 (43.8) | 72.9 (40.0) | 0.067 |
| Bodily Pain | 60.7 (29.5) | 73.0 (26.4) | 0.009 | 60.0 (30.6) | 70.4 (24.7) | 0.025 |
| General Health | 56.0 (24.3) | 61.7 (22.7) | 0.140 | 56.6 (24.9) | 58.6 (22.0) | 0.613 |
| MCS1: | 70.7 (32.9) | 63.4 (33.2) | 0.178 | 68.5 (31.3) | 70.2 (23.2) | 0.708 |
| Mental Health | 69.5 (29.1) | 69.8 (24.3) | 0.945 | 67.5 (28.2) | 68.6 (20.2) | 0.793 |
| Role-Emotional | 67.0 (42.7) | 62.4 (43.7) | 0.518 | 64.6 (43.7) | 77.7 (36.7) | 0.051 |
| Social Functioning | 76.9 (30.3) | 75.7 (27.9) | 0.809 | 73.7 (29.2) | 81.2 (23.2) | 0.085 |
| Vitality | 66.2 (26.8) | 68.7 (27.3) | 0.576 | 61.2 (26.5) | 68.7 (22.7) | 0.068 |
| CHANGES IN HEALTH | 62.4 (23.1) | 70.0 (24.2) | 0.052 | 61.3 (24.3) | 76.1 (19.5) | <0.001 |
| **CT:** | | | | | | |
| PCS1: | 55.7 (27.6) | 67.9 (25.8) | 0.025 | 51.9 (28.3) | 62.2 (29.0) | 0.068 |
| Physical Functioning | 65.2 (27.0) | 80.5 (20.9) | 0.001 | 60.5 (31.8) | 77.4 (24.8) | 0.002 |
| Role-Physical | 59.2 (43.8) | 77.3 (37.2) | 0.022 | 58.3 (45.2) | 64.4 (46.8) | 0.498 |
| Bodily Pain | 66.7 (28.1) | 71.5 (25.1) | 0.377 | 64.8 (28.5) | 62.2 (31.6) | 0.648 |
| General Health | 59.2 (22.8) | 64.2 (21.2) | 0.262 | 50.4 (25.7) | 62.3 (25.3) | 0.021 |
| MCS1: | 73.8 (28.9) | 79.6 (24.8) | 0.302 | 69.9 (27.0) | 69.0 (28.9) | 0.875 |
| Mental Health | 71.8 (24.5) | 78.3 (20.9) | 0.167 | 69.5 (24.3) | 70.7 (22.1) | 0.811 |
| Role-Emotional | 73.4 (39.1) | 84.7 (27.9) | 0.068 | 69.0 (41.4) | 74.1 (37.1) | 0.520 |
| Social Functioning | 79.1 (28.1) | 87.1 (22.0) | 0.136 | 74.8 (29.0) | 73.7 (27.0) | 0.851 |
| Vitality | 66.0 (24.9) | 73.8 (23.0) | 0.110 | 60.7 (26.8) | 65.8 (24.6) | 0.325 |
| CHANGES IN HEALTH | 64.3 (21.0) | 71.5 (20.6) | 0.084 | 61.4 (23.2) | 66.7 (21.6) | 0.249 |

RPP: Renal Protection Program. CT: Conventional treatment PCS1: Physical health summary score. MCS1: Mental health summary score. SD: Standard deviation

Table 4. Distribution of HRQOL scores, by age, in patients with chronic renal failure in predialysis before and after an intervention. Medellín, 2007-2008.

| Domains and summary scores | Mean adjusted for initial HRQOL | | Mean adjusted for gender | | Mean adjusted for age | |
|---|---|---|---|---|---|---|
| | RPP | CT: | RPP | CT: | RPP | CT: |
| PCS1: | 58.2 | 54.9 | 58.7** | 51.0** | 56.0 | 57.1 |
| Physical Functioning | 65.3 | 64.9 | 65.5 | 59.8 | 61.5* | 68.7* |
| Role-Physical | 66.7 | 59.4 | 66.2 | 56.1 | 64.3 | 61.7 |
| Bodily Pain | 65.3 | 64.0 | 64.8 | 60.0 | 63.6 | 65.6 |
| General Health | 58.0* | 52.8* | 57.6 | 52.6 | 56.6 | 54.2 |
| MCS1: | 70.5 | 68.6 | 69.2 | 66.6 | 69.2 | 69.9 |
| Mental Health | 68.7 | 69.1 | 67.9 | 67.2 | 67.7 | 70.2 |
| Role-Emotional | 72.5 | 68.6 | 70.7 | 65.1 | 69.2 | 71.9 |
| Social Functioning | 78.0 | 73.8 | 77.2 | 72.1 | 76.3 | 75.6 |
| Vitality | 65.0 | 61.8 | 64.6** | 57.7** | 63.5 | 63.3 |
| CHANGES IN HEALTH | 68.5* | 62.6* | 68.5 | 63.0 | 67.2 | 64.0 |

RPP: Renal Protection Program. CT: Conventional treatment PCS1: Physical health summary score. MCS1: Mental health summary score.
The underlined values correspond to significant difference by intervention type and by adjustment variable. P value: * $p<0.05$ ** $p<0.01$.

Table 5. Distribution of health-related quality of life scores in patients with chronic renal failure in predialysis after one year of treatment. Scores are adjusted for initial health-related quality of life, gender, and age. Medellín, 2007-2008.

### 3.6 Reasons for not participating in the study

The reasons for the unreachability of the remaining 118 patients during the first measurement were: wrong phone number = 43 (40% RPP), occupation = 33 (45% RPP), being out of geographical reach = 17 (35% RPP), and exclusion criteria = 14 (57% RPP). Only 11 patients (36% RPP) were excluded due to concomitant disease or death, which is associated with a decrease in HRQOL. One year later, of the missing RPP patients: 6 refused to participate (2 due to disease), 6 couldn't be contacted, and 3 had died. In CT: 5 refused to participate (1 due to disease), 4 couldn't be contacted, and 6 had died.

## 4. Discussion

This is the first report in Colombia to provide an account of the factors affecting HRQOL in patients with mild to moderate renal impairment. It is also the first to point out the advantages that a renal protection program may have over conventional treatment regarding its impact on patient HRQOL. This study's results are presented to comply with the demands that appear in international literature regarding the need to determine the impact on HRQOL in early stages of renal impairment (Chandban et al., 2003; Perlman et al., 2005) and to insist that current interventions must emphasize the preservation of renal functioning in order to decrease the negative impact of kidney failure on HRQOL (Chandban et al., 2003; Fukuhara et al., 2007; Valdebarrano et al., 2001).

The study's data were collected from 293 patients in the early stages of CRF. Patients followed two kinds of medical treatment during one year. The groups showed no differences for the main comorbidities, but it was evident that the RPP collected more patients in earlier stages of CRF due to its active search. The higher proportion of male patients in CT could be due to the faster progression of CRF in males (Silbiger & Neugarten, 1995). This could explain the gender and age disparities found between the groups at the start of the study.

One year later, the RPP group's scores for the different HRQOL domains were slightly lower, but these differences were not significant. Conversely, the CT group showed a significant decrease in four of the eight domains after the same time. This accounts for the effect of the RPP even in a short follow-up period. It is worth noting that general health was the most affected domain in both groups. After one year, the initial value for the RPP remained unchanged, but decreased drastically for CT.

The results obtained from data collected from predialysis patients confirm that HRQOL is affected from the early stages of CRF and continues to decrease as the condition evolves. Even after only one year, the scores for most domains decreased. This conclusion is shared by other studies whose patients lacked RRT. The population assessed in such studies was Japanese (Fukuhara et al., 2007), African-American (African American Study of Kidney Disease and Hypertension Trial Group [AASK], 2002), Australian (Chandban et al., 2005), Korean (Chin et al., 2008), and Dutch (Korevaar et al., 2000).

In this study, the physical health of predialysis patients was found to be more affected than their mental health. This was true for both study groups. These findings are in accordance with the conclusions reached in other publications on the same topic (Chandban et al., 2005; Fukuhara et al., 2007; AASK, 2002; Korevaar et al., 2000; Hopman et al., 2000). Regarding mental health, CT patients initially showed significantly superior values compared to the RPP patients. This result is consistent with the ideas exposed in other studies, which suggest that older patients —or those with an older diagnosis— have better mental health. This proves that mental health is worse in young or recently diagnosed individuals (Hopman et al., 2000). Nevertheless, one year later, the scores for the mental component of HRQOL increased within the RPP group, whereas CT scores decreased, and the initial differences between the RPP and CT disappeared.

Gender was a key factor for the SF-36 scores since its first application. It was observed that the scores for women were lower and had significant differences regardless of the group. However, these differences disappeared within the RPP group one year later. In CT, however, the differences remained and values in men decreased statistically. Other researchers also recognized this affectedness of HRQOL by gender. They also proposed that women may be particularly more vulnerable (Yepes et al., 2008). This was also done in the AASK study (AASK, 2002), which focused on the need for exploring the mechanisms allowing HRQOL in female CRF patients to decrease quickly. In studying the HRQOL of the Australian population suffering from kidney failure Chandban (Chandban et al., 2005) described similar worsening patterns for both genders.

After one year, women's HRQOL in most domains continued to be worse than that of men. However it is worth noting that differences between the values obtained at the start of the study and after one year could be indirectly considered as clinically important in the vitality values for the RPP (ES=0.69) and the bodily pain values for CT (ES=0.61).

Regarding age, patients older than 65 had a lower HRQOL. Physical functioning was the most affected domain for the two groups both at the start of the study and one year later. This could be explained by the strong negative association between the state of physical health and old age. Such association was reported in literature by studies on this and other chronic diseases (Chandban et al., 2005; Hopman et al., 2000; Yepes et al., 2008). The RPP patients younger than 65 showed an increase in four of the domains one year after the start of the study. The rest of the domains also decreased, but not significantly, except for the role-physical domain. For the CT group, all the domains values decreased in the second measurement, and four of them did so significantly. The difference found in physical functioning between the age groups in CT according to the effect size (> 0.60) can be considered to be clinically important. This must be corroborated for each case with the medical staff.

It is imperative to adjust the differences found in the final HRQOL scores for the variables that can influence such results. As for general health and change in health, upon adjusting for the respective value of the initial score, an increase of more than five points of HRQOL was generated in the difference that favors the RPP over CT in both domains. In the PCS1 and vitality domains, adjusting scores for gender yielded an important increase of the difference in favor of the RPP in both cases (Yepes et al., 2008). In physical functioning, adjusting scores for age increased the difference in HRQOL scores, favoring CT (Yepes et al., 2008).

In short, exposure to a RPP has a positive impact on the HRQOL of CRF patients from the early stages of their condition. The initial HRQOL score, gender, and age are fundamental characteristics to take into account for measuring the HRQOL of patients upon exposure to an intervention. It seems that early detection of CRF patients and interdisciplinary control of risk factors have a significant influence in the outcome of both physical and mental HRQOL measurements.

HRQOL values have been proposed as an important outcome in patients with high death, hospitalization, and depression risks. Measuring the HRQOL with validated instruments such as the SF-36 allows it to become a strong indicator of the health-related quality of life in ambulatory patients. In fact, it is considered a mortality and morbidity predictor in elderly and CRF patients (DeOreo, 1997; Han et al., 2009; Kalantar-Zadeh, 2005; Mapes et al., 2003). Assessing the well-being of CRF patients periodically with the SF-36 is important for measuring response to treatment and for improving healthcare. In fact, improving the HRQOL of CRF patients is a key objective in the U.S (Kalantar-Zadeh, 2005).

This study's main limitation is its short follow-up period, which could not provide an appropriate account of the characteristics of a slow, progressive disease while explaining that many changes are not significant enough. Another limitation is that demographic variables like marital status, socioeconomic level, occupation, educational level, income, etc., were disregarded. Some studies state that both PCS1 and MCS1 are closely associated with demographic characteristics that are likely to have a deeper impact than clinical characteristics themselves (AASK, 2002; Fukuhara et al., 2007).

Data loss due to patient death and other causes was expected for the second application of the SF-36 one year later. Like many other health scales, the SF-36 has no clear directions regarding how deaths within a studied population should be analyzed. This has limited the analysis in research. This issue is most frequently addressed by excluding these cases from the study or by analyzing these data separately. Paradoxically, if two study groups are compared, the group with more diseased individuals seems to obtain better results. This is because most individuals have died and have been thus excluded from the results and from the analysis.

Due to the negative impact of CRF on HRQOL, it is necessary to determine potential areas for research and clinical intervention. Such areas include: psychological support for the most vulnerable population (women, young people, recently diagnosed patients, patients in early stages of the condition), early prescription of nephroprotectors, and complete physical therapy programs focusing on older patients and on those with high deterioration rates.

## 5. Acknowledgment

The authors would like to thank University of Antioquia, Colciencias and Sura EPS for sponsoring this research. We are also very grateful for the patients' cooperation, for the support provided by José Miguel Abad and José Ignacio Acosta, for the advice provided by Professors Rubén Darío Gomez and Juan Luis Londoño, and for Andrés Felipe Quintero Rave's thoughtful translation of this text.

## 6. References

Allison PD. (2001). *Missing data.* Sage University Papers on Quantitative Applications in the Social Sciences, series 07-136. ISBN: 0-7619-1672-5 (p) Thousand Oasks, CA: Sage.

Amoedo M, Egea J, Millán I, Gil M, Reig A & Sirvent A. (2004). Evaluación de la calidad de vida relacionada con la salud mediante láminas COOPWONCA en una población de hemodiálisis. *Nefrología,* Vol. XXIV, No. 5, 2004, p.p 470-479. ISSN: 0211-699

Atkins RC. (2005). The epidemiology of chronic kidney disease. *Kidney International,* Vol. 67, No. 94, Apr 2005, p.p S14-S18. EISSN: 1523-1755

Atkins RC. (2005). The changing patterns of chronic kidney disease: the need to develop strategies for prevention relevant to different regions and countries. *Kidney International Supplement.* Vol. 98, Sep 2005, p.p 83-85. EISSN: 1523-1755

Cardona D, Estrada A & Agudelo H. (2003). *Envejecer nos toca a todos.* Facultad Nacional de Salud Pública Universidad de Antioquia; 2003. p.p 33 -38, ISBN: 9586557138, Medellín, Colombia.

Cardona D & Agudelo HB. (2005). Construcción cultural del concepto calidad de vida. *Revista Facultad Nacional de Salud Pública.* Vol. 23, No. 1, 2005, p.p 79-90. ISSN: 0120-386

Chandban SJ, Briganti EM, Kerr PG, Dunstan DW, Welborn TA, Zimmet PZ & Atkins RC. (2003). Prevalence of kidney damage in Australian adults: the AusDiab Kidney Study. *Journal of the American Society of Nephrology.* Vol. 14, 2003, p.p s131–s138. EISSN: 1533-3450

Chin HJ, Song YR, Lee JJ, Lee SB, Kim KW, Na KY, Kim S & Chae DW. (2008). Moderately decreased renal function negatively affects the health-related quality of life among the elderly Korean population: a population-based study. *Nephrology Dialysis Transplantation.* Vol. 23, No. 9, 2008, p.p 2810-2817. EISSN: 1460-2385

Cohen J. (1988). The t Test for Means. In: *Statistical Power Analysis for the Behavioral Sciences. Second Edition.* Academic Press, p.p 20 – 27, ISBN: 0805802835, New York, retrieved from: <http://www.questia.com/PM.qst?a=o&d=98533106>

De Alvaro F, López K & García F. (1997). Salud percibida, estado funcional y mortalidad en pacientes diabéticos en tratamiento renal sustitutivo: diseño del estudio Calvidia. *Nefrología.* Vol. XVII, No. 4, 1997, p.p 296-303. ISSN: 0211-6995

DeOreo PB. (1997). Hemodialysis patient-assessed functinal health status predicts continued survival, hospitalization, and dialysis-attendance compliance. *American Journal of Kidney Disease*. Vol. 30, No. 2, Aug, 1997, p.p 204–212. EISSN: 1523-6838.

Fleury E, Lana Da Costa C. (2004) Qualidade de vida e saúde: aspectos conceituais e metodológicos. *Cadernos de Saúde Pública*. Vol. 20, No. 2, Mar-Abr 2004, p.p 580-588. EISSN 1678-4464

Frison L & Pocock SJ. (1992). Repeated measures in clinical trials: analysis using mean summary statistics and its Implications for design. Statistics in Medicine. Vol.11, No.13, Sep 1992. p.p 1685-704. EISSN: 1097-0258.

Fukuhara S, Yamazaki S, Marumo F, Akiba T, Akizawa T & Fujimi T. (2007). The Predialysis CRF Study Group in Japan. Health-Related Quality of Life of Predialysis Patients with Chronic Renal Failure. *Nephron Clinical Practice*. Vol. 105, No.1, 2007, p.p c1-8. ISSN: 1660-2110

García M, Sánchez M, Liébana A, Pérez V, Pérez P & Viedma G. (2993). Calidad de vida relacionada con la salud en pacientes ancianos en hemodiálisis. *Nefrología*. Vol. XXIII, No. 6, 2003, p.p 528- 537. ISSN: 0211-6995

Han SS, Kim KW, Na KY, Chae DW, Kim YS & Chin HJ. (2009). Quality of life and mortality from a nephrologist's view: a prospective observational study. *BMC Nephrology*. Vol. 10, 2009, p.p 39. ISSN: 1471-2369

Hopman WM, Harrison M B, Coo H, Friedberg E, Buchanan M & VanDenKerkhof EG. (2000). Associations between chronic disease, age and physical and mental health status. *Chronic Diseases in Canada*. Vol. 29, No. 3, 2000, p.p 108-116. EISSN: 1481-8523

Kalantar-Zadeh K & Unruh M. (2005) Health related quality of life in patients with chronic kidney disease. *International Urology and Nephrology*. Vol. 37, No. 2, 2005, p.p 367–378. EISSN: 1573-2584

Korevaar JC, Jansen MA, Merkus MP, Dekker FW, Boeschoten EW & Krediet RT. (2000) Quality of life in predialysis end-stage renal disease patients at the initiation of dialysis therapy. *Peritoneal Dialysis International*. Vol. 20, Jan 2000, p.p 69–75. EISSN: 17184304

Kusek, JW; Greene, P; Wang, SR; Beck, G; West, D; Jamerson, K; Agodoa, L; Faulkner, M; Level, B. (2002). Cross-Sectional Study of Health-Related Quality of Life in African Americans with Chronic Renal Insufficiency: The African American Study of Kidney Disease and Hypertension Trial. *American Journal of Kidney Disease*, Vol. 39, No. 3, March 2002, p.p 513-24. EISSN: 1523-6838.

Leanza H, Giacoletto S, Najún C & Barreneche M. (2000) Niveles de hemoglobina y probabilidad de mejor calidad de vida en hemodializados crónicos. *Nefrología*. Vol. XX, No. 5, Sep 2000, p.p 440-444. ISSN: 0211-6995

Leese M, Schene A, Koeter M, Meijer K, Bindman J, Mazzi M, Puschner B, Burti L, Becker T, Moreno M, Celani D, White IR & Thonicroft G. (2008). SF-36 scales, and simple sums of scales, were reliable quality-of-life summaries for patients with schizophrenia. *Journal of Clinical Epidemiology*. Vol 61, No. 6, Jun 2008; p.p 588-596. ISSN: 0895-4356

Lugo LH, García HI & Gómez CR. (2006) Confiabilidad del cuestionario de calidad de vida en salud SF-36 en Medellín, Colombia. *Revista Facultad Nacional de Salud Pública*. Vol. 24, No. 2, Jul-Dec 2006; p.p 37-50. ISSN: 0120-386

Mapes DL, Lopes AA, Satayathum S, McCullough KP, Goodkin DA, Locatelli F, Fukuhara S, Young EW, Kurokawa K, Saito A, Bommer J, Wolfe RA, Held PJ & Port FK. (2003). Health-related quality of life as a predictor of mortality and hospitalization: the Dialysis Outcomes and Practice Patterns Study (DOPPS). *Kidney International.* Vol. 64, 2003, p.p 339–349. EISSN: 1523-1755

Martínez F, Valencia M. (2005) *Modelo de prevención y control de la enfermedad renal crónica. Componente de un modelo de Salud Renal.* Fedesalud, p.p 17-55, ISBN: 978-958-44-0734-4, Bogotá.

National Kidney Foundation. (2000) K/DOQI Clinical Guidelines for Chronic kidney disease. In: N*ational Kidney Foundation.* Access in July, 2007. Available from: <http://www.kidney.org/professionals/kdoqi/guidelines_ckd/toc.htm>

Organización Mundial de la Salud. (2002). Programa de envejecimiento y ciclo vital. Envejecimiento activo: un marco político. *Revista española de geriatría y gerontología.* Vol. 37, No. 2, Aug 2002, p.p 104-105. EISSN: 1578-1747

Pérez M, Martín A, Díaz R & Pérez J. (2007}9 Evolución de la calidad de vida relacionada con la salud en los trasplantados renales. *Nefrología.* Vol. XXVII, No. 5, 2007, p.p 619-626. ISSN: 0211-6995

Perlman R, Finkelstein F, Liu L, Roys E, Kiser M, Eisele G, Burrows-Hudson S, Messana JM, Levin N, Rajagopalan S, Port FK, Wolfe RA & Saran R. (2005). Quality of Life in Chronic Kidney Disease (CKD): A Cross-Sectional Analysis in the Renal Research Institute. *American Journal of Kidney Disease.* Vol. 45, No. 4, Apr 2005, p.p 658-666. EISSN: 1523-6838.

Rebollo P, Ortega F, Bobes J, Gónzalez M & Saiz P. (2000). Interpretación de los resultados de la calidad de vida relacionada con la salud en terapia sustitutiva de la insuficiencia renal terminal. *Nefrología.* Vol. XX, No. 5, Sep 2000, p.p 431-439. ISSN: 0211-6995

Rebollo P, Ortega F, Bobes J, Gónzalez M & Saiz P. (2000). Factores asociados a la calidad de vida relacionada con la salud (CVRS) de los pacientes en terapia renal sustitutiva (TRS). *Nefrología.* Vol. XX, No. 2, Mar 2000, p.p 171-181. ISSN: 0211-6995

Rebollo P, Ortega F, Badía X, Álvarez-Ude F, Baltar J & Álvarez J. (1999). Salud percibida en pacientes mayores de 65 años en tratamiento sustitutivo renal (TSR). *Nefrología.* Vol. XIX, (Supl. 1), 1999, p.p 73-83. ISSN: 0211-6995

Sanz D, López J, Jofre R, Fort J, Valderrábano F, Moreno F, Vázquez MI & Fort. J (2004). Diferencias en la calidad de vida relacionada con la salud entre hombres y mujeres en tratamiento con hemodiálisis. *Nefrología.* Vol. XXIV, No. 2, 2004, p.p 167-178. ISSN: 0211-6995

Silbiger S & Neugarten J. The impact of gender on the progression of chronic renal disease. *American Journal of Kidney Disease.* Vol. 25, No. 4, Apr 1995; p.p 515-533. EISSN: 1523-6838.

Tazeen H. (2006). The growing Burden of Chronic Kidney Disease in Pakistan. *New England Journal of Medicine.* Vol. 354, No. 10, Mar 2006, p.p 995-7. ISSN 1533-4406

Valderrabano F, Jofre R & López JM. (2001). Quality of life in end-stage renal disease patients. *American Journal of Kidney Disease.* Vol. 38, No. 3, Sep 2001, p.p 443-464. EISSN: 1523-6838.

Yepes CE, Montoya M, Orrego BE, Cucllar MH, Yepes JJ, López JP, et al. Calidad de vida en pacientes con enfermedad renal crónica sin diálisis ni trasplante de una muestra aleatoria de dos aseguradoras en salud. Medellín, Colombia, 2008. *Nefrología.* Vol. 29, No. 6, 2009, p.p 548-556. ISSN: 0211-6995